Fourth Edition

Language and Communication Disorders in Children

Deena K. Bernstein
Lehman College
City University of New York

Ellenmorris Tiegerman-Farber
School for Language and Communication Development
and Adelphi College

Allyn and Bacon
Boston • London Toronto • Sydney • Tokyo • Singapore

Executive Editor: Stephen D. Dragin
Series Editorial Assistant: Christine Svitila
Senior Marketing Manager: Kathy Hunter
Production Coordinator: Christopher H. Rawlings
Editorial-Production Service: Walsh & Associates, Inc.
Composition and Prepress Buyer: Linda Cox
Manufacturing Buyer: Suzanne Lareau
Art Director: Linda Knowles
Photo Researcher: Susan Duane

Library of Congress Cataloging-in-Publication Data
Bernstein, Deena K. (Deena Kahan)
    Language and communication disorders in children / Deena K.
    Bernstein, Ellenmorris Tiegerman-Farber. — 4th ed.
        p.   cm.
    Includes bibliographical references and index.
    ISBN 0-205-19894-5
    1. Language disorders in children.   2. Communicative disorders in
children.   I. Tiegermann-Farber, Ellenmorris.   II. Title.
RJ496.L35B47   1996
618.92'855—dc21   96-48262
                                                           CIP

Printed in the United States of America
10 9 8 7 6 5 4 3 2   00 99 98

Contents

Preface

Language and Communication Disorders has proceeded through four editions in the past decade. The reflected changes within this textbook are indicative of a range of professional and clinical changes that have occurred in American education. Children with language and communication disorders need to be recognized as a distinct population. Our professional discipline of speech-language pathology needs to be recognized as a primary contributor to special education and educational decision making. Parents need to be recognized as primary teachers and facilitators of their children's growth and development. The population of language communication disordered, our discipline, and the rapid changes in educational reform create a challenging synergy in the field of education. The changes within the textbook involve greater emphasis on early intervention programs, family ecology, multicultural assessment measures, clinical and educational accountability, and educational efficacy. Clearly, there appears to be a trend in redefining special education programs within educational settings. The discussion related to inclusive education has become much more intense over the past several years. The general education classroom has been defined as the least restrictive environment. Schools throughout the United States are attempting to develop inclusive models for children with special needs. The child with language and communication disorders will be affected by the modifications in classroom programming and the de-emphasis on individual therapeutic services. The question for us as speech-language pathologists will be to face the challenge of the future with an understanding of the needs of the children and families that we serve. This edition is organized to provide you with the most up-to-date information in this rapidly changing field.

The goal of this book is to introduce you to the dynamic areas of speech-language pathology and special education. These areas of study touch the heart of human experience—the ways children learn language and ways to help children who do not. Studying children's language and communication disorders will challenge you to apply theories of child development, speech and hearing science, and language development and disorders for the rewarding experience of providing language intervention to communicatively disordered children.

This book is divided into three sections. Part I presents the fundamentals of language and communication development; Part II describes the general principles of assessment and best practices for intervention; and Part III focuses on four language-disordered populations—

children with learning disabilities, mental retardation, autism, and hearing impairment. Included in Part II and Part III are examples that illustrate how to apply clinical constructs to the actual evaluation and remediation of children with language disorders.

A number of new improvements highlight this edition. In Part I, Chapters 2 and 3 present a new framework for viewing the prerequisites for language development in terms of the ecology of the family. In Chapter 4 the reader is introduced to the concept of emerging literacy, while in Chapter 5 increased attention is given to the language development of school-age children.

Part II (Chapters 6 to 11) bridges the gap to clinical application. In this section new information on language assessment of school-age children has been contributed by Elaine Silliman and Sharon James, and a new chapter (Chapter 10), written by Dolores Battle, focuses on the delivery of services to multicultural populations.

Communication disorders is an exciting area to study because it is constantly changing. We sincerely hope this book will motivate you to keep abreast of new research and the results of clinical procedures.

Acknowledgments

Acknowledging those who help make a text a reality is a risky venture because a person deserving thanks inadvertently may be omitted.

Thanks to Kris Farnsworth and Steve Dragin, and also Christine Svitila, at Allyn & Bacon who helped this edition see the light of day; thanks also to Christopher Rawlings for his assistance with the production of the book.

Our reviewers (Ellen Meyer Gregg, University of Northern Colorado; Carole Gorenflo, Eastern Michigan University; and Carol Strong, Utah State University) offered suggestions and comments that substantially improved this edition. Additionally, all the contributors to this text deserve special thanks for their flexibility during the reworking of the manuscript. New contributors Elaine Silliman and Dolores Battle deserve a special thanks for working under the constraints of tight deadlines.

I appreciate the help of the staff of Walsh & Associates who so thoroughly and conscientiously edited this edition.

Last, I am grateful to my husband and friend Josh for his invaluable support over the years, and to my children—Ariella Bernstein-Losice, Chaim Zanvil, and Yakov—who have taught me the lessons of patience and perseverence.

To the memory
of two of my dearest friends,
my parents, Julius and Pearl Kahan,
for whom the love and understanding
of children were overriding values.

and

In honor of their great granddaughters
Chaya Peryl Bernstein and Bracha Josepha Losice

D.K.B.

Over the past several years my lessons have been drawn from those that I love. To my husband Joseph Farber, there are no words to express my deep love and devotion. You remain to be the very center and core of who I am.

To my children, you have taught me a great deal about myself as a mother, a parent, and a teacher. I thank my children Jonathan, Jeremy, Andrew, Douglas, Dana, and Leslie—from whom I have learned more than any course or textbook could teach. The most important lesson is that we are a family.

My deepest appreciation goes to the Honorable Dean G. Skelos, Deputy Majority Leader, New York State Senate, 9th District, and Nassau County Executive Thomas S. Gulotta for making "The Dream" into a reality for the School for Language and Communication Development. I thank you both for your commitment over the years to families and children with special needs. In all of these years you have never lost your patience with me—I am grateful.

My love, devotion, and respect go to Dr. Christine Radziewicz, Dr. Stephen Cavallo, Mrs. Madeline Mando, Mrs. Rosemarie King, Mrs. Andrea Rieger, Mrs. Marie Dalli, Dr. Helene Mermelstein, and Mr. Andrew Plastrik for being the support, the heart, and the soul of the SLCD mission.

To the parents of SLCD—the words are worth the struggle! Be grateful for your child's words, never forget the time of silence, and advocate, advocate, advocate.

To the professionals at SLCD, I give you the spirit and the future of education. I hope that your experiences at SLCD will remain as a cornerstone in your personal and professional lives. Never forget what you have learned at SLCD, and never lose the challenge of excellence.

Special thanks must go to SLCD's Board of Directors—Paul Rosen, Joseph Gnesin, Mark Weinstein, Toya Davis, Bonnye Kaufman-Fuks, and Mario Fischetti—for their strength, suggestions, and SUPPORT.

Finally, to my parents, Morris and Rita Jacobs, I give my love and gratitude for all of their years of giving—to me.

E.T.-F.

Part I

The Nature of Language and Language Development

Chapter 1
The Nature of Language and Its Disorders

Chapter 2
Social Cognition: The Communication Imperative

Chapter 3
The Ecology of the Family: The Language Imperative

Chapter 4
Language Development: The Preschool Years

Chapter 5
Language Development: The School-Age Years

The Nature of Language and Its Disorders

DEENA K. BERNSTEIN
Lehman College
City University of New York

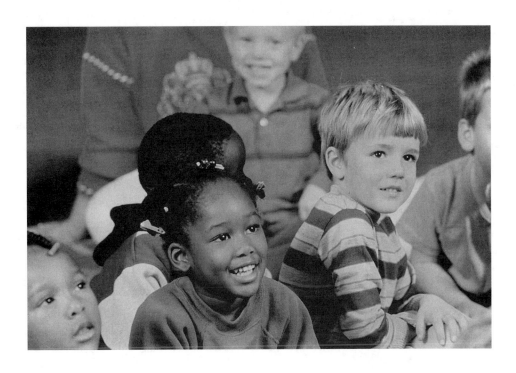

Most children acquire language naturally and, for the most part, without any formal instruction. Some children, however, experience serious difficulties in their acquisition of language. These children are language disordered. To overcome their disorders, such children require the assistance of various professionals, including speech-language pathologists, psychologists, and, in the school setting, special educators and resource room teachers.

The multidisciplinary nature of the study of language disorders is one reason for the complexity of the discipline. Speech-language pathology, special education, sociolinguistics, linguistics, psycholinguistics, and psychology, the disciplines that study language, have their own respective inventories of terms and methods. Diversity of terms, constructs, and even attitudes and biases pervades the study of language and its disorders. A cursory perusal of the writings in this field is enough to convince the student of this diversity.

A second reason for the complexity in studying language disorders relates to the complexity of language itself. Although in this decade of the 1990s we program computers to process information so that they can control a factory, cook a meal, and even fly a plane, we have not yet succeeded in programming a computer to simulate the generative nature of human language. This may happen someday, but, for the present, language remains too complex for reduction to a simpler format by programming. Comprehending language, theoretically, is a formidable task. Applying theories pragmatically to assess and to provide remediation to individuals who are language disordered is even more complex.

The centrality of language in the human experience is a third factor that complicates the study of language disorders. Language is crucial to all social and educational functioning. Parents are most concerned that their children acquire language because they recognize that a language deficiency may have a serious effect on future educational, social, and vocational opportunities. "Language," it has been said, "may be the most distinctive attribute of human beings; its acquisition is an integral part of human development. It is not surprising that how language is learned and taught are major issues in education and other human service fields" (McCormick & Schiefelbusch, 1984, p. 2).

This first chapter consists of fundamental information on three interrelated subjects relevant to language: the components or elements of language, perspectives on language acquisition, and approaches to language disorders in children. These areas were chosen because speech-language pathologists and special educators must possess a clear understanding of the nature of language and how it is acquired if they are to provide appropriate interventions for children with language and communication disorders.

We will begin, however, by exploring the differences between three seemingly similar but in reality different terms—*communication, speech,* and *language.* We will then further explain the notion of *language* by providing an explanation of its components.

Communication, Speech, and Language

To the average person, the terms *communication, speech,* and *language* are synonymous. Professionals in the field of speech-language, who spend years studying and treating language disordered children, often must go into lengthy descriptions of their chosen field of specialization to explain why their area of interest does not include correcting stuttering or improving diction. Confusion about the focus of speech-language specialists probably results from confusion of these terms. To the specialist these terms are very different and denote different aspects of development.

Communication

Communication is the process by which individuals exchange information and convey ideas (Owens, 1990). It is an active process requiring a sender who encodes, or formulates, a message. It also requires a receiver who decodes, or comprehends, the message. Each partner must be alert to the needs of the other to ensure that messages are effectively conveyed and understood.

Although we may primarily use speech and language to communicate, other aspects of communication may enhance or distort the linguistic code. Paralinguistic cues, which include intonation patterns, stress, and speech rate, can signal the attitude and emotions of the speaker and alter the linguistic information. Consider the difference that stress makes in the meaning a speaker wishes to convey when uttering the following:

> She *grabbed the money from him.*
> *She grabbed the* money *from him.*
> *She grabbed the money from* him.

Or consider the effect a rising intonation would have on the following sentence:

> *John kissed her on the lips.*

In addition to paralinguistic cues, nonlinguistic cues also contribute to the communication process. Nonlinguistic cues include gestures, body movements, eye contact, and facial expression, which can add to or detract from the linguistic message. All of us are familiar with the individual who looks at us as we talk and may intermittently nod his head, indicating to us that he is actively involved in the communication process. Conversely, the individual who does not make eye contact often communicates a lack of interest or involvement in the communicative interaction, and we in turn may diminish our communication with him.

Speech

Speech is one of the modes that may be used for communication. It is the oral verbal mode of transmitting messages and involves the precise coordination of oral neuromuscular movements in order to produce sounds and linguistic units.

Although we primarily use speech for the purpose of communication, it is not the only means available to us. Writing, drawing, and manual signing are other modes of communication. Individuals select a mode depending on the context, their needs, the needs of the decoder, and the message they wish to transmit.

For some children with disabilities acquiring speech is not a realistic goal. The limited physical control these children have over the speech mechanism makes it unlikely that they could learn to produce recognizable speech. However, many of these children can acquire the ability to communicate if given alternative means. In recent years, a number of alternative and/or augmentative communication systems have been designed for them. These systems allow the child to transmit messages without using speech. Beukelman and Mirenda (1992) describe a number of these systems (Blissymbolics, American Sign Language, computer-operated systems, etc.). In addition, Owens (Chapter 12), Tiegerman (Chapter 13), and Radziewicz and Antonellis (Chapter 14) also discuss the use of nonspeech modes in the intervention programs for mentally retarded, autistic, and hearing-impaired individuals.

Language

Language is a socially shared code, or conventional system, that represents ideas through the use of arbitrary symbols and rules that govern combinations of these symbols. There are hundreds of languages, each with its own particular symbols and rules. Language exists because language users have agreed on the symbols and rules to be used. Because these symbols are shared, the language user can employ them to exchange information and ideas. The linguistic code allows the language user to represent an object, an event, or a relationship with a symbol or a combination of symbols.

Language encompasses complex rules that govern sounds, words, sentences, meaning, and use. These rules underlie an individual's ability to understand language (language comprehension) and his or her ability to formulate language (language production). An individual's implicit knowledge about the rules of his or her language is called linguistic competence. A person who possesses linguistic competence has the knowledge needed to be a language user. He or she knows the rules about sounds and their combination; he or she knows what makes sense and what doesn't. He or she can understand and create an infinite number of sentences and can use language in a variety of social settings. Even though he or she cannot explicitly state the rules, the language user behaves in a way that demonstrates that he or she knows them. Although children give evidence of knowing the rules of language at quite an early age, how this rule-learning occurs is still being investigated.

In sum, native speakers/listeners of a language learn a linguistic rule system. This rule system can be divided into three major components: form, content, and use. These components are described more thoroughly in the next section.

The Components of Language

Language is a complex combination of several component rule systems. Bloom and Lahey (1978) have divided language into three major components: form, content, and use.

Form

Form includes the linguistic elements that connect sounds and symbols with meaning. Included in linguistic form are rules that govern sounds and their combination (phonology), rules that govern the internal organization of words (morphology), and rules that specify how words should be ordered to produce a variety of sentence types (syntax).

Phonology

Phonology is the system of rules that govern sounds and their combination. Each language has specific sounds, or **phonemes,** that are characteristic of that language. Phonemes are combined in specific ways to form linguistic units known as words.

A phoneme is the smallest linguistic unit of speech that signals a difference in meaning. The words *bat* and *pat* differ from each other in only one way—their initial sound. Because this initial sound difference produces two different words, the difference is a meaningful one. Therefore, /b/ and /p/ are, by definition, two different phonemes.

Phonemes are classified by their acoustic properties (the pattern of their sound waves), their articulatory properties (where in the oral cavity they are produced, or place of articulation), and their production properties (manner of articulation).

The use of phonemes is governed by two sets of rules. One set describes how sounds can be used in various word positions. These are called distributional rules. In English, for example, the *ng* sound, as in the word *long,* is a single phoneme that never appears at the beginning of a word. The second set of rules determines which sounds may be combined. They are called sequencing rules. In English, for example, the sound sequence *rs* may not appear in the same syllable. In sum, phonological rules govern sounds and their distribution and sequencing within a language.

Morphology

The second component of language—**morphology**—governs word formation. Morphological rules are concerned with the internal structure of words and how they are constructed from morphemes. **Morphemes** are the smallest linguistic unit with meaning (and cannot be broken into any smaller parts that have meaning). Words consist of one or more morphemes. Each of the words *ball, toy,* and *play* consists of one morpheme that can stand alone. Morphemes that can stand alone are called free morphemes. Bound morphemes cannot stand alone and are always found attached to free morphemes. They are affixed to free morphemes as prefixes (*un*happy) or suffixes (tall*est*). Bound morphemes that modify tense, person, or number are called inflectional morphemes. Examples of inflectional morphemes include the plural *s* (cat*s*), the past tense *ed* (play*ed*), and the possessive *'s* (Joan*'s*).

Bound morphemes can also be used to change one word into another word that may be a different part of speech. For example, *ness* changes the adjective *sad* into the noun *sadness.* In this case, bound morphemes are called derivational morphemes because they are used to derive new words.

One task for the student of language development and disorders is to determine whether children have knowledge of morphology and to what extent it resembles the rule system of adults.

Syntax

Syntax is the rule system that governs the structure of sentences. It specifies the order words must take and the organization of different sentence types. It allows the individual to combine words into phrases and sentences and to transform sentences into other sentences.

A competent language user can take a basic sentence like "The boy hit the ball" and transform it into a number of different sentence types.

> *Did the boy hit the ball? (interrogative)*
> *The ball was hit by the boy. (passive)*

Knowledge of the syntactic system allows a speaker to generate an almost infinite number of sentences (from a finite group of words) and to recognize which sentences are grammatical ("The boy hit the ball") and which sentences are not ("Ball the boy the hit").

Syntactic rules have two additional functions: They describe parts of speech (noun—*house;* verb—*hit;* adjective—*red*) and sentence constituents (noun phrases, verb phrases).

> *Lightning* hit *(verb) the* red *(adjective)* house *(noun).*
> *The boy (noun phrase)* hit the ball *(verb phrase).*

As children produce longer sentences, they begin to build sentences according to syntactic rules. They learn how to construct negative sentences, questions, and imperatives. Later, they add complex structures like compound sentences and embedded forms. The development of syntax begins at about 18 months and continues for many years. Chapters 5 and 6 discuss syntactic growth during the preschool and school years.

Content

The **content** component of language involves meaning. It maps knowledge about objects, events, and people, and the relationship among them. Included are the rules governing **semantics,** that subsystem of language that deals with words—their meanings and the links that bind them. It encompasses meanings conveyed by individual words and the speaker's or listener's mental dictionary (called a lexicon).

Words are used differently by young children than they are by adults. A very young child may use a word that occurs in the adult linguistic system, but that word may not mean the same thing to him as to the adult. A 2-year-old may say the word *doggie,* but his word may refer to sheep, cows, and horses as well as to a dog. Alternatively, a 2-year-old may use the word *doggie* to refer to a particular dog without knowing it refers to a whole class of animals. Studying children's semantic system involves, in part, examining their understanding and use of words. Early lexical acquisition is discussed more fully in Chapter 4.

The content component of language maps an individual's knowledge of not only objects (*big car*) but also the relationship that exists between objects, events, and people. Note the use of the following semantic relations in the utterances of three 18-month-old toddlers, Tim, Yakov, and Judy:

Context	*Utterance*	*Semantic Relation*
Mother and child sitting on the floor. Child pushes car and says:	"Push car"	Action-Object
Mother and child are sitting in the kitchen. Mother is eating a cookie. Child says:	"Mommy eat"	Agent-Action

Mother and child are in the kitchen. The
child has just finished the milk in her cup.

She points to the milk container on the table and says:	"More milk"	Recurrence

A more complete account of the meanings (semantic relations) children convey in their early utterances is discussed in Chapter 4.

Although most meaning is literal, it can sometimes be nonliteral. For example, if we talk about the *dance of life,* we do not mean *dance* in the literal sense. Our meaning is figurative; that is, we are speaking of life in terms of patterns, grace, movement, and change.

Similarly, if I said, "I had a ball," you might infer that I had a good time. The word *ball* is used here in its nonliteral sense. However, note that a literal meaning is also possible (e.g., "I possessed a volleyball," baseball, basketball, etc.). Which meaning is appropriate will depend on the context and what has already been said.

In sum, meaning in language is conveyed through the use of words and their combinations. Content maps an individual's knowledge about objects, relationships, and concepts. This knowledge is derived from experiences and is a result of one's cognitive development. Lastly, it is important to remember that meaning can be both literal and nonliteral and is dependent on linguistic and nonlinguistic contexts.

Use

The **use** component of language encompasses rules that govern the use of language in social contexts. These rules are also called **pragmatics** and include rules that govern the reason(s) for communicating (called communicative functions or intentions) as well as rules that govern the choice of codes to be used when communicating (Bloom & Lahey, 1978).

The functions of language relate to the speaker's intention or goal. Greeting, asking questions, answering questions, requesting information, giving information, and requesting clarification are examples of language functions.

In addition to coding communicative intentions, a speaker must use information regarding the listener and the nonlinguistic context to achieve his communicative intention. He must choose from alternative forms of a message the one that will best serve his communicative intention. The speaker must take into account what the listener already knows and does not know about a topic, as well as information about the context. The selection of the words and sentences to use to formulate a message depends upon this information. For example, knowing the age and occupation of different listeners influences the choice of words to greet them. It is appropriate to say "Hi ya" to a 3-year-old and "How do you do?" to a school principal. The form of the message is also influenced by whether the topics of the message are present in the situation in which the utterance is used. For example, whether a speaker says "The doll is on the floor" or "It's over there" depends on whether the doll and the floor are in the immediate situation.

Lastly, pragmatics encompasses rules of conversation or discourse. Speakers must learn to organize their conversations to make them coherent. They must learn how to enter, initiate, and maintain conversations. They must learn how to take turns, how to respond appropriately, and how to tell a cohesive narrative. Armed with these skills, an individual is said to be an effective communicator.

Correspondence and Integration of the Components of Language

We began this introductory chapter by defining language and by discussing the components that constitute it. The components of language and their subsystems are depicted in Table 1-1. Although the components of language appear as distinct entities, Bloom and Lahey (1978) have pointed out that they are indeed interrelated (see Figure 1-1).

How a child integrates linguistic components is best exemplified by the 2½-year-old child who looks through a window into the yard while her mother sits in the same room reading a book. As the child sees a kitten in the yard, she says to her mother, "Look, baby cat." As a result of this statement, the child has accomplished three things. First, she has linguistically coded two communicative intentions (getting attention and describing) by saying "look" and by describing what she sees. Next, she has linguistically coded knowledge about the animal she sees. Finally, she has expressed an utterance containing an acceptable word order. In sum, the child has successfully communicated by integrating pragmatic, syntactic, and semantic rules.

By taking the example a step further to a 3-year-old, we are able to demonstrate the child's integration of phonology and morphology with pragmatic, syntactic, and semantic rules. Both mother and her 3-year-old child are gazing through a window as two puppies are playing in the yard.

Mother: What do you see?

Child: Two puppies.

As in the previous case, the utterance codes knowledge about the animals and contains appropriate word order. In addition, the latter utterance contains the morphological ending that codes plurality. Using phonological rules, the child "knows" that the *s* in *puppies* is pronounced as a *z* because it follows a vowel, in contrast to the *s* in *cats,* which is pronounced as *s.*

TABLE 1-1   Language Is

Components	Linguistic Subsystems
Form	*Phonology* Rules that govern speech sounds and their combination
	Morphology Rules that govern the organization of words
	Syntax Rules that govern word order, sentence structure, and organization of different sentences types
Content	*Semantics* Rules that govern meaning (words and their combinations)
Use	*Pragmatics* Rules relating to the use of language in social contexts

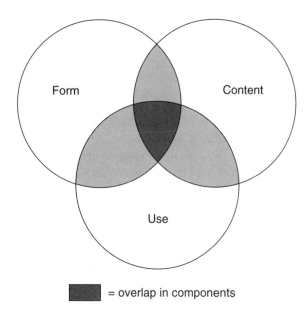

**FIGURE 1-1   Bloom and Lahey's model
of language.**

Reprinted with the permission of Macmillan Publishing Company
from *Language Development and Language Disorders* by Bloom, L.
and Lahey, M. Copyright © 1978 by Macmillan Publishing Company.

Whereas the integration of form, content, and use is observed in the language of non-disabled children, a disruption of the components is often found in the language of children with disabilities. For example, many hearing impaired youngsters produce language that possesses content but may be deficient in linguistic form. Their vocabulary and their communicative ability may be age appropriate, but their phonological, morphological, and syntactic skills often lag behind. Note the errors (indicated by bracketing) in the sample of David, a 5-year-old who is hearing impaired.

*"Ye[s]terday I give it to ... to ... What['s] hi[s] name? Oh, Bob? Right. He['s] not
in my cla[ss]. He's on my bu[s]. Why he can't come with me?"*

Or consider the following utterances produced by Sean, an 11-year-old child with autism. Note the inappropriateness of his utterances and the lack of meaning in his sample. Also note the lack of errors in linguistic form.

Clinician: Sean, how are you today?

Sean: Fine, oh so fine, so very very fine and on my mind.

Clinician: Your class went on a trip yesterday. Tell me about it.

Sean: A trip, a trip. Yesterday, today, tomorrow. Hot dogs dogs—all kinds of dogs—bow-wow. It's October and Halloween. Pepsi the choice of a new generation; Coca-Cola red, white, and blue . . . and soup is good food, too.

The terms and concepts outlined thus far are basic to the study of language and its disorders. Because an understanding of normal language development is crucial to the student who will undertake intervention with language disordered children, the following section outlines four theoretical perspectives on language acquisition. As this review is merely introductory, the beginning student is strongly urged to supplement it with references noted in the text.

Perspectives on Language Acquisition

Four multidisciplinary approaches to the study of language acquisition have predominated the literature in the past two decades: the behavioral, the psycholinguistic/syntactic, the semantic/cognitive, and the pragmatic. Each approach is summarized in terms of essential elements, emphasizing background, limitations, and contributions. Owens (1996), Nelson (1993), Bohannon and Warren-Leubecker (1993), Berko Gleason (1993), James (1990), and McCormick and Schiefelbusch (1990) provide a more detailed description of these approaches for interested readers.

Behavioral Approach

Background.   The behavioral approach to language development was first presented by B. F. Skinner (1957) in *Verbal Behavior.* Language learning, according to this approach, depends on environmental variables, which are mastered by imitation, practice, and selective reinforcement. The result is the acquisition of language through the gradual accumulation of vocal symbols and sequences of symbols. Within the process, parents and significant others are crucial because they model the appropriate utterances that children imitate and practice. By rewarding children's correct productions, parents shape children's utterances until they are grammatical and acceptable. In short, children learn language because their verbal behavior is selectively rewarded by others in the environment (Skinner, 1957). Variations on this theme are provided by Osgood (1963), Mowrer (1954), and Staats (1963).

Limitations.   Chomsky (1959) faulted Skinner on four counts, the first being that Skinner attempted to explain the process of language acquisition while ignoring the content being learned. Chomsky said, "There is little point in speculating about the process of acquisition without a much better understanding of *what* is acquired" (p. 55).

Second, Chomsky pointed out that children seem to acquire a verbal repertoire far too quickly to depend on environmental conditioning mechanisms alone. Third, Chomsky argued that children produce utterances they never heard adults use—utterances such as "I goed," and "mouses." A fourth criticism of the behaviorist model has come from research that has shown that parents rarely, if ever, correct or punish children's grammatical errors (Brown & Hanlon, 1970). Hence, the role of parental reinforcement is, at best, limited and not crucial to language acquisition as described by Skinner.

Contributions.   Although in the early 1960s criticism was leveled at the behavioral school for overemphasizing parental input, recent researchers have revised their thinking to acknowledge its importance in language development. Studies by Snow (1972), Newport (1976), and others have clearly shown the positive effects of parental linguistic input to children's language development. Another contribution made by the behaviorists to the field of speech-language pathology has been to delineate "systematic training designs and their applications to nonspeaking individuals" (McCormick & Schiefelbusch, 1984; Schiefelbusch & Bricker, 1981). Structured behavioral techniques are commonly used in speech-language therapy and provide a basis for many intervention programs used with language disordered children.

Psycholinguistic/Syntactic Approach

Background.   In the late 1950s and early 1960s, linguists, particularly Noam Chomsky, hypothesized that the human brain contains a mental plan to understand and generate sentences (Chomsky, 1957, 1965). This mental plan incorporates the necessary "electronic circuitry" for children to internalize the knowledge necessary for deriving sentences.

Proponents of the psycholinguistic/syntactic approach hold that children have an innate predisposition to apply linguistic rules and that the human infant is "prewired" for language acquisition. According to Chomsky, a baby is born with an innate linguistic mechanism (called the language acquisition device [LAD]) that is activated by exposure to linguistic input. The LAD contains two parts: a set of rules or general principles for forming sentences, and procedures for discovering how these principles are to be applied to the child's particular language.

The child's LAD processes information from the linguistic environment and generates hypotheses about the rules of his language. Using the concept of the preprogrammed LAD, Chomsky was able to explain the seemingly miraculous ability of very young children to acquire language easily and rapidly and to produce an infinite number of novel yet grammatical utterances.

More recently, Chomsky (1981) revised his ideas of grammar and syntax to account more for language rules and well-formedness as well for language learnability. The result is called government-language binding theory (GB theory). Chomsky's goal was to present a theory that could account for the constraints on the kinds of hypotheses a child can form about the structure of his or her language no matter what language the child is learning. Government-binding theory attempts to account for the diversity of human languages and to explain the development of grammar by children on the basis of limited input. The resultant principles Chomsky (1981) called universal grammar. (For a more complete account of GB theory see Berko Gleason, 1993; Cairns, 1995; Leonard & Loebb, 1988; Nelson, 1993; and Owens, 1996).

Limitations.   Child development specialists (Schlesinger, 1977; Sinclair-deZwart, 1973) argue that Chomsky treats language learning as if it occurred independently of cognitive development. Citing Piaget's work, Sinclair-deZwart (1973) said that language development is dependent on cognitive development. Schlesinger (1977) pointed out that it is very difficult to ascertain from Chomsky's model precisely what children are born "knowing" as opposed to what they "come to know" and how this knowledge eventually gets linked to words and phrases.

Semanticists (Fillmore, 1968) fault Chomsky by arguing that language depends more on underlying semantic representation than on syntactic rules. Sociolinguists challenge Chomsky's assertion that linguistic input is too fragmented, confused, and unsystematic to facilitate children's acquisition of language. Their data (Nelson, 1973b; Newport, 1976; Phillips, 1973; Snow, 1972) show that parental input enhances language learning. In Chapter 3 we detail the nature of parental input and its facilitating effect on language development.

Contributions.   Although the psycholinguistic/syntactic approach is currently viewed as being inadequate to explain language development, Chomsky's work provided the impetus for much in depth research on the language acquisition process. Investigators began to search for developmental patterns that crossed cultural boundaries. More important, they began to realize the value of naturalistic observations (McCormick & Schiefelbusch, 1984). A host of studies on both normal and disordered language were published in the 1960s (Braine, 1963; Brown & Bellugi, 1964; Brown & Fraser, 1964; Menyuk, 1964), and studies comparing normal and language disordered children's acquisition of morphology and syntax continue to be published (Fletcher, 1991, Hansson & Nettelbladt, 1995, Johnston & Shery, 1976, Leonard, 1992). Last, an alternative view of language learning evolved in contrast to the behaviorists' view, with the result that we currently view the child as being active and creative, rather than passive, in the language acquisition process.

Semantic/Cognitive Approach

Background.   With the publication of Bloom's *Language Development: Form and Function of Emerging Grammars* (1970), there appeared a new focus in the study of language development: the meanings conveyed by children's utterances rather than their syntax.

In her study of children's language at the early multiword stage, Bloom (1970) found that one of her subjects used "Mommy sock" on two different occasions. She used it once while she was picking up her mother's sock and once while her mother was putting a sock on her (the child's) foot. Although the form of the child's utterance was the same in both contexts, the *meanings* the child conveyed were clearly different. On the first occasion, she conveyed possession. The sock she was holding belonged to her mother. On the second occasion, the child's utterance conveyed a meaning found between an actor (Mommy) who was doing an action and an object (sock). Bloom concluded that children's language maps meanings. The meaning categories that children use to code relationships among entities found in the world were termed *semantic relations* by Bloom.

Bloom further postulated that children express meanings long before they know anything about syntax and that the meanings they convey are based on their cognitive knowledge.

Following Bloom, the cognitive prerequisites for language acquisition became the subject matter of much research. The works of Piaget (1952, 1954, 1964) were reexplored, and the search began for linkages between the concepts attained in early cognitive development and early linguistic constructions (Sinclair-deZwart, 1973).

The evidence (Nelson, 1973a) tends to show that children begin to use language expressively to talk about what they know and that this knowledge is related to their sensorimotor experiences. A fuller account of the cognitive prerequisite for language acquisition is found in Chapter 3. Rees (1980) best captured the essence of the semantic/cognitive approach when she said that "children say only what they know how to mean" (p. 21).

Limitations. The semantic/cognitive approach to language development highlights the importance of meaning and cognition. However, it does not explain why some children, in spite of age-appropriate cognitive abilities, lag in their linguistic development (Cromer, 1974). It would seem that conceptual abilities are not the only abilities important for language learning but that these other abilities are not accounted for in the semantic/cognitive approach.

Three other criticisms of the semantic/cognitive view have been offered. Bowerman (1978) pointed out that the semantic/cognitive approach does not answer the question of *how* children acquire language, nor does it explain the relationship between later developing cognitive abilities and corresponding linguistic attainments. Schlesinger (1977) observed that the semantic/cognitive approach ignores the role of linguistic input to the language acquisition process. How could language be learned if the child is not exposed to it? Last, McLean and Snyder-McLean (1978) argued that an adequate description of language acquisition must include formulations about the nature and purposes of children's social communicative interactions. They maintained that the social environment of the child is crucial to language development.

Contributions. The semantic/cognitive approach to language development is set against a background of overall development; hence, it gave impetus to multifaceted research on (a) the cognitive prerequisites of language (Bowerman, 1974; Sinclair-deZwart, 1973), (b) the universality of children's cognitive experiences resulting in a universality in their coding of meaning, and (c) the relationship between language and thought (Cromer, 1974; Miller, 1981; Rice, 1983). The role of imitation and play was reexamined (Bates, Benigni, Bretherton, Camaioni, & Volterra, 1979; Sinclair-deZwart, 1973; Westby, 1980) because scholars believed it was rooted in children's symbolic functioning. Last, the importance of contextual support (that is, the nonlinguistic context) was highlighted as being important to understanding the meanings children convey.

The Pragmatic Approach

Background. Because communicative intentions are expressed in social contexts, the pragmatic approach views language development within the framework of social development. According to Bruner (1974/1975), children learn language in order to socialize and to direct the behavior of others. Social interaction and relationships are deemed crucial because they provide the child with the framework for understanding and formulating linguistic content and form.

Within the pragmatic model, caretaker-child interactions are considered to be the originating force for language learning (Rees, 1978). As caretakers respond to infants' early reflexive behaviors and their gestures, the infant learns to communicate intentions. Infants refine these communication skills through repeated communicative interactions with caretakers.

McLean and Snyder-Mclean (1978) summarized the pragmatic model in four major statements:

1. Language is acquired if and only if the child has a reason to talk. Herein it is assumed that the child has learned that he can influence his environment through communication.
2. Language is acquired as a means of acknowledging already existing communication functions.
3. Language is learned in dynamic social interactions involving the child and the mature language user in his environment. The mature language user facilitates this process.
4. The child is art active participant in this transactional process and must contribute to it by behaving in a way which allows him to benefit from the adult's facilitating behavior. (p. 28)

The pragmatic model spawned a range of new research efforts. Expanding on the work of Searle (1965), Dore (1975), Halliday (1975), and Bates (1976) formulated a classification system for categorizing children's communicative intentions, and Bruner (1974/1975), Bates (1976), and others examined the role of parents and caretakers in the language acquisition process.

Limitations.   The explanation of language acquisition by the pragmatic approach leaves two major questions unanswered:

1. How do communicative intentions get linked to linguistic structures?
2. How do children acquire symbols for referents?

Two further limitations relate to the newness of the pragmatic view. One, present researchers cannot agree on a common system for classifying communicative intentions, and two, a system for assigning a specific intention to children's utterances has not yet emerged.

Contributions.   The pragmatic view highlights the social aspect of language and places language use in center stage. It specifies the contribution of environmental linguistic input and the role of caregiver modeling and feedback. In addition, it has stimulated research on the conditions and contexts in which communication develops, (Bates, 1976; Bruner, 1974/ 1975), and has identified the social prerequisites of language acquisition (See Chapter 2). All of these contributions are aspects of a general communication background, established well before children learn to use language expressively.

Approaches to Language Acquisition Revisited

The four approaches to language acquisition—behavioral, psycholinguistic/syntactic, semantic/cognitive, and pragmatic—contribute to our understanding of language development and enable us to appreciate the complexity of language in the absence of a full-blown model. The need for a complete model of language acquisition, however, remains. Future research may indeed provide it, pending the successful integration of constructs developed in the four approaches reviewed here. This need for integration is best summarized by McLean and Snyder-McLean (1978):

> *By nature of its content, language carries within it the products of the cognitive developmental domain; by nature of its function, language carries within it the products of social development; by nature of its form, language carries within it the complex products of all the inputs identified . . . plus the effect of the nature and functions of human physiological and neurological systems. (p. 43)*

For the present, without a full model of language, we may view each approach as best describing one or more of the phases in development. As the normal child passes through these phases, different aspects of language acquisition may be emphasized. In the earliest stage of development (infancy), emphasis may be on pragmatic development. In the early preschool years, emphasis may be on syntactic development. Understanding the process of normal language acquisition provide the reader with a firm basis for understanding language disorders.

Approaches to Language Disorders

There are two major approaches to the study of language disorders in children: the etiological-categorical and the descriptive-developmental. In this section, we define each approach and identify the respective strengths and limitations of each. In conclusion, we present a working definition of language disorders as proposed by the American Speech-Language-Hearing Association (ASHA, 1980).

Etiological-Categorical Approach

The traditional approach to child language disorders involves the classification of disorders by their causes, or etiology. Each etiological category summarizes a cluster of behaviors that differentiates the language disordered child from his normally developing peers.

The use of etiological typologies grew out of the early work of McGinnis (1963) and Myklebust (1954). The etiological categories used by Myklebust (1954) included: (a) mental retardation, (b) deafness and hearing impairment, (c) emotional disturbance and autism, and (d) childhood aphasia and neurologically based disorders. A fifth category, culturally and socially deprived, was later added, reflecting on the political-social climate of the 1960s (Kamhi, 1990).

McCormick and Schiefelbusch (1984) classified language disorders into five etiological categories:

1. Language and communication disorders associated with motor disorders. Included in this category are children who possess motor deficits, as well as language disorders due to brain pathology (e.g., cerebral palsy) or damage to the nervous system (e.g., spina bifida). Children in this category possess motor difficulties and may be mentally retarded, visually and hearing impaired, and in possession of seizure disorders. Because of the simultaneous multiple disabilities of these children and the space constraints of this text, we will not discuss this category. Instead, the reader is referred to Cruickshank (1976), McDonald and Chance (1964), and Mysack (1971) for a fuller account of this group.

2. Language and communication disorders associated with sensory deficits. Included in this category are children who possess hearing and visual impairments. Because the data on the language deficits of the blind are very scanty (Bernstein, 1978), we will discuss only hearing impairments as they relate to language disorders (see Chapter 14).
3. Language and communication disorders associated with central nervous system damage. Damage may be either mild or severe. Children are generally classified as learning disabled when the damage to the central nervous system is mild. When the damage to the central nervous system is severe, however, they are classified as developmental aphasics. Differentiating the aphasic from other severely language disordered children is both difficult and complex (McCormick & Schiefelbusch 1984). Hence, we limit our discussion to the language disorders associated with learning disabilities (see Chapter 11).
4. Language and communication disorders associated with severe emotional-social dysfunctions. Included in this category are children who are classified as psychotic, schizophrenic, and/or autistic. These children experience a profound disruption in the development of their verbal and nonverbal interaction skills. Considerable research on this disruption has been carried out in the area of autism and is reported in Chapter 13.
5. Language and communication problems associated with cognitive disorders. Included in this category are children who are classified as mentally retarded. The cognitive disabilities of children in this group vary according to the level of retardation. Chapter 12 discusses mental retardation and the language deficits associated with it.

Strengths of the Etiological-Categorical Approach.   Etiology is a convenient way of comparing and distinguishing autistic, learning disabled, mentally retarded, and hearing impaired children. Each classification is like a label that summarizes how a child is similar to, or different from, other children both within and across the disability categories.

A second and practical advantage of the etiological-categorical classification is that often a diagnostic label is needed for a child to receive appropriate services in schools. In many states today, children are placed in special education programs for speech, language, and resource services based on their diagnostic label. Furthermore, special education programs often are tailored to the etiology of a language disorder. Thus, one finds programs for the autistic, hearing impaired, or mentally retarded child. In this context, it is understandable that a child must be so labeled in order to be admitted to the most appropriate program.

Some advocacy groups have argued vociferously for the continuance of a categorical classification because they believe that it is better to be labeled and to receive attention and services than to be ignored. This has been especially true of advocacy groups for the severely developmentally delayed: the autistic and the mentally retarded.

A third advantage of the etiological-categorical approach is that it provides speech and language pathologists with clues as to what type of remediation might be indicated and the modalities to be used during intervention. For example, knowing that a child possesses cognitive deficits, as in mental retardation, suggests remediation that focuses on teaching the concepts that language codes and on providing the child with redundant and repetitive cues to support the language being taught. Knowing that a child is hearing impaired may lead the speech-language pathologist to search for alternative or augmentative systems to teach language. This may involve teaching some form of manual communication (e.g., sign language) or combining manual and spoken language (e.g., total communication).

Because much of the research concerned with language and communication disorders has focused on groups of children within etiological categories, four chapters—11, 12, 13, and 14—are devoted to explaining these findings. This information should be helpful to the speech-language pathologists working in educational or clinical settings in which diagnostic labels are used.

Caution, however, is called for on two accounts: (a) There exists considerable overlap among categories and (b) not all children within a diagnostic category possess similar abilities.

Limitations of the Etiological-Categorical Approach.   Drawbacks of the etiological-categorical approach were highlighted by Bloom and Lahey (1978), who pointed out that a particular diagnostic label does not tell the speech-language pathologist what the child really knows about *language* and what he or she needs to learn. Moreover, they stated, it is rare to find a child who neatly fits into one diagnostic category. For example, it is not uncommon to find a child who is both mentally retarded and hearing impaired or a child who is mentally retarded and also possesses autistic characteristics. In a similar vein, they maintained that a categorical label implies that there is only *one* cause of the language disorder. This is rarely the case. Although a single factor may appear in large part responsible for a language disorder, there are almost always several contributing factors.

A second critique of the etiological-categorical approach has been made by Naremore (1980), who argued that assessment and intervention are not helped by categorizing. She stated that it would be difficult to find a procedure to assess a group of children defined as either mentally retarded or hearing impaired. Within the group, assessment must be "customized" to each child with the aim of maximizing the resulting information and the understanding of that child's linguistic system and performance. The goal is to describe the child's linguistic behavior and to prescribe the specific methods and materials for improving his or her linguistic skills.

A third critique of the etiological-categorical model has been made by Kamhi (1990). He noted that an unfortunate outcome of this approach is that it serves "to divide treatment domains" (p. 73). Mentally retarded, autistic, and emotionally disturbed children are considered the province of the psychologist or special educator, whereas hearing impaired children are the domain of educators of the deaf. This leaves developmentally aphasic and culturally deprived children to be served by speech-language pathologists. Kamhi (1990) pointed out that, in most instances, "speech-language pathologists are the most qualified professionals to treat language disorders regardless of etiological type" (p. 73).

The Descriptive-Developmental Approach

The descriptive-developmental approach *describes* rather than classifies language disorders in children. It involves comparing the language disordered child's ability to comprehend and formulate language with that of nondisabled children. It assumes that a child with a language disorder needs to learn what the nondisabled child needs to learn at some point in development (Naremore, 1980). McCormick and Schiefelbusch (1984) summarized this point of view:

> There is every reason to think that children with deficient language: (a) need language learning experiences as rich as those provided normal language users,

(b) will attend to, understand and talk about many of the same objects, events and relations as typical learners, and (c) want and need to experience the same control over their environment as their more competent peers at the same stage of development. (p. 36)

According to the descriptive-developmental approach, a language disorder is "any disruption in the learning or use of the conventional system of arbitrary signals used by persons in the environment as a code for representing ideas about the world for communication" (Bloom & Lahey, 1978, p. 290). Disruptions occur in either form, content, or use, or in the interactions among them. Based on this construct, Bloom and Lahey (1978) differentiated five types of language disorders in children:

1. Children who exhibit difficulties in learning linguistic form. Included are children whose primary difficulty is in understanding and using phonological, morphological, and syntactic rules.
2. Children who exhibit difficulty in conceptualization and formulation of ideas about objects, events, and relations. Their primary difficulty is related to the semantic component—language content.
3. Children who exhibit difficulties in language use. Included are children who cannot adjust their language to meet listeners' needs, who do not use language to convey a range of communicative functions, and who have difficulties in understanding and speaking in certain contexts. Their primary deficit is in the area of pragmatics.
4. Children who exhibit difficulties in integrating form, content, and use. Bloom and Lahey (1978) termed this group of children as having association problems.
5. Children who exhibit language and communication skills that are similar in all ways to those of younger, normally developing children. Delayed language development is their primary disability.

Strengths of the Descriptive-Developmental Approach.   The descriptive-developmental approach focuses on identifying the strengths and weaknesses of children with language deficits. It allows the speech-language pathologist to describe children's language behaviors and to target those areas needing remediation.

Rather than labeling a child, this noncategorical approach is instructionally relevant. It zeroes in on those areas of language that pose difficulty for the child and gives the speech-language pathologist a teaching plan and sequence.

Limitations of the Descriptive-Developmental Approach.   Although the descriptive-developmental approach overcomes some of the limitations of the etiological-categorical approach, three problems still prevail:

1. It does not present the clinician with clear-cut procedures as to how to teach those areas needing remediation. Although form, content, and use are useful constructs for understanding language and its disorders, the therapeutic contexts and procedures in which form, content, and use should be taught are not delineated.

2. It assumes that the administration of therapy to a language disordered child is based on his linguistic disability and is irrelevant to his age or total environment. The descriptive-developmental approach has been criticized by Brown, Nietupski, and Hamre-Nietupski (1976), who have questioned whether it is useful to teach a 16-year-old mentally retarded adolescent who has the developmental skills of a 2-year-old the same vocabulary as one might teach a nondisabled 2-year-old. A strict adherence to the developmental approach without regard to the domestic, community, and vocational settings in which the child must ultimately function is to Brown and his colleagues not educationally sound.

   Brown et al. (1976) advocated an ecological perspective to intervention. The clinician is asked to search the relevant environments in which the child must function for clues as to what to teach. This might be considered the epitome of "customized therapy."

3. The descriptive-developmental approach ignores the practical problems faced by educators who require a disability label for a child prior to assignment to a special class or special services (Hobbs, 1978).

Language Disorders: A Definition

Because of the limitations described in both the traditional etiological-categorical approach and the descriptive-developmental approach, it is obvious that neither provides a complete definition. We present, then, ASHA's definition of language disorders as an alternative:

> *A language disorder is the abnormal acquisition, comprehension or expression of spoken or written language. The disorder may involve all, one, or some of the phonologic, morphologic, semantic, syntactic, or pragmatic components of the linguistic system. Individuals with language disorders frequently have problems in sentence processing or in abstracting information meaningfully for storage and retrieval from short and long term memory. (ASHA, 1980, pp. 317–18)*

According to the definition, impairment is in language comprehension (understanding), expression (formulation), or a combination of both. These deficits may be noted in listening and speaking or in reading and writing. Children who have language disorders may have difficulty in processing linguistic information, organizing and storing it, or retrieving it from memory. In short, ASHA's definition informs us about three important guidelines for considering language disorders: the components of language that might be impaired, the modalities that might be impaired, and the processes that might be impaired.

Summary

In this chapter we have described the nature of language and its subsystems. After defining language, we went on to explain the various approaches to language acquisition. The discussion began with the behavioral approach and proceeded through the approaches of the psycholinguistic/syntactic, semantic/cognitive, and the pragmatic. Lacking a full-blown model, we integrated the several approaches to language acquisition by suggesting that normal language acquisition is a temporal process emphasizing different dimensions of language development at different stages of chronological development. Apropos is the comment of Owens (1984), who concluded his monograph on language development by saying that "A teacher or speech-language pathologist has to rely upon many sources of information" (p. 334). These sources of information equate with the various approaches to language development. On a practical level, this means that the speech-language pathologist "should be a behaviorist, a pragmatist, a cognitivist, a linguist, a developmentalist, and an optimist in order to put together an effective means of teaching language to children" (Schiefelbusch, 1978, p. 461).

A discussion of language disorders followed, with a review of two different approaches to language disorders: the etiological-categorical and the descriptive-developmental. Each approach was shown to have advantages as well as disadvantages. Unable to reconcile the differences, we presented an alternative, ASHA's approach to defining language disorders, attempting to summarize those impairments in the linguistic system that account for language disorders.

The following thirteen chapters will elaborate and detail the preliminary discussions and definitions presented here. As you study them, do not hesitate to refer to the terms and definitions outlined in this introductory chapter. This will significantly contribute to a better understanding of communication acquisition and its disorders.

Study Questions

1. List at least five ways of communicating that you have used. Be specific.
2. What is the relationship of speech to language? Is language part of speech or speech part of language?
3a. Define each of the following systems of language:
    a. phonology
    b. morphology
    c. syntax
    d. semantics
    e. pragmatics
3b. How do each of the above subsystems fit into Bloom and Lahey's model of form/content/use?
4. Define *phoneme* and *morpheme* in your own words. How does each relate to meaning?
5. Discuss the strengths and weaknesses of each of the following perspectives in language acquisition:
    a. the behavioral perspective
    b. the psycholinguistic/syntactic perspective
    c. the semantic/cognitive perspective
    d. the pragmatic perspective
6. Compare and contrast the etiological-categorical classification of language disorders with the descriptive-developmental approach. What are the contributions and limitations of each approach?

References

The ASHA Committee on Language, Speech and Hearing Services in the Schools. (April, 1980). Definitions for communicative disorders and differences, *Asha, 22,* 317–318.

The ASHA Committee on Language. (June, 1983). Definition of language, *Asha, 25,* 44.

Bates, E. (1976). *Language and context: The acquisition of pragmatics.* New York: Academic Press.

Bates, E., Benigni, L., Bretherton, I., Camaioni, L., & Volterra, V. (1979). *The emergence of symbols: Cognition and communication in infancy.* New York: Academic Press.

Berko Gleason, J. (1993). The development of language. New York: Macmillan.

Bernstein, D. K. (1978). *Semantic development of congenitally blind children.* Unpublished doctoral dissertation, City University of New York.

Beukelman, D. R. and Mirenda, P. (1992). *Augumentative and alternative communication: Management of severe communication disorders in children and adults.* Baltimore, MD: Paul H. Brookes.

Bloom, L. (1970). *Language development: Form and function of emerging grammars.* Cambridge: MIT Press.

Bloom, L., & Lahey, M. (1978). *Language development and language disorders.* New York: Macmillan.

Bohannon, J., & Warren-Leubecker, A. (1993). Theoretical approaches to language acquisition. In J. Berko Gleason (Ed.), *The development of language* (3rd ed). New York: Macmillan.

Bowerman, M. (1974). Discussion summary—Development of concepts underlying language. In R. Schiefelbusch & L. Lloyd (Eds.), *Language perspectives—Acquisition, retardation and intervention.* Baltimore: University Park Press.

Bowerman, M. (1978). The acquisition of word meaning: An investigation in some current conflicts. In N. Waterson & C. Snow (Eds.), *The development of communication.* New York: Wiley.

Braine, M. (1963). The ontogeny of English phrase structure: The first phrase. *Language, 39,* 1–13.

Brown, L., Nietupski, J., & Hamre-Nietupski, S. (1976). The criterion of ultimate functioning and public school services for severely handicapped students. In M. A. Thomas (Ed.), *Hey, don't forget about me!* Reston, VA: The Council for Exceptional Children.

Brown, R., & Bellugi, U. (1964). Three processes in the child's acquisition of syntax. *Harvard Educational Review, 34,* 133–151.

Brown, R., & Fraser, C. (1964). The acquisition of syntax. In U. Bellugi & R. Brown (Eds.), *The acquisition of language. Monographs of the Society for Research in Child Development, 92.*

Brown, R. J., & Hanlon, C. (1970). Derivational complexity and order of acquisition. In J. Hayes (Ed.), *Cognition and the development of language.* New York: Wiley.

Bruner, J. (1974/75). From communication to language: A psychological perspective. *Cognition, 3,* 225–287.

Cairns, H. (1996). *The Acquisition of Language.* Austin, TX: Pro-ed.

Chomsky, N. (1957). *Syntactic structures.* The Hague: Mouton.

Chomsky, N. (1959). A review of Skinner's "Verbal Behavior." *Language, 35,* 26–58.

Chomsky, N. (1965). *Aspects of the theory of syntax.* Cambridge: MIT Press.

Chomsky, N. (1981). *Lectures on government and binding: The Pisa lectures.* Dordrecht: Foris Publications.

Cromer, R. (1974). The development of language and cognition: The cognitive hypothesis. In D. Foss (Ed.), *New perspectives in child development.* New York: Penguin Education.

Cruickshank, W (1976). *Cerebral palsy: A developmental disability.* Syracuse, NY: University Press.

Dore, J. (1975). Holophrases, speech acts, and language universals. *Journal of Child Language, 2,* 21–40.

Fillmore, C. (1968). The case for case. In E. Bach & R. Harmes (Eds.), *Universal in linguistic theory.* New York: Holt, Rinehart & Winston.

Fletcher, P. (1991). Evidence from syntax for language impairment. In J. Miller (Ed.), *Research on child langua3ge. A decade of progress* (pp. 169–187). Austin: Pro-ed.

Halliday, M. (1975). *Learning how to mean: Explorations in the development of language.* New York: Edward Arnold.

Hansson, K., & Nettelbladt, U. (1995). Grammatical characteristics of Swedish children with SLI. *Journal of Speech-Hearing Research. 38,* 559–598.

Hobbs, N. (1978). Classification options: A conversation with Nicholas Hobbs on exceptional child education. *Exceptional Children, 44,* 494–497.

James, S. (1990). *Normal language acquisition.* Boston: Allyn & Bacon.

Johnston, J., & Schery, T. (1976). The use of grammatical morphemes by children with communication disorder. In D. Morehead & A. Morehead (Eds.), *Normal and deficient language* (pp. 239–258). Baltimore: University Park Press.

Kamhi, A. (1990). Language disorders in children. In M. Leahy (Ed.), *Disorders of Communication.* London: Whurr.

Leonard, L. (1992). The use of morphology by children with specific language impairment: Evidence from three languages. In R. Chapman (Ed.), *Processes in language acquisition and disorders* (pp. 186–201). Chicago: Mosby-Yearbook.

Leonard, L. B., & Loebb, D. F. (1988). Government binding theory and some of its applications: A tutorial. *Journal of Speech and Hearing Research,* 31, 515–524.

McCormick, L., & Schiefelbusch, R. (1990). *Early language intervention* (2nd ed.). Columbus, OH: Merrill/Macmillan.

McCormick, L., & Schiefelbusch, R. L. (1984). *Early language intervention.* Columbus, OH: Merrill/Macmillan.

McDonald, E. T., & Chance, B., Jr. (1964). *Cerebral palsy.* Englewood Cliffs, NJ: Prentice Hall.

McGinnis, M. (1963). *Aphasic children: identification and education by association method.* Washington, DC: Alexander Graham Bell Association for the Deaf.

McLean, J., & Snyder-McLean, L. (1978). *A transactional approach to early language training.* Columbus, OH: Merrill/Macmillan.

Menyuk, P. (1964). Syntactic rules used by children from preschool through first grade. *Child Development, 35,* 533–546.

Miller, J. (1981). *Assessing language production in children.* Baltimore: University Park Press.

Mowrer, O. (1954). The psychologist looks at language. *American Psychologist, 9,* 660–694.

Myklebust, H. (1954). *Auditory disorders in children: A manual for differential diagnosis.* New York: Grune & Stratton.

Mysack, E. (1971). Cerebral palsy speech syndromes. In L. E. Travis (Ed.), *Handbook of speech pathology and audiology.* Englewood Cliffs, NJ: Prentice Hall.

Naremore, R. (1980). Language disorders in children. In T. Hixon, L. Schriberg, & J. Saxman (Eds.), *Introduction to communication disorders.* Englewood Cliffs, NJ: Prentice Hall.

Nelson, K. (1973a). Some evidence for the cognitive primacy of categorization and its functional basis. *Merrill-Palmer Quarterly, 19,* 21–39.

Nelson, K. (1973b). Structure and strategy in learning to talk. *Monographs of the Society for Research in Child Development, 38.*

Nelson, N. W. (1993). Childhood language disorders in context: Infancy through adolescence. New York: Macmillan.

Newport, E. (1976). Motherese: The speech of mothers to young children. In J. Castellan, D. Pisoni, & G. Potts (Eds.), *Cognitive theory* (Vol. 2). Hillsdale, NJ: Lawrence Erlbaum Associates.

Osgood, C. (1963). On understanding and creating sentences. *American Psychologist, 18,* 735–751.

Owens, R. E. (1984). *Language development: An introduction.* Columbus, OH: Merrill.

Owens, R. E. (1990). Communication, language and, speech. In G. Shames & E. Wiig (Eds.), *Human communication disorders* (3rd ed.). Columbus, OH: Merrill/Macmillan.

Owens, R. E. (1996). *Language development: An introduction* (4th ed.). Needham, MA: Allyn & Bacon.

Phillips, J. (1973). Syntax and vocabulary of mothers' speech to young children: Age and sex comparisons. *Child Development, 44,* 182–185.

Piaget, J. (1952). *The origins of intelligence in children.* New York: International Universities Press.

Piaget, J. (1954). *The construction of reality in the child.* New York: Basic Books.

Piaget, J. (1964). Three lectures. In R. Ripple & U. Rockcastle (Eds.), *Piaget rediscovered.* Ithaca, NY: Cornell University Press.

Rees, N. (1978). Pragmatics of language. In R. Schiefelbusch (Ed.), *Bases of language intervention.* Baltimore: University Park Press.

Rees, N. (1980). Learning to talk and understand. In T. J. Hixon, L. D. Shriberg, & J. H. Saxon (Eds.), *Introduction to communication disorders.* Englewood Cliffs, NJ: Prentice Hall.

Rice, M. (1983). Contemporary accounts of the cognition-language relationship: Implications for language clinicians. *Journal of Speech and Hearing Disorders, 48,* 347–359.

Schiefelbusch, R. (1978). Summary and interpretation. In R. Schiefelbusch (Ed.), *Bases of language intervention.* Baltimore: University Park Press.

Schiefelbusch, R. L., & Bricker, D. D. (Eds.). (1981). *Early language: Acquisition and intervention.* Baltimore: University Park Press.

Schlesinger, I. (1977). The role of cognitive development and linguistic input in language acquisition. *Journal of Child Language, 4,* 153–169.

Searle, J. (1965). What is a speech act? In M. Black (Ed.), *Philosophy in America.* New York: Allen & Unwin; Cornell University Press.

Sinclair-deZwart, H. (1973). Language acquisition and cognitive development. In T. E. Moore (Ed.), *Cognitive development and the acquisition of language.* New York: Academic Press.

Skinner, B. R. (1957). *Verbal behavior.* New York: Appleton-Century-Crofts.

Snow, C. (1972). Mothers' speech to children learning language. *Child Development, 43,* 549–566.

Staats, A. W. (1963). *Complex human behavior.* New York: Holt, Rinehart & Winston.

Westby, C. (1980). Assessment of cognitive and language abilities through play. *Language, Speech and Hearing Services in Schools, 111,* 154–168.

Social Cognition: The Communication Imperative

ELLENMORRIS TIEGERMAN-FARBER
School for Language and Communication Development
and
Adelphi College

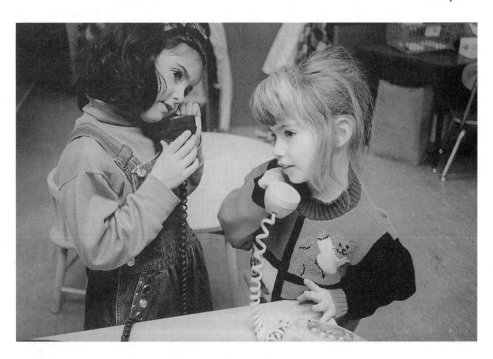

The next two chapters utilize a model proposed by Bronfenbrenner (1979, 1989) that views child development in terms of an ecological system (see Figure 2-1a). Individual aspects of development occur as a function of the child's experiences within broadening social contexts: the microsystem of the family to the exosystem of the external environment to the macrosystem of the cultural society. Bronfenbrenner proposes that the family constitutes a social microsytem in which the child has direct experiences with significant caregivers. The family in turn is affected by a range of variables as individual members themselves interact outside of the microsystem and within other environments that constitute the exosystem. Although the child does not directly experience the exosystem, he or she is affected by it. Economic and social changes in the exosystem impact upon his or her parents, their job employment and family lifestyle decisions. As a result, parents often bring their fears, frustrations, hopes, and aspirations back into the family context—the child's primary context for learning.

Several research theorists have suggested that in order to understand the needs of the child, it is important to take into consideration his or her family and how it functions within the framework of broader social contexts (Simeonsson & Bailey, 1988). The final social network involves a macrosystem that includes the ethnic community and the larger cultural society. The relationship between the child and his or her environment suggests a bidirectional learning process (see Figure 2-1b). The qualitative and quantitative dynamics within the microsystem define the child, but these dynamics are in turn defined by events within the exo- and macrosystems. Child development problems are often symptomatic of broader social issues. The child's social context, the quality of his or her parent-child relationships, and his or her economic status, his or her community environment are all influenced by society's network system of support services to children and families.

The next two chapters discuss child development by means of a systems theory that incorporates family variables as part of the learning process (Sameroff, 1983). The two chapters are also linked together by a theory referred to as the contextualist paradigm (Szapocznik & Kurtines, 1993). This theory emphasizes the social context within which child development is embedded. The social context creates a schematic model for child development. The development of communication, which is discussed in this chapter, and language, which is discussed in the next chapter, are described in terms of a highly complex process that is bidirectional; the child impacts on the family and is in turn influenced by contextual variables that affect family functioning (see Figure 2-1b).

Within the micro system, the infant develops his or her earliest relationships. These interactional relationships are part of a relatively new area of research development called social cognition. This chapter describes social cognition in terms of the child's primary imperative—communication development. Within the microsystem of the family, the child learns about people, interaction, and communication behaviors; this establishes a basis for the development of a representational model that allows the child to compare and reference his or her behaviors. Social cognition enhances the child's understanding of self, peers, physical objects, and organizational rules that are generated from experiential learning. Social knowledge and event knowledge develop contextual scripts that allow for learning about the social-physical world, the interactional rules that define contextual environments, and the social behaviors that allow the child to establish himself or herself as a primary agent of change. The social cognition process provides a mechanism for the developing

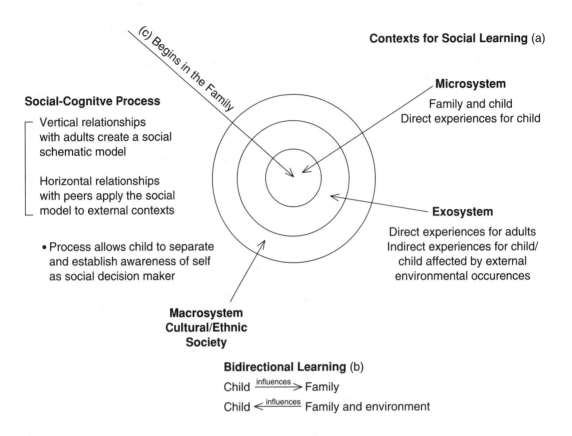

Social-Cognitve Process

┌ Vertical relationships
│ with adults create a social
│ schematic model
│
│ Horizontal relationships
│ with peers apply the social
└ model to external contexts

• Process allows child to separate
  and establish awareness of self
  as social decision maker

(c) Begins in the Family

Contexts for Social Learning (a)

Microsystem
Family and child
Direct experiences for child

Exosystem
Direct experiences for adults
Indirect experiences for child/
child affected by external
environmental occurences

Macrosystem
Cultural/Ethnic
Society

Bidirectional Learning (b)

Child ──influences──> Family

Child <──influences── Family and environment

FIGURE 2-1   Ecological systems approach to child development.

child to integrate and to generalize the rules established within the family microsystem in order to make social decisions within broadening contextual environments as he or she gets older. Social cognition maps out the development of social independence, which requires an awareness of self as a decision maker.

Hartup (1989) suggests that the child needs to experience two different types of relationships: vertical and horizontal (see Figure 2-1). The vertical relationship involves the interactional process with someone who has greater social power or knowledge, such as a parent or a teacher. This relationship is described as being complementary rather than reciprocal, since the behaviors exhibited by adult and child are quite different. Horizontal relationships are reciprocal in nature and provide the young communicator with experiences involving social peers who have equal social status. These two relationships serve highly different functions; both are necessary for the child to acquire effective social-communicative skills. It is interesting to note that Hartup suggests that within the framework of vertical relationships the young communicator acquires an internal social schematic model that acts as a reference and standard for the development of fundamental social skills. In horizontal relationships with peers, the child applies the skills that he or she has learned in order to develop an understanding of relationship variables such as cooperation, competition, and intimacy—variables critical to maintaining relationships throughout life.

The discussion of social cognition in this chapter highlights the following theoretical and developmental issues.

1. Attachment theory is a central theory in research concerning infant-parent relationships.
2. Relationships with adults and peers are of central importance in the child's social development.
3. Children's relationships with peers become increasingly more important for their social development.
4. Peer interactions are focused on common activities and create the framework for early friendships.
5. Social interaction provides the framework for communication learning.
6. Social cognition involves an ongoing and active learning process.
7. Interactive experiences with people stimulate conceptual learning about social knowledge. Interactive experiences with objects in the environment stimulate conceptual learning about event knowledge.

Vertical Relationships

Socio-affective Attachment

The parent's bond to the child provides an opportunity for the development of mutuality and attachment behaviors. During infancy the formation of such a parent-child bond creates a social interactional exchange that is affectively, communicatively, and emotionally satisfying for both parents and infants (Bowlby, 1988; Ainsworth, 1989). The interactional exchange provides a practice process in which a whole series of social behaviors are acquired, emitted, and perfected. Social behaviors as they are practiced over time create interactional patterns between adults and infants. These interactional patterns establish a mutually satisfying affective schematic framework in which young communicators learn to initiate and to respond to other social communicators. Interacting with people and contexts provides the infant communicator with "on-the-job training." The child learns how to achieve different purposes through communication. He or she learns about the effects and contingencies of different communication purposes as well as the differences in communication consequences across different situations. The context in which communication takes place becomes an important variable. The child also learns that there are communication variables related to the person to whom he or she is speaking. The child quickly learns to modify behavior given the listener and the context.

The quality of attachment is directly related to the pattern of social interaction between parent and infant (Bretherton, 1992a, b). The interactional relationship provides a framework for the child to develop a model for self as communicator and a model of others with whom he or she interacts, socializes, communicates, and plays. The child attempts to recreate in each new relationship a pattern of behavior that is familiar and secure. Ongoing interactional experiences allow the infant to develop a social referencing model—an internal schemata that provides a mechanism for infants to socially explore relationship parameters. For securely attached infants, the contingency and responsiveness from parents play a key role. The affective security that adults within the environment respond consistently to the infant's needs provides the child with a viewpoint about his or her world. Within the framework of this parent/infant relationship, the child learns to communicate his or her needs by combining and recombining the social behaviors that have achieved a contextual result or change.

The pragmatic approach to language learning emphasizes the social-communicative functions of language. The primary motivation for language development is thought to be effective communication (Bates, 1976; McLean & Snyder-McLean, 1978). The child learns to choose the form and content that will best achieve his or her intentions within a given situation. According to this communication perspective, the primary context for language learning is the caretaker-child dyad. Adult-child dyadic interaction is highly specialized for language learning. During interaction, the adult and the child negotiate the topic and purpose of communication. Although there is asymmetry in skill between the participants, there is ample evidence of reciprocity of interaction. Features of the child's behavior affect the language and the communication input of the adult. The attunement of the adult to the child provides the opportunity for regulated levels of learning. The processes of language learning are developed and enhanced within the parameters of interactive relationships. Although the social environment facilitates the communication learning process, the child's organizational preprogramming imposes a bias that selects, modifies, and reorganizes the information provided within the environment (Gleitman, Newport, & Gleitman, 1984).

Adult Input and Motherese

Several research studies have indicated that adults regulate and attune their language according to a child's level of comprehension and that adult-child conversational exchanges are different from adult-adult conversational exchanges. This regulated language input—which is child-centered, child-oriented, and child-sensitive—has come to be called motherese (Newport, 1977; Snow & Ferguson, 1977). The characteristic features common to motherese indicate an interactional learning process that may be child-motivated or culturally determined. Several cross-cultural studies have indicated that motherese is sensitive to differences in cultural styles (Brice Heath, 1983; Pye, 1986). As a result, the input provided to the young language learner will vary in certain critical aspects as a function of cultural determinants. Another important issue related to motherese is its role in language learning; this role is sometimes referred to as the motherese hypothesis. Duchan (1986) referred to the way in which the adult alters her input to what the child is thinking or doing as fine-tuning. The assumption made is that the closer the fine-tuning of the adult input to the child's activities, "the better the conditions" for child language learning. In the fine-tuning process, the adult has to make a decision about what the child knows in a particular activity. Part of the decision-making process involves the adult's choice of one label or description (e.g., house, jump) over another (mansion, leap). The adult also decides what is important or relevant for the child to know at a particular point in developmental time.

The term motherese was coined to describe language a mother regulates and attunes according to her baby's needs but has come to refer to any such child-oriented language by an adult. Investigators have researched many features that relate to baby talk or caretaker register (Furrow, Nelson, & Benedict, 1979; Newport, 1977; Newport, Gleitman, & Gleitman, 1977 Olson, Bates, & Kaskie, 1992;). Bernstein Ratner and Pye (1984), described pitch elevation as a prominent expressive feature in mothers addressing their infants. They suggested that characteristics of motherese probably vary from class to class and from sociolinguistic culture to sociolinguistic culture. Aspects of maternal input and regulation may include universal characteristics as well as culturally specific aspects. The maternal linguistic differences indicate that language is ultimately the result of social interaction within specific speech communities. Bernstein Ratner (1984) analyzed vowel patterns in conversational speech to adult and to child listeners in the speech provided by nine mothers. The data indicate "an emerging pattern of content word clarification" when speaking to children. The study provides support for the notion that mothers modify their speech for children and that this modification may vary at different child stages and rates. According to Ratner, "Mothers do, either consciously or unconsciously, produce speech sounds when speaking to children which share features of highly intelligible speech" (p. 574). According to Snow (1972), mother-child interaction represents a communication process that is also sensitively attuned to the language skills of child communicators. For example, Snow suggested that the routine daily experiences of mother and child (e.g., washing, dressing, playing, and feeding) teach the child language. Within these experiences, the mother orients and regulates her speech to enhance the child's acquisition of language. Several communication and language factors provide the child with "language lessons" (Cross, 1977; Dunham, Dunham, & Curwin, 1993; Phillips, 1973; Remick, 1976; Snow, 1977). The findings of these researchers are discussed in the next section.

Complexity

A mother's language is child-sensitive in terms of its complexity; it is regulated to the child's level of comprehension. Maternal utterances, therefore, are short. They usually consist of a single clause, are clearly enunciated, and rarely contain a true grammatical error. Part of the facilitative effect of adult input involves the tuning of the adult's speech to the child's level of language development. As the linguistic structure of the child's language develops, the mother increases the syntactic complexity of other input (Snow, 1972).

Semantic Relatedness

Maternal language is child-focused and contextually based. The topic of conversation and the content of the interaction are determined by the child within the context. Mothers speak about the context in which the child is the focus of attention and about the child's activities. For example, if a mother sees her child playing with a large stuffed dog, she might say "Nice doggie," Big doggie," or "Jimmy is playing with the doggie." This is called semantic relatedness. Snow (1977) noted that approximately 70 percent of mothers' speech is directly related to children's vocal, verbal, and nonverbal behavior.

Redundancy

Because maternal input relates to ongoing contextual occurrences, it tends to be redundant. A mother's linguistic message is an explanation of, clarification of, and/or comment about the child's environmental experiences (Harris, 1992). The overlapping of the linguistic with the nonlinguistic provides the young language learner with an extension of other syntactic and semantic knowledge. By coding what is occurring in the child's immediate frame of reference, the mother is providing the child with a bridge between the form and the content of language. First, a mother's input provides the child with a formal code that can be used to communicate about what is happening in the context. Second, a mother's input directs the child's attention to the relevant aspects of ongoing events (e.g., agents, actions, and objects), which extends the child's semantic knowledge. Thus, by being directly related to the events in the environment, maternal input teaches the child about the overlapping relationship between the linguistic message and the nonlinguistic context. For example, if the child is pointing to a cookie that is out of reach, a mother might say, "Maria wants a cookie?"

Maternal Responsiveness

Another variable that contributes to the child's development of communicative behavior is the consistency of the adult's responses to the child's vocal, verbal, gestural, and/or action performances. The young communicator learns about his or her relationship to the environment by noting the changes created by his or her behavior. The consistent response or behavior of an adult or object enables the infant to note that its own behavior has a predictable effect (Beckwith, Cohen, Kopp, Parmalee, & Marcy, 1976; Bradley & Caldwell, 1976). Consider the following incident with Jeremy, a 6-month-old:

> *Jeremy is seated in a baby-tender in the kitchen with Nana and Aunt Sue, who is a physician. Jeremy's mother is in another room of the house when she hears Nana scream. She runs into the kitchen and finds Aunt Sue delivering a deliberate back blow to Jeremy as he rests on her forearm.*

Nana: He's choking!

Aunt Sue: Don't get hysterical, everything is under control.

Jeremy: (Choke)…(choke)…(choke)…

Nana: Do something!

Aunt Sue: What does it look like I'm doing?

In the interim, Jeremy spits up whatever is lodged in his throat. He is relaxed and returned by his mother to the baby-tender, while Aunt Sue takes care of a distraught Nana. Nevertheless, Jeremy continues to cough even though apparently nothing is wrong with him. Everyone's response is to turn to him. For the next several months, Jeremy continued to cough, especially in the presence of Nana, who responded consistently with additional attention and care. Nana's behavior provided the reinforcement of Jeremy's continued predictable behavior. The child's development of communication was a function of the adult response provoked by his behavior.

Bruner (1975) noted that the adult actively attempts to interpret the child's behaviors within the context that "an enormous amount of consequent behavior flows from the nature of these interpretations" (p. 12). He noted that mothers provide two types of interpretations of the infant's behavior, both of which involve joint attention and reference. One interpretation of the child's behavior involves the adult as a mediator. The adult perceives the infant's behavior as an intention to perform some action. The adult's role is to assist the infant in achieving an outcome (e.g., holding an object so the child can manipulate it). Another form of interpretation is more concerned with the child's attention than with his or her action. The child's gaze at an object signals the adult to look where the child is looking; the adult then provides the child with the object.

Joint attention and adult interpretation of the child's behavior help the child develop communicative behavior. The consistency of the mother's actions with objects and her actions oriented to the child teaches the child to anticipate; Bruner (1975) described this as the child's predictions of the mother's intentions. The child is thus enabled to develop ways of signaling his or her own intentions. By consistently functioning as a responder/mediator when the infant initiates some behavior, the adult teaches the infant to control behavior and function as an initiator. Ongoing interaction provides the scaffolding for communicative learning.

Reciprocity

Maternal language is sensitive to the child's independent communications. Much of the mother's behavior is directed toward eliciting responses from the infant. In treating the infant as a partner in the communication process, the mother interprets a broad range of infant behavior as communicative (e.g., yawns, sneezes, burps, and hiccups). By being responsive, the mother provides the child with role experience as a speaker. By interacting as a speaker, the mother provides the child with experience as a listener. For the infant to function as a speaker, he or she must learn when the conversational turn has been passed to him or her. The mother stimulates this learning process by making turn-taking pauses between utterances much longer than the pauses within utterances. The mother provides these temporal lapses so that the infant learns about the speaker-listener roles (Stern, Spieker, Barnett, & MacKain, 1983). Further, the mother greatly exaggerates the terminal pitch, clearly marking the end of an utterance. This additional cue develops the infant's turntaking behavior, later evident in conversation.

Infant studies report that the conversational nature of the mother-infant exchange occurs as early as *4* months of age (Penman, Cross, Milgrom-Friedman, & Meares, 1983; Stern, 1974; Stern, Jaffe, Beebe, & Bennett, 1975; Stern et al., 1983). The development of communication behaviors so early in life emphasizes their importance to the language learning process. The child's ability to interact as a speaker and a listener forms the basic framework of communication learning. Thus, the fact that the mother modifies her speech style to encourage interaction helps us to understand the cues used by infants in language learning. She interacts with the infant with a conversational perspective and expectation. Her speech is directly related to the infant's behavior and is specifically oriented to eliciting a response.

D'Odorico and Franco (1985) analyzed maternal input in terms of semantic and syntactic features. The authors noted that, when talking to their children, mothers use a linguistic register that differs from the language they use with other adults. One factor that appears to affect maternal input is the context. Different types of contextual activities elicit different types of maternal language, which suggests that conversational constraints are operating in interactions between mother and infant (Penman et al., 1983; Snow, Arlmann-Rupp, Hassing, Jobse, Joosten, & Vorster, 1976). Their results indicate that contextual aspects influenced the semantic input provided by mothers. The interactive context determined the transmission of informational content to children. The relationship between context and content underscored "a specific conversational constraint operating on the linguistic interaction between mother and infant" (p. 569). In addition, the authors proposed a hierarchy of determinants that progresses from context to syntactic variables; context affects maternal content, and content in turn influences structural linguistic properties of motherese.

Murray, Johnson, and Peters (1990) described gross-tuning and fine-tuning processes that occur between a mother and infant during the first year of life. During the early part of the first year, maternal input consists of shorter utterances with an affective qualitative function. Maternal adjustments during this early period relate to a gross-tuning process to social and affective responsiveness in the infant. In the second half of the first year, mothers begin to fine-tune their utterances due to three developmental changes in the infant. First, at around 9 to 10 months, infants begin to show some early understanding of words. Second is the infant's development of intentional communication and the use of interactional combinations of gaze, vocal, and gestural behaviors. The third developmental change relates to object manipulation abilities. As the infant becomes more object oriented, the mother shifts from affective speech to informative referential speech. The data from Murray et al. (1990) also indicate individual differences in the degree to which mothers fine-tuned their speech. These differences in maternal behavior relate to social class and to attitude differences that have an impact on later language skills. Specifically, maternal speech adjustments and higher levels of verbal input were predictive of receptive language development nine months later. The finding appears to support the "motherese hypothesis that simpler input contributes to more advanced receptive language development" (p. 522).

Farrar (1990) noted that specific links between input and language acquisition can be established. His research findings support the position that adult input assists the child in acquiring language-specific characteristics, such as grammatical morphemes, compared to language-universal characteristics. Specific relationships between morphology present in parental speech and children's acquisition of those morphological forms were established. The research suggests that environmental factors along with discourse variables can provide greater insight into the child's learning strategies in the language learning process.

In summary, four major implications can be drawn regarding adult language as a variable in language acquisition. First, an adult's speech to the infant learner has a much simpler structure than speech to the older language learner. An adult matches the complexity of his or her speech to the child's level of understanding. As the child's level of understanding becomes more sophisticated, the adult's input becomes more linguistically complex. Second, an adult's speech to the young language learner is highly redundant. Third, an adult talks about what is present in the infant's immediate surroundings. Furthermore, the adult gives the child new and relevant information about objects and events that are directly observable to both of them. And fourth, the adult's speech encourages conversational communication.

Horizontal Relationships

Child-Initiated Communication

Interaction is a reciprocal process. Several studies confirm the view that even the young infant is an active communicator in the interactive language learning process. Analyses of the behaviors of infants during the first three months of life indicate that infants can finely attune their responses to the adults' communication. In addition, the infants' response behaviors are not only complex but well organized in relation to adult input changes (Murray & Trevarthen, 1985). The infant, even at this early stage, influences the communication process and contributes to the nature of the interactions that occur. Mothers frequently describe their infants as responsive communicators and, given that underlying presumption, interact freely with them. Videotape analyses indicate that Mother is filling in gaps in the interactive process to maintain the timing and the flow of the exchange. Several researchers have commented that what looks like a two-way process is really an artifact of mothers' contributions and timing (Hoff-Ginsberg, 1990; Fernald, 1989). Although researchers may not, at this point, agree on the nature and the degree of the infants' contribution to the interactional process, it is clear that mothers enter the dyadic exchange with certain perceptions of their infants. Researchers do agree, however, that a high degree of mutual coordination and responsiveness exists between the partners. At present, the behaviors and/or qualitative aspects that mothers are responding to may be difficult to identify and quantify, even with videotaped analyses in naturalistic contexts; nonetheless, mothers' speech is sensitive to a wide range of infant variables (Murray & Trevarthen, 1986).

Stylistic Differences

Lieven (1977) noted a significant difference in the way two mothers communicated with their children. She showed that the mothers accommodated readily and almost naturally to the language conditions imposed by their infants. With the child whose style was "conversation oriented" the mother used questions to keep the conversation going. With the child whose speech was object and event oriented, the mother commented on the child's environment and focused on what he or she was saying. This attunement of the adult communicator to the young language learner is also discussed in Barnes, Gutfreund, Satterly, and Wells (1983), who reported that young children demonstrate different styles of language use. Although inadequately documented, these stylistic differences influence the input provided by adult communicators. Barnes et al. (1983) concluded, therefore, that children facilitate changes in adult language and this establishes an ongoing cyclical process that is regulated to the child's developing abilities. This has important implications for handicapped language learners and the cyclical patterns of communication interaction established with their parents/caregivers.

Platt and Coggins (1990) suggested that two different types of comprehension mechanisms may be operating in children at the sensorimotor stage of development. The first is an analytic stylistic approach that segments information into component elements, and the second is a holistic approach that chunks entire units of information. The authors noted that children who rely on the analytic style of processing information have a "flexible" use of object and action object and action words and gestures across contexts, as well as a larger comprehension vocabulary. Children with a holistic processing style lack contextual flexibility, which means that they have difficulty understanding the verbal message independent of the contextual situation. The authors proposed that an analytically oriented child would show an earlier ability to use conventional behaviors in social-action games than a child with a holistic processing style. The early use of the analytic style allows the young child to recombine language structures based on his knowledge of the basic building blocks of the system. Platt and Coggins also noted that mothers exhibited different interaction styles in attempting to elicit participation in social games. Among the different behavioral techniques mothers used to engage and to maintain their child's interaction were exaggerated facial expressions, stress and intonation, well-defined pauses, and various attention-getting devices.

Gaze Behavior

One of an infant's earliest communicative acts is gazing at another human being. Mother and infant make eye contact and thereby communicate. In this first communication, both mother and child have equal control over their gaze behavior (Rutter & Durkin, 1987). To initiate and terminate interaction, both adults and infants effectively regulate their gaze toward or away from each other. While gazing at the infant, the mother engages in behavior unique to communication with the infant and quite different from adult communicative exchanges. Mothers sit very close to their infants—almost nose to nose—producing rapidly changing and exaggerated vocal variables such as rhythm, pitch, loudness, rate, and vowel production. They emphasize these vocal extremes with dramatic changes in facial expression. The infant is not passive in this interaction. A baby's gaze has a strong effect on the mother. By regulating the gaze, the infant learns to "turn" his or her mother "on and off." While the infant gazes at the mother, the mother does not look away. In fact, the infant is very much in control of the interaction with his or her mother; more than 90 percent of all these interactions are ended by the infant (Stern, 1974). The mother acts as if the infant were talking and responds by continuously gazing and listening. Jaffe, Stern, and Peery (1973) proposed that gazing is a prototype conversation involving mother and infant decisions on when to look at or look away from one another. Gaze conversation, therefore, is present long before linguistic communication is achieved. The research of Murray and Trevarthen (1986) further indicates that when the infant is no longer responsive, the form and content of his or her mother's speech change. Usually relaxed and effortless, the mother's speech now indicates an increase in negative statements and anxious comments. The researchers noted that these responses in mothers were largely determined by "the amount of time the infant's eyes were directed to her face" (p. 27).

Gaze and Vocal Behaviors

Adult-infant conversation has been compared structurally to adult-adult conversation. As with adult conversations, there is nearly constant eye communication and intermittent, alternating vocal communication. Thus, the mother and child maintain gaze interaction for long periods of time and alternate their vocal interchanges. In this communication interplay between the mother and infant, the mother-child communication process begins before the infant's fourth month and can be viewed as a "proto-conversation" that has definite consequences in later conversational exchanges (Bateson, 1975; Rutter & Durkin, 1987).

Patterns of Vocal Interaction

Another factor in child-motivated variables is vocal interaction with two structurally and functionally different patterns: the simultaneous and the alternating. Mothers and infants vocalize simultaneously during the expression of extremely positive or negative feelings. In the alternating mode, which looks and functions like a conversational exchange, the mother and child alternate as speaker and listener. The presence of these two distinct patterns of vocal exchange indicates that mothers and infants engage in complex communication exchanges very early in life (Stern et al., 1975). Research further suggests that these modes may represent some universal formal property of communication (Jaffe et al., 1973). Flax, Lahey, Harris, and Boothroyd (1991) noted that intonation has been considered one of the earliest linguistic features acquired by infants. Mothers are highly aware of their infants' sensitivity to intonational variations. As a result, mothers use variations as a means of establishing and maintaining infants' attention. The Flax et al. research suggests that the use of intonation by mothers and infants during interaction underscores the possibility that intonation is the "first association of language form with aspects of meaning. Such early associations may lead the child to later inductions of lexico-grammatical means of coding similar aspects of meaning" (p. 4).

In short, research shows that infants themselves are active contributors to the acquisition process through interaction with their mother and other adults. During these early interactions, the infant learns about the communication process, including the rules for interacting with another person. The infant learns to be a speaker and a listener and to coordinate gaze, vocal, and gestural behavior into a fairly complex, patterned exchange that follows the structure of adult-adult conversation (i.e., simultaneous gaze-vocal behavior followed by gaze behavior alone). We may conclude that prelinguistic patterns of behavior can be traced to early infancy and that patterns established in this period are reflected in later adult communicative exchanges.

The Child's Relationships with Peers

As stated earlier, peer relationships play a significant role in a child's social development. The definition of horizontal relationships involves the equality and interdependence of mutual interaction between equal partners. These reciprocal interactions and relationships can only be learned with peers. Peer relationships provide a transition from dependence to independence as the child develops an awareness of self as a communicator (Dunn, 1993). The child's relationships with his or her peers become increasingly more important to long-term social learning. The vertical relationships that a child establishes with parents and other adults provide a framework and backdrop to the roles and rules involved with personal responsibility as a social communicator. Adults continue to assist the child to understand social complexities and to resolve ongoing interactional problems by supporting and assisting the child in decision making. It is, however, within the framework of horizontal relationships that children apply the understanding that they have acquired from the adult-child interactions to the "new world" experiences of mutual partners and peers. Beginning as early as two years of age, children begin to show an interest in other children. Howes and Matheson (1992) describe children in the first year of life as indicating preferences for particular peer partners. Children not only express preferences during play but also indicate the ability to maintain ongoing relationships with particular peers. Although these early friendships are not quantitatively or qualitatively different than the relationships engaged in by older children, preschool friendships indicate the same emerging parameters that occur in other developmental areas. These early friendship relationships include the following characteristics: partner preference, mutual liking, reciprocal exchange, extended communicative and play interactions, and positive pro-social behavior (Berndt, 1992, 1986, 1983; Berndt, Hawkins, & Hoyle, 1986).

Cognitive Trends in Development

Viewing language as part of a social cognition model implies that the various developmental areas interface with one another, that developmental changes in one area affect occurrences in other areas, and that behaviors are shared across developmental areas. In attempting to discuss how children integrate their social learning experiences in order to construct a developmental model, several questions need to be addressed. How is information shared across learning domains? Are domain areas separate and distinct? Can all areas of learning be integrated within a single developmental model? The model in Figure 2-1 suggests that children possess a general learning system that resembles a DNA molecule. What does this model suggest about the sequence of development? What are the implications concerning the relationship between areas such as cognition, social interaction and language? How does this developmental processing model compare with some of the other models that are described later in the text (i.e., shared base model or direct causal model)?

Developmental Components

In Figure 2-2, the individual strands represent various developmental components (cognition, play, pragmatics, etc.). The components intertwine, share information, and continue to develop by incorporating the shared information. In addition, during the course of the child's development, the components continue to interface. The development of a component (e.g., pragmatics) involves integrating information from other components (e.g., social interaction, play, cognition). Thus, the manipulation of objects in play, for example, affects children's cognitive development. In addition, early social interactions and exchanges affect the development of pragmatic intentions. Cognition, pragmatics, play, and semantics are viewed as interrelated aspects of development. Consequently, deficits in any one area may negatively affect changes in other areas of learning.

Component Relationships

In the model in Figure 2-3, the individual learning components are operative at birth as separate and distinct areas, but they interface during development. Any two components, such as cognition and pragmatics, can be described as interdependent; that is, all of the components are separate areas derived from and mapped onto a more basic system instead of being dependent on, or derived from, one another. This interdependence suggests that language and cognition are derived from broader capacities—a shared base (see Figure 2-2). Thus, in a shared base model cognitive ability would not be a more basic and primary process than language. Contrast this model with Piaget's model (Piaget's theories are discussed later in this chapter), in which language is derived from broader cognitive capacities. In Piaget's model, cognitive ability would be a more basic and primary process than language, providing the foundations for language development and ultimately directing language development. Piaget's model is called a direct causal model (see Figure 2-3).

Certainly, further research will provide insight into the language learning process from birth. The purpose of the present discussion is to emphasize the function and significance of a developmental model. The models we have presented indicate different relationships between components, this in turn has important implications for the way in which the theorist describes the developmental process. Keep in mind that our developmental framework or viewpoint affects therapeutic programming and decision making. Several issues are next presented to highlight possible differences in the relationship between cognition and language.

Cognition and Language

Various cognitive theories propose that the normally developing child comes to the learning environment with different types of structural and processing equipment. Common to these

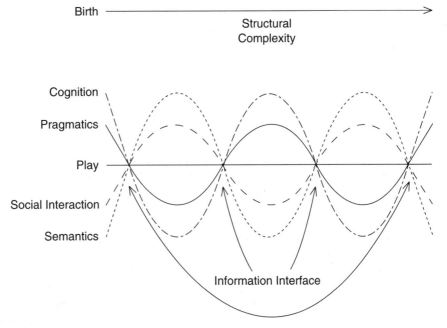

FIGURE 2-2   The interchange of information at various points in development.

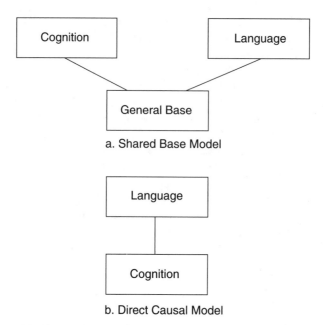

a. Shared Base Model

b. Direct Causal Model

FIGURE 2-3   Shared base and direct causal models.

differing cognitive theories is the need to explain how children organize and code environmental experiences. This gradual process codes perceptual and conceptual patterns of social interaction into linguistic forms. Children learn to use a representational form of behavior that enables them to interact with other communicators in society. In the following section, one theory is presented for discussion to highlight the complex interaction among developmental processes in the normally developing learner. It is important to focus on the various parts of a theory of development without losing sight of the theoretician's general orientation to and viewpoint of development.

The Strong Cognition Hypothesis

Cognition has been defined as the process of knowing and includes factors such as awareness, perception, conceptualization, and judgment. The relationship of language development to cognitive development has been an area of debate among child development specialists. Some claim that cognition is both necessary and sufficient for language development. This viewpoint, termed the strong cognition hypothesis (or cognition-first hypothesis), is discussed more fully by Rice (1980a, b). Evidence for this point of view has been provided by many researchers, including Piaget (1962), Slobin (1973), Sinclair-deZwart (1973), and Morehead and Morehead (1974). The strong cognition hypothesis proposes that language development is directed by perceptual-conceptual structures. The underlying contention is that language is a subsystem within a broader symbolic capacity. This symbolic capacity, in turn, depends on the development of sensorimotor intelligence. As a result, the strong cognition hypothesis proposes that (a) language depends on cognitive development and (b) cognitive abilities precede linguistic abilities.

Developmental Processes

Piaget (1962) hypothesized that cognitive development proceeds as children interact with their environment. The theory stresses the child's active role in organizing the environment. For Piaget, intellectual development parallelled the stages of mental development. He described intelligence as twofold, comprising adaptation and organization. The two processes of adaptation are assimilation and accommodation. Assimilation involves incorporating the environment into present patterns of behavior. When children carry out an action sequence, such as grasping a cup, they have assimilated reality into the action scheme. Accommodation involves a change in scheme as a function of the environment. When a child changes the action scheme to conform to the environment (grasping the cup more tightly when the child is lifted from the high chair), he has modified his behavior to fit reality. These processes enable children to adapt their performance to environmental and contextual changes, which are in turn incorporated for use in other situations. These processes also help children develop a complex repertoire of behaviors for solving problems as social contexts change. Intelligence is a system of hierarchical organizations that do not become fully operational until the end of a long developmental process. Finally, according to Piaget, cognitive development results from interaction among genetic programming, physical maturation, environmental experience, and self-regulation.

Piagetian Principles

Some important aspects of Piaget's theory include:

1. Distinct periods of development are postulated to be universal and sequentially invariant.
2. Biological structures focus and direct the infant's learning.
3. The child learns through experience and interaction with the environment.
4. The child must learn to act upon and transform the environment to know reality.
5. Physical knowledge is acquired by experiencing actions and object characteristics.
6. Perception (i.e., sensory processing, sensory reorganization, sensory exploration) is an active rather than a passive learning process.
7. Perceptual development permits the development of symbolic representational systems.
8. Language is part of and is one form of symbolic functioning.
9. Cognitive structures and their development underlie the acquisition of language.
10. Symbolic functioning includes all mental behavior concerned with aspects of reality that are not immediately present.
11. Language differs from other forms of symbolic functioning because it is a social communication system rather than an isolated internal system such as imagery.
12. Language as a social system is the end result of communicative, cognitive, social, play, and imitative development.
13. Language, as a symbolic function, represents the child's reality—the child's experiences (Morehead & Morehead, 1974).

Piaget described four stages of cognitive development and their associated developmental ages (see Table 2-1).

TABLE 2-1   Piaget's Stages of Development

Stages of Cognitive Development	Corresponding Chronological Age
I Sensorimotor	Birth to 24 months
II Preoperational	2 to 7 years
III Concrete operations	7 to 11 years
IV Formal operations	11 to 14 years

The Principle of Distancing

The principle of distancing underlies the developmental changes that occur during Piaget's sensorimotor period (birth to 24 months). Piaget described the development of language as being based within the sensorimotor period. The distancing principle provides an explanation for the unique progression of accomplishment in which children learn to control their actions and the actions of others by acquiring a language code—a system of symbols.

At first, only reflexes are manifested. These reflexes undergo modifications with experience as movements are brought under the infant's voluntary control. During this period, children free themselves from the physical constraints of gravity, maturation, space, and time. They gradually learn to overcome these constraints of space and time to develop the ultimate form of distancing, symbolic or representational behavior. Actions are directed toward objects and events, and gradually intentionality of action emerges. Children learn and use means-end sequences to explore new objects and situations. New means are invented in goal-oriented activities. The ability to represent the environment or reality in another form, such as deferred imitation, symbolic play, imagery, or language, enables children to separate an object or event from its referent in the immediate context. Representation allows children to symbolically remove the object or event from its time and physical place, an ability that also permits children to free themselves from the immediate present. Language provides children with the means of changing events and consequences within their environments. Language becomes a powerful tool for children to talk about themselves and their social experiences. The language system expands as children continue to develop language. The more language children acquire, the more sophisticated they become as language learners and users. Social experiences change—qualitatively and quantitatively—as language becomes more abstract and complex. Eventually, language allows children to share their thoughts and feelings about relationships and experiences in daily life.

Sensorimotor Period (birth to 24 months)

The sensorimotor period consists of six substages:

Substage 1:   Reflexive (birth to 2 months). Infants' behavior is controlled by involuntary reflexes. As these reflexive behaviors begin to change, children develop more voluntary control of their behavior. The infants are active learners; as they gain more motor control, they attempt to apply patterns of movements directly to the environment.

Substage 2: Primary circular reaction (2 to 4 months). These applications of movement to the environment often bring an unanticipated result that provides an important source of learning for the infants. To recreate the environmental response, infants repeat their behavior over and over. In directing their behavior to the environment, infants also learn to coordinate visual, auditory, and tactile sensations with motor activity such as sucking, crying, and grasping.

Substage 3: Secondary circular reaction (4 to 8 months). Infants' ability to crawl and stand gives them a new perspective of their environment. In directing their behavior to objects, infants begin to note the effect created by their actions. They develop an object class and differentiate themselves from other objects in their environment. The development of an object concept eventually results in an understanding of object permanence. Thus, when an object leaves the infants' sight, they will look for it.

Substage 4: Anticipatory/intentional (8 months to 1 year). Infants coordinate their actions in different ways to develop new action patterns, eventually becoming able to determine which action (means) results in a particular goal (end). The infants learn to direct their behavior to achieve a goal; the means now precedes the end. Becoming increasingly mobile, children develop intentional and anticipatory behaviors as they interact with objects and people. They learn that other people can be an important source of action, further differentiating themselves from others.

Substage 5: Exploration and experimentation (1 year to 18 months). Children actively pursue novelty, exploring objects in their environment to discover their properties. To expand this physical knowledge, they vary their actions on objects and observe the effects. By the end of this stage, the child exhibits adultomorphisms, relational knowledge enabling them to use objects in a way that is similar to adult use (Morehead & Morehead, 1974).

Substage 6: Transitional (18 months to 2 years). This stage marks the end of the sensorimotor period and the transition to the next stage. By representation, children now can manipulate reality internally. They become able to achieve a goal not only by external or physical activity, but also by internalized processes. They may achieve a goal by sudden comprehension or insight (Piaget & Inhelder, 1969). The ability to represent objects or events and their related action patterns is the onset of symbolic behavior (Piaget, 1962).

In summary, during the sensorimotor period, the child progresses from reflexive, involuntary behavior to physically generated intentional behavior to internally generated (i.e., symbolic) intentional behavior.

An incident involving 18-month-old Jeremy illustrates this process. (Piaget described the development of relational knowledge at the end of Substage 5, as children's ability to manipulate objects in ways that they observe others in their environment manipulating those objects. This relational knowledge is evident in the children's adultomorphisms.)

Jeremy had a babysitter who spoke to him only in Spanish. When she scolded him, she would shake her head and finger at him and say, "No toca [touch]! No toca!" One evening, Jeremy's mother heard some noise in the kitchen and proceeded to look for Jeremy. She peeked into the kitchen to see Jeremy open a drawer and take out two cooking mitts, which he put on. Chattering away, he opened the oven, took out a pan, and slammed the door shut. He put the pan on the stove, then took off the mitts and threw them back into the drawer. While shaking head and finger, he said, "No! No! No!"

This is a typical incident for the child at this substage of development. What does it indicate? The adultomorphism indicates that the child has the ability to integrate, within his world and his experience, complex sequences of behavior that he has observed in his environment. Here Jeremy was recreating a situation he had experienced with his babysitter that was both meaningful and memorable to him.

Language during the Sensorimotor Period

If language is one form of representational behavior, what are its other forms? Language is a social system; it serves a social and interactional function. Language enables children to distance themselves in time and space by referring to objects and events that are not immediately present. According to Piaget, language development depends on underlying cognitive structures. Several components are important to understanding children's language abilities during the first twenty-four months of life. First, from a cognitive perspective, children's language is concrete, or contextually based, because their mental operations are concrete. During the sensorimotor period, children tend to talk about the here and now. Their cognitive abilities, according to the strong cognition hypothesis, determine their language abilities. Children who cannot talk about past or future events cannot cognitively separate themselves, objects, or actions from the immediate context. At this stage, children can talk about only what is happening and what they are doing right now. Changes in language development, therefore, reflect changes in cognitive abilities. As children conceptually learn to reconstruct past actions, they use words to refer to those actions and to evoke their recurrence in the present and immediate context. Thus, children talk initially about their own actions and eventually about the performance of other agents outside the boundaries of the present place and time.

Reviewing the Language-Cognition Relationship

Piaget's theory has been around for a long time, and many professionals have become comfortable with its theoretical terms and their relationships. In fact, educational programs throughout the United States have developed curricula based upon Piaget's cognitive constructs. One serious problem with this, however, is that the definition of language has changed during the past two decades. Piaget's cognitive hypothesis states that language as a representational system is acquired at the end of Substage 6 of the sensorimotor period. It is possible that this rigid relationship is based in part on the limited definition of language in terms of syntax. With the advent of the semantic and the pragmatic revolutions, the definition of language changed dramatically.

Child language is now viewed as a social learning process; language use is a social event carried out by interactants in naturalistic communicative contexts. This view credits children with communicative intentions long before they evidence syntactic abilities. In addition, many researchers have described children who, as early as 9 months of age, develop wordlike utterances that are embedded within sentence-like structures. Between 9 and 24 months, the child develops linguistic abilities, although he or she is clearly at a presyntactic level. These wordlike and word structures are used consistently, meaningfully, and appropriately by the child when referring to an object. The research of Bates, Benigni, Bretherton, Camaioni, and Volterra (1977) indicates the problem inherent in Piaget's theory: Substage 6 is not a necessary prerequisite for language. Bates et al. indicate that by 13 months of age children have discovered that "things have names." The word becomes a symbolic vehicle when it names or stands for a referent. This symbolic representation means that the child can substitute the symbol for its referent while "realizing that the symbol is not the same thing as its referent" (p. 38). Children evidence symbolic abilities before the end of Substage 6; they can certainly talk about objects and events that are not present within the immediate context (Karmiloff-Smith, 1993). In addition, several researchers indicated other developmental occurrences that appeared earlier than Piaget described. Piaget did not think that deferred imitation could occur before the end of the sensorimotor period, because it requires internal symbolic representation. Hanna and Meltzoff (1993) and Meltzoff (1988) indicated that deferred imitation occurred in children as young as 14 months; this suggests again a much earlier developmental use of some kind of internal representation to remember actions and events. How does this affect the relationship between cognition and language? How would the development of symbolic representational behavior at Substage 4 alter Piaget's theory?

Rovee-Collier (1993) investigated memory in infants. She demonstrated that infants as young as 3 months could remember objects and their actions over periods as long as a week. These studies contradict Piaget's view of the sensorimotor infant. The infant appears to be cognitively more sophisticated than Piaget described. The suggestion that infants may be capable of some forms of internal/symbolic representation before the end of the sensorimotor period raises important questions about their abilities. The infant seems to be functioning at a higher level of skill organization than Piaget proposed (Karmiloff-Smith, 1993).

Interaction Hypothesis

The interaction hypothesis proposes that the relationship between language and cognition is bidirectional. According to this hypothesis, developments in the linguistic domain inextricably alter the child's cognitive developments. The child's linguistic behaviors interact with his or her nonlinguistic meanings, and this exchange process provides a mechanism for systematic adjustments in and modifications of categories and concepts. This contrasts with Piaget's theoretical position, which argues that cognitive structures direct linguistic developments and that linguistic expression reflects "what" the child already "knows." As already noted, theorists now place more of an emphasis on the role of the social context and communication in child development. The interaction hypothesis also argues that the relationship between nonlinguistic and linguistic meanings is not isomorphic. Linguistic structures cannot be directly mapped on top of cognitive structures; there is not a one-to-one relationship between cognitive and linguistic organization, categories, and concepts (Rice & Kemper, 1984). Vygotsky described a different relationship between cognition and language; specifically, that language influences thought:

> *The relation of thought to word is not a thing but a process, a continual movement back and forth from thought to word and from word to thought. In that process, the relation of thought to word undergoes changes that themselves may be regarded as development in the functional sense. Thought is not merely expressed in words; it comes into existence through them. (Kozulin, 1987, p. 218)*

Weak Cognition Hypothesis

The Piagetian and interaction hypotheses propose that there is a direct relationship between cognition and language. The weak cognition hypothesis argues that children exhibit various kinds of linguistic knowledge and structures that do not directly relate to their cognitive abilities. Child language studies have shown that as children acquire formal linguistic structures there is not necessarily a developmental synchrony between nonlinguistic meanings (concepts) and the linguistic structures used to express those underlying meanings. Linguistic errors indicate that even when children "have mastered the nonlinguistic notions—the underlying meanings; they are still sorting out the formal linguistic devices available for the expression" of meaning (Rice & Kemper, 1984, p. 39). In addition, cross-linguistic investigations have shown that although young children may acquire cognitive concepts at relatively stable stages, their mastery of syntactic and morphosyntactic structures varies across different languages. This research suggests that a linguistic complexity factor determines when linguistic structures are acquired within a given language. In fact, the acquisition sequence also varies, indicating that specific linguistic forms are easier to express in certain languages and therefore are acquired earlier. The hierarchical differences across languages lend support for the notion of linguistic processing strategies. So, although cognition determines a relatively stable order for the development of specific concepts, "there are language-specific departures from this order because of the interaction of linguistic variables" (Rice & Kemper, p. 40).

Language-Specific Processing

If cognition cannot account for all of the child's language learning skills, then it is reasonable to consider the possibility of language-specific processing abilities. This position was originally proposed by Chomsky (1988, 1986) in his innateness hypothesis. Language ability is part of the biological programming of humans and therefore is unique to human physiological structures. Chomsky argued that linguistic competencies represent tacit knowledge that is induced by social interactional experiences. The strength of this position relates to the similarities across languages in terms of linguistic structures and patterns of acquisition in young children.

To the extent that language is independent of cognitive representations, children with developmental deficits may exhibit specific language learning disorders. Rice and Kemper

(1984) noted that a causal relationship among perceptual, cognitive, and linguistic processes has not been established. In addition, a return to the innateness hypothesis suggests that environmental factors play a diminished role in learning. This leads to a rather skeptical view of intervention approaches for the developmentally disabled because environmental change is a cornerstone for remediation. Clearly, if knowledge is innate, then how can the language-disordered child be "taught" these specific processes or abilities? The issue of language-specific abilities in children may have to be viewed apart from the premises of the innateness hypothesis. As Rice and Kemper (1984) observed, "The recent recognition of cognitive factors has balanced the earlier enthusiasm for behaviorism, in that it has returned the clinical focus to the internal capacities of children as well as environmental events" (p. 47).

Communicative Competence

An alternative to the cognitive-linguistic theories involves communicative competence and its role in child language learning. The theoretical premise is that linguistic structures cannot be viewed outside of a social context and that linguistic rules vary as a function of contextual variables. Before the child acquires linguistic rules, he or she must learn about his or her role as a social communicator. Communicative intentions, speaker-listener roles and rules, socially based adjustments, listener's perspective, and regulatory and revision behaviors are just some of the variables that underlie social knowledge or communicative competence. Rice and Kemper (1984) suggested that person knowledge, social categories, and event knowledge provide a nonlinguistic framework for language learning not considered previously. An understanding of social knowledge might alter not only the relationship between cognition and language but also our perception of the contribution of each domain area to child development.

Perceptual Bases for Language Development

The infant is bombarded with input from his or her senses. What he or she sees, hears, and feels must be identified, categorized, and integrated so that he or she can make sense out of his or her noisy and stimulating environment. At this stage, the infant explores his or her environment through his or her senses. The earliest sensory system to come under the infant's control is the visual system. By 3 months of age, the infant has developed control of his or her eye movements to the extent that he or she can regulate the level of visual stimuli he or she receives. The infant indicates this ability by orienting his or her gaze to, or averting his or her gaze from, the adult. Gaze, incidentally, also serves a signal function for the infant, because it indicates his or her willingness to interact by its presence or absence. By looking, the infant discovers a great deal about his or her environment. He or she notices different colors, shapes, sizes, patterns, and movements in his or her world. In addition to visual skills, the infant has auditory abilities that were present before birth. Although the middle and inner ears are functioning at birth, the immaturity of the auditory cortex and the central nervous system limits the child's ability to integrate sound at this time. The infant can distinguish sound variables such as loudness, pitch, and duration. He or she can also discriminate between sounds (Fernald, 1993).

The infant, even at this age, indicates certain visual and auditory preferences. These preferences can be determined by measuring changes in respiration, eye movements, general changes in activity level, and startle reactions (Walton, Bower, & Bower, 1992). The infant is visually attracted to objects that move, that have designs or patterns, and that have contrasting colors (Haith, 1990). And, in terms of auditory stimulation, he or she clearly prefers the human voice, learning very early to recognize his or her mother's voice. By 9 months of age, infants learning English prefer to listen to words that have English stress and intonation patterns. Infants apparently indicate a preference for listening to the typical patterns—features of their own cultural language (Jusczyk, Cutler, & Redanz, 1993). As the infant develops greater voluntary muscle control, he or she gains new perspectives on people and objects in his or her environment. The infant's world certainly looks very different when he or she is sitting or crawling. The ability to coordinate his or her movements allows greater freedom, independence, and control. He or she can move toward an object that interests him or her and explore "nooks and crannies" more aggressively. Looking becomes coordinated with movements such as reaching, grasping, and pointing. There is a vital interaction between sensory input and movement. The infant learns to discriminate, integrate, and categorize his or her perceptions by interacting with and changing his or her environment. The infant "moves from perceiving reality as a continuousness of undifferentiated sights, smells, sounds, tastes, and tactile sensations impinging on his sense organs at birth, to perceiving reality as separate entities, actions, and people in space" (Lindfors, 1987, p. 167).

Infants learn to organize their perceptions and experiences into distinct categories. This enables them to establish some order in their world by arranging entities, actions, and people into categories and by identifying relationships that are shared by members of the group. Organization and order are critical to normal cognitive and language development. In accomplishing this process, infants learn to attend to a stimulus selectively by blocking out competing stimuli. Incoming stimuli must be stored in memory and compared with other stimuli to determine their organizational relationship. Information is stored in short-term and long-term memory to record events for later retrieval. Several theories propose ways in which children organize their perceptions. Stern (1977) described two types of stimulation: perceptual and cognitive. Perceptual stimulation, also called sensory stimulation, involves receiving a stimulus and identifying its characteristics. Cognitive stimulation refers to the relationship between a stimulus and its referent. The infant organizes perceptual stimulation and later uses these perceptual organizations to establish a relationship between a stimulus and its referent. Initially, infants may establish broad categories based upon what is salient to them. The infant does not attend to all aspects of a situation equally. An important factor that seems to affect what information the infant will process is environmental change. Objects move, people move, and infants move and are themselves moved by others. Movement involves change around the infant. In perceiving change and the results of movement, infants begin to learn about people and objects. They learn about the relationship between object and object, and people and objects. This information about objects, people, and events is coded symbolically. The ability to identify constant and predictable aspects within the environment provides the basis for conceptual development.

Cognitive Bases for Language Development

Object Permanence

Object permanence is the development of an object concept. It is indicated by a child's knowing that an object exists even though he or she cannot currently see it. At about 6 months of age, an infant can locate an object that is completely covered or hidden behind a screen. If the object is hidden a second time in a different location, however, the infant will return to the first location to find it. By 12 months of age, the infant will no longer be bound to this original placement. As long as he or she sees where the object is hidden, the infant will locate it, even if the location is changed each time. The limiting factor at this stage involves a change in placement after the object has disappeared. If the child tracks the object to its point of disappearance, he or she will look for it only there and not search any other location. By 18 months, the child will persist in the search for the disappearing object by checking several different places. Spelke (1991) proposes that infants are preprogrammed with certain assumptions about the nature of objects. She describes a connected surface principle that states that when two surfaces are connected together they belong to the same object. She also showed that infants were aware of how objects moved even when they were out of sight. Infants showed surprise if objects violated expected performance outcomes—that is, moved in unanticipated ways. Spelke suggests that infants have some built-in notions-rules about objects, actions and object-action relationships.

Children's concepts indicate that they have certain expectations about an object and the way it will function (Bloom & Lahey, 1978). Brown (1973) has noted that object permanence is sufficient by 12 months of age for the development of single words that children use to refer to objects present in the context. Several researchers suggest that object permanence involves the children's knowledge of objects and, ultimately, the content of language. As children develop an understanding of objects and their relationships to one another, they also acquire relational knowledge and the "concepts of relations between object concepts" (Bloom & Lahey, 1978, p. 82).

Tomasello and Farrar (1984) found that in Substage 5 of Piaget's sensorimotor period, object permanence is a sufficient cognitive prerequisite for the child to learn relational words that refer to objects perceived as present. In Substage 6, object permanence is a sufficient cognitive prerequisite for the child to learn relational words that refer to objects perceived as absent. The authors' research suggests that there must exist in the sensorimotor period some conceptual basis for lexical acquisition; however, "there is no fundamental reason why cognitive task performance should developmentally precede language performance" (p. 489). The Piagetian concept of horizontal "decalage" proposed that both object permanence and task performance and relational word production rely on the same underlying competence, but one precedes the other developmentally because of the child's differential experiences with the separate domain areas. Tomasello and Farrar (1984) have argued that the sensorimotor experience is the cognitive framework from which the child creates a linguistic reality. The sensorimotor scheme occurs before the linguistic symbolization—both logically and psychologically, "a case of vertical, not horizontal, decalage" (p. 490). The relationship between cognition and language learning remains a central controversy underlying many research investigations in child language.

Object Concepts and Relational Knowledge

By exploring and interacting with the environment, the child comes into contact with many different objects. As he or she manipulates each object, his or her senses are challenged by the sight, taste, smell, sound, and feel of the object. Certain aspects of the object might be striking or surprising to the child—the popping action of a jack-in-the-box or the movement and noise of a choo-choo train—and, therefore, are memorable. Each time a child explores an object, he or she processes additional information about his or her physical world. As object experiences are added to his or her knowledge base, the child recognizes similarities and differences. He or she codes the perceptual information and stores it so that he or she will be able to remember and retrieve it later.

Looking, tracking, and searching behaviors are tools of exploration and, eventually, independence. Exploration allows the child to acquire knowledge about and strategies for dealing with specific objects and classes of objects. The child's task is to determine which objects are related and on what basis they are related. The ability to establish categories involves processes of discrimination and generalization. Children must be able to recognize perceptual and functional characteristics so that general parameters for categories can be established. Based on these categorical criteria, the child will make a decision about whether an individual item or member (e.g., a four-legged animal) is assigned to one category (e.g., cat) or another (e.g., dog). Learning about objects enables the child to develop categories of objects and, then, concepts of objects. Sapir (1921) described an object concept as an "average" of one's experiences with the individual items in the category. The child's image, schema, or concept is a composite representation or prototype of all of the objects in the category. The child learns that there is a prototype cookie that represents all of the various members of the cookie category. The child develops the concept of "cookie-ness."

Learning words that represent object concepts requires that the child have a physical knowledge of the object. The child learns to refer to the object by using a word. The word is used to represent the object as a symbol, but the word is not the object. Just as the child learns about the object, he learns about object relations and relational concepts. Again, through direct interaction with objects, actions, and people, the child learns how people affect objects, how objects relate to other objects, and how actions affect objects. The child must acquire the conceptual foundation for these relationships before he or she can code them with symbolic word forms. In child language, the "semantic relations between words that are coded in messages reflect underlying conceptual relationships"(Bloom & Lahey, 1978, p. 82).

Gopnik and Meltzoff (1992) proposed that there is a strong relationship between the acquisition of particular types of meanings and particular cognitive developments. Children appear to acquire words that encode concepts they have just developed or are in the process of developing. They suggested a specific relationship between the acquisition of words that encode the concept of disappearance, the word gone, and the development of the object concept. The notion here is that the child needs to solve simple invisible displacement tasks. The authors suggested that object-related experiences provide the child with trial-and-error learning. The knowledge acquired from object manipulations involves problem solving and planning. Bruner (1973) described the child's ability to reflect on action alternatives, which underlies the development of insight at the end of the sensorimotor period. When the child "rehearses" possible outcomes and plans before he or she actually acts, he or she can make comparisons to ultimately choose a successful solution without the need for the trial-and-error experience.

Although people share perceptual and cognitive systems, the differences in environment and experience across cultural groups often reflect differences in language, organization, and meaning. Different cultures organize their realities differently. English speakers have a single category for snow. Eskimos have many different words for snow, depending upon the kind of snow that is present. This difference indicates how cultural differences can result in different categories of word meaning. Speakers of a particular language share a common reality and, therefore, a similar organization of that reality into categories and relationships. Consequently, "the words of their language reflect their categories (dog, wolf, loud) and relations (bigger, less, because)" (Lindfors, 1987, p. 37). Speakers of a language share a similar semantic knowledge. This suggests that speakers of a language share similar words and word meanings due to shared experiences.

Causality

Causality relates to the child's realization that he can be the agent of change. Aspects of causal development require knowledge of action as well as of the consequence of that action in relation to an object. Bates (1993) noted that causal development is an important indicator of social and communicative developments. The child becomes aware of himself or herself as a mover and doer; his or her actions create change and have consequences that are immediately observable. The child's experiences in creating change permit him or her to make predictions about the consequences resulting from his or her own actions. The child's ability to express a range of communicative intentions relates to the development of causality in social behavior (Sexton, 1980). Bates (1993) also reported that causality with people and causality with objects appear to develop differently.

Means-End

Means-end refers to the developing problem-solving ability in children at 9 months of age. The child approaches a problem with an anticipation of outcome. He or she chooses a means (a behavior or behavioral sequence) that will permit him or her to achieve a desired end (result or object). Initially, an action performed by a child is quite accidental, producing an unanticipated result in the environment. As the child acquires more fine-tuned motor skills, he or she repeats the means (the action) so that the end (the consequence) can be observed and reobserved. Eventually, the child learns that a variety of means can result in a single end. He or she then chooses from among a number of means to attain his or her goal. In the natural course of events, it is quite usual for a means not to result in the desired end. At this point the child indicates an adaptive skill by modifying the means; the child learns to accommodate his or her own behavior to meet the minute changes that can occur across contexts. This strengthens and broadens his or her social and manipulative repertoire. The development of gestural and communicative behavior is frequently described in terms of means-ends. The child must learn to select the form of a behavior that will produce a desired result in a listener. The child must also expand his or her repertoire of communicative forms to meet individual idiosyncrasies of listeners. Eventually, communicative gestures become early wordlike and word utterances. These word forms are used with gestural forms in a complex sequence to achieve the child-speaker's communicative intention or goal.

Cause and Effect

The traditional notion of prerequisites to language development focuses on a causal relationship between cognition and language. A causal relationship would indicate a pattern in which linguistic developments could be directly tied to nonlinguistic developments. For example, children come to use names (e.g., bed) as they develop object permanence. In fact, the relationship of object permanence to language has been questioned by several investigators (Cornell, 1978; Gratch, 1979). At this point, causality has been difficult to prove. In order to determine whether cognitive development provides the underpinnings for language development, cognitive skills must be identified in the child's behavior. So, for object permanence to play a role in the development of language, object permanence must, at the very least, appear as a skill in the child's repertoire before language appears. For many years, the relationship between object permanence and language was assumed. As noted earlier, several researchers have suggested that object permanence may not be a necessary prerequisite for the early development of words (Bates, 1993; Brown, 1973). The use of words seems to appear before Piaget's Substage 6 object permanence; this issue underscores the ongoing discussion concerning the developmental relationship between cognitive abilities and linguistic skills.

Considering Children with Disabilities

In this chapter we have discussed the development of communication within the framework of social cognition and broader social relationships. It has been stressed that the social interactional process is critical to normal language development. There are many infants and preschoolers who are entering educational programs because they have not acquired these prerequisite communication skills and therefore have been labeled as handicapped. Although their diagnostic labels may vary—autistic, hearing impaired, cerebral palsied, visually impaired, or mentally retarded—these children share a basic and a primary problem: a language disorder. They also share many language learning characteristics and needs. In later chapters it will become much more evident that a disruption in communication development imposed by a handicapping condition or factor results in many similar problems.

Let us consider some of the characteristic problems that might be indicated in a child at this stage of development. Diagnostic evaluation of 18-month-old Alyssa could not be accomplished through formal testing and evaluation, so informal evaluation was attempted through play. Alyssa was totally nonverbal. The only sounds she emitted were guttural grunts. She was not able to remain seated at a small table, so play interaction was attempted in an infant stimulation classroom. The diagnostician offered a number of toys in succession in an effort to establish some kind of interaction between peers. Alyssa did not respond to either verbal or gestural forms of communication. Although attempts were made to establish gaze interaction with the child by using various objects, Alyssa moved erratically from object to object about the room, without responding to any of the diagnostician's initiations. During the session, the child did not initiate any interactions with the peers in the room. Alyssa's responses to peers indicated a rather limited repertoire of social interactional behaviors. Alyssa wandered about the room engaging in highly repetitive self-stimulatory behaviors.

Consider the social cognitive capabilities of children during their first 6 to 9 months of life, and compare Alyssa's behavior. It is important to note that Alyssa is not an unusual child. It is also interesting that Alyssa received a number of different diagnoses; she was placed in a special education program. Two different reports were received from independent practitioners. A psychiatric evaluation indicated that the behavioral symptomatology was characteristic of a child at risk for autism. Alyssa was described as a child with poor social interactional skills and severely impaired object relational skills. She used people as objects and manipulated objects without regard for their functional usage. Her object performances were repetitive and self-stimulatory. An important means for learning about objects is play, and Alyssa did not know how to play. Play is also an avenue for learning adult-child and child-child interaction. Alyssa did not indicate the range of social communicative functions necessary for the development of language. She could not establish or maintain a social exchange by using gaze, vocal, or gestural behaviors. Alyssa was isolated from her social as well as her physical world. What were Alyssa's perceptions of her environment? How could these perceptions affect her cognitive development?

Another report was received two days later indicating that Alyssa had a profound hearing loss. In addition, the report indicated that medical testing could not determine whether Alyssa had functional vision, because she did not respond consistently to any of the stimuli presented. This information about Alyssa's severe perceptual weaknesses in possibly two sensory areas further explained her behavioral and interactional performances. It is not unusual for children who are experiencing sensory deprivation to exhibit autistic-like behaviors.

The Role of Parents in Early Intervention Programs

The role of parents in normal language development has changed during the past decade due to the broadening understanding of the interactive process that occurs in early child development. In this chapter, we have discussed the importance of social interactional exchange and how each partner contributes to the communication process. We have also noted that the adult makes an important assumption about the child's potential to interact in the dyadic interaction. What happens, however, when the infant does not respond to the adult's initiations? What happens in the peer-Alyssa dyad? Tiegerman and Siperstein (1984) noted that approximately 60 percent of the utterances presented by mothers to their children with language disorders in a dyadic interaction were not semantically related to the child's vocal, verbal, or nonverbal behavior. The research stressed the fact that mothers were not able to effectively attune themselves to the interactional and language needs of the children. The findings across a number of studies suggest that children with language disorders may receive a limited range of semantic information, which is quite different from the variety provided to normally developing children. Clearly, the child with a language disorder cannot be of much help in facilitating interaction with adults and peers. Parents and peers do not have the formal knowledge or the skills to repair problems in the communication process. There is clear evidence and agreement that social interactional exchange is critical to communication learning and language development (Tiegerman-Farber, 1995a).

In recognizing the importance of parents to children's early language learning, educational and clinical programs must establish parent training programs that provide information about content and procedure: language development, language disorders, and language intervention (McDade & Varnedoe, 1987). The content of such training programs for parents must be determined; specifically, what should parents know about development, disorders, and intervention or facilitation procedures? Professionals must also decide how they are going to train parents to acquire this knowledge base (Tiegerman-Farber, 1995b). Will parent training programs consist of lectures, formal classes, classroom observations, or videotapes? Finally, professionals must come to terms with the issue of outcome. What do professionals want parents to do with their language-disordered children, and how will parent as well as child changes be measured? It is important to keep in mind that the educational process has traditionally excluded parents from the classroom. This is not productive or reasonable with children who have language disorders, given their extensive need for services and the mandate for inclusive programming. Given the constraint that traditional education takes place only between 9 A.M. and 3 P.M., there is clearly a need and an opportunity to enlist parents in the educational process for the remainder of the day. The result should be to generalize education to the home environment and expand education to include other facilitators, such as fathers, siblings, and grandparents. Public Law 99-457 extends the provision of educational services to 3- to 5-year-old children with disabilities and provides early intervention opportunities.

Although increased sensitivity to and awareness of the importance of early identification and intervention exists, a rather glaring piece of the educational puzzle still remains neglected. Parents of normally developing and gifted children have not been included in parent training or facilitation programs (Clark, 1992). Research indicates that child development issues are relevant for all parents. The educational system must, from a broad based philosophical perspective, begin to include parents in collaborative decision making. Child development and parenting skills should be systematically presented to all parents, not just to parents whose children have disabilities (Tiegerman-Farber, 1995b). Parent training programs should be evaluated to determine the efficacy of content and procedural variables so that more consistent programming can be developed and used across settings and populations.

Summary

A variety of developmental models describe the interdependence of language, cognition, and social development in the attempt to show how these components interact. These models share an underlying assumption that the components do, indeed, interact. Interaction of components, as noted earlier, may occur in several different ways. Interaction in a model in which there is an interdependent relationship between components suggests separate areas that interface and are derived from a more basic area (the shared base model; see Figure 2-2).

Interaction in which there is a dependent relationship between components suggests that one area requires input from another (the direct causal model; see Figure 2-3). The strong cognition hypothesis proposes a developmental dependence between language and cognition: that language as a system requires input from cognition. Many researchers argue that early social and cognitive developments prepare children for later developments in language (Bloom & Lahey, 1978; Bruner, 1975). Developmental continuity can explain the emergence of symbols and, thus, the acquisition of language.

A prerequisite to language development is defined as a "structure in one system that provides input to the structure of a second system" (Bates, Benigni, Bretherton, Camaioni, & Volterra, 1979, p. 14). The notion that certain skills or structures are prerequisite to language echoes the strong cognition hypothesis that cognitive underpinnings precede developments in language. The issue of prerequisites presents interesting insights in light of recent research investigations. Several researchers have suggested the existence of prerequisite cognitive and social schemes that gradually combine into complex communicative sequences (Sugarman, 1977). Bruner (1973) suggests that the semantic structure of language is derived from the nature and structure of social interaction and relationships. That is to say that the child learns about speaker-listener roles during social interactional exchanges with adults and peers. The language used to express social knowledge is based on, or mapped onto, the child's social-cognitive experiences.

Study Questions

1. How do vertical and horizontal relationships play a role in social development?
2. Children's relationships with peers become increasingly significant; discuss how peer interactions facilitate communication learning.
3. How does Piaget describe the child as an active agent in his or her own development?
4. Describe the developments that occur during the sensorimotor period and the changes that occur as a function of the distancing principle.
5. Discuss the changing relationship between language and cognition. How has the change in the definition of language contributed to a reconsideration of the strong cognitive hypothesis?
6. How does the child's interaction with his environment facilitate knowledge about objects and events?
7. Discuss the child's development of an internal schematic representation of his or her interactional and interpersonal experiences with his or her world.
8. What behaviors exhibited by infants during their first six months of life affect their mothers' interactional behaviors?
9. How does a mother regulate her input when talking to the young language learner? How does a mother's input change as the child becomes a more sophisticated communicator?
10. Describe the relationship between cognition and language according to Piaget.
11. Discuss the controversy concerning the relationship between cognition and language given the changing definition of language during the past decade.

12. Describe the development of language during the sensory motor period.
13. Why is it important to approach the area of communication development from a social cognitive perspective?

References

Ainsworth, M. D. S. (1989). Attachments beyond infancy. *American Psychologist, 44*, 709–716.

Barnes, S., Gutfreund, M., Satterly, D., & Wells, G. (1983). Characteristics of adult speech which predict children's language development. *Journal of Child Language, 10*, 65–84.

Bates, E. (1976). Pragmatic and sociolinguistics in child language. In D. Morehead & A. Morehead (Ed.), *Normal and deficient child language.* Baltimore: University Park Press.

Bates, E. (1993). Commentary: Comprehension and production in early language development. Monographs of the Society for Research in Child Development, 58 (3–4, Serial No. 233), 222–242.

Bates, E. Benigni, L., Bretherton, I., Camaioni, L., & Volterra, V. (1977). From gesture to the first word: On cognitive and social prerequisites. In M. Lewis & L. Rosenblum (Ed.), *Interaction conversation and the development of language* (pp. 247–307). New York: Wiley.

Bates, E. Benigni, L., Bretherton, I., Camaioni, L., & Volterra, V. (1979). *The emergence of symbols: Cognition and communication in infancy.* New York: Academic Press.

Bateson, M. D. (1975). Mother-infant exchanges: The epigenesis of conversational interaction. In D. Ironstone & R. Ribber (Eds.), *Annals of the New York Academy of Sciences: Vol. 263. Developmental psycholinguistics and communication disorders* (pp. 101–113).

Beckwith, L., Cohen, S., Kopp, C., Parmalee, A., & Marcy, T. (1976). Caregiver-infant interaction and early cognitive development in preterm infants. *Child Development, 47*, 579–587.

Berndt, T. J. (1983). Social cognition, social behavior, and children's friendships. In E. T. Higgins, D. N. Ruble, & W. W. Hartup (Eds.), *Social cognition and social development. A sociocultural perspective* (pp. 158–192). Cambridge, England: Cambridge University Press.

Berndt, T. J. (1986). Children's comments about their friendships. In M. Perlmutter (Ed.), Cognitive perspectives on children's social and behavioral development. *Minnesota Symposia on Child Psychology* (Vol. 18, pp. 189–212). Hillsdale, NJ: Erlbaum.

Berndt, T. J. (1992). Friendship and friends' influence in adolescence. *Current Directions in Psychological Science, 1*, 156–159.

Berndt, T. J. Hawkins, J. A., & Hoyle, S. G. (1986). Changes in friendship during a school year: Effects on children's and adolescents' impressions of friendship and sharing with friends. *Child Development, 57*, 1284–1297.

Bernstein Ratner, N. (1984). Patterns of vowel modification in mother-child speech. *Journal of Child Language, 11*, 557–578.

Bernstein Ratner, N., & Pye, C. (1984). Higher pitch in B is not universal: Acoustic evidence from Quiche Mayan. *Journal of Child Language, 11*, 515–522.

Bloom, L., & Leahy, M. (1978). *Language development and language disorders.* New York: Wiley.

Bowlby, J. (1988). *A secure base: Parent-child attachment and healthy human development.* New York: Basic Books.

Bradley, R., & Caldwell, B. (1976). The relation of infants' home environments to mental test performance at 54 months: A follow-up study. *Child Development, 47*, 1172–1174.

Bretherton, I. (1992a). Attachment and bonding. In V. B. V. Hasselt & M. Hersen (Eds.), *Handbook of social development: A lifespan perspective* (pp. 133–155). New York: Plenum Press.

Bretherton, I. (1992b). The origins of attachment theory: John Balboa and Mary Ainsworth. *Developmental Psychology, 28*, 759–775.

Brice Heath, S. (1983). *Ways with words: Language, life and work in communities and classrooms.* New York: Cambridge University Press.

Bronfenbrenner, U. (1979). *The ecology of human development.* Cambridge, MA: Harvard University Press.

Bronfenbrenner, U. (1989). Ecological systems theory. *Annals of Child Development, 6*, 187–249.

Brown, R. (1973). *A first language: The early stages.* Boston: Harvard University Press.

Bruner, J. S. (1975). The ontogenesis of speech acts. *Journal of Child Language, 2,* 1–19.

Bruner, J. S. (1973). Organization of early skilled action. *Child Development, 44,* 1–11.

Chomsky, N. (1986). Knowledge of language: Its nature, origin and use. New York: Praeger.

Chomsky, N. (1988). *Language and problems of knowledge.* Cambridge, MA: MIT Press.

Clark, B. (1992). *Growing up gifted.* New York: Merrill/Macmillan.

Cornell, E. (1978). Learning to find things: A reinterpretation of object permanence studies. In L. Siege & C. Brained (Eds.), *Alternatives to Piaget.* New York: Academic Press.

Cross, T. (1977). Mothers' speech adjustments: The contribution of selected listener variables. In E. G. Snow & C. B. Ferguson (Eds.), *Talking to children.* New York: Cambridge University Press.

D'Odorico, L., & Franco, F. (1985). The determinants of babytalk: Relationship to context. *Journal of Child Language, 12,* 567–586.

Duchan, J. (1986). Learning to describe events. *Topics in Language Disorders, 6,* 27–36.

Dunham, P. J., Dunham, F., & Curwin, A. (1993). Joint attentional states and lexical acquisition at 18 months. *Developmental Psychology, 29,* 827–831.

Dunn, J. (1993). Young children's close relationships. Knobbier Park, CA: Sage.

Farrar, M. (1990). Discourse and the acquisition of grammatical morphemes. *Journal of Child Language,* 607–624.

Fernald, A. (1989). Intonation and communicative intent in mothers' speech to infants: Is the melody the message? *Child Development, 60,* 1497–1510.

Fernald, A. (1993). Approval and disapproval: Infant responsiveness to vocal affect in familiar and unfamiliar languages. *Child Development, 64,* 657–674.

Flax, J., Lahey M., Harris, K., & Boothroyd, A. (1991). Relations between prosopic variables and communicative functions. *Journal of Child Language, 18,* 3–19.

Furrow, D., Nelson, K., & Benedict, H. (1979). Mothers' speech to children and syntactic development: Some simple relationships. *Journal of Child Language, 6,* 423–442.

Gleitman, L., Newport, E., & Gleitman, H. (1984). The current status of the motherese hypothesis. *Journal of Child Language, 11,* 43–70.

Gopnik, A. (1984). The acquisition of gone and the development of the object concept. *Journal of Child Language, 11,* 273–292.

Gopnik, A., & Meltzoff, A. N. (1992). Categorization and naming: Basic-level sorting in eighteen-month-olds and its relating to language. *Child Development, 63,* 1091–1103.

Gratch, G. (1979). The development of thought and language in infancy. In J. D. Osofsby (Ed.), *Handbook of infant development* (pp. 439–461). New York: Wiley-Interscience.

Haith, M. (1990). Progress in the understanding of sensory and perceptual processes in early infancy. *Merrill-Palmer Quarterly, 36,* 1–26.

Hanna, E., & Meltzoff, A. N. (1993). Peer imitation by toddlers in laboratory, home and daycare contexts: Duplications for social learning and memory. *Developmental Psychology, 29,* 701–710.

Harris, M. (1992). *Language experience and early language development: From input to uptake.* Hove, England: Erlbaum.

Hartup, W. A. (1989). Social relationships and their developmental significance. *American Psychologist, 44,* 120–126.

Hoff-Ginsberg, E. (1990). Maternal speech and the child's development of syntax: A further look. *Journal of Child Language, 17,* 85–99.

Howes, C., & Matheson, C. C. (1992). Sequences in the development of competent play with peers: Social and pretend play. *Developmental Psychology, 28,* 961–974.

Jaffe, J., Stern, D., & Peery, J. (1973). Conversational coupling of gaze behavior in prelinguistic human development. *Journal of Psycholinguistic Research, 2,* 321–329.

Jusczyk, P. W., Cutler, A., & Redanz, N. J. (1993). Infants' preference for the predominant stress patterns of English words. *Child Development, 64,* 675–687.

Karmiloff-Smith, A. (1993). Neo-Piagetians: A theoretical misnomer? *Society for Research in Child Development Newsletter, 3,* 10–11.

Kozulin, A. (Ed.) (1987). Thought and language. Cambridge, MA: MIT Press.

Lieven, D. V. M. (1977). Conversations between mothers and young children: Individual differences and their possible implications for the study of language learning. In E. G. Snow & C. B. Ferguson (Eds.), *Talking to children: Language input and acquisition.* New York: Cambridge University Press.

Lindfors, J. W. (1987). *Children's language and learning.* Englewood Cliffs, NJ: Prentice Hall.

McDade, H. L, & Varnedoe, D. A. (1987). Training parents to be language facilitators. *Topics in Language Disorders,* 7, 19–31.

McLean, J., & Snyder-McLean, L. (1978). *A transactional approach to early language training.* Columbus, OH: Merrill/Macmillan.

Meltzoff, A. N. (1988). Infant imitation and memory: Nine-month-olds in immediate and deferred tasks. *Child Development,* 59, 217–225.

Morehead, D., & Morehead, A. (1974). From signal to sign: A Piagetian view of thought and language during the first two years. In R. R. Schiefelbusch & L. P. Lloyd (Eds.), *Language perspectives—Acquisition, retardation, and intervention* (pp. 153–190). Baltimore: University Park Press.

Murray, A., Johnson, J., & Peters, J. (1990). Fine tuning of utterance length to proverbial infants: Effects on later language development. *Journal of Child Language,* 17, 511–526.

Murray, L., & Trevarthen, C. (1985). Emotional regulations of interactions between 2 month odds and their mothers. In T. V. Field & N. C. Fox (Ed.), *Social perception in infants.* Neuroid, NJ: Able.

Murray, L., & Trevarthen, C. (1986). The infant's role in mother-infant communications. *Journal of Child Language,* 13, 15–31.

Newport, E. (1977). Motherese: The speech of mothers to young children. In N. C. Castellan, D. B. Pacini, & G. Poets (Eds.), *Cognitive theory* (Vol. 2). Hillsdale, NJ: Lawrence Erlbaum Associates.

Newport, E., Gleitman, H., & Gleitman, L. (1977). Mother, I'd rather do it myself: Some effects and non-effects of maternal speech style. In E. G. Snow & C. B. Ferguson (Eds.), *Talking to children: Language input and acquisition.* New York: Cambridge University Press.

Olson, S. L., Bates, J. E., & Kaskie, B. (1992). Caregiver-infant interaction antecedents of children's school age cognitive ability. *Merrill-Palmer Quarterly,* 38, 309–330.

Penman, R., Cross, T., Milgrom-Friedman, J., & Meares, R. (1983). Mothers' speech to prelingual infants: A pragmatic analysis. *Journal of Child Language,* 10, 17–34.

Phillips, J. (1973). Syntax and vocabulary in mothers' speech to young children: Age and sex comparisons. *Child Development,* 44, 182–185.

Piaget, J. (1962). *Play, dreams and imitation in childhood.* New York: Norton.

Piaget, J., & Inhelder, B. (1969). *The psychology of the child.* New York: Basic Books.

Platt, J., & Coggins, T. (1990). Comprehension of social-action games in prelinguistic children: Levels of participation and effect of adult structure. *Journal of Speech and Hearing Disorders,* 55, 315–326.

Pye, C. (1986). One lexicon or two? Interpretation of early bilingual speech. *Journal of Child Language,* 13, 591–594.

Remick, H. (1976). Maternal speech to children during language acquisition. In W. von Raffler-Angel & Y. Lebrun (Eds.), *Baby talk and infant speech.* Lisse: Swets & Zeilinger.

Rice, M. (1980a). *Cognition.* Baltimore: University Park Press.

Rice, M. (1980b). *Cognition to language: Categories, words, meanings and training.* Baltimore: University Park Press.

Rice, M., & Kemper, (1984). *Child language and cognition.* Baltimore: University Park Press.

Rovee-Collier, C. (1993). The capacity for long-term memory in infancy. *Current Directions in Psychological Science,* 2, 130–135.

Rutter, D. R. and Durkin, K. (1987). Turn-taking in mother-infant interaction: An examination of vocalizations and gaze. *Developmental Psychology,* 23, 54–61.

Sameroff, A. J. (1983). Developmental systems: Contexts and evolution. In W. Keesen (Ed.), *Handbook of child psychology: Vol. 1, History, theory, and methods* (pp. 237–294). New York: Wiley.

Sapir, E. (1921). *Language.* New York: Harcourt, Brace & World.

Sexton, H. (1980). *The development of the understanding of causality in infancy.* Paper presented at the International Conference on Infant Studies, New Haven, CT.

Shatz, M. (1982). On mechanisms of language acquisition: Can features of the communicative environment account for development? In E. Wanner & L. Gleitman (Eds.), *Language acquisition: The state of the art.* New York: Cambridge University Press.

Simeonsson, R. J., & Bailey, D. B. (1988). *Family assessment and early intervention.* Columbus, OH: Merrill.

Sinclair-deZwart, H. (1973). Language acquisition and cognitive development. In T. E. Moore (Ed.), *Cognitive development and the acquisition of language.* New York: Academic Press.

Slobin, D. (1973). Cognitive perspectives for the development of grammar. In C. B. Ferguson & D. A. Slobin (Eds.), *Studies of child language development* (pp. 175–208). New York: Holt, Rinehart & Winston.

Snow, C. (1972). Mothers' speech to children learning language. *Child Development,* 43, 549–565.

Snow, C. (1977). Mothers' speech research: From input to interaction. In C. Snow & C. B. Ferguson (Eds.), *Talking to children: Language input and acquisition* (pp. 31–50). New York: Cambridge University Press.

Snow, C., Arlmann-Rupp, A., Hassing, Y., Jobse, H., Joosten, J., & Vorster, J. (1976). Mothers' speech in three social classes. *Journal of Psycholinguistic Research,* 5, 1–20.

Snow, C., & Ferguson, C. (1977). Talking to children: Language input and acquisition. New York: Cambridge University Press.

Spelke, E. S. (1991). Physical knowledge in infancy: Reflections on Piaget's theory: In S. Carey and R. Gelman (Eds.), *The epigenesis of mind: Essays on biology and cognition* (pp. 133–169). Hillsdale, NJ: Erlbaum.

Stern, D. (1974). Mother and infant at play: The dyadic interaction involving facial, vocal and gaze behaviors. In M. Lewis & L. Rosenblum (Eds.), *The effect of the infant on its caregiver* (pp. 187–213). New York: Wiley.

Stern, D. (1977). *The first relationship.* Cambridge: Harvard University Press.

Stern, D., Jaffe, J., Beebe, B., & Bennett, S. (1975). Vocalizing in unison and in alternation: Two modes of communication within the mother-infant dyad. In D. Ironstone & R. Ribber (Ed.), *Annals of the New York Academy of Sciences:* Vol. 263. *Developmental psycholinguistics and communication disorders* (pp. 89–100).

Stern, D., Spieker, S., Barnett, R., & MacKain, K. (1983). The prosody of maternal speech: Infant age

and context-related changes. *Journal of Child Language,* 10, 1–16.

Sugarman, S. (1977). A description of communicative development in the prelanguage child. In I. Markova (Ed.), *The social context of language.* New York: Wiley.

Szapocznik, J., & Kurtines, W. M. (1993). Family psychology and cultural diversity: Opportunities for theory, research and application. *American Psychologist,* 48, 400–407.

Tiegerman-Farber, E. (1995a). The changing role of the family. In *Language and communication intervention in preschool children* (pp. 37–60). Needham Heights, MA: Allyn & Bacon.

Tiegerman-Farber, E. (1995b). Training the parent as facilitator. In *Language and communication intervention in preschool children* (pp. 155–184). Needham Heights, MA: Allyn & Bacon.

Tiegerman, E., & Siperstein, M. (1984). Individual patterns of interaction in the mother-child dyad: Implications for parent intervention. *Topics in Language Disorders,* 4, 50–62.

Tomasello, M., & Farrar, M. (1984). Cognitive bases of lexical development: Object permanence and relational words. *Journal of Child Language,* 11, 477–494.

Vygotsky, L. (1976). Play and its role in the mental development of the child. In J. S. Bruner, A. Jolly, & K. Sylvan (Eds.), *Play: Its role in evolution and development.* New York: Basic Books.

Vygotsky, L. (1987). Thought and word. In A. Kozulin (Ed.), *Thought and language.* Cambridge, MA: MIT Press.

Walton, G. E., Bower, N. J. and Bower, N. J. (1992). Recognition of familiar faces by newborns. *Infant Behavior and Development,* 15, 265–269.

Westby, C. (1980). Assessment of cognition and language abilities through play. *Journal of Language, Speech and Hearing Services in the Schools,* 11, 154–168.

Chapter 3

The Ecology of the Family: The Language Imperative

ELLENMORRIS TIEGERMAN-FARBER
School for Language and Communication Development
and
Adelphi College

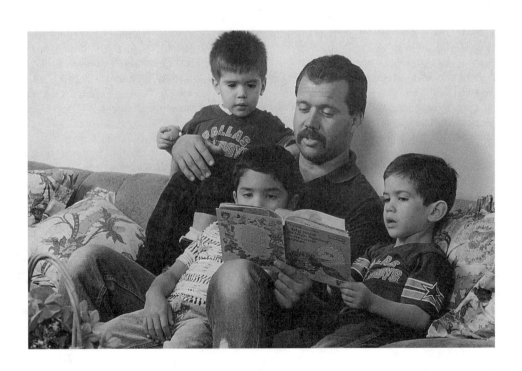

The traditional American family no longer consists of a working father, a mother who stays at home, two children, and a dog. The concept of the traditional family has been replaced by many alternative relationships. The assessment of family needs and of children with disabilities has taught us a great deal about the family as an ecological system (Trout & Foley, 1989). The family today is faced with many problems—financial, cultural, religious, and educational—that have created additional stress and fragmentation for all of its members. Several statistics highlight the significant changes within the family:

1. Almost 45 percent of preschool children will be raised by single parents before they reach the age of 18; half will experience one or more family breakups.
2. Fifty-five percent of preschool children currently have mothers who work outside the home. By 1995, 75 percent of their mothers will work outside the home, most in a full-time capacity (Barona & Garcia, 1990).

An Ecological Approach to Understanding Family Issues

In the last chapter we discussed that in order to understand child development issues within the framework of our complex social society, it is important to consider all of the child's social networks. Bronfenbrenner (1989) describes an ecological system in which the child develops within a series of contextually related environments (see Figure 3-1). The inner context, which he refers to as the microsystem, refers to the contextual settings in which the child has direct experience; the family, the school, the child-care center, and the play group fall within this central circle. The next circle, called an exosystem, includes a range of contexts and experiences with which the child is not directly involved but that may influence the child within the microsystem. This broader context highlights a distancing principle described as a progressive extension between the child and the environment; the qualitative aspect of a child's development is influenced by experiences that impact upon members of his or her family. When parents go to work and siblings attend school, their individual experiences impact positively and/or negatively on the nature of family interaction. Finally, Bronfenbrenner describes a macrosystem that represents the larger cultural context in which the micro- and exosystems are embedded.

A child's development is a function not only of the nurturance within the framework of the family system, but is also affected by the economic status of the family, the community within which he or she lives, the social and mental health of each of the family members, the social services provided within the community, and all of the economic factors that create emotional and financial stress in today's complex society. Family interaction patterns influence the qualitative nature of the child's attachment to the family, his or her peers, and later to the community. A child's development represents a complex interaction between his individual characteristics and the environmental experiences that challenge his individual learning. Szapocznik and Kurtines (1993) propose a contexualist paradigm that suggests that child development is a function of the individual child within layers of contextual challenges. This suggests that in order to understand the child, the theorist, the teacher, and the therapist must also assess the family interactional patterns, as well as the child's contextual

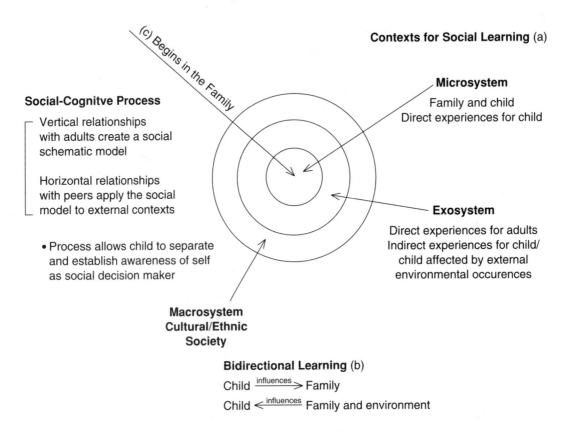

Social-Cognitve Process

┌ Vertical relationships
│ with adults create a social
│ schematic model
│
│ Horizontal relationships
│ with peers apply the social
└ model to external contexts

 • Process allows child to separate
   and establish awareness of self
   as social decision maker

Contexts for Social Learning (a)

Microsystem
Family and child
Direct experiences for child

Exosystem
Direct experiences for adults
Indirect experiences for child/
child affected by external
environmental occurences

(c) Begins in the Family

Macrosystem
Cultural/Ethnic
Society

Bidirectional Learning (b)
Child ──influences──> Family
Child <──influences── Family and environment

FIGURE 3-1   Ecological systems approach to child development.

experiences. This approach proposes that child learning occurs within the framework of a family system that is itself embedded within the larger social environment of community and culture. Child language learning represents a dynamic, embedded, and contextualized process. In order to understand how children develop language, it is important to consider the interacting systems that network to affect the child's language and communication learning. The purpose of this chapter is to discuss the development of early child language in terms of a systems theory, in this case the family as an ecological system. The following principles apply within the contextualist model. How would these principles affect child language learning (Bee, 1995)?

1. The family represents an adaptive social system; as a system any change experienced by one member of the family affects every other member.
2. Within the family microsystem, parental behavior toward the child is significant to an infant's emotional, social, and language development.
3. Families that establish rules and standards and relatively high levels of expectation and are consistent but loving, have children with high self esteem and social competence.

4. Parents who facilitate language in their infants and who are highly responsive to child communicative initiation have children who develop language more rapidly and also have more positive relationships with parents and peers.

5. The ecological system within the family is affected by cultural influences and economic factors.

6. The family system is affected by child-related variables such as temperament, gender, position within the family, and social adaptability.

7. The changing structure of the family has a significant affect on the relationship between the adults and the parent-child relationships.

8. Divorce and melded family structures, as well as nontraditional adult relationships, alter family patterns and dynamics.

9. The working mother faces many challenges inside and outside of the family context. The working mother changes the family system by altering how she functions within the family.

10. Environmental factors that change the structure of the family create stress for parents and children who are struggling to understand themselves and their social environment.

What Is Language?

Language codes human interaction within the social environment. During the first two years of life, children learn many behaviors that they integrate and use to communicate. Communication gradually changes from the use of personal and idiosyncratic forms within the family to the use of conventional forms within society (Bates, 1993; deVilliers & deVilliers, 1992; Harris, 1992). Children learn about the communicative function of language long before they learn about its linguistic structure.

Language is a system of symbols that has a highly complex form and structure. In normal language development, young children learn that an idea can be expressed by manipulating and combining these linguistic forms. Embedded within the sound, the word, and the sentence is meaning. Language has structure and meaning, but it also has purpose. Although people use language to communicate, it is not the only means or mechanism available to them. Mime, dance, and sign are communication forms that can be used by adults and children.

Language is used by people when they want to communicate with one another. Just as there are many languages, there are many forms of communication. Children learn that language, particularly spoken language, is an extremely efficient and effective means of communication. The language code provides the speaker with a tremendous ability to express an infinite number of ideas rapidly as well as universally to speakers within a sociolinguistic community.

Language has a purpose—communication. Language may be used to accomplish many different communication purposes. A mother may use language to comfort her crying infant. She may use language to comment about ongoing events in their environment. She may use language to direct her infant to perform or not to perform some action with toys.

Language learners acquire a knowledge of the structure of language, the ideas that can be expressed through the language code, and the function of language-communication.

Children first acquire the ability to communicate, which provides a foundation for the later acquisitions of ideas and structure. Children learn to communicate in a social context whenever they interact with adults and peers.

From a developmental perspective, it is important to understand that communication precedes and facilitates speech and language behavior, discussed in the last chapter. The motive for language learning is effective communication. During the first 24 months of life, communicative intentions are coded by a variety of forms; gradually, these early intentions attain a linguistic form. Language is a system that codes the social process in which communicative forms of exchange are learned; that is, it is a system that is learned in the social context (Dunn, 1993). The infant's conquest of the social context involves a pursuit of efficient and effective forms of interactional behavior. Children learn first about the conventions that code social interaction, then about social communication, and, finally, about linguistic communication. The focus of this chapter is how the infant functions as an active language learner in pursuit of rule-governed knowledge given the ecological dynamics of his or her family.

How Does Language Develop?

Communication Development

Research has shown that communicative intent appears before the development of speech. The infant expresses interactional intentions initially by combining gaze, gesture, and vocal behaviors. Gradually these communicative forms of behavior become wordlike utterances, as the infant acquires the speech forms of his linguistic environment. Bates (1976) suggested that semantics and syntactics are derived from pragmatics: "Semantics emerges, developmentally and logically, from pragmatics, in much the same way that syntax has been shown to emerge from semantic knowledge" (p. 420). Pragmatics involves the use of language within context. The infant learns to use various forms of behavior to carry out a communicative function. Thus, the early appearance of communicative acts provides a developmental time line across which various components of language are acquired.

Communicative Intentions

Greenfield and Smith (1976) noted that children's first words are not referential in that they do not refer to or name an object or event. The word accompanies an act but does not represent or stand for a particular object "any more than the act of pointing itself represents the thing to which it refers" (p. 425). As already discussed, according to Piaget, words become symbolic and representational at the end of the sensorimotor period (Substage 6, 18 to 24 months). But children are using words long before they develop symbolic skills. How are these words used? From birth to 24 months of age, children use many forms of behavior (vocal, gestural, and lexical) to signal interaction. At first, infants are aware of no communicative purpose for their actions. However, over time they learn to use behaviors to create an effect within the social context; these intentional signals of interaction can be called **speech acts.** The speech act refers to the act that the speaker intends to carry out. Children may express many different intentions—request, command, question, and so forth—within the social context. During the first 24 months, the important issue is the acquisition of speech acts, specifically, how the infant learns to code various intentions (see Table 3-1).

TABLE 3-1   Acquisition of Speech Functions

Substages	Intention to Communicate; Communicative Functions	Conventional Coding of Ideas; Semantic Functions	Conventional Coding of Forms and Structures; Syntactic Structures
I	No	No	No
II	Yes	No	No
III	Yes	Yes	No
IV	Yes	Yes	Yes

Adapted with permission of Macmillan Publishing Company from *Language Development and Language Disorders* by L. Bloom and M. Lahey (New York: Macmillan, 1978).

Table 3-2 illustrates some of the intentions communicated by the 9-month-old infant. Notice how the infant is able to indicate a variety of communicative intentions by combining vocal, gestural, and gaze behaviors. Bates, Benigni, Bretherton, Camaioni, and Volterra (1979) pinpointed 9 months of age as a developmental turning point:

> *We can infer the onset of intentionality from at least three types of evidence: changes in eye contact and checks for feedback, alterations in signaling until the goal is reached, and changes in the shape of signals toward a form that is appropriate only for communication. . . . It is sufficient to note that the relatively sudden onset of intentional, conventional communication around 9 months seems to be related to some other developments in learning how to get things done in the world. (p. 38)*

The infant's ability to communicate intentions precedes the development of linguistic language structures, which are symbolic-representational forms. During this period of prelinguistic behavior, the context plays an important role in helping the mother interpret the infant's intentions. The change from prelinguistic to linguistic forms can be viewed as a transition from idiosyncratic communication to symbolic communication (Bates, Benigni, Bretherton, Camaioni, & Volterra, 1977). Once children develop linguistic structures, the conventional form of the language of their society, they can be understood with less and less contextual support (Bruner, 1974).

In her study of linguistic and nonlinguistic vocalizations of children between 14 and 22 months of age, Marcos (1987) found a relationship between intonational patterns and communicative functions. She noted that a higher pitch and rising tones signaled requests, whereas a lower pitch and falling tones accompanied labeling. Flax, Lahey, Harris, and Boothroyd (1991) noted that children exhibited individual differences in the intonational patterns they established for specific communicative functions and that these prosodic variables remained relatively constant for each infant from the prelinguistic period through the

TABLE 3-2   **Prespeech Communication at 9 Months**

Communicative Intentions	Behavioral Form
Request	Vocal: *eh;* reaches hand out in direction of object; alternates gaze back and forth from object to adult
Demand	Vocal: *eh, eh, eh* (staccato vocalization getting progressively louder and higher); alternates gaze between object and adult; reaches hand in direction of object, opening and closing hand
Attention getters	Coughs; gazes at adult Vocal *eh* (drawn-out production); pulls an adult leg; gazes at adult
Rejection	Pushes object away with hand; averts gaze
Initiating ritual play	Pokes chest and gazes toward adult (X-marks-the-spot game) Claps hands and gazes toward adult (pat-a-cake game) Puts hands up and gazes toward adult (hurrah game)

single-word-utterance phase. In addition, the rising contour was more often used with utterances that required a response, such as requests and protests, whereas the falling contour was more often used with functions that did not require a response. This research suggests that the differences across children may be related to stylistic differences in parental responses to the infants' use of contour patterns.

Early Sound Production

Although infants are uniquely attuned, or perhaps preprogrammed, to perceive various phonemes in language, they cannot produce a wide range of speech sounds (Eimas, Siqueland, Jusczyk, & Vigorito, 1971). The structure of an infant's mouth and throat simply does not permit it. A relatively large tongue fills the oral cavity, limiting its movement and, therefore, the production of sounds.

The earliest sounds are vowels or are vowellike in quality. At 6 months of age, the baby utters and repeats syllable sequences, initiating the babbling period. Jakobson and Halle (1956) noted that the babbling stage begins with undetermined sounds that are neither consonants nor vowels, and it ends with a distinct separation. During the first 12 months, the form of sound production changes to express communicative intentions. Children learn to use sounds as well as gestures to communicate their intentions.

With the development of the semantic system comes the use of phonemic structures. Phonology is part of the infant's developing linguistic system. It is rule-governed as the other components of language are rule-governed. The phonetic abundance of babbling gives way to phonemic restriction with the onset of the semantic stage. The phonological system interfaces with the semantic and syntactic components to result in language—a symbolic social system. The infant's earliest words are limited in number and type of syllables and in phoneme types, restraints that gradually disappear. Greater complexity and diversity in production result as the infant's production becomes governed by phonological rules. Kiparsky and Menn (1977) have suggested that production is the result of underlying phonological rules rather than the result of word or sound development. The infant acquires rule-governed patterns that are based on higher-level linguistic organization.

Kent and Bauer (1985) described the acoustic-phonetic properties of vocalizations in infants 13 months of age. At this developmental stage, the utterances can be described as babbling and grunts with underlying but productive communicative abilities. The authors noted that the vocal tract of the infant is not a miniature version of the adult tract. The infant's tract differs substantially in physiological proportions and configuration, therefore effecting sound production differences. Kent and Bauer suggested that the theories describing phonological development generally predict a gradual conformation with the adult production system, "when in fact phonological acquisition is characterized by both regression and overgeneralization" (p. 493). Phonological theories need to incorporate cognitive developments because the infant takes an active, problem-solving approach to acquisition. The cognitive-based theory of phonological development proposes that the infant builds more complex structures from the revisions of the child's hypotheses. Kent and Bauer categorized the sound productions of infants in their study as vocants or closants. Vocants are vowellike sounds that are precursors of vowels, and closants are consonant like sounds thought to be precursors of consonants. Their results indicate a continuity in early phonetic development. The vocalizations of the 13-month-olds fell along a production continuum, with the younger babbling infant at one end and the more linguistically sophisticated 2-year-old at the other end. It is the development of the first words that disrupts this continuity. Thus, "it remains an interesting question if early words are essentially a phonetic outgrowth of babbling vocalizations and vocables, or if they represent the emergence of a separate phonology that shares only general features with preceding vocalization categories" (p. 522).

Elbers and Ton (1985) suggested that the study of infant phonology seems to be moving away from an emphasis on linguistic processing toward a more cognitive viewpoint: "In Piagetian terms: the babbling system may accommodate to forms selected by the talking system, whereas the talking system may assimilate forms developed by the babbling system" (p. 563). Their results demonstrate a relationship between the infant's phonological preferences and changes in babbling behaviors, highlighting that the phonological repertoire results from this interactive interplay. The authors proposed that babbling provides the infant with a learning strategy that stimulates phonological problem-solving.

Elbers and Ton (1985) described the possible relationship between babbling and linguistic word development, and several investigators have proposed that early babbling is a speech-related behavior (de Boysson-Bardies, Sagart, & Durand, 1984; Elbers, 1982). Infants do not stop babbling when they initially produce wordlike structures. However, the relationship between postlinguistic or speech-concurrent babbling and early word forms is not so clear. Early word forms tend to be highly variable and idiosyncratic within and across young language learners. According to Elbers and Ton (1985), early word production and concurrent babbling are related through an ongoing interactive process. During this continuous interactive interplay, "a new word may influence and change the character of babbling, whereas babbling in turn may prepare the ground for the production of other new words" (p. 552). Although at times babbling may not be communicative or interactive in nature, it represents a language behavior that provides a practice experience for the infant to act upon his or her phonological hypotheses and preferences.

Communication Stages

The development of language use results from the interaction of infant and context. The infant learns how to create change within the context by combining and recombining behaviors in different ways. Bloom and Lahey (1978) hypothesized three chronological levels in the development of language use. The first stage, infancy, involves gradual change in reflexive types of behavior, such as crying, to achieve ends; these types of behavior are called **primary forms.** Infant behavior is initially directed by basic biological and psychological needs. These physiological states determine the strength, form, and direction of the behavioral acts. Gradually, involuntary reflexive behaviors become voluntary motor acts, permitting infants to control their behavior more directly. But the infant's repertoire does not yet include a variety of communicative behaviors. One particular behavior, such as crying, can be used to meet several different needs. Crying signals several affective states or needs: hunger, distress, and fatigue.

At the second stage, although using some of their culture's vocalizations, gestures, and movements, children still have only a limited repertoire of forms. However, they demonstrate the ability to combine and recombine those forms to express varied communicative functions. They begin to show awareness of the conventional forms that signal intentionality and result in communication with the adult. For example, pointing is a conventional form of behavior—a single behavior—that can be used to convey several different messages, such as "Give me that" (a request) or "Look at that cup" (an attention directive).

At the third stage, children express the same message in different ways. They take into consideration the social variables—listener, context, and so forth—that affect the form of the message. At this stage, children learn that there are alternative means to achieve the same purpose; they "learn when and how to say what to whom" (Bloom & Lahey, 1978, p. 203). They learn to suit the message to the social requirements of the listener, the situation, and the purpose of the interaction. The extent to which children adapt their use of language to the rules of the social context defines their skill as effective communicators (Tomasello & Mannle, 1985).

Consider the following incident with Jeremy (48 months) and Jonathan (15 months), in which Jeremy shares his observations on social interactional rules.

Monday—Jonathan is playing with Super Dog.

Jeremy: Jonathan, gimme that.

Jeremy pulls Super Dog away from Jonathan.

Jeremy: Say "Please."

Jonathan: Eh.

Jeremy: Okay, here.

Tuesday—Jonathan goes to Nana and points to Super Dog on the shelf.

Nana: You Want Super Dog?

Jonathan: Eh. (continues pointing)

Jeremy: Yes, he wants Super Dog. He can have it; he said "Please."

Nana leaves the room. Jeremy and Jonathan are alone together.

Jeremy: Jonathan looks at Jeremy.

Jeremy: Jonathan, when you talk to Nana you have to remember to say "Please." She turns her ears off if you don't say "Please."

The last dialogue highlights certain aspects of the social and pragmatic learning that occurs during the third communication stage. At 48 months, Jeremy was very aware of the how-to part of talking to adults. He had already mastered several conventional forms of the same message. In his experiences and interactions with Nana, he had learned that certain forms of a message achieved certain effects, whereas other forms did not. Notice that he did not use the desired form with Jonathan, with whom he did not perceive a need to say "please." It is also clear that Jeremy was passing on his knowledge to Jonathan. And, more, Jeremy was able to interpret Jonathan's intentions from Jonathan's vocal and gestural behavior. Therefore, in addition to providing Jonathan with some advice about Nana, Jeremy also interpreted Jonathan's behavioral intentions for Nana.

Also highlighted by the dialogue are some differences between the 48-month-old and the 15-month-old. Although his repertoire of vocal and gestural performances was very limited, Jonathan could nevertheless express a variety of intentions. At 48 months, Jeremy could analyze and interpret differences in listeners and contexts to alter the form of his message. Thus, Jeremy exercised alternative means for achieving the same purpose in different situations (Bloom & Lahey, 1978), whereas Jonathan's goal was simply to achieve his purpose (Bates, O'Connell, & Shore, 1987).

Characteristics of Early Communicative Acts

Bates, Camaioni, and Volterra (1975) suggested that there are three stages in the development of communication that correspond to Austin's (1962) perlocutionary, illocutionary, and locutionary functions. In the **perlocutionary stage,** from birth to about 10 months, children are not aware of the communicative impact of their behaviors. When they point at or reach for an object, they do not look at the adult for assistance, nor do they use objects to get the adult's attention. Their signals are perlocutions that create an effect but are not recognized by the speaker and the listener as a communicative act.

In the **illocutionary stage,** from 10 to 15 months, children develop prototypes of communicative acts. The protoimperative is the intentional use of an adult as a mediator to obtain a desired object. The protodeclarative is the intentional use of an object to gain an adult's attention. The signals children use to achieve these intentions are illocutions, conventional social acts (combined vocal and gestural performances) that are recognized by the speaker and the listener as communicative acts. The infant's intention and awareness, in relation to the adult, shift the nature of the infant's act from perlocution to illocution. These intentional communications do not necessarily involve speech. The cognitive prerequisite for intentional communication is Piaget's sensorimotor Substage 5. Particularly relevant to the development of these gestural performances is the development of means-end relations in which the infant acquires new action schemas to achieve specific goals.

The **locutionary stage** begins when the infant uses words to refer to environmental objects and actions. The appearance of words corresponds to Piaget's sensorimotor Substage 6, which involves the capacity for mental representation and the use of symbols. Thus, the referential use of words coincides with the nonlinguistic developments of Substage 6. The locutionary stage represents the final stage of functional communication development. It is the stage in which conventional word forms are used with or without gestures to achieve communicative intentions. Where, initially, these communicative functions had been accomplished by gestures or wordlike sounds and gestures, gradual transition from one stage to the next brings development of language's conventional forms—phonology, pragmatics, and syntax—into the infant's capability.

Finally, the infant must learn about the effect, planned or unplanned, of his or her utterance, by means of the listener's reaction. The speaker's intention is a speech act, a performative or illocutionary force associated with an utterance (i.e., a question, a command, or a request). The infant must learn how the listener responds to the speech act or illocutionary force in order to understand the relationship between the utterance and the changes it creates in his or her environment; social interaction provides the scaffolding for communication learning.

Social Functions of Language

Children learn in infancy that vocalizations and gestures can perform certain functions for them. Although these vocalizations and gestures do not conform to the sounds and structures of the adult model, they have meaning in the functions they serve for children. Children evidence functions of language long before they develop conventional form and structure. Halliday (1975) noted that "from the functional point of view, as soon as there are meaningful expressions there is language" (p. 6).

The first function Halliday identified in his son of 9 months was the interactional, or "me and you," function of language, as the infant used sounds and gestures to interact with others in the environment (Table 3-3). The personal function, also identified at 9 months, allowed the infant to express feelings such as interest, annoyance, and anger.

TABLE 3-3   Halliday's Phase I Function

I	Interactional	The "me and you" function
II	Personal	The "here I come" function
III	Instrumental	The "want" function
IV	Regulatory	The "do as I tell you" function
V	Heuristic	The "tell me why" function
VI	Imaginative	The "let's pretend" function

Adapted from Halliday (1975).

By 10 months, two more language functions could be identified, still without the infant using the forms and structures of conventional language. The infant's creative and idiosyncratic sounds, gestures, and movements, although lacking conventional form, conveyed meaning and communicative intention. These two functions were the instrumental function, whereby the infant obtained objects and actions, and the regulatory function, whereby the infant manipulated the behavior of others. The distinction between the instrumental and the regulatory functions concerns the individual providing the service for the infant. The regulatory function requires that a specific person provide the object and act for the infant; anyone can provide the object or action in the instrumental function. In the heuristic, or "tell me why,'" function, the infant used language to explore the environment. In the early stages of this function, children demand to be told the names of objects. In the imaginative, or "let's pretend," function, children use language to create their own environment, for sound play, and for storytelling.

Motherese Revisited

The focus on the social interactional process opened the door to new research into adult-infant interaction and its role in infant language development. The mother attempts to expand the infant's limited linguistic abilities by providing utterances that are several morphemes longer than the infant's. The expansion process also includes a **semantic contingency,** in which the adult repeats the semantic relations (the ideas) expressed by the infant. The adult also comments on what the infant is doing or saying. In a sense, the infant sets the topic of conversation, and the adult follows the infant's conversational interests and directions. The mother may attempt to provide the infant with additional information about ongoing events during shared interaction. Whenever she does, the mother must be aware of her infant's interests at that moment as well as the infant's knowledge of the environment. Fine-tuning involves the mother's decisions to regulate the linguistic, semantic, and cognitive complexity of her input. Research on the motherese hypothesis suggests that adult input can promote or hinder infant language learning. Several research investigations have analyzed the characteristics of maternal speech in terms of its facilitative qualities during adult-infant interaction (Masataka, 1992). Certain characteristics, such as expansions, have been shown to facilitate infant language development; other characteristics, such as maternal directiveness, may negatively affect vocabulary development.

Akhtar, Dunham, and Dunham (1991) found that vocabulary development at 13 months of age correlated positively with adult responsiveness to the infant's focus of attention. Their data provide positive support for the **attention regulation hypothesis,** which proposes that the way in which an adult regulates a infant's attention can facilitate language learning. Although directiveness was shown to have negative effects in other research, the authors noted that adult directiveness *in the context of joint attention and focus* may promote early lexical development in the infant. Mother-infant joint focus provides a framework for the adult to regulate the nature and quality of input relative to the objects and events that the infant is focused on. The mother's input is prescriptively determined by the infant's attention and interests. This maternal fine-tuning "fosters understanding of the words used in the utterance, but also enables the infant to respond appropriately" (Akhtar et al., 1991, p. 48). The infant's responsiveness will further reinforce the mother's perception that the infant "understands" her input. This adult-rich interpretation that the infant understands provides a scaffolding for the regulatory attunement of adult to infant during interaction.

As discussed in Chapter 2, motherese tends to be facilitative, redundant, and repetitive. Pegg, Werker, and McLeod (1992) describe an interesting phenomenon in child language learning—expansion or recasting. When a mother provides a child with linguistic communicative information, she can utilize the child's production as a reference. The mother could develop the child's utterance providing more sophisticated structural information on language form (i.e., Child: "Two cookie." Mother: "There are two cook*ies*."). The mother could also develop the child's utterance by extending his or her ideas about relevant contextual information (i.e., Child: "Cookie." Mother: "You want the cookie? Mommy made cookies. The cookie is hot."). Ferrar (1992) indicated that 2-year-old children seem to attend more closely to recast sentences. They are twice as likely to imitate the adult's more sophisticated productions after they hear their mothers recast their own utterances. The adult's recasting of the child's productions seems to facilitate the rate of linguistic development. The recasting process uses the child's language as the critical reference point for further learning.

Context and Interpretation

The context also plays a role in facilitating the mother-infant interaction. The context serves to disambiguate the infant's limited linguistic productions. In addition, adult input or correction (e.g., "That's a cow, not a dog") provides children with new semantic or criteria information that they can use to define and identify the object. Given the fact that adults and children have different semantic systems (words have different meanings for adults and children), how do they understand each other? The environment and context play an important supporting role in establishing, maintaining, and clarifying communication between adults and children. In developing word meanings, children rely on the perceptual and functional characteristics of an object. Relying on the context permits the adult to understand the infant's meaning of the word. Thus, in attempting to understand children's meanings, adults analyze what children say within the framework of what is happening. This dependence on context lasts until children develop the ability to ask questions (e.g., "What's that?") about their new experiences.

The adult's perception of the infant as an active participant is critical to their communication. An interpretive process occurs with the adult's assumption that the infant is an active communicator: The adult attempts to determine the infant's meaning by fitting together the limited pieces of context, gesture, vocalization, intonational pattern, and word in the infant's utterances. This interaction facilitates and stimulates further exchange between the adult and the infant. That a parent of a language disordered infant has an entirely different perception of the infant as a language learner and communicator will affect the quantity and the quality of their adult-infant interaction.

Social Play Routines

Consistencies in the child's environment (objects and related actions) and the routines established in social interactional exchanges further facilitate the language learning process.

Ratner and Bruner (1978), in analyzing early children's games and routines such as peek-a-boo, revealed a highly structured pattern of mother-infant exchanges containing rules that teach the infant about communication. Games such as X-marks-the-spot, one potato, pat-a-cake, and peek-a-boo incorporate these rules and may be considered to be of the same genre. Consider the game of X-marks-the-spot:

> *X marks the spot with a dot, dot, dot (tap on infant's chest),*
> *And a dash, dash, dash (draw lines across infant's chest),*
> *And a wiggle, wiggle, wiggle,*
> *And a tickle, tickle, tickle,*
> *And a hug*
> *And a squeeze*
> *And a cool mountain breeze (blow in infant's face).*

Four rules enhance the infant's language acquisition:

1. The use of a restricted semantic format, with the adult presenting a limited number of words and semantic relationships.
2. The close relationship between what is said and what is done. When Mother says, "hug," she hugs the infant; when she says, "squeeze," she squeezes the infant. The word and the action are paired.
3. The repetition of the same words and actions each time the game is performed. The infant learns the sequence of events and eventually predicts the next event or action.
4. A clearly defined role structure that provides for the development of speaker and listener roles.

The mother functions initially as an actor or speaker, and the infant functions as a recipient or listener. The mother does all of the actions to the infant as she produces the verbal sequences. Ratner and Bruner (1978) reported that, as the infant continues to play the game with his or her mother, the infant's behavior changes from passive recipient to active initiator. Between 5 and 9 months old, the infant learns to be a partner in a communicative exchange, having mastered rules that include how to take turns in the exchange process and how to combine gaze, gesture, and vocal behaviors to establish, maintain, and terminate interaction. In short, the infant has become a communicator, aware of the structures of turn-taking, role differentiation, and discourse components. The infant's behavior sharply contrasts with that of the autistic language disordered infant who is discussed later. Platt and Coggins (1990) noted that social games provide a structure and predict ability for interaction. From 9 to 15 months old, an infant's changes within the framework of the social game indicate development of conventionalized structures. As the infant progresses through this period, he or she moves from a context-dependent to a context independent state. According to the authors' research, most children acquire the criteria action sequences within social games early in the second year of life. In general, children demonstrated (a) increased responsiveness, (b) greater number of initiations, (c) increase in explorations of objects, and (d) greater motor control over nonverbal performances. In the present study, although infants were observed in an unfamiliar clinical situation, the results were similar to those observed in familiar settings. In addition, children used greater numbers of behaviors in games where their parents paired gestural and physical cues with their verbal requests. These results lend support to the notion that "children rely on parental cuing to produce situationally appropriate behaviors while their understanding of the game is being formed" (p. 323).

Learning to Mean

Integrating Language Components

As children develop, the forms they use to express the functions of language become more conventional in that they more closely approximate the linguistic structures of other language users. During infancy, babies use gaze and vocal behaviors to interact and communicate with adults and other children. By the end of the first 12 months, children are adding gestures and wordlike utterances to their repertoire. When they finally produce and combine words, children use their language's conventional forms and structures. Children's ability to interface form, content, and use—the three components of language—is critical to normal language development. This is an important issue to keep in mind as you consider the infant with a language disorder. Table 3-4 provides a description of Jeremy's language abilities at 28 months. Notice the variety of forms and functions and the way he uses the environment and Mommy to accomplish his communicative goals. Children with a language disorder may indicate developmental difficulties in one or all of the language components. As a result, the quality and the quantity of language acquired by the disordered infant will be significantly different from that acquired by a normal learner. Use Table 3-4 to consider the implications of a infant using only one communicative function—how it would affect the infant's communication process and how the communicative difficulty would affect the form and content areas of the infant's language.

Children's earliest intentions to communicate relate to themselves; they talk about themselves and their needs. As they experience the world, they come to learn about other agents, actions, and objects. They develop broad categories that reflect the relationships

TABLE 3-4   Interfacing Form, Content, and Use

Pragmatic Function	Form	Gesture/Action	Context
I Interactional	"Hi"	Gestures with hand and approaches adult	Greets Mommy as she enters room
II Personal	"No like bed"	Shakes head repeatedly	Jeremy placed in crib
III Instrumental	"Cookie"	Points to object	Points to cookie jar
IV Regulatory	"Open"	Gives object	Gives closed jar of bubbles to Mommy
V Heuristic	"Pig?"	Points to picture	Mommy and Jeremy looking at a book

they see among these agents, actions, and objects: possession ("Jeremy book"), negation ("No juice"), and recurrence ("More cookie"). At this point, children can talk about occurrences that do not concern their own needs (Jeremy: "Jonathan hat"). The next step is the gradual development of linguistic structure and form to match those of others in the cultural environment. From communicating intentions, children gradually progress to communicating ideas and, then, to learning the structural forms to express those ideas:

1. Pragmatic intentions (pointing to cookie)
2. Semantic ideas (pointing to and saying "Cookie")
3. Linguistic structures (pointing to and saying "I want that cookie")

The normal language learner is an integrated learner.

The Embedded Word

During the linguistic stage, children use words but are presyntactic insofar as they use only one word at a time. At this point, the content of the communicative act is expressed by a word form combined with other forms. The word forms are clarified and supported by gestures, intonational patterns, and context. The word forms are embedded within a broader communication schema. Table 3-5 describes the infant's single-word utterance, that is, form, in terms of its content and use. Early in the infant's language development (12 to 24 months of age), the single-word message represents a complex ability to integrate various aspects of language. The word ("Cookie") conveys a message ("More cookie") for a social purpose ("You give me"). Between 18 and 24 months some children show rapid vocabulary growth (Goldfield & Reznick, 1990).

Barrett, Harris, and Chasin (1991) found that during the second year of life children use two different types of internal representation: event representations and prototypes. The model of early lexical development attempts to explain the developmental changes that occur in the use of context-bound, nominal, and non-nominal words. A context-bound word is related to an event representation; the infant uses the word only in the context of the event. A nominal or non-nominal word is related to a prototype; the infant uses this type of word to designate objects, actions, or relations that resemble the prototype. Children acquiring early lexical forms can use both kinds of internal representation. The subsequent developments that occur in the use of early words stem from the further processing by the

TABLE 3-5　Single-Word Utterance in Terms of Content and Use

Pragmatic Functions	Form	Content
I Interactional	"Hi"	Greeting
II Personal	"No!"	Rejection
III Instrumental	"Cookie"	Recurrence
IV Regulatory	"Open"	Action
V Heuristic	"Pig?"	Object

infant of these two different kinds of initial underlying representations (processing that can ultimately yield both principal and contrastive features as further information about word meanings for the infant to add to his or her lexical entries for words) (Barrett et al., 1991, p. 22).

Veneziano, Sinclair, and Berthoud (1990) presented a possible explanation for how children progress from one-word to multiword utterances. The authors noted an interim phase that Dore, Franklin, Miller, and Ramer (1976) referred to as "something more than one word and something less than syntax" (p. 26). Children in this transitional stage use chaining and relating as aspects of coordination in language learning. Chaining is "the ability to utter more than one word in close temporal contiguity" (Veneziano et al., 1990, p. 646). Relating is "the ability to utter more than one word to express one single intention" (p. 646). At the one-word stage, the infant conveys sentential intent—the integration of linguistic word, gesture, vocalization, intonational contour, and event occurrences. At the syntax stage, the infant attempts to "hold in mind," and to talk about temporally, more than one aspect of the situation. The authors proposed that when the young infant in the one-word stage uses self-repetition as an expressive pattern or device, the infant is attempting to understand the linearity of language production. Repetition facilitates language learning because it stimulates further interaction during communicative exchange. In addition, repetition allows the infant to maintain interaction with the adult but reduces the demand on infant processing. The development of two-word utterances (in chaining and then relating) appears to signal "the beginnings of a simultaneous or temporally overlapping processing mechanism" (p. 648), whereas the infant's use of repetition indicates an overlapping between conceptualizing and verbalizing. The authors also suggested that repetition may help the infant "build" multiword productions by providing a level of conceptualization beyond the single-word form.

Reference and Referents: Theories

Which comes first, the concept or the word? As discussed in Chapter 2, this issue concerns the relationship between language and cognition. Gopnik and Meltzoff (1992) suggest that the vocabulary spurt occurs just after or at the same time as a new concept is acquired. Once children understand that relationships among objects, actions, and agents provide the basis for categories, reference labels follow. Waxman and Hall (1993) propose that the acquisition of a label influences a child's cognitive organizational schema. As children acquire labels, new categories are generated. New labels change the child's thinking about the world by altering his or her ability to reference a new relationship. The new label allows the child to reorganize old knowledge. This suggests that there is a bidirectionality in language learning. Old concepts—new labels and new concepts—old labels are dynamically reorganized to accommodate ongoing child language experiences. Several interesting theories attempt to explain how children learn about meaning and how they learn to mean. Olson (1970) suggested that meaning consists of concepts or knowledge about the world, noting that children must learn about signs (words and symbols that represent environmental objects and events), reference (meaning), and referents (objects and events). Olson stated that "everything has many names and every name has many things . . . something mediates between the word and the thing, this thing is called meaning" (p. 262). Children must learn to organize their world and experiences by developing categories that reflect how objects and events are related. In establishing these categories, children must determine a basis by which to group objects and events, for example, by identifying salient factors or common characteristics. The following child language theories have been proposed in the literature.

Semantic-Feature Hypothesis

Semantic development relates to the rules that govern the meaning or content of words or grammatical units. Meaning is an arbitrary system; the actual words or forms used by speakers represent ideas or concepts about objects and events, not the objects or events themselves. The **semantic-feature hypothesis** proposes that children establish meaning by combining features (characteristics) that are present and observable in the environment. As children continue to experience reality, their ideas and concepts about objects and events change.

Clark (1987, 1983) described how referential word meanings develop. A word that names an object or referent in the environment has referential meaning. The object consists of many features and characteristics. Children must determine which features are critical or criteria in establishing a category for this referent. During the first language learning year—12 to 24 months—children make errors in referent identification. These errors, often referred to as overextensions, result when the infant recognizes a limited set of semantic features. An **overextension** is a meaning that is broader than the adult's meaning. Children identify only the most salient characteristic(s) or feature(s) and determine that this is what the word refers to or means, a problem universally exemplified by children who call all men *Dada* or all four-legged creatures *doggie*. For *doggie* to mean four-leggedness to a infant indicates that the infant is using fewer semantic features than the adult in defining the word, that *doggie* means something different to the infant than it does to the adult.

Initially, children use one or two features in defining a word and gradually add semantic features until their meaning for the word matches the adult meaning. Overextensions are noticeable between 12 and 30 months of age; their occurrence relates to vocabulary development. When children note a new object, they assign a label based on their established semantic system. If an adult provides the infant with a word or label for the new object, such as doggie, the word may not indicate to the infant which characteristic to attend to: shape, color, size, texture, movement, sound, or four-leggedness. Let's consider an incident that occurred quite frequently with Jeremy:

Jeremy: (looking at animal pictures) Mommy, a big pig.

Mommy: No, that is an elephant. See, the elephant has a long trunk. (pointing to the elephant's trunk in the picture)

Jeremy: Like a long nose! (pointing to Mommy's nose)

Mommy: Yes, the elephant has a long nose. (squeezing Jeremy's nose)

Jeremy: Little pig no has long nose.

Mommy: That's right.

Jeremy: No worry little piggy, you get bigga, you get bigga nose like Mommy.

In the process of developing meaning, children formulate certain hypotheses about underlying concepts and apply their concepts to new examples. Throughout this application procedure, children acquire knowledge about objects that belong and do not belong within a particular conceptual category. Overextension in infant language has been more frequently cited than underextension. An **underextension** is a meaning that is more restricted than the adult's meaning (e.g., /bibi/ referring to one and only one pacifier) (Harris, 1992). Woodward and Markman (1991) suggest that children may approach the language learning process with some built-in biases or constraints. The child's hypothesis may be that a word refers to an object or an event but not both. Clark (1990) proposes another built-in constraint, referred to as the principle of contrast. This child hypothesis supposes that every label refers to a different referent (i.e., has a different meaning), so when the child is provided with a new word, it must refer to a different object.

Bloom (1973) suggested that the extension process follows a developmental pattern. Initially, the infant forms a concept loosely associated with the referent, resulting in unsystematic overextensions. This is followed by a period of underextension in which the infant applies the concept correctly but in a very restricted manner.

Functional-Core Hypothesis

Nelson (1974) proposed another theory that described the development of infant meaning. According to the **functional-core hypothesis,** children base their word concepts on active or functional characteristics of the object rather than basing them on perceptual features. Children's definitions of objects are based on what they do with the objects (e.g., something they wear or eat). Nelson suggested that perceptual features (as in the semantic feature hypothesis) represent static components that are too abstract for young children. This hypothesis complements Piaget's theory concerning the development of physical knowledge. The functional-core hypothesis suggests that children's early explorations of object functions through direct manipulation provide the basis for concept formation. Cognitive aspects of early infant development are related to semantic language development. During Piaget's sensorimotor period, children develop prototypical preconcepts based on the principle that objects that can be manipulated in the same way are similar.

Prototype Hypothesis

Bowerman (1978) has summarized problems related to both the semantic-feature and functional-core hypotheses. She suggested that each hypothesis is too limited to explain the infant's development of meaning. Her **prototype hypothesis** proposes that children construct meaning by developing a prototype against which all other exemplars are compared. The prototype represents an underlying concept of, for example, "chairness," and other objects are contrasted with this stored mental representation. The closer the exemplar is to the prototype concept, the greater the likelihood that it will be called by that name.

In summary, children learn word meanings gradually. Their initial use of a word is often at variance with the adult's use, reflecting their narrow frame of reference. Several hypotheses describe how children attempt to define a word within new contexts. The semantic-feature hypothesis proposes that all referents can be defined by a universal set of semantic features, or perceptual attributes. As the infant develops, word meaning changes as features are added and deleted. The functional-core hypothesis proposes that meaning is based upon knowledge of the object and the way it is used in the environment; as experience expands, meaning develops. The prototype hypothesis supports the development of a prototype against which objects are compared. No single theory adequately addresses the complexities related to the development of meaning in the young language learner, the levels of which include word, sentence, text, and sound conceptualizations.

Strategies

N. Nelson (1986) suggested that more than one theory may be needed to explain that children use different strategies to acquire semantic concepts and that they may use all of the strategies but at different times. K. Nelson (1974), however, asserted that children indicate a preference for one language strategy over another. Choosing a referential strategy, some children use language to talk about things. Other children use an expressive strategy to express social-interactional meanings. N. Nelson (1986) also noted that these strategy preferences result in a stylistic difference in children's language.

Several researchers have commented on the language processing styles used by children with and without language disorders. Peters (1983) described the use of a gestalt processing style in nonimpaired children. With gestalt processing, children reproduce whole chunks or segments of language without appreciating their components or understanding their organizational relationship. Underlying this approach is the hypothesis that gestalt patterns in language and interaction are important to cognitive and communicative development. Research has demonstrated that children use interactive rituals and routines to facilitate participation in social interaction. Gestalt processing provides children with the framework to develop more complex communication skills. The unanalyzed chunk permits the infant to use language by viewing the communication process through "one end of a telescope." The language chunk is applied as a whole to achieve a specific communicative function (Boskey & Nelson, 1980; Folger & Chapman, 1978). N. Nelson (1986) noted that children who "use expressive strategies tend to be relatively more holistic, in that they primarily use strategies for making unanalyzed sentence-like utterances that refer to social interactions" (p. 5). Children who use referential strategies tend to be more analytic in their language learning style. Peters (1977) described a continuum of nonimpaired language users who used varying proportions of both strategies.

Nonimpaired language learners use a variety of strategies to acquire their language structures and concepts. In contrast, many children with language disorders indicate a preference for one processing strategy over the others. Prizant (1982) noted that children with autism tend to learn language as unanalyzed chunks that relate to particular experiences. These language chunks are then applied to other, dissimilar situations. The result is language production that is either unrelated or only partially related to the immediate context.

The inability to use analytical strategies means that the infant with autism cannot formulate new utterances that relate to specific contextual meanings.

Semantic Bootstrapping Hypothesis

The **semantic bootstrapping** hypothesis proposes that the infant uses semantic notions as underpinnings for the development of grammatical structures. The names of persons, places, and things may be described as signaling nouns and the names of actions as indicating verbs. Because many nouns do not refer to objects just as many verbs do not refer to actions, semantic bootstrapping has a limited application. The theoretical premise, however, is that semantic bootstrapping provides an organizational framework for prototypical entries to be categorized. The nonprototypical items are contrasted against and compared with items that have semantic-syntactic correspondence.

Evidence for semantic bootstrapping may be found in the speech of young children or in the parental input provided to them (Rondal & Cession, 1990). That is, parents may present a semantic-syntactic correspondence by filtering out nonprototypical grammatical relations. The semantic bootstrapping hypothesis predicts that, as the infant's language becomes more sophisticated, input by parents and others no longer contains this close semantic-syntactic correspondence. When adults stop filtering their language, the infant is able to develop nonprototypical forms. The results of Rondal and Cession's (1990) research indicate that parents appear to filter nonbasic sentences out of the input to their young children. The semantic-syntactic correspondence posited by the semantic bootstrapping hypothesis appears to be an operational strategy.

> *The relevant semantic notions (action, physical object, agent, etc.) reliably corre-late in parental speech with the syntactic element canonically paired with it in the grammar of the language. This correspondence may indeed make the infant's con-struction of grammatical categories easier (p. 716).*

Semantic Development

The development of meaning has been described in terms of semantic characteristics, which are closely related to children's perceptual and functional notions of the environment. Children's experiences with agents (people), actions (doing and manipulating), and objects enable them to develop relationships between and among these basic components. The similarities across environmental contexts—people, their manipulation of objects, and the objects they manipulate—have been highlighted by many theorists in infant language development. Children's variegated experiences result in the development of semantic relationships that express how an object relates to an agent (possession) or how an object or action is noted again and again (recurrence). Because there is such consistency across environments, children of various cultures, although they speak different languages, develop the same semantic relationships. The result is that all children learn to express the same ideas about agents, actions, and objects. There are, of course, certain experiential differ-ences across cultures and environments that might explain why different children code different occurrences within their environment, therefore highlighting individual differences in learning.

Table 3-6 illustrates how different environments and experiences can affect the content of a infant's language. Notice that although Jeremy and his friend Jason (both 30 months of age) have different-looking lexical corpora, they are expressing the same semantic functions. Table 3-6 does not represent complete corpora for these children either in the semantic categories developed by 30 months of age or in the lexical entries in each category. It is important to note that these two children came from rather different environments. They were, therefore, coding different objects, actions, and agents while developing the same semantic relations or categories. Children talk about, or code, their immediate experiences; children talk about what they know. Whereas Jason's put-put is his father's private plane, put-put for Jeremy is a piggy bank: The boys are using the same form for different referents. In contrast, Jeremy's Nana and Jason's Grandmother are different forms used for the same referent. Although there may be many different lexical entries within each semantic category, the general categories that children learn are universal across languages and cultures. In addition, the ideas about the world that are expressed by these semantic relationships are universal. It is important to remember that what is happening in the immediate social context helps the adult determine what the infant means. By combining children's lexical productions with their vocal and gestural behaviors within a context, the adult formulates a gestalt about what they are talking about.

Form and Function: Interaction and Integration

Between 12 and 24 months of age, children express semantic relationships by integrating phonology with pragmatics, a complex process because the sounds of the language are being acquired at the same time that lexical items are being added to semantic categories. Note Jeremy's semantic categories and his phonological system at 14 months (Table 3-7). In this stage, the infant's phonological system begins to include wordlike vocalizations that add to the context of language and contribute to communication clarification. Without this

TABLE 3-6   Universality of Semantic Functions

Semantic Function	Jeremy's Words	Jason's Words
Object	Ball, shoe, binky, cup, boat, car, put-put (piggy bank)	Snoopy (cup), ball, yacht, Mercedes, put-put (plane; i.e., family's airplane)
Action	Up, throw, open, give	Fly, throw, swim, ski, give
Agent	Mommy, Nana, Poppy, Mimi	Miss Ann (governess), Henny (maid), Mother, Father, Grandmother
Recurrence	More	Again, another
Negation		
Rejection	No	No
Cessation	No	Stop

contextual support, the infant's speech productions are difficult to understand for an adult unfamiliar with the infant's phonological system. This difficulty is frequently evident when an adult interacts with a 14-month-old. Consider the following exchange with Jeremy:

Jeremy: /Da/ (Grandpa)

Grandpa: (no response)

Jeremy: /Da/ (louder and more insistent)

Grandpa: (no response)

Jeremy: /Da/ (plus a yank on Grandpa's arm)

Grandpa: Hmm? (looking at Jeremy)

Jeremy: /Gi bibi/ (pointing to Binky pacifier on a cluttered table)

Grandpa: What does he want?

Mommy: (answering from another room) He wants his pacifier.

Jeremy: /Bibi, bibi, bibi, bibi/ (jumping up and down)

Grandpa: Where is it?

Mommy: Dad, where is he pointing?

Grandpa: Oh, I see it.

Is there a first word? The one-word stage really represents a combination of lexical, vocal, and gestural forms that are used to communicate a message (Table 3-8). Given the gradual changes in form and function, there is not an isolated first word but, rather a progressively integrative process. As children acquire their language's phonemes, their speech production more closely approximates the phonological system and they become more in-

TABLE 3-7   Semantic and Lexical Systems at 14 Months

Semantic Function	Lexical Entries Described Phonologically	
Object	/ba/	ball
	/bibi/	Binky pacifier
	/da/	dog
	/g g/	cup
Action	/bi/	up
	/fo/	throw
Agent	/mama/	Mommy
	/papa/	Poppy
	/n~en~e/	Nana
Recurrence	/m l/	more

**TABLE 3-8   Progression toward Combining Lexical,
Vocal, and Gestural Forms**

Developmental Period	Descriptive Form	System
0–12	Vocal behavior	Suprasegmental
	Gestural behavior	Kinesis
	Pragmatic functions	Communication
12–24	Phonemes	Phonological
	Lexical items	Semantic
24–36	Lexical combinations	Syntactic

telligible. The phonological system interfaces with the semantic system, and the one-word stage highlights this interface.

As noted earlier, adults interpret children's messages as complex wholes; they rely on a combination of lexical, vocal, and gestural behavior and context to understand the message. Adults' sometimes liberal or rich interpretations of children's meanings usually involve the assumption that children mean more than they actually say. Children are viewed as active communicators who have something meaningful to contribute to the social exchange process. The following interaction between Grandpa and Jeremy demonstrates the multifaceted nature of communication even during this developmental stage:

Jeremy: /Da/ k< ... INVE/V>m/

Grandpa: Jeremy wants Grandpa to come?

Jeremy: /K<...INVE/V>m, k<.. INVE/V>m/ (Jeremy gesturing for Grandpa to approach)

Grandpa: Okay, what do you want?

Jeremy: /Mi du<PHO/TH>/ (pointing to refrigerator)

Grandpa: You want me to give you something? (Grandpa does not understand what /du<PHO/~H>/ is.) Show Grandpa what you want. (Grandpa opens the refrigerator.)

Jeremy: /Du<PHO/TH>/

Grandpa: Jeremy wants milk?

Jeremy: /NO du<PHO/TH> du<...PHO/TH> du<...PHO/TH>I (pointing)

Grandpa: Oh, you want some juice! (taking the container out and pouring juice into a cup) Here's the juice. (giving the cup to Jeremy)

Jeremy: /Du<PHO/TH>I (pointing to the cup that he now holds)

What seems to occur first is the development of a communication system. Children learn about the interactional exchange process and learn progressive forms to code the communicative exchange. During the first period (birth to 12 months of age), they learn to combine vocal and gestural forms to communicate a message. During the second stage (12 to 24 months of age), they begin to code some of their ideas and experiences by using the phonemes within the language. Finally, from age 24 to 36 months, they learn to combine lexical items (Table 3-8). This gradual progression indicates children's ability to develop the conventional structures of their language system. As they learn to approximate the sounds and words of their language more closely, they learn to express an idea by using a more conventional or sophisticated form.

Meaning and Sentence Structure

Nelson described the multiword process this way: "meaning is not the exclusive province of individual words" (1986, p. 7). Even at the single-word stage, children augment their limited linguistic productions with gestures to express broader semantic understanding of relational concepts. Children must learn how to express their ideas by learning to encode meaning syntactically in the form of phrases, sentences, and, finally, texts. Just as there are rules that govern the way in which words are constructed within a language, there are rules that determine how words are arranged in sentences; linguistic form serves semantic function. Learning to mean has a primacy in language; the child identifies a linguistic structure or form that expresses his or her idea or meaning.

Word order is one strategy used in some languages such as English. By following these word-order rules or arrangement rules for words, children can go beyond the meaning expressed by the individual words "to express the relationships holding between them" (deVilliers & deVilliers, 1979). Bloom and Lahey (1978) have described these early combinations as semantic-syntactic. They are semantic in that their bases for combination are the meaning relations; they are syntactic in that children make use of the word-order rules in generating them.

Word order is a powerful strategy that controls language production and comprehension for several years. Not until the infant is a sophisticated language user can he or she manipulate the form or structure of a complex sentence in order to derive its meaning. (Consider the development of passive sentences in production and comprehension.) After children begin to express the basic semantic-syntactic relations, they learn to express the relations between the events that contain those basic relations. Children begin to connect two occurrences or events by using *and, and then, when,* and *because* by 33 months of age.

Schemata and Narratives

Schemata are representations of the infant's experiences and knowledge as they are stored in memory (Kintsch, 1974). The infant's daily experiences are organized around certain events that are "action-sequenced." Common events become organized scripts over time. These scripts come to have anticipated outcomes and recognizable sequences that assist the language learner in making predictions and inferences about the sequence of events.

As children begin to understand the organization of events and learn to conceptualize the event as well as its sequence, they start to code elements linguistically within the experience or schema. Yoshinaga-Itano and Downey (1986) noted that children develop narratives or stories when they are able to embed one schema within another. Duchan (1986) noted that schema descriptions "require knowledge of how common events ordinarily take place, the ability to use language to convey the essentials of the event schema, and linguistic strategies for taking into account the speaker's and listener's perspectives on the event" (p. 32).

The narrative process is probably facilitated through natural conversational exchange. During conversational interaction with an adult, a infant describes events, their sequence, and their outcomes. The adult asks the infant questions about the event sequence, which further expands the infant's perception of the linguistic-descriptive relationship. Thus, during conversational exchange the infant learns to function as both a speaker and a listener, roles that require critical responsibilities if the dyadic, interactional exchange is going to continue. In addition to learning about speaker/listener roles, the infant must also learn how to remain on topic by providing information that is relevant to both the listener and the topic. The infant must learn to adjust his or her behavior and message to individual communication partners. The give-and-take of information during conversational interaction provides the infant with important language learning skills. Foster (1985) has noted that the infant's ability to handle topics of conversation involves an interaction of linguistic, cognitive, and social factors.

As children acquire new knowledge, schemata are restructured and reorganized to incorporate additional elements. Children acquire a great deal of knowledge by observing as well as interacting with the environment. Unimpaired children acquire a vast amount of information incidentally from a variety of situations. The infant's knowledge base affects the development and organization of schemata, which in turn affect the quantity and the quality of the narrative. As Yoshinaga-Itano & Downey (1986) noted, "Knowledge is used to understand narratives, but individuals may use knowledge gained through narratives to help organize their world" (p. 49). The development of narrative provides the basis for further language learning and interaction with other communicators.

Theory of Mind

Production and comprehension skills represent primary abilities in children. Metalinguistic skills represent a higher conceptual understanding of production and comprehension skills with which the infant can stand back and "talk about talking." This indicates an awareness of the language rules and how they can be applied.

Mommy: Mommy taked the car to the mechanic.

Jonathan: Taked? You mean took. Mommy took the car to the mechanic. Mommy, is this a game?

The infant is aware of language structures and can make judgments about the integrity of the production. Just as the infant can make judgments about the acceptability of utterances because of his or her increasing ability, he or she also can revise and repair structural aspects at the sound, word, and sentence levels. Metalinguistic abilities usually develop after the infant has mastered a linguistic structure. After the infant both comprehends and produces the form integratively within his or her language system, he or she can stand back and talk about the form, judge its acceptability, and, finally, revise its use. Metalinguistics involves the ability of the infant to reflect upon his or her knowledge of language. Hakes

(1982) suggested that there is a strong relationship between cognitive and metalinguistic abilities. Metalinguistic abilities are similar to metapragmatic, metacomprehension, and metacognition in terms of the knowledge of process.

Phonological Processes

In early theories of sound acquisition, emphasis centered on the infant's learning of sounds and features. Another theory focuses on rules for learning words—phonological processes. Strategies or rules for learning words were originally described by Francescato (1968). Building on this early work, other researchers elaborated phonological rules or processes that account for the sound sequences that children produce in their first words (Ingram, 1974; Klein, 1978; Smith, 1973). Children learn the sounds of a language not as separate entities, but in relation to one another within the framework of the word. Phonological processes have been identified as regularities in the ways in which children change the target production of syllables in their attempts to produce words.

Menn (1976) suggested that phonological development involves the infant's active discovery of patterns in linguistic input. Children use these patterns to attempt new words and to analyze adult input for new structures. Phonological development is the interaction between the infant's inventory of stored perceptual and productive strategies with the ongoing incidental input. This interactionist-discovery theory assumes that children invent a set of phonological rules that reduce the linguistic input to a manageable and predictable level. Fey and Gandour (1982) hypothesized that the form of the rules used by children reflects the specific developmental relationship between a developing phonological system and articulatory control. Thus, children's phonological knowledge must be viewed in terms of phonetic output and production limitations. Correct phonological output and production finally occur when children possess both the necessary control over the articulatory mechanism and the perceptual awareness that a phonological contrast must be coded.

Since the need to study phonology from a cognitive perspective became apparent in the 1980s, more recent research shifted to this arena (Elbert, 1983). (The focus of many theoretical approaches had been on motor skill, motor planning, and articulatory constraints during development). The work of Kent and Bauer (1985) and Elbers and Ton (1985) was discussed in the section on prelinguistic sound production. This research focuses on the infant's development of a conceptual or cognitive understanding of the phonological structure of his language. The infant formulates hypotheses about categories, recognizes patterns, and develops rules based on those patterns. As the infant acquires more knowledge of his or her phonological system, he or she reformulates hypotheses. Interestingly enough, just as children are beginning to indicate preferred styles of learning in cognitive, pragmatic, and semantic areas, individual differences in their phonological development are appearing (Ferguson & Macken, 1980). Individual differences have been explained as a preference for a specific articulatory pattern, a particular class of sounds, or a particular syllable structure (Ingram, 1979). An understanding of individual styles of phonological acquisition would explain how each infant uniquely conceptualizes his or her language's phonological system into working hypotheses.

Many children indicate methodological ways of replacing sounds in adult words. As mentioned, these infant changes and regularities are called **phonological processes:** The changes or phonological processes may be (1) substitution, in which segments are modified, often depending on their position in a word; (2) assimilation, in which adjacent phonemes or features become more alike; or (3) syllable structure changes, in which the number of syllables or the consonant-vowel patterns of syllables is systematically changed (Lund & Duchan, 1988, p. 108). Children appear to develop sound sequences, not just sounds. An infant's regularities may be described in terms of **canonical forms,** abstract patterns that represent sets of words. The canonical form is marked by specific differentiating features that allow for contrastive analysis and demarcation (Menn, 1983). Each word that conforms to that abstract pattern is described as an instance of that canonical form. These abstract patterns suggest that children generate individual word forms based upon a broader conceptual sound sequence pattern. An understanding of canonical forms provides insight into the infant's rules and regularities. These rules indicate how the individual infant adjusts the adult word forms to fit his or her conceptual pattern.

In summary, phonological development is rule-governed and consistent. All children learning a language acquire the phonemes of the language in an ordered and predictable sequence. Phonemes are not acquired until the semantic component is operative. Thus, the sounds produced during the babbling period are not phonemes and are not indicative of phonological progression, although they serve a communicative function, a function that remains controversial. The relationship between the sounds produced during the babbling period and those produced during the phonological acquisition period is not clear. Phonological acquisition is accomplished over several years; therefore, substitutions appear as part of the normal acquisition process. Finally, recent theories suggest that phonological processes underlie the development of phonemes. An understanding of the normal phonological process is necessary if phonological impairments are to be identified.

How Do Contextual Factors Influence Child Language Development?

The Working Mother

For a whole variety of reasons, more mothers are working today than ever before. The mother's role has changed dramatically from being a primary homemaker to a wonder woman, having a job in the house and a job in the office. The mother's employment has also changed her relationship with her primary partner, her husband. The role of father thus has shifted, with many more men assuming responsibilities in the home and for child care. Girls and boys perceive their parents differently within the framework of the family because the roles of mother and father involve more interchangeable responsibilities. More egalitarian role concepts have shifted family relationships. Important within the framework of this process is the mother's own reasons for working and her self-esteem. How the mother perceives herself as an independent individual influences her interactions with her adult partner and her young children. Bronfenbrenner (1989) has noted that working mothers provide more positive messages to their young daughters than do nonworking mothers. As a result, it appears that working mothers stimulate positive developmental outcomes for young girls who are themselves developing their own personal identities.

The mother's employment creates significant changes in daily activities, household routes, and complicated interactional patterns. In a household with two working parents, who comes home when the baby is sick? Who gets home first to relieve the babysitter? Who makes dinner? What impact does the mother's job have on the family? What relationship changes occur when the mother is not available during the day? How are chores and responsibilities reassigned to other family members? How does the mother's employment affect her relationship with the father? Perhaps the most important issue is how the mother feels about herself and what impact her employment has on members of the family. Has the mother chosen to work? The mother's changing role creates a change in traditional expectations, rules, and responsibilities within the family. The change in the responsibilities at home impacts on the nature of the interaction between the adults. When the stresses of the environment and the culture force parents to make changes in their roles, child and relationship conflicts often arise. Clearly, parents provide a role model for their young children. The working mother provides a distinctive role model in today's changing family. Mothers have entered the labor force at an ever-increasing rate over the past two decades and the resulting social problem in many communities throughout the United States involves the high demand for day care. How the mother feels about herself has a direct impact on the quality of her child rearing and her responsibilities with all of the other members of the family. How does the mother-child relationship change when the mother's role changes within the family? How do changes in family interaction patterns affect child language development?

Changing Family Dynamics

Much of the research investigating the role of parents in education has related to issues concerning children with developmental disabilities. Parents of nondisabled children are often faced with many of the same problems, concerns, and issues. Parents of disabled and nondisabled children need to realize that they share many issues in education and child care. Quality child care for working parents is a critical issue for families across the United States. Parents who work need to feel comfortable about the fact that their infants and preschoolers will be placed in a stimulating, safe environment. Researchers investigated the elements of child care that are associated with quality programs. These factors include stimulating early childhood environments that have small group instruction, low child-to-staff ratios, low staff turnover, age-appropriate materials, and contextual settings that are safe and regulated by governmental agencies. Quality child care has been identified as critical to the child's linguistic, physical, cognitive, emotional, and social development (Andersson, 1992). Educators argue that child care must refocus its mission on early childhood education. Many of the social problems that we face with school-age disabled children can be addressed by means of early stimulation and remediation. Research has shown over the past several decades that for the child with special needs, the longer it takes to intervene, the more serious the developmental deficits and the more expensive the remediation. Quality child care provides a mechanism for early intervention, socialization, stimulation, and support for working parents and families. Clearly, the infant who is placed in an early stimulation program is provided with an early childhood opportunity that facilitates development (Scarr & Eisenberg, 1993). Early stimulation theory has its roots in the recognition of the critical period for the child's development of normal language. (Hurford,

1991). It is incumbent upon programs and local government to ensure that early childhood programs are centers of stimulation and learning since they represent a critical support service for working families. Many communities have worked diligently to change social welfare programs and provide job training as well as parent education. Often the only way in which families can receive such training support and networking is if infants and preschoolers are provided with child care. Parents cannot look for jobs or be involved with educational programming if children are not appropriately taken care of. There is a crying need for the development of early child care programs in most communities throughout the United States (Cherlin, 1992).

Some of the literature appears to indicate that early childhood developmental experiences within day care programs enhance children's intellectual functioning. Studies also show that children who have been in day-care programs may display more aggressive behaviors with peers, and are less compliant with teachers and parents as they develop (Belsky & Eggebeen, 1991). Other studies provide support for the fact that children who have had early childhood experiences in various kinds of preschool programs are more social interpersonally with peers as they develop (Clarke-Stewart, 1992). The conflicting results may be a function of differences in methodological approaches as well as multicultural differences across the populations investigated. The reality, however, is that the working requirements of single parents and working mothers have created a dramatic demand for extended-day programming and day-care services for infants and preschoolers. Perhaps further investigations need to be done; future studies need to focus on qualitative issues in child care and educational instruction (Field, 1991). Early child-care models need to be developed and studied in terms of their program components. As more mothers enter the work force and spend more time meeting the responsibilities outside of the home, the dynamics within the family begin to change. How do day-care and early stimulation programs change family interaction patterns? How do these programs affect child language development? How do the resulting changes in family interaction patterns affect child language development?

Family Support System: Inclusive Parent Programming

A parent education process should begin with parents of an infant—a new family member. Historically, parent education has only been a consideration for families who have a disabled child. Parents of disabled and nondisabled children share many of the same problems and concerns and should be involved with community-based social programs that provide *all* parents with support services (Tiegerman-Farber, 1995a). It is in the best interest of communities and society in general to support the goals of families. The research literature on parents of disabled children provides a wealth of information on the importance of parent empowerment and parent education. Being a parent involves a great deal of on-the-job training. Parents often comment to their children, "You did not come with an instruction manual." Parents need to understand that there is a partnership, a long-term collaboration between themselves and their children. Preschool programs should provide educational support to *all* parents on child development issues as well as parent networking. The time invested in young families and parents who are beginning the long child-rearing passages process is an investment that pays off for society in the long run.

Parents need to learn to assert their role in the educational system. They need to become partners in the educational process (Wiese, 1992). In order to do this, however, parents need to receive training on parenting skills, children, and family problems. Perhaps the greatest gift that educators can provide to parents is in helping them to define their roles as facilitators and teachers of their children. Parents do not come equipped with the knowledge of effective parenting skills. All parents learn through the trials and tribulations of on-the-job training. Parents of disabled children often have the benefit of early childhood programs. Parents of nondisabled children are left adrift in our society until their children reach school-age level; even then most schools throughout the United States do not provide parent education programs. Early childhood intervention programs should expand their services to include all parents within a local community. This would provide educational training for parents of disabled children and sensitize other parents to the early warning signs of possible delay and disorder. When parents are educated and empowered, they become part of the educational system (Tiegerman-Farber, 1995a). The educated parent is better equipped to manage ongoing issues in child care. A parent with high self-esteem who has the tools to understand developmental change in his or her child and his or her family is also much better equipped to manage family problems. Early childhood education provides a mechanism to support children and families; schools need to make a commitment to early childhood development and child-care services. How does parent training change family interaction patterns? How do changes in family interaction patterns affect child language development?

Parental Concerns

Parents have their own perceptions and expectations of their children. The parental process suggests a life cycle of change in perceptions and expectations as infants acquire language and begin to assert themselves as individual communicators. The challenges today for young families given the complexities within our social environment suggest that parents must learn to capitalize on looking within the framework of the family itself for support. One instance of challenge and stress represents the realization that the infant who is planned and long awaited has a developmental disability. Parents proceed through a grieving process in which they are angry, depressed, and overwhelmed by this realization (Tiegerman-Farber, 1995b). Parents of disabled children often ask, "Why me?" All of the parental expectations related to the future—the child graduating from college, getting married, and having children—appear to be shattered in the instant of diagnosis.

Today there are many more immigrant families establishing homes within urban environments than ever before (Edwards, 1990). It is difficult enough raising "normal children." Raising a developmentally disabled child or a child in an environment in which English is not the primary language is even more stressful. Several researchers have indicated that the complexities of today's urban environment have created children who are more behaviorally and socially at risk for exhibiting aggressive and violent behavior (Barona & Garcia, 1990). When parents perceive that children must behave in specific ways and satisfy unresolved adult expectations, parents and children often have behavioral conflicts. The uncertainty of our economic environment creates profound emotional difficulties for the parent and the entire family. The economically and/or emotionally frustrated, angry, and depressed parent often cannot nurture or meet the needs of the young developing child (Healy, Keesee, & Smith, 1989). The developmental history and individual characteristics of each parent creates a highly individualized interactive family system. No two families are the same because parents and children contribute their own individual behaviors. Just as the infant contributes to the interactional dynamics within the family, the child is in turn affected by the behavior of parents and siblings. In attempting to understand the individual learning needs of the infant, it is important to focus on family and cultural variables. How do parental attitudes and concerns affect family interaction patterns? How do changes in family interaction patterns affect child language development?

Changing Family Structure

The structure of the family—the traditional family—has changed. Hofferth (1985) has indicated that only 30 percent of the children in the United States will be living with two natural parents by the time they turn age 17; this figure drops to 6 percent for black children. What is particularly interesting to researchers involves the different family structures that have been created as a function of today's changing society and the high rate of divorce: live-in relationships, melded families, and alternative families. The majority of children in the United States today experience several different family systems (Hunter & Ensminger, 1992).

In a recent landmark case in New York State, the highest court ruled in favor of adoptions by unmarried couples, including nontraditional couples (Slackman, 1995). The controversial decision makes New York State the third state whose highest court recognized such adoptions. The court expressed the fact that the ruling recognized the reality of New York families and American families in general. The court indicated that the law had to be applied in a way in which it best served the interest of children who have married as well as unmarried parents.

Structural changes within the family such as divorce and/or remarriage create a great deal of stress. Young children often react negatively by acting more aggressively. There appears to be some disagreement about the long-term negative effects of divorce as a function of the age of the child. Some researchers suggest differences as to whether the divorce occurs in a child under or over the age of five. The disruption in the family is compounded by emotional difficulties, changes in lifestyle, economic problems, changes in domicile, and moving from one community to another. Children respond to divorce as a loss of one member of the family. The ongoing conflict between parents who are in the process of divorce often creates a fear and depression in children because of the uncertainty, lack of control, and heightened helplessness. Divorce creates significant changes in the microsystem; the resulting changes in roles, rules, and responsibilities alter the relationships among all of the family members. The loss must be experienced also in terms of a grieving process, and here again parental attitudes affect the parent-child communication process. How do these changes in family interaction patterns influence child language development?

Considering Children with Disabilities

In the last chapter, Alyssa was brought by her mother to a community preschool program for diagnostic evaluation. Since Alyssa was an infant at the time of assessment, the multidisciplinary team generated an IFSP (individual family service plan-program). During the course of the family assessment, Alyssa's mother indicated to the social worker that she and her husband were in the middle of a divorce. The mother indicated that the ongoing stress within the family finally reached a breaking point when it was clear that Alyssa had severe developmental disabilities. Part of the recommendation for service provision involved family counseling for the parents. Alyssa's mother indicated that she was not sure if the father would attend these conjoint sessions. The mother's primary concern was to identify a special education program for Alyssa that provided an opportunity for full-day child care. Alyssa's mother expressed the fact that given the divorce situation within her family she was going to be involved in a welfare training program for single mothers. Alyssa's mother was also deeply concerned about the quality of care that Alyssa would be receiving in a child-care program. She expressed the fact that the special education program was clearly equipped to deal with Alyssa's developmental disabilities. Past experience, however, had left a rather negative impression in this parent's mind that day care was nothing more than babysitting. The complex needs of this child required a child-care program that had a professional staff of educators who could understand the educational needs of this developmentally disabled infant in an integrated setting. Although there was a range of special education programs available for Alyssa, the identification of an appropriate child-care program became an ongoing and problematic issue. Alyssa had to be transported from one end of the community to another in order for her to receive the appropriate services and programs.

The history of PL94-142 and PL99-457 has created a range of special education programs nationally. Today's emphasis on inclusive educational programs provides an extraordinary opportunity for special education preschools to expand programming to include nondisabled children. The inclusion of nondisabled infants and preschoolers within traditional special education preschools would allow communities to (1) provide inclusive opportunities for handicapped infants and preschool children, (2) address the mandate of Least Restrictive Environment, and (3) provide full-day child care opportunities for working families.

Summary

In this chapter we have discussed the development of language by means of a contextualist paradigm. Since language is a social learning process and represents a social symbolic system, the child acquires language within the framework of a microsystem. In this chapter we have also discussed many of the contextual factors that influence family interactional patterns. In order to understand how children develop language, it is important to take into consideration the interacting systems that network to affect the child's learning environment. Child language learning represents a dynamic, embedded, and contexualized process; the child embedded within the family and the family embedded within a larger social environment—community and culture.

Study Questions

1. Explain the viewpoint that children are communicative long before they are linguistic.
2. Describe the relationship between intentionality and reference. How do children express their intentions during the prelinguistic period? How does this change during the linguistic period?

3. Explain how children's meanings are closely related to their experiences with objects and events. How do their meanings change over time?
4. What is the difference between pragmatic and semantic functions?
5. Describe how form and function interface during the first 24 months.
6. Describe child language within the context of the family as a microsystem.
7. How does the contextualist paradigm provide a universal explanation for language development as a dynamic, embedded, and contextualized process?
8. How do the exo- and macrosystems affect the interactional patterns within the family?
9. How do changes in family interactional patterns affect child language development?

References

Akhtar, N., Dunham, F., & Dunham, P. (1991). Directive interactions and early vocabulary development: The role of joint attentional focus. *Journal of Child Language, 18,* 41–49.

Andersson, B. (1992). Effects of day-care on cognitive and socioemotional competence of thirteen-year-old Swedish school children. *Child Development, 63,* 20–36.

Austin, J. (1962). *How to do things with words.* London: Oxford University Press.

Barona, A., & Garcia, E. (Eds.) (1990). *Children at risk: Poverty, minority status, and other issues in educational equity.* Washington, DC: National Association of School Psychologists.

Barrett, M., Harris, M., & Chasin, J. (1991). Early lexical development and maternal speech: A comparison of children's initial and subsequent uses of words. *Journal of Child Language, 18,* 21–40.

Bates, E. (1976). Pragmatics and sociolinguistics in child language. In E. M. Morehead & A. E. Morehead (Eds.), *Normal and deficient child language.* Baltimore: University Park Press.

Bates, E. (1993). Commentary: Comprehension and production in early language development. *Monographs of the Society for Research in Child Development, 58* (3–4, Serial No. 233), 222–242.

Bates, E., Benigni, Bretherton, I., Camaioni, L., & Volterra, V. (1977). From gesture to the first word: On cognitive and social prerequisites. In M. Lewis & L. Rosenblum (Eds.), *Interaction, conversation, and the development of language* (pp. 247–307). New York: Wiley.

Bates, E., Benigni, L., Bretherton, I., Camaioni, L., & Volterra, V. (1979). *The emergence of symbols: Cognition and communication in infancy.* New York: Academic Press.

Bates, E., Camaioni, L., & Volterra, V. (1975). The acquisition of performatives prior to speech. *Merrill-Palmer Quarterly, 21,* 205–226.

Bates, E., O'Connell, B., & Shore, C. (1987). Language and communication in infancy. In J. D. Osofsky (Ed.) *Handbook of infant development* (2nd ed.; p. 149–203). New York: Wiley-Interscience.

Bee, H. (1995). *The Developing Child.* New York: HarperCollins College Publishers.

Belsky, J., & Eggebeen, D. (1991). Early and extensive maternal employment and young children's socioemotional development: Children of the National Longitudinal Survey of Youth. *Journal of Marriage and the Family, 53,* 1083–1110.

Bloom, L. (1973). *One word at a time.* The Hague: Mouton

Bloom, L., & Lahey, M. (1978). *Language development and language disorders.* New York: Wiley.

Boskey, M., & Nelson, K. (1980, October). Answering unanswerable questions: The role of imitation. Paper presented at the Fifth Annual Boston University Conference on Language Development, Boston.

Bowerman, M. (1978). The acquisition of word meaning: An investigation in some current conflicts. In N. Waterson & C. Snow (Eds.), *The development of communication.* New York: Wiley.

Bronfenbrenner, U. (1989). Ecological systems theory. *Annals of Child Development, 6,* 187–249.

Bruner, J. (1974). From communication to language—A psychological perspective. *Cognitive, 3,* 255–287.

Cherlin, A. (1992). Infant care and full-time employment. In A. Booth (Ed.), *Child care in the 1990s:*

Trends and consequences (pp. 209–214). Hillsdale, NJ: Erlbaum.

Clark, E. V. (1983). Meanings and concepts. In J. H. Flavell & E. M. Markman (Eds.), *Handbook of child psychology.* Vol. 3: *Cognitive development* (pp. 787–840). New York: Wiley.

Clark, E. V. (1987). The principle of contrast: A constraint on language acquisition. In B. MacWhinney (Ed.), *Mechanisms of language acquisition* (pp. 1–34). Hillsdale, NJ: Erlbaum.

Clark, E. V. (1990). On the pragmatics of contrast. *Journal of Child Language, 41,* 417–431.

Clarke-Stewart, A. (1992). Consequences of child care for children's development. In A. Booth (Ed.), *Child care in the 1990s: Trends and consequences* (pp. 63–82). Hillsdale, NJ: Erlbaum.

de Boysson-Bardies, B., Sagart, L., & Durand, C. (1984). Discernible differences in the babbling of infants according to target language. *Journal of Child Language, 11,* 1–17.

deVilliers, J., & deVilliers, P. (1979). *Early language.* Cambridge, MA: Harvard University Press.

deVilliers, P. A., & deVilliers, J. G. (1992). Language development. In M. H. Bornstein & M. E. Lamb (Eds.), *Developmental psychology: An advanced textbook* (3rd ed.; pp. 337–418). Hillsdale, NJ: Erlbaum.

Dore, J., Franklin, M., Miller, R., & Ramer, A. (1976). Transitional phenomena in early language acquisition. *Journal of Child Language, 3,* 13–28.

Duchan, J. (1986). Learning to describe events. *Topics in Language Disorders, 6,* 27–36.

Dunn, J. (1993). *Young children's close relationships.* Newbury Park, CA: Sage.

Edwards, P. (1990). Strategies and techniques for establishing home-school partnerships with minority parents. In A. Barona & E. Garcia (Eds.), *Children at risk: Poverty, minority status, and other issues in educational equity.* Washington, DC: National Association of School Psychologists.

Eimas, P., Siqueland, E., Jusczyk, P., & Vigorito, J. (1971). Speech perception in infants. *Science, 171,* 303–306.

Elbers, L. (1982). Operating principles in repetitive babbling: A cognitive continuity approach. *Cognition, 12,* 45–63.

Elbers, L., & Ton, F. (1985). Playpen monologues: The interplay of words and babbles in the first words period. *Journal of Child Language, 12,* 551–565.

Elbert, M. (1983). A case study of phonological acquisition. *Topics in Language Disorders, 3,* 1–10.

Ferguson, C., & Macken, M. (1980). Phonological development in children's play and cognition. In K. E. Nelson (Ed.), *Children's language,* Vol. 4. New York: Gardner Press.

Ferrar, M. J. (1992). Negative evidence and grammatical morpheme and acquisition. *Developmental Psychology, 28,* 90–98.

Fey, M., & Gandour, J. (1982). Rule discovery in phonological acquisition. *Journal of Child Language, 9,* 71–82.

Field, T. M. (1991). Quality infant day-care and grade school behavior and performance. *Child Development, 62,* 863–870.

Flax, J., Lahey, M., Harris, K., & Boothroyd, A. (1991). Relations between prosodic variables and communicative functions. *Journal of Child Language, 18,* 3–19.

Folger, J., & Chapman, R. (1978). A pragmatic analysis of spontaneous imitations. *Journal of Child Language, 5,* 25–38.

Foster, S. (1985). The development of discourse topic skills by infants and young children. *Topics in Language Disorders, 5,* 31–45.

Francescato, G. (1968). On the role of the word in first language acquisition. *Lingua, 21,* 144–153.

Goldfield, B. A., & Reznick, J. S. (1990). Early lexical acquisition: Rate, content, and the vocabulary spurt. *Journal of Child Language, 17,* 171–183.

Gopnik, A., and Meltzoff, A. N. (1992). Categorization and naming: Basic-level sorting in eighteen-month-olds and its relation to language. *Child Development, 63,* 1091–1103.

Greenfield, P., & Smith, J. (1976). *The structure of communication in early language development.* New York: Academic Press.

Hakes, D. (1982). The development of metalinguistic abilities: What develops? In S. Kuczaj (Ed.), *Language, cognition, and culture.* Hillsdale, NJ: Lawrence Erlbaum Associates.

Halliday, M. A. K. (1975). *Learning how to mean: Explorations in the development of language.* London: Edward Arnold.

Harris, M. (1992). *Language experience and early language development: From input to uptake.* Hove, England: Erlbaum.

Healy, A., Keesee, P., & Smith, B. (1989). *Early services for children with special needs: Transactions for family support.* Iowa City: University Hospital School.

Hofferth, S. L. (1985). Updating children's life course. *Journal of Marriage and the Family,* 47, 93–115.

Hunter, A. G., & Ensminger, M. E. (1992). Diversity and fluidity in children's living arrangements: Family transitions in an urban Afro-American community. *Journal of Marriage and the Family,* 54, 418–426.

Hurford, J. R. (1991). *The evolution of the critical period for language acquisition cognition,* Vol. 40, 159–201.

Ingram, D. (1974). Phonological rules in young children. *Journal of Child Language,* 1, 97–106.

Ingram, D. (1979). Phonological patterns in the speech of young children. In P. Fletcher & M. Garman (Eds.), *Language acquisition.* Cambridge: Cambridge University Press.

Jakobson, R., & Halle, M. (1956). *Fundamentals of language.* The Hague: Mouton.

Kent, R. & Bauer, H. (1985). Vocalizations of one-year-olds. *Journal of Child Language,* 12, 491–526.

Kintsch, W. (1974). *The representation of meaning in memory.* Hillsdale, NJ: Lawrence Erlbaum Associates.

Kiparsky, P., & Menn, L. (1977). On the acquisition of phonology. In J. Macnamara (Ed.), *Language learning and thought.* New York: Academic Press.

Klein, H. (1978). The relationship between perceptual strategies and productive strategies in learning the phonology of early lexical items. Doctoral dissertation, Columbia University, New York.

Lund, N., & Duchan, J. (1988). *Assessing children's language in naturalistic contexts.* Englewood Cliffs, NJ: Prentice Hall.

Marcos, H. (1987). Communicative function of pitch range and pitch direction in infants. *Journal of Child Language,* 14, 255–268.

Masataka, N. (1992). Motherese in a signed language. *Infant Behavior and Development,* 15, 453–460.

Menn, L. (1976). Evidence for an interactionist-discovery theory of child phonology. *Papers and Reports on Child Language Development,* 12, 169–177.

Menn, L. (1983). Development of articulatory phonetic and phonological capabilities. In B. Butterworth (Ed.), *Language production: Vol. 2.* London: Academic Press.

Nelson, K. (1974). Concept, word and sentence: Interrelations in acquisition and development. *Psychological Review,* 81, 267–285.

Nelson, N. (1986). What is meant by meaning (and how can it be taught)? *Topics in Language Disorders,* 6, 1–15.

Olson, D. (1970). Language and thought: Aspects of a cognitive theory of semantics. *Psychological Review,* 77, 257–273.

Pegg, J. E., Werker, J. F., & McLeod, P. J. (1992). Preference for infant-directed over adult-directed speech: Evidence from 7-week-old infants. *Infant Behavior and Development,* 15, 325–345.

Peters, A. (1977). Language learning strategies: Does the whole equal the sum of the parts? *Language,* 53, 560–573.

Peters, A. (1983). *The units of language acquisition.* Cambridge, MA: Cambridge University Press.

Platt, J., & Coggins, T. (1990). Comprehension of social-action games in prelinguistic children. Levels of participation and effect of adult structure. *Journal of Speech and Hearing Disorders,* 55, 315–326.

Prizant, B. (1982). Gestalt language and gestalt processing in autism. *Topics in Language Disorders,* 3, 16–23.

Ratner, N., & Bruner, J. (1978). Games, social exchange, and the acquisition of language. *Journal of Child Language,* 5, 391–402.

Rondal, J., & Cession, A. (1990). Input evidence regarding the semantic bootstrapping hypothesis. *Journal of Child Language,* 17, 711–717.

Scarr, S., & Eisenberg, M. (1993). Child care research: Issues, perspectives, and results. *Annual Review of Psychology,* 44, 613–644.

Slackman, M. (1995). The right to adopt: Unmarried partners win ruling from top New York court. *Newsday,* Friday, November 3.

Smith, N. V. (1973). *The acquisition of phonology: A case study.* Cambridge, MA: Cambridge University Press.

Szapocznik, J., & Kurtines, W. M. (1993). Family psychology and cultural diversity: Opportunities for theory, research and application. *American Psychologist,* 48, 400–407.

Tiegerman-Farber, E. (1995a). Training the parent as facilitator. In *Language and communication intervention in preschool children.* Needham Heights, MA: Allyn & Bacon.

Tiegerman-Farber, E. (1995b). The changing role of the family. In *Language and communication intervention in preschool children.* Needham Heights, MA: Allyn & Bacon.

Tomasello, M., & Mannle, S. (1985). Pragmatics of sibling speech to one-year-olds. *Child Development,* 56, 911–917.

Trout, M. and Foley, G. (1989). Working with families of handicapped infants and toddlers. *Topics in Language Disorders,* 10, 1, 57–68.

Veneziano, E., Sinclair, H., & Berthoud, I. (1990). From one word to two words: Repetition patterns on the way to structured speech. *Journal of Child Language,* 17, 633–650.

Waxman, S. R., & Hall, D. G. (1993). The development of a linkage between count nouns and object categories: Evidence from fifteen- to twenty-one-month old infants. *Child Development,* 64, 1224–1241.

Wiese, M. R. (1992). A critical review of parent training research. *Psychology in the Schools,* 29, 229–236.

Woodward, A. L., & Markman, E. M. (1991). Review. Constraints on learning as default assumptions: Comments on Merriman & Bowman's "The mutual exclusivity bias in children's word learning." *Developmental Review,* 11, 137–163.

Yoshinaga-Itano, C., & Downey, D. (1986). A hearing-impaired child's acquisition of schemata: Something's missing. *Topics in Language Disorders,* 7, 45–57.

Chapter 4

Language Development:
The Preschool Years

DEENA K. BERNSTEIN
Lehman College
City University of New York

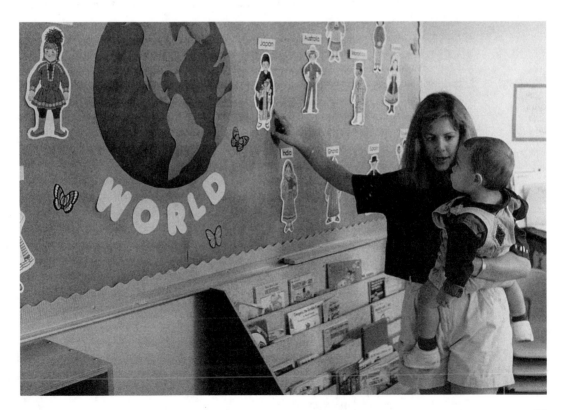

The previous chapters traced the origins of early communicative functions and the coding of early semantic relationships. Maternal input, social interaction, play, and cognitive development all play a dynamic role in early language development. Although children come to the language acquisition process biologically equipped to learn language, the role they play is an active one. Their eye-gaze behaviors, gestures, interactions with caretakers, and attempts to affect the behavior of others are significant for understanding the origins of early child language as well as for later language learning.

Although a large body of literature focusing on children's development of syntax emerged in the 1960s, more recent research emphasizes the influence of semantics and pragmatics on syntactic development. Researchers argue against viewing syntactic development in isolation (Bloom & Lahey, 1978; deVilliers & deVilliers, 1978). Attention to the meanings children convey in their utterances and to the social purposes of child language is considered crucial (Bates, 1979; Bloom & Lahey, 1978; McLean & Snyder-McLean, 1978; Rees, 1978). Syntax, semantics, and pragmatics essentially operate together and must be treated as such in the theoretical description of language development and in assessing and planning language intervention programs (Bloom & Lahey, 1978; Lund & Duchan, 1983; McLean & Snyder-McLean, 1978). However, for the purpose of analysis and study, I will treat each separately and point out their interrelationships where appropriate.

Five aspects of preschool language learning are the focal points of this chapter:

1. Development of syntactic forms, including increased use of morphological endings and various sentence types
2. Phonological growth
3. Development of meaning
4. Elaboration of pragmatic skills
5. Emergence of literacy skills

The section that follows presents a general overview of language development during the preschool period. it is followed by a review that highlights the linguistic forms, meanings, and communicative functions acquired by preschoolers. For a more detailed discussion of preschool language development, the reader is referred to Berko Gleason (1992), James (1990), Nelson (1993), and Owens (1996).

Preschool Language Development: An Overview

What changes are observable in children's language in the preschool years? As children advance from simple one- and two-word utterances, their utterances become longer and more complex. Children gradually elaborate the way they say things by adding more detail. in terms of syntactic development, they add and fill in words and word endings that were missing in their early utterances. These take the form of articles (*a, the*), prepositions (*in, on*), pronouns (*I, he*), auxiliary verbs (*is, are*), noun endings (such as -*s* to indicate plurality), and verb endings (such as -*ed* to indicate past tense). The inclusion of these forms into children's speech makes their utterances seem more like adults' and less like a telegram. For example, they progress from "More milk" to "I want more chocolate milk," or "Mommy car" to "Mommy is going in the car."

In the early preschool years, children's vocabulary continues to grow, and children learn many new word meanings. They learn new concepts and how to code these concepts linguistically. They also learn how to transform their ideas into sentences, and they begin to use a variety of sentence types. By age 4, most children's syntax is adultlike (Menyuk, 1977). Their utterances contain expanded noun and verb phrases ("Gimmie the big red ball," "He pushed me down the steps"), negative sentences ("I won't do it"), yes/no questions ("Can you cut the cake?"), and *Wh-* questions ("What will I do later?"). Causal constructions ("He didn't get a prize because he was bad"), conditional constructions ("If I'll do my homework, I'll get to watch TV"), and temporal constructions ("When he will come, he'll get a surprise") are also evident. Children learn more complex ways to use language socially, and they begin to develop discourse skills such as participating in conversations; giving instructions; providing descriptions about objects, events, and people; and relating personal experiences and simple stories. By the time they enter the first grade, they are able to use language for a variety of functions: to contribute new information on a topic (Bloom, Rocissano, & Hood, 1976); to describe objects, events, past experiences, and plans (Moerk, 1975); and to use language to demonstrate, instruct, and reason (Tough, 1977).

In the preschool years, children progress from talking about events in the here-and-now to talking about events in the "there and then" (Lucariello & Nelson, 1982). Young children generally talk about events and objects in the immediate environment; for example, they refer to what they are doing or what another person is doing. Also, maternal input to younger children focuses on events and objects in the immediate environment. As children develop cognitively, they begin to refer to people, objects, actions, and events that are displaced in terms of time and place. They talk about past and future events and about objects and activities in the absence of external props or contextual support.

Last, during this period children begin to learn about the nature of print. The emergence of preliteracy skills during the preschool years lays the foundation for their development of reading and writing.

Although children's language has reached a measure of complexity by age 5, much communicative development is yet to come. Vocabulary continues to grow throughout the school years (McGhee-Bidlack, 1991; Johnson & Anglin, 1995). Children begin to use nonliteral language such as jokes, riddles, and metaphors (Bernstein, 1986; Bernstein, 1987; Nippold, Leonard, & Kail, 1984) in middle childhood and to comprehend sentences that contain verbs such as *promise* or *ask* (Chomsky, 1969). Ambiguous sentences that allow for more than one interpretation, such as "The lamb is too hot to eat," are understood a bit later, during middle childhood and early preadolescence (Schultz & Pilon, 1973; Wiig, Gilbert, & Christian, 1978).

In addition, during the school-age years, children expand their pragmatic and discourse skills. Their conversational abilities become refined, and they are better able to plan, organize, and sequence their ideas into more complex narratives, or stories. Last, during this period children develop the ability to think and talk about language (called metalinguistic ability) and master language in another mode by learning to read and write. These abilities are discussed more fully in Chapter 7.

Although language development continues as children mature cognitively and socially, a good deal of language learning has already been mastered by the time the child enters the first grade. Just how complex a 5-year-old's language can be is underscored in the following incident:

In a course entitled Language Development and Disorders of Children, students were asked to observer record, and analyze the language of a 2- to 2½-year old nondisabled child. The assignment included two parts: (a) computing the average number of morphemes used by the child (called MLU—mean length of utterance) and (b) recording the language forms and functions used by the child. Both of these measures were to be used by the college student as an index of the subject's overall language development. (Greater detail about MLU is provided later in this chapter. In addition, Chapter 7 discusses how to compute an MLU and how to analyze the language sample of a child with a language disorder).

The students followed the instructor's advice and studied 2- to 2½-year-old subjects, with the exception of one student who had a 5-year-old brother and chose him as her subject. At the end of the semester when the assignment was due, the student approached the instructor in desperation and exclaimed, "This assignment has been very difficult. I never realized how complex a 5-year-old's language could be. I should have chosen to do my report on a 2-year-old!"

The student in this incident was overwhelmed by three things: first, the sheer volume and length of the language produced by a normal 5-year-old; second, the complex syntax of her subject's language sample; and third, the variety of pragmatic functions evidenced by the 5-year-old, necessitating analysis using a variety of taxonomies.

Syntactic Development

This section deals with the question of what linguistic forms, meanings, and communicative functions children learn in the preschool years. The order in which children acquire linguistic forms is examined first.

Brown's Stages

Brown's pioneering work, *A First Language* (1975), demonstrated that children's acquisition of syntactic structures is not as much a function of their chronological development as it is a function of the average number of morphemes per utterance that they produce. This measure is called an MLU (mean length of utterance) (How to calculate an MLU is described in Chapter 7). In a longitudinal study of three children, Adam, Eve, and Sarah, Brown found that utterance length and the mastery of grammatical forms varied greatly with age. For example, Sarah and Adam progressed from an MLU of less than 2.0 to an MLU of 4.0 in 15 months. It took Eve less than 8 months to make this progress. Eve achieved an MLU of 2.75 morphemes at age 2. Adam was 3 years old and Sarah was 3 years and 5 months when their utterances reached that length. In contrast, the three children were remarkably consistent with each other in one very important way: the order in which morphological endings and function words were acquired.

Brown noted that major linguistic changes took place as MLU increased. By identifying these developments, he could characterize certain MLU stages. These stages are outlined in Table 4-1. According to Brown, Stage I is characterized by single-word utterances and early multiword combinations that follow semantic rules. Examples of utterances during this period include "More" "Drink Milk," "Gimme juice," "Push car," and "Mommy." Stage II is characterized by the appearance of grammatical morphemes. During this stage children expand and modify their linguistic productions by including morphological endings such as *-ing,* the plural *-s,* and the prepositions *in* and *on.* Utterances such as "Jimmy eating," "Put ball in," and "See cats" are characteristic of this stage.

A burst of development occurs in Stage III. Utterance length continues to grow as children begin to use simple declarative sentences as well as imperatives, *wh-* questions, and simple negative sentences. During this period we see children beginning to use a variety of sentence types. Examples of utterances characteristic of this stage include "Jimmy hit the ball," "Will I eat?," "The boy is not eating," and "Push the truck."

Stage IV is marked by the emergence of complex construction, although mastery continues beyond this stage. Children exhibit the use of noun- and verb-phrase elaborations as well as compound and complex sentences. Examples of utterances produced at Stage IV and beyond include "Daddy is cooking and Mommy is writing," "The first boy is nice." "Jill wants to buy the dress with the green band," "She likes to eat chocolate ice cream," and "I want to push the red truck."

Although Brown's study included only three subjects, his findings were confirmed by deVilliers and deVilliers (1978), who studied a significantly larger number of children.

The Acquisition of the 14 Grammatical Morphemes

At Brown's Stage II (at approximately 2 to 2½ years of age), children begin filling out their short, immature sentences by incorporating one or more of the 14 grammatical morphemes studied by Brown. it should be noted that grammatical morphemes begin to emerge in Stage II, but many are not mastered (used correctly 90 percent of the time) until after Stage V. Table 4-2 lists the order of emergence of these 14 grammatical morphemes.

TABLE 4-1   Brown's Stages

Linguistic Stage	MLU	Approximate Chronological Age (months)	Characteristics
I	1.0–2.0	12–26	Use of semantic rules
II	2.0–2.5	27–30	Morphological development
III	2.5–3.0	31–34	Development of a variety of sentence types: negative, imperative, interrogative
IV	3.0–3.75	35–40	Emergence of complex constructions: coordination, complementation, relativization
V	3.75–4.5	41–46	
VI	4.5+	47+	

Adapted from Brown (1975).

The 14 morphemes studied by Brown were those that were within obligatory contexts. When morphological use is obligatory, its absence means it has not been acquired. Thus, the absence of an obligatory morpheme indicates nonacquisition and can be of concern if observed in a child whose linguistic stage indicates that mastery should have been obtained. (Morphological development is one area that is assessed both formally and informally during a language evaluation; it is discussed more fully in Chapter 7.)

Researchers have studied early grammatical morphemes other than those studied by Brown. These morphemes begin to develop in Brown's Stage II and continue developing until Stage V. They include the pronouns and noun and adjective suffixes described in the following sections.

TABLE 4-2   Order of Emergence of 14 Grammatical Morphemes

Grammatical Morphemes	Examples	Age of Mastery* (months)
1. Present progressive verb ending *-ing*	Mommy push*ing*. Johnny throw*ing*.	19–28
2. Preposition *in*	Put *in* box.	27–30
3. Preposition *on*	Put *on* table.	27–30
4. Plurals (regular) (*-s*)	Eat cookie*s*. More block*s*.	24–33
5. Past irregular verbs (*came, fell, broke, went*)	He *went* outside. Johnny *broke* it.	25–46
6. Possessive noun (*'s*)	Jimmy*'s* car. Mommy*'s* coat.	26–40
7. Uncontractible copula (*be* as the main verb: *am, is, are, were, was*)	He *was* bad. They *are* good.	27–39
8. Articles (*a, the*)	Billy throw *the* ball. Give me *a* big one.	28–46
9. Past regular (*-ed*)	He jump*ed*. She push*ed* me.	26–48
10. Third person singular regular	He cook*s*. Johnny goe*s*.	26–46
11. Third person singular irregular	He *has* books. She *does* work.	28–50
12. Uncontractible auxiliary (*be* verbs preceding another verb: *am, is, are, was, were*)	The boys *are eating*. The baby *is crying*.	29–48
13. Contractible copula	I*'m* good. She*'s* nice.	29–49
14. Contractible auxiliary	I*'m* eating. She*'s* jumping. They*'re* playing.	30–50

Adapted from Brown (1975).

*Used correctly 90% of time in obligatory contexts.

Pronoun Acquisition

Learning the English pronominal system is a very complex process (Haas & Owens, 1985; Trantham & Pedersen, 1976). It requires the understanding that one word—the pronoun—refers or is equivalent to a word or a group of words previously mentioned. In fact, the meaning of a sentence that contains a pronoun often cannot be understood without referring to the preceding sentence. To decipher the meaning of she and it in the sentence "She bought it," one would have to know what preceded that sentence in the discourse. Knowing that "Sue loved the dress" was previously uttered allows one to understand the referents of *she* and *it*. The use of a pronoun to refer to what has come before is known as anaphoric reference. It is discussed more fully later in this chapter in the section on contextual, or intersentence, meaning.

Some pronouns appear in Brown's Stage II, whereas others emerge much later. In general, the earliest pronouns to emerge usually involve the child as subject (*I, mine, my, me*). Other subjective pronouns emerge later (*he, she, they*). Objective pronouns (*him, her, them*) follow and are acquired earlier than possessive pronouns (*his, her, theirs*). Reflexive pronouns (*himself, herself, themselves*), the last to emerge, are usually not mastered until after age 5. Table 4-3 presents the general order of pronoun acquisition.

Adjective and Noun Suffixes

During the preschool years, children acquire a few additional suffixes for adjectives and nouns. The adjectival comparative -*er* and the superlative form -*est* are mastered during this period. Children learn to add these forms to adjectives to create the words nic*er*, bigg*est*, and small*est*. The superlative is understood by children by 3½ years of age and the comparative at about age 5 (Carrow, 1973). Comparatives and superlatives that are exceptions to the rule (*better, best*) usually take longer to acquire.

Derivational noun suffixes are usually understood by children by age 5 and mastered somewhat later. Thus, by age 5 children understand and produce such words as *hitter* and *teacher* (which contain the derivational noun suffix -*er*), whereas they acquire words that contain the derivational -*ist* morpheme somewhat later (*pianist, cyclist*).

TABLE 4-3   Development of Pronouns within Brown's Stages

Brown's Stages	Pronouns
I	I, mine
II	My, me
III	He, she, we, you, your
IV	They, his, hers
V	Their, our, ours, theirs
V+	Herself, himself, themselves

Adapted from Haas and Owens (1985) and Owens (1988).

Phrase and Clause Development

Whereas words are made up of morphemes, sentences are composed of phrases and clauses. There are two major types of phrases: noun phrases and verb phrases. Noun phrases must contain a noun and may contain optional elements that modify the noun. In the sentence "The girl in the red dress is pretty," there are two noun phrases: *The girl* (*girl* is the main noun) and *in the red dress,* a noun phrase that modifies the main noun.

There are four types of noun phrase modifiers:

1. *Determiners*—include articles (*a* and *the*), possessive pronouns (*my, your*), demonstratives (*this, that*), and qualifiers (*any, some*). They are always the first element in a noun phrase (e.g., *the* boy, *my* book, *some* toys).
2. *Adjectivals*—include adjectives (*little, big*), ordinals (*first, last*), and quantifiers (*two, few*). They modify nouns (e.g., *two* dresses, *big* boy).
3. *Initiators*—include *all, only, both,* and *just,* which limit or quantify nouns and must precede a determiner (e.g., *only* the boy, *all* the girls).
4. *Postmodifiers*—modifiers that follow the main noun. They may include prepositional phrases (e.g., the toy *on the floor* is broken) and clauses (e.g., the boy *who came to my house*).

Although noun phrases emerge at Brown's Stage II, the greatest surge in their development occurs at Stage IV (Miller, 1981). Early modifier types are determiners and adjectivals; initiators and postmodifiers are noted later in development. By late Stage IV, noun phrase elaboration appears both in subject and object positions and includes the use of almost all the modifier types mentioned previously.

In addition to noun phrases, sentences also contain verb phrases. Verb phrases must contain a main verb and may contain some optional elements. In the sentence "The girl is pushing the boy," *is pushing* is the verb phrase. It contains the main verb *push* and the optional present progressive forms *is* and *-ing*. Optional elements of verb phrases include progressive constructions (e.g., *is* eat*ing*), modals (words that indicate mood or attitude, e.g., *may, must*), and perfective constructions (used to specify certain types of action, e.g., *has seen*). Verb phrase elaboration emerges at Brown's Stage II (with the marking of the present progressive) and continues through Stage V (Miller, 1981). Modals emerge at Stage IV and perfective constructions at Stage V.

In contrast to a phrase, a clause is a group of words that contains both a subject and a predicate. Some clauses can stand alone and can function as simple sentences (*Billy walks, Mary ate*). Sometimes a sentence contains more than one clause. Sentences that are made up of two or more main clauses joined as equals are called compound sentences ("John drank, and Mary ate"). They usually emerge at Brown's Stage IV (Miller, 1981).

Complex sentences are made up of one main clause (that can stand alone) and one subordinate clause. Although a subordinate clause contains both a subject and a predicate, it cannot stand alone. Note the embedding of the subordinate clause *that we bought yesterday* into the sentence "The dress that we bought yesterday was pretty." The embedding of subordinate clauses appears late in language development, usually at early Stage V. (The use of clauses in compound and complex sentences is discussed in later sections.)

Clauses can also be classified according to the nature of the verb contained in the clause (Crystal, Fletcher, & Garman, 1976). Generally, intransitive clauses (clauses containing a verb that cannot take a direct object, such as *The girl walked*) appear in children's declarative sentences before transitive clauses (clauses that take a direct object, such as *The boy drank milk*). The last type of clause to emerge is equative clauses (Dever, 1978), which contain a copula and a complement (*He is the teacher*).

Sentence Development

One of the most basic and elemental syntactic rules states that every sentence must contain a noun phrase and a verb phrase. Thus, the only required syntactic elements of a sentence are the subject and the predicate. By the end of Brown's Stage II or early Stage III, children have mastered this rule, enabling them to understand and produce simple, active declarative sentences such as "The boy hit the ball." Children then begin to modify this basic sentence pattern. They develop a variety of sentence types, including the negative, interrogative, and imperative sentence forms. Although the initial development of these sentence types appears much earlier, the emergence of these in adultlike form is evident within Brown's Stage III. Table 4-4 presents the acquisition of sentence forms within Brown's stages of development. A more detailed account of the development of each sentence type follows the table.

The Development of Negative Sentence Forms.   Bloom (1970) found that children at the one- and two-word utterance stage express three semantically distinct types of negation: (a) **nonexistence** ("Allgone juice"—when there is no more juice in the cup), (b) **rejection** ("No milk"—as the child rejects the offer of milk), and (c) **denial** ("Not a book"—as mother points to a truck and says, "This is a book"). Mastery of the rules that change a declarative sentence into a negative sentence, however, does not emerge until Brown's Stage III.

Klima and Bellugi (1966) traced the development of negation in Adam, Eve, and Sarah. Three phases in the acquisition of the negative construction were identified. In Phase I, the appearance of the negative element *no* at the start of the sentence indicates that children have acquired the deep structure for negation and apply it primarily for negating affirmative sentences. In Phase II, children learn to transfer the *no* marker to its correct position before the verb in the sentence. The negative form, *not,* also appears. In Phase III, the negative contractible forms *can't* and *don't* emerge. Table 4-5 illustrates the development of the negative sentence form.

Although most negative forms are mastered within the preschool period, indefinite negative forms such as *nobody, no one,* and *nothing* are difficult even for older school-age children. Utterances such as "I don't got no books" or "Nobody don't goes there" are often heard in the speech of older children (and even some adults).

The Development of the Interrogative Sentence Form.   There are two types of questions: yes/no questions and *wh-* questions. Yes/no questions ("Do you want a cookie?") require that the listener simply answer the question with either a *yes* or a *no* word. *Wh-* questions (questions that begin with *who, what, when, where, why,* or *how*) are more com-

TABLE 4-4   Acquisition of Sentence Forms Within Brown's Stages of Development

Stage	Negative	Interrogative	Embedding	Conjoining
Early I (MLU: 1–1.5)	Single word—*no, all gone, gone;* negative + X	Yes/no asked with rising intonation on a single word; *what* and *where*		Serial naming without *and*
Late I (MLU: 1.5–2.0)	*No* and *not* used interchangeably	*That* + X; *What* + noun phrase + (doing)?	Prepositions *in* and *on* appear	*And* appears
Early II (MLU: 2.0–2.25)		*Where* + noun phrase + (going)?		
Late II (MLU: 2.25–2.5)	*No, not, don't,* and *can't* used interchangeably; negative element placed between subject and predicate	*What* or *where* + subject + predicate	*Gonna, wanna, gotta,* etc., appear	
Early III (MLU: 2.5–2.75)				*But, so, or,* and *if* appear
Late III (MLU: 2.75–3.0)	*Won't* appears; auxiliary forms *can, do, does, did, will,* and *be* develop	Auxiliary verbs begin to appear in questions (*be, can, will, do*)		
Early IV (MLU: 3.0–3.5)			Object noun phrase complements appear with verbs like *think, guess, show*	Clausal conjoining with *and* appears (some children cannot produce this form until late V); *because* appears
Late IV (MLU: 3.5–3.75)	Adds *isn't, aren't, doesn't,* and *don't*	Begins to invert auxiliary verb and subject; adds *when, how, why*		
Stage V (MLU: 3.175–4.5)	Adds *wasn't, wouldn't, couldn't,* and *shouldn't*	Adds modals; stabilizes inverted auxiliary	Relative clauses appear in object position; multiple embeddings by late V; infinitive phrases with same subject as the main verb	Clausal conjoining with *if* appears
Post-V (MLU: 4.5+)	Adds indefinite forms *nobody, no one, none,* and *nothing;* has difficulty with double negatives		Relative clauses attached to the subject; embedding and conjoining appear within same sentence above an MLU of 5.0	Clausal conjoining with *because* appears with *when, but,* and *so* beyond MLU of 5.0; embedding and conjoining appear within same sentence above an MLU of 5.0

From *Language Development: An Introduction* by R. Owens, 1988, Needham, MA: Allyn & Bacon. Reprinted by permission.

TABLE 4-5   **Development of the Negative Sentence**

Phase	Description	Example
I	The negative marker appears outside the sentence.	*No* the girl running.
II	The negative marker occurs before the verb.	The girl *not* running.
III	The auxiliary is added and complete the transformation to the adult form	The girls is *not* running.

plicated. They require that the listener provide further content to the speaker based on the question word that specifies the information being requested. For example, *where* questions demand information about location; *when* questions demand temporal information; and *who* questions demand information about people.

To form correct yes/no questions, children must learn to invert the subject and the auxiliary verb ("Is the boy eating?"). To form correct *wh-* questions, they must learn to (a) transpose the subject and the auxiliary verb and (b) add the *wh-* form at the beginning of the sentence ("*What* is the boy eating?").

Klima and Bellugi (1966) found that children go through four phases as they develop the ability to formulate questions.

- *Phase 1*—use of rising intonation and some *wh-* forms (MLU 1.75 and 2.25). In this first phase, children typically ask yes/no questions by adding a rising intonation to the end of their utterances. Examples of such question forms are "Johnnie eat?" "Baby drinking?" and "Go outside?" To ask *wh-* questions, children simply attach a *wh-* word to an assertion and produce questions like "Where doggie?" and "What dat?" These *wh-* questions are used only in routines in which children generally ask for names of objects, actions, or locations of previously present objects. The more prominent *wh-* questions used during this phase are *where* and *what* questions. At this stage, however, children do not respond appropriately to any of the *wh-* questions.
- *Phase 2*—use of greater variety of *wh-* questions (MLU 2.25 to 2.75). Children at this stage continue to ask yes/no questions by using rising intonation. Children ask *wh-* questions by adding the *wh-* form at the beginning of the question but fail to use the auxiliary verb. Examples of *wh-* questions that characterize this period are:

Where my truck?
Why you pushing it?
What the man doing?

Children can give appropriate answers to *what, who,* and *where* questions.

- *Phase 3*—limited use of inversion (MLU 2.75 to 3.5). At this phase, children regularly invert the subject and verb to produce yes/no questions but fail to do so in all *wh-* questions. Examples of questions that characterize this period are:

Will I go?
What the boy is riding?

- *Phase 4*—use of inversion in positive *wh-* question (MLU 3.5+). In this last stage, children invert the subject and the auxiliary verb when asking positive *wh-* questions but still have difficulty with negative *wh-* questions. Examples of *Wh-* questions of this period are:

What is the boy eating?
Where are you going?
Why I can't do that?

Ervin-Tripp (1970) analyzed the specific order of emergence of the *wh-* form. Her data show that children comprehend *what, where,* and *who* questions before *when, why,* and *how*—a correspondence to the production of these forms in their own speech. Ervin-Tripp explained that *what, where,* and *who* forms code cognitively simple ideas involving person, place, and identity *when, why,* and *how* forms code the cognitively more complex ideas of temporal and causal relationships. The order of acquisition of questions is summarized in Table 4-6.

Another explanation for the emergence of *wh-* questions was offered by Wotten, Merkin, Hood, and Bloom (1979). They suggested that the semantics of the verb influences children's comprehension and production of *wh-* questions. For example, the verb *eat* is more clearly linked with the question form *what* than with *where* or *who.* Similarly, the verb *drive* is most logically linked with the question form *where.* A verb that codes time, such as *finish,* would logically have as its expected question marker *when.* Wotten et al. (1979) suggested that certain verbs are expected with certain *wh-* markers and that the development of syntactically correct *wh-* questions is closely related to semantic considerations.

The Development of Imperative Sentence Forms.   The imperative sentence requests, demands, commands, and insists that the listener perform some action. In imperative sentences, the subject *you* is understood and not included in the surface form of the sentence, and the verb is uninflected. Examples of imperative sentences are "Gimme milk," "Push the truck," and "Pass the butter, please."

At the prelinguistic level, infants request and demand by pointing and gesturing. As they develop into toddlers, they begin to employ the imperative form to request, demand, and command. At Brown's Stage I, children produce forms that sound like imperatives be-

TABLE 4-6   Order of Acquisition of *Wh-* Questions

Type	Example
What	What is the girl eating?
Where	Where is the ball?
Who	Who is pushing the truck?
When	When will you go?
Why	Why is it dark?
How	How did it break?

cause they often omit the subject even from sentences that require one. These early forms are not the true imperatives that begin to appear at Brown's Stage III, when the omission of the subject in the surface form reflects the mastery of the rule of subject deletion for imperative sentences rather than the omission of the subject due to processing limitations.

The Development of Complex Sentences

Children begin to combine more than one semantic/syntactic relation in a single utterance when their MLU increases beyond 3.0. Their utterances reflect the elaboration or specification of agent-action-object interactions, and sentence construction advances from a linear ordering of words to a hierarchical ordering within and among sentence elements. Children learn to use complex sentences allowing the expression of old functions and new ideas with increasing clarity (Tyack & Gottsleben, 1986).

Coordination.   The complex construction that emerges first in children's language is **coordination.** There are two types of coordination constructions: sentential coordination and phrasal coordination. In sentential coordination, two events are combined into one sentence by the conjunction *and* ("John went to the doctor, *and* his sister stayed home"). No redundant elements are expressed in either phrase. In phrasal coordination, the connective *and* is also used, allowing the speaker to delete a redundant element. In the sentence, "Jane went to the movies and ate popcorn," the word *and* allows for the deletion of *Jane* from the second phrase ("...and [Jane] ate popcorn.")

The earliest use of coordination by children is in stereotypic phrases (*bread and jam, milk and cookie*) that are present in young children's utterances as responses to routine questions like, "What do you want to eat?" Researchers in the early 1970s believed that sententials were less complex than phrasal coordinated sentences and were therefore acquired first. Recent studies do not confirm this order of emergence. DeVilliers (1982) found that children 2½ to 3 years of age used both sentential and phrasal coordinations appropriately when the communicative context was set up to elicit them.

Bloom, Lahey, Hood, Lifter, and Fiess (1980) focused on semantic considerations in children's acquisition of coordinated sentences. They found the following order of acquisition of *and* coordinations:

1. *Additives*—the use of *and* to connect two propositions that go together ("Mother is baking a cake *and* Daddy is reading").
2. *Temporal*—the use of *and* to designate a sequential ordering of events ("Mommy will mix the batter *and* put it in the oven").
3. *Causal*—the use of *and* to indicate that one event led to another ("She put a bandage on *and* it made her feel better").
4. *Adversitive*—the use of *and* to indicate a contrast relationship ("This goes in here *and* that goes there"). Often the connective used in this instance is *but.*

The sequence of acquisition of coordinate constructions proposed by Bloom, Lahey, Hood, Lifter, and Fiess (1980) suggested that the level of cognitive development determines their use. DeVilliers (1982), however, suggested that children's learning of adaptive social strategies determines their use of coordinate constructions. Bloom's and deVilliers's views are not mutually exclusive. The learning of syntactic structures may be a function of cognitive/semantic *and* social/pragmatic constraints.

Complementation.   There are several types of complement structures in English. Examples of sentences with complement constructions are "I want to buy a *red lollipop,*" "Show me *where this one goes,*" and "Look at *what she's doing.*" In each of these sentences, the main portion of the sentence is coupled with a clause that in some way modifies the verb.

Bloom, Lifter, and Hafitz (1980) studied complement constructions and found that their order of emergence was based on the semantics of the verb. The first complements to emerge in children's speech are with state verbs, verbs that express a feeling or intention. *Like, want,* and *need* are state verbs and take the complement *to.* Examples of sentences using state verb complements are "I want *to go home*" and "I like *to get dirty.*"

The next complement to emerge is attached to notice verbs. Notice verbs like *see, look,* and *watch* are followed by the complement *what,* as in "Look at *what he's doing.*"

The third complement to emerge is attached to knowledge verbs like *know* and *think.* These are followed by the complement *that* or *what,* as in "I know *what to do*" or "I think *that one is good.*"

The last complement to emerge is attached to the speaking verbs—*ask, tell,* or *promise.* Speaking verbs require the complement construction *to* plus a verb. Sentences like "Ask Mary *to come inside*" or "John promised *to leave*" are examples of sentences with speaking verb complements. In keeping with an earlier hypothesis, Bloom, Lifter, and Hafitz concluded that the acquisition of complement constructions is a function of semantic constraints.

Relativization.   Complex sentences can be formed by adding relative clauses, which restrict or qualify the meaning of another portion of the sentence. Relative clauses are of two types: objective and subjective. Objective relative clauses modify the object of the sentence, as in "That picture is about some birds *that got all smeared up.*" An example of a sentence with a subject relative clause is "The girl *who lives down the block* is my cousin." Menyuk (1977) reported that object relative clauses emerge before subject relative clauses. The object relative clause develops after 5 years of age, whereas the subject relative clause is rare even at 7 years. DeVilliers, Tager-Flusberg, Hakuta, & Cohen (1979), remaining consistent with their social context/pragmatic approach, maintained that children use both subject and object relative clauses if the context is structured to demand specification of the referent. Accordingly, if several similar objects, such as toy people, are placed in an array and each has a distinguishing feature such as hair color, clothing style, or body shape, the child will produce a sentence with a subject relative clause specifically describing each object. DeVilliers et al. concluded that the pragmatic context influences children's use of relative clauses.

Phonological Development

Children produce their first words with recognizable meaning between 1 and 1½ years of age. But toddlers' ability to make themselves understood is often limited by inadequate production of the sounds and the sound sequences that constitute these words. Without know-

TABLE 4-7   Age at Which 75 Percent of Children Produced Consonant Sounds

Sound	According to Templin (based on testing in initial, medial, and final positions)		According to Prather (based on testing in initial and final positions only)	
	Years	Months	Years	Months
m	3		2	
n	3		2	
h	3		2	
p	3		2	
ŋ (as in sing)	3		2	
f	3		2–4	
j (as in *yes*)	3–6		2–4	
k	4		2–4	
d	4		2–4	
w	3		2–8	
b	4		2–8	
t	6		2–8	
g	4		3	
s	4–6		3	
r	4		3–4	
l	6		3–4	
ʃ (as in *sh*oe)	4–6		3–8	
tʃ (as in *ch*urch)	4–6		3–8	
ð (as in fa*th*er)	7		4	
ʒ (as in gara*g*e)	7		4	
ʤ (as in *j*udge)	7		4+	
θ (as in *th*umb)	6		4+	
v	6		4+	
z	7		4+	

Adapted from Templin (1957) and Prather, Hedrick, and Kern (1972).

ing the child or something about the nonlinguistic context, it would be difficult to recognize /doti/ for *doggie* or /dut/ for *juice.*

To master the sound system of the language, children must acquire an inventory of sounds. The sequence of English consonant acquisition is listed in Table 4-7.

In addition to acquiring individual sounds, children must also learn the rules that govern the position of sounds in words, **distributional rules,** and the rules for sequencing these sounds, **sequential rules.** They must learn to determine which speech sounds make a difference in meaning (Ingram, 1974). These rules are learned gradually, beginning in the early preschool years and continuing into early elementary school.

Phonological Processes

As with morpho-syntactic development, children formulate and discard hypotheses regarding the rules of the sound system of the language. In examining the phonological rules used by children, linguists have noted that children simplify adult productions of a target word. The simplification "rules" used by children are called phonological, or natural processes. They reduce the complexity of the consonant structure of a word or syllable that the child attempts to say. These are evident in children's first words and are discarded or fade out of children's speech by age 4. Some of the phonological processes used by children are described in the following sections (Edwards & Shriberg, 1983; Lund & Duchan, 1983).

Syllable Structure Processes

Children frequently simplify words by reducing them to either the basic consonant-vowel (CV) syllable or to CVCV structure. Four processes that accomplish this simplification are reduplication, final consonant deletion, cluster reduction, and deletion of unstressed syllables.

- *Reduplication*—a well-known childlike pattern that usually occurs in nondisabled children's first words. Using this process, children repeat the first syllable (which is usually the stressed syllable) and substitute it for subsequent syllables in multisyllabic words. Examples of reduplication are /kæ kæ/ for *cracker* or /dada/ for *Daddy*.
- *Final consonant deletion*—a syllable structure process in which the final consonant of a word is deleted. The result of this simplification is the production of a CV structure for a CVC word, such as /bɛ/ for *bed* or /fI/ for *fish*. Normally, this process completely disappears by the time the child is 3 to 3½ years old.
- *Cluster reductions*—a structural simplification in which one or more consonants from a target consonant cluster are deleted. For example, the word *stop* becomes /top/ and the word *please* becomes /piz/. Cluster reduction is evident in children's speech until they are about 3 years of age.
- *Deletion of unstressed syllables*—a simplification resulting in words like /næna/ for *banana*.

Substitution Processes

A number of rule-governed substitutions are common in the speech of preschoolers. These substitutions are classified according to the place or manner of production of the speech sounds. Among the substitution processes are fronting, stopping, and gliding. Substitution processes are those in which one sound is substituted for another, depending on the sound's position in a word.

- *Fronting.* One of the best known patterns in early childhood speech, this process occurs when children replace palatal and velar sounds (made in the back of the mouth) with alveolar sounds (made in the front of the mouth). Examples of fronting are the production of /t∧p/ for *cup* or /d∧n/ for *gun*. Fronting of velars is usually suppressed by 2½ to 3 years of age, and velar consonants are usually established in children's speech by age 4 at the latest.
- *Stopping.* Instead of producing fricatives (sounds that are made by passing air through a narrow constriction, thereby creating a hissing sound) or affricates (sounds that com-

bine a popping sound and a fricative), children substitute a plosive (a popping sound). The use of the stopping process results in productions such as /dut/ for *juice* or /ban/ for *van*. Stopping begins to disappear for most fricatives and affricates by 2½ to 3 years of age, but the emergence of the correct pronunciation of these sounds is gradual (Grunwell, 1982).

- *Gliding*. Children substitute glides (sounds that are produced during the movement of articulators from one vowel position to another) for liquids (sounds with vowellike quality of little air turbulence). Examples of gliding are the production of /wabɪt/ for *rabbit* or /yaɪt/ for *light*. This process may persist for many years.

Assimilation Processes

Another group of processes are those in which two phonemes within a word become alike. Two assimilation processes are consonant harmony and prevocalic voicing.

- *Consonant harmony*—process in which consonants within a word become more alike in terms of place or manner of articulation. An example of consonant harmony is the production of /gɔgi/ for *doggy*.
- *Prevocalic voicing*—process in which unvoiced consonants are affected by the following vowel and take on the voicing feature of the vowel. The result is the production of /dʌb/ for tub.

Summary

Children's development of linguistic form can be traced in the directions of (a) lengthier utterances and (b) increased phonological, morphological, and syntactic complexity. There are both semantic and pragmatic considerations to children's development of various sentence types. It is important to note that the elaboration of children's linguistic form is the result of their need to express more complex ideas in a greater variety of social situations.

Attention is now turned to children's semantic and pragmatic development during the preschool years, with emphasis on how the meanings children express become more complex and on how they expand their repertoire of linguistic use.

Semantics: The Development of Meaning

Semantics is the component of language concerned with meaning. Without meaning, there would be no point to language. People talk in order to express meaning, and they listen in order to discover the meaning of what others say.

Meaning can be conveyed through language at the word, sentence, and discourse levels. The meaning of some words can also be derived from the nonlinguistic context.

Lexical Meaning

The most familiar sense of meaning is **lexical meaning.** It is concerned with the meanings of words and the characteristics of the category to which a word belongs. The preschool period is one of rapid lexical growth. Carey (1978) estimated that the child adds approximately five words to his lexicon every day between 1½ and 6 years of age. Children's lexical growth continues steadily during the preschool years; by age 8, children's receptive vocabulary is said to be between 6,000 and 8,000 words, whereas their expressive vocabulary ranges from 2,500 to 2,800 words (Berry, 1969).

As children develop, they become better able to define words as semantically unique by including different types of information and by using different approaches to organize both the words and the information. For example, during the late preschool period and into the early school years, children's definitions are concrete—primarily descriptions of the referent's appearance and function. As children progress through elementary school, their definitions are gradually joined by more complex, abstract types of responses: synonyms, explanations, and specifications of categorical relationships (Litowitz, 1977). Lexical growth is a gradual process and continues for many years (Johnson & Anglin, 1995; McGhee-Bidlack, 1991).

Relational Meaning

In addition to acquiring lexical knowledge that specifies referents, children acquire meanings that code relationships among people, objects, and events. These relationships can be conveyed at the word level and the sentence level (also called **intrasentence meaning**). The early relational meanings (or semantic content categories) of existence, nonexistence, and recurrence evident in children's language are coded, using single word and multiword combinations. (They were discussed in Chapter 3.) Later, these relationships are coded in children's simple sentences. As children develop cognitively, the relationships they map and the forms they use to express these relationships become increasingly complex. In addition to coding the early semantic relations, their utterances reflect the coding of more complex concepts. Thus, the semantic relations expressed by preschool children include the coding of concepts of space, time, causation, and sequencing of action, using more complex linguistic forms and a variety of sentence types. Table 4-8 lists the semantic relations expressed by

TABLE 4-8 Semantic Relations (Intrasentence Meanings) Expressed by 2- to 4-Year-Olds

Semantic Relation	Age	Example
Coordination	2.0	My car... truck.
Sequence	2.0	Bye-bye, Mommy, Daddy, Joey.
Causality (logical)	2.0	I can't do it. It too long.
Reasons	2.4	You hit me because you don't like me.
Temporality	2.8	Now I wash my hands, then I eat. When he goes to school he goes on the bus.
Conditionality	3.4	I wear this while walking.
Temporal sequence	3.5 to 4.0	I will make a tree after I finish this.

Adapted from Miller (1981).

children between 2 and 4 years of age. Note not only the more advanced relationships pre-schoolers are mapping but also the complex syntax they are using to express them.

While word and sentence meanings expand during the preschool years, contextual meanings also develop. That is, the child learns (a) how to discern meanings from the linguistic and nonlinguistic context and (b) how to use linguistic forms to glue discourse together. The development of contextual meaning continues during the school-age period. The contextual meanings that emerge during the preschool period are discussed in the next section.

Contextual Meaning: The Role of Discourse

Context affects many aspects of language. The linguistic context, or discourse, provides information necessary to derive intersentence meaning. The influence of the linguistic context on meaning can be understood by examining the following sentence:

> *He bought it.*

Is it possible to derive the meaning of this sentence without knowing something about the previous linguistic context? Who is *he* and what is *it?* If the sentence occurs within the context of the following discourse, however, the meaning of *he* and *it* becomes clear.

Tom: John saw a red Jaguar at a car dealer yesterday.

Susan: What happened?

Tom: He bought it.

In the discourse, the pronouns *he* and *it* are used to refer to something that had already been identified linguistically. The use of a pronoun to refer to a previously mentioned referent is called **anaphoric reference.** Anaphoric reference, as well as other linguistic devices, helps bind discourse so that it is better understood. Collectively, these are called **cohesive devices** because they provide the glue for intersentence meaning. They are included within the semantic component of language to highlight how meaning is derived from the linguistic context. Table 4-9 defines some cohesive devices and gives examples of each.

There is little information about the development of children's use of cohesive devices. In a seminal study, Bloom, Lightbown, and Hood (1975) found that 2-year-olds do not use pronouns anaphorically. The children in their study used pronouns when the context gave the listener no clues about the referent (and when the use of a noun would have been more appropriate). At the same time, the children used nouns (instead of pronouns) when the referent was obvious from the context. It was concluded that the ability to recognize when it is appropriate to use pronouns anaphorically is a developmental achievement related to children's cognitive and social awareness of the linguistic context. In a related study, Tanz (1980) found that although children of 3 years of age understood the pronoun *it* when used anaphorically, the age at which they used pronouns anaphorically was not clearly determined.

Although some investigators have examined the use of anaphoric reference, ellipsis, and lexical cohesion in young children (Fine, 1978; Warden, 1976), the data on children's acquisition of discourse cohesive devices are presently limited. Nevertheless, Silliman and

James (Chapter 7) suggests that an examination of children's use of discourse cohesion devices presents the clinician with valuable information regarding children's ability to express intersentence meaning.

Contextual Meaning: The Role of the Nonlinguistic Context

In addition to the linguistic context, the nonlinguistic context gives clues about the meaning of words whose referents shift with the perspective of the speaker and the timing of the utterance. Consider the sentence, "I want you to go there tomorrow." The meanings of *I, you, there,* and *tomorrow* depend on who is speaking, who is listening, where the speaker is when the sentence is uttered, and when the sentence is spoken. Words whose meaning shifts as the nonlinguistic context changes are called **deictic terms.** Thus *I, you, here, there,* and *today, tomorrow* are words that express the deictic relationship of person, place, and time, respectively.

Some studies have examined children's development of person, place, and time deixis. The limited data in this area indicate that it takes considerable time to master deictic terms. Although the exact ages for deictic acquisition are not specified, developmental sequence is (Tanz, 1980). Tanz found that children tend to acquire person deixis first; deixis involving prepositions (*in back of, in front of*) usually develops next. Temporal deixis (*today, tomorrow*) is the last to emerge.

Summary

The acquisition of words, their meanings, and the links between them is a process that requires time. During the preschool period, children acquire new words and gradually develop an understanding of the nature of words, sentences, and their relationship. The meanings that children learn are the result of their encounters with the physical and social world and are dependent on their cognitive and social development.

TABLE 4-9   Cohesive Devices

Type	Definition	Example
Anaphoric reference	The use of pronouns or definite articles that refer to a previously established entity	Gina is sick today. *She* has the flu.
Cataphoric reference	The use of pronouns or demonstratives that direct the listener to coming elements	After *he* warms up, John will be unbeatable.
Ellipsis	The deletion of information available in an immediately preceding portion of the discourse	Do you like to paint? I do. (like to paint)
Lexical cohesion	The use of synonyms that refer to previously noted referents	Suddenly a lion appeared. The *beast* let out a terrifying roar.

Adapted from Halliday and Hasan (1976).

Pragmatic Development

As noted in previous chapters, language is learned within a social context. As children interact with their caretakers (and later with their peers), the uses to which they put language continually multiply. The intentions they code increase, and they learn to become more aware of social settings and the interactors within those social setting.

During the preschool years, children learn to describe objects and events removed from the immediate context. They talk about objects not within the immediate environment and about events both past and future. They relate some personal occurrences that were meaningful to them during their daily routine. They use language effectively to convey their wants and needs and ask as well as answer a variety of questions. In addition, they become more aware of the general conditions governing cooperative conversations. They learn to take turns in a conversation, to stick to the conversational topic, and to contribute new and relevant information to the discourse (Bloom, Rocissano, & Hood, 1976). Although these abilities emerge in the preschool period, they continue to grow through the years as children mature cognitively and socially.

The development of language use in the preschool years sets the stage for later changes. During the school years, children learn to be skilled conversationalists and more effective communicators as they become increasingly sensitive to what their listeners need to know. They learn to organize and plan narratives and can relate stories in a coherent and cohesive manner. Last, they add to their repertoire various means for conveying their intentions, including indirect expression. Consider the different uses of language by a 2-year-old, a 4-year-old, and a 9-year-old in the same context:

CONTEXT: a plate of cookies

2-year-old to adult: Gimme cookie.

4-year-old to adult: Can I have a cookie, please?

9-year-old to adult: My, those cookies look good!

The 2-year-old directly requested the object, the 4-year-old indirectly and politely requested it, and the 9-year-old hinted at the request.

This section discusses three aspects of pragmatic development during the preschool years: the elaboration of communicative functions, the emergence of conversational skills, and the beginning of children's ability to produce narratives. Later developing pragmatic abilities will be discussed in Chapter 5.

The Elaboration of Communicative Functions

Several studies have explored children's use of language during the preschool years. In addition to using the early communicative function outlined in Chapter 3, children expand their repertoire of language use (Dore, 1978). The communicative intentions they express include:

1. *Requesting information* by asking a variety of questions ("Can I go now?" "Is he eating candy?" "Where are you going?" "Why can't I have it?")
2. *Responding to requests* by answering questions or supplying information ("It's in my closet," "I wasn't the one who broke the cup," "I don't want to")
3. *Describing events, objects, or properties* ("There's a red truck," "He's building it slowly," "That's a truck with a crane")
4. *Stating facts, feelings, attitudes, and beliefs* ("It happened yesterday," "I feel sick," "I don't like her," "Ghosts are not real")

Moerk (1975) outlined nine language functions that 2- to 5-year-olds use as they interact with their caretakers. These include:

1. Imitating (*Mother:* Buckle up! *Child:* Buckle up!)
2. Asking a question ("What's that?")
3. Expressing a need ("I want a drink")
4. Answering a question ("It's on the chair")
5. Encoding from picture books ("And the boy and girl got into the car and the car took them to the train")
6. Describing objects or events ("My balloon is big and red")
7. Describing own actions ("I'm building a house")
8. Describing plans ("First I'll make a fence . . . then a house")
9. Describing a past experience ("David pushed me so hard I fell off the swing")

The internal cognitive and social changes that take place in children influence the ways they use language. For example, young preschoolers use language to direct themselves and to instruct others, as well as to report on present and past experiences. Older preschoolers, however, add more complex communicative functions; they use language to reason, think, and solve problems (Tough, 1977). Consider the following samples:

Ari (age 5): If the roof isn't strong enough, he'll fall in.

Dani (age 5): I think the tape will fix it. Yep, I'll get the tape.

Sheri (age 5½): If you put your block here and I put my block there, it will hold everything up.

Last, during the preschool years children use language to tease, annoy, complain, criticize, and threaten. These communicative functions are observed not only as children interact with caretakers and siblings but also as children interact with their peers (Dore, 1978; Miller, 1981; Tough, 1977).

Teasing:	You're a fatso!
Annoying:	I'll do it again and again!
Complaining:	You always give the big one to him!
Criticizing:	Your picture is yukky!
Threatening:	Give it back or I'll tell the teacher!

Thus, during this period we see children expressing a wide variety of communicative intentions and simultaneously expanding linguistic forms.

Conversational Skills

In general, children learn language within a conversational context. The preschool child acquires many conversational skills, but much of his conversation concerns the here-and-now, and he has much to learn about the conventional routines of conversation. Although he has learned to take turns in a conversation (see Chapter 2), the conversations are short and the number of turns is very limited. These skills will be refined during the school-age years.

The young child (2½ to 3) is very good at introducing new conversational topics in which he is interested, but he has difficulty sustaining that topic beyond one or two turns. Although he learns to acknowledge his partners, taking his conversational turn and building a bridge for the next speaker's turn are especially difficult. As the child advances during the preschool years, he gains the ability to maintain a topic, resulting in fewer new topics being introduced within a given conversation. Garvey and Hogan (1973) maintained that 50 percent of 5-year-olds can sustain certain topics through about a dozen turns, occasionally filling their turns with *yeah* and *uh-huh.*

Between 3 and 4 years of age the child seems to gain a better awareness of the social aspects of conversation. He begins to adapt his language to the needs of his listeners. With the realization that other people's perspective must be taken into account (called **presuppositional ability**) comes language that is well adapted to the listener. That is not to say that the preschooler is always successful in getting his message across. He is often unable to reformulate his message in response to a facial expression of noncomprehension and must be specifically asked to clarify his message. The most common way preschoolers clarify or repair their messages is by simply repeating what they have said.

Child (age 3½): (*to mother*) He took it away from me!

Mother: What?

Child: He took it away from me!

Mother: What?

Child: He took it away from me!

Mother: Who did what?

Child: Jimmy took my boat.

The inability to respond to a nonspecific request for clarification is characteristic of preschoolers. The ability to respond more appropriately does not develop until the school-age years (Owens, 1996).

Throughout the preschool years children learn to become fuller conversational partners by using a greater variety of linguistic forms to attain their ends. Although they take their conversational turns without being prompted, they still tend to make more coherent contributions to a conversation if they are discussing an ongoing activity in which they are engaged actively. Children are more aware of social roles at 5 than at 2 and can adjust their speech to younger children (Shatz & Gelman, 1973); but they still lack many of the subtleties of older children.

In the next section we will examine children's development of a different discourse skill—their emerging ability to tell narratives.

The Development of Narratives

The narrative is a form of discourse. It is an uninterrupted stream of language modified by the speaker to capture and hold the listener's attention (Owens, 1996). Narratives differ from conversations in a number of ways. When producing a narrative, the speaker produces a monologue throughout and must presuppose the information needed by the listener. In addition, the speaker must present all the information in an organized way, and must introduce and organize sequences so that events are related and lead to some conclusion.

There are a number of different types of narratives. Narratives include sharing and recounting of personal events and experiences, self-generated stories, telling and retelling of familiar tales, and the retelling of stories from movies, books, and television shows.

Research has shown that 2-year-olds incorporate dialogue that accompanies familiar everyday routines into their speech. This type of narrative is called a script and is used by young children to talk about events that occurred to them (Owens, 1996; Tiegerman-Farber, 1995). However, it is not until the age of 4 that they are able accurately to describe event sequences, called a plan (Karmiloff-Smith, 1986).

In general, two types of strategies are used by preschool children for organizing their narratives: centering and chaining (Applebee, 1978). Centering is the lending of entities to form a story nucleus. Chaining is the sequencing of events (that share some attributes) and lead directly from one event to another.

Most of the stories of 2-year-olds are organized by centering. The child's story centers on certain highlights in his or her life. It may have a vague plot, but does not have an easily identifiable beginning, middle, or end. By age 3, 50 percent of typical children use centering and chaining when producing a narrative and by age 5, 75 percent of normal children use both strategies. (See Table 4-10 for examples of narratives of typical preschoolers.)

TABLE 4-10 Narratives of Typical Preschoolers

Narrative	Description
Child: Rivky, age 3	Descriptive statements
Context: Retelling a story	No causal or temporal link.
There was this magician. He had a hat and rabbits come from the hat. The end.	
Child: Chaim, age 5	Action sequence with chronological order.
Context: Recounting a birthday experience	No causal relations.
I had a birthday party. All the children came to my party. Everybody sang "Happy Birthday to You." I got presents. We ate cake.	

By the time most children enter school, they have acquired the basic elements of narratives and can share their experiences and recount sequentially familiar events. However, these narrative skills are not always well developed by minority or bilingual children (Heath, 1986). In the school-age years, as children's linguistic abilities and their knowledge of the world continue to develop, they will learn to understand and produce more complex narrative forms.

Summary

In our review of pragmatic development we have seen that preschool children elaborate their use of language to suit a variety of social contexts and begin to gain competence in their use of different discourse skills (i.e., conversations, narratives). During this period they also begin to learn about print. The next section discusses the research in this new area of preschool language development.

Emergent Literacy

Recent research from diverse disciplines have begun to highlight the importance of the preschool year in laying the foundation for children's later development of reading and writing (van Kleeck, 1995). There are strong indications that listening/speaking and reading/writing share, at least in part, a common linguistic base, although they differ in other ways. The importance of this information for speech-language pathologists and special educators who work with preschool children lies in the fact that delays in the comprehension and formulation of oral language often foreshadow difficulties in reading and writing that will appear during the school years (Butler, 1988; Maxwell & Wallach, 1984; Weiner, 1985; Nelson, 1993).

The term that has often been used for the knowledge that preschoolers learn about print before the actually learn to read is *emergent literacy*. Attention to the concepts of emergent literacy should help parents and professionals in facilitating preschool children's knowledge of what print is, how it works, and why it is used.

Studies of emergent literacy research have taken numerous directions. One focus has been on the knowledge that preschool children acquire about formal print before learn to read. Investigators have concluded that during this period, children:

- Master the convention of print (how to hold a book, awareness that the organization of English print is from left to right and top to down, scribble writing)
- Learn to name and write letters
- Recognize that print represents meaningful ideas
- Acquire an understanding of the structure of written language (that stories are organized in a particular way)
- Develop a print-related vocabulary (understanding and using words such as read, write, story, page)
- Acquire the rudimentary skills of phonological awareness (that words consist of discrete units)

Other researchers have focused on the print literacy environment of the young child, particularly in the child's home. Researchers have found that the availability of print in the home (books, magazines, newspapers, postcards, nameplates) as well as the presence of print artifacts (paper, pencils, pens, crayons, markers) had a positive impact on children's later literacy development (Thorndyke, 1976; Leichter, 1984). In addition, various literacy events that occurred within the child's family also influenced the child's later reading development. These included:

- Entertainment activities such as reciting nursery rhymes, reading books and stories, playing card games, coloring and drawing, playing computer and video games involving print
- Activities of daily living including creating shopping lists, reading product labels, reading street signs
- Using print for interpersonal communication including writing notes to family members, sending greetings as well as birthday and holiday cards

Most of the literacy events that occur in the lives of preschool children are embedded in ongoing real life family experiences. However, there is a need for guidance and support by a literate individual (usually a parent), who uses such techniques as semantic contingency (staying on a topic introduced by a child), scaffolding (structuring the linguistic and nonlinguistic context to facilitate the child's success), and routines (highly predictable situations that occur frequently), to help facilitate an appreciation for literacy experiences (Snow, 1983).

Most of the research in parental roles in literacy acquisition has focused on middle-class mainstream families (regardless of ethnicity). Not all families, however, are alike even when they have similar cultural and sociolinguistic histories (Lieven, 1984). When families come from diverse cultural backgrounds, there may be culturally based differences in the literacy environments, literacy events, parental guidance, and the preliteracy expectations of those parents for their preschool children (Nelson, 1993).

In sum, normal preschoolers develop literacy skills and absorb a wealth of knowledge about print prior to learning to read through family literacy events that assist them in developing an understanding of this form. The school years will see the blossoming of children's ability to use print as they are formally taught to read and write (Butler, 1995).

Summary

Children's language development is indeed a multifaceted and complicated process. Although there are common developmental patterns, there are variances in children's language acquisition that account for their respective differences. Children have unique predispositions from birth and different cognitive, social, and linguistic experiences. In a similar vein, the rate of learning linguistic forms differs among children.

This chapter analyzed the process of language development. Children's utterances are observed to increase in length and complexity. From an MLU of 2.0 and continuing beyond an MLU of 4.0, children simultaneously learn several linguistic subsystems. The develop grammatical morphemes, acquire a variety of sentence types, and master the phonological system. They acquire more abstract meanings and the ability to map these onto linguistic structures. In addition, they elaborate their use of language to suit a variety of social contexts and describe events and personal experiences as well as sequences and outcomes. Finally, they begin to gain knowledge about print, even though they may not learn how to actually decode print until they are formally taught to do so in school. Although each component of language was discussed separately, in the real world, language form (phonology, morphology, and syntax), content (semantics), and use (pragmatics) are interrelated in development.

I conclude this chapter on preschool language development with a quotation from Rees (1980).

> *For professionals in the area of communication disorders, it is recognized that only the most complete understanding possible of the nature and growth of child language will suffice as basic information with which to approach clinical problems. Normal language development provides not only the base of reference against which to evaluate the communicative functioning of the clinical subject, but also guidelines for assessment and intervention. (p. 38)*

Information about normal language development provides the speech-language pathologist with a framework for understanding the assessment and remediation of language disorders in children. Because new knowledge is continuously emerging about the stages, strategies, and processes of normal language development, what we "do today will be replaced tomorrow by wiser principles and improved techniques" (Rees, 1980, p. 38).

Study Questions

1. What are the main characteristics of each of Roger Brown's stages of language development?
2. List and briefly explain the grammatical morphemes studied by Brown.
3. Describe the order of acquisition of negative and interrogative sentences.
4. Describe the phonological processes observed in preschoolers' language.
5. What are some of the pragmatic skills of preschool children?
6. Discuss narrative development during the preschool years.
7. Of what value is the research on emergent literacy for the communication specialist?

References

Applebee, A. N. (1978). *The child's concept of story.* Chicago: University of Chicago Press.

Bates, E. (1979). *The emergence of symbols.* New York: Academic Press.

Berko Gleason, J. (1992). *The development of language.* Columbus, OH: Merrill/Macmillan.

Bernstein, D. K. (1986). The development of humor: Implications for assessment and intervention. *Topics in Language Disorders, 4,* 65–73.

Bernstein, D. K. (1987). Figurative language: Assessment strategies and implications for intervention. *Folia Phoniatrica, 39,* 130–144.

Berry, M. F. (1969). *Language disorders of children.* Englewood Cliffs, NJ: Prentice Hall.

Bloom, L. (1970). *Language development: Forms and functions of emerging grammars.* Cambridge, MA: MIT Press.

Bloom, L., & Lahey, M. (1978). *Language development and language disorders.* New York: Wiley.

Bloom, L., Lahey, M., Hood, L., Lifter, K., & Fiess, K. (1980). Complex sentences: Acquisition of syntactic connectives and the semantic relations they encode. *Journal of Child Language, 7,* 235–262.

Bloom, L., Lifter, K., & Hafitz, J. (1980). Semantics of verbs and the development of verb inflection in child language. *Language, 56,* 386–412.

Bloom, L., Lightbown, P., & Hood, L. (1975). Structures and variation in child language. *Monographs of the Society for Research in Child Development, 40.*

Bloom, L., Rocissano, L., & Hood, L. (1976). Adult-child discourse: Developmental interaction between information processing and linguistic knowledge. *Cognitive Psychology, 8,* 521–552.

Brown, R. (1975). *A first language: The early stages.* Cambridge, MA: Harvard University Press.

Butler, K. (1988). Preschool language processing performance and later reading achievement. In R. Masland (Eds.), *Preschool prevention of reading failure.* Parton, MD: York Press.

Butler, K. (1995). Preface to *Best practices II: The classroom as an intervention context* (pp. v–xi). Gaithersburg, MD: Aspen Press.

Carey, S. (1978). The child as word learner. In M. Halle, J. Bresnan, & G. Miller (Eds.), *Linguistic theory and psychological reality.* Cambridge, MA: MIT Press.

Carrow, E. (1973). *Test of Auditory Comprehension of Language.* Austin, TX: Urban Research Group.

Chomsky, C. (1969). *The acquisition of syntax in children from 5 to 10.* Cambridge, MA: MIT Press.

Crystal, D., Fletcher, P., & Garman, M. (1976). *The grammatical analysis of language disability: A procedure for assessment and remediation.* London: Edward Arnold.

Cullinan, B. E. (1989). Literature for young children. In D. S. Strickland and L. M. Morrow (Eds.) *Emerging literacy: Young children learn to read and write* (pp. 35–51). Newark, DE: International Reading Association.

Dever, R. (1978). *TALK: Teaching the American language to kids.* Columbus, OH: Merrill/Macmillan.

deVilliers, J., Tager-Flusberg, H., Hakuta, K., & Cohen, M. (1979). Children's comprehension of relative clauses. *Journal of Psycholinguistic Research, 8,* 499–518.

deVilliers, J. G., & deVilliers, P. A. (1978). *Language acquisition.* Cambridge: Harvard University Press.

deVilliers, P. (1982). Later syntactic development: The contribution of semantics and pragmatics. Paper presented at New York State Speech-Language-Hearing Association Convention.

Dore, J. (1978). Requestive systems in nursery school conversations: Analysis of talk in its social context. In R. Campbell & P. Smith (Eds.), *Recent advances in the psychology of language: Language development and mother-child interaction* (pp. 271–292). New York: Plenum Press.

Edwards, M. L., & Shriberg, L. (1983). *Phonology: Applications in communicative disorders.* San Diego: College-Hill Press.

Ervin-Tripp, S. (1970). Discourse agreement: How children answer questions. In J. R. Hayes (Ed.), *Cognition and the development of language* (pp. 79–107). New York: Wiley.

Fine, J. (1978). Conversation, cohesive and thematic patterning in children's dialogues. *Discourse Processes, 1,* 247–266.

Garvey, C., & Hogan, R. (1973). Social speech and social interaction: Egocentrism revisited. *Child Development, 44,* 562–568.

Grunwell, P. (1982). *Clinical phonology.* Rockville, MD: Aspen Publications.

Haas, A., & Owens, R. (1985, November). Preschooler's pronoun strategies: You and me make us. Paper presented at the American Speech-Language-Hearing Association Annual Convention, Washington, DC.

Halliday, M., & Hasan, R. (1976). *Cohesion in English.* London: Longman.

Health, S. (1986). Taking a cross-cultured look at narratives. *Topics in Language Disorders, 7* (1), 84–94.

Ingram, D. (1974). Phonological rules in young children. *Journal of Child Language, 1,* 97–106.

James, S. (1990). *Normal language acquisition.* Boston: Allyn & Bacon.

Johnson, C. J., and Anglin, J. M. (1995). Qualitative development in the content and form of children's definitions. *Journal of Speech and Hearing Research, 38,* 612–625.

Karmiloff-Smith, A. (1986). Some fundamental aspects of language development after age 5. In P. Fletcher and M. Garman (Eds.), *Language Acquisition* (2nd Ed.). New York: Cambridge University Press.

Klima, E., & Bellugi, U. (1966). Syntactic regularities in the speech of children. In J. Lyons & R. Wales (Eds.), *Psycholinguistic papers* (pp. 183–208). Edinburgh: Edinburgh University Press.

Leichter, H. (1984). Families as environments for literacy. In H. Goelman, A. Oberg, and F. Smith (Eds.), *Awakening to literacy.* Exeter, NH: Heinemann Educational Books.

Lieven, E. (1984). Interactional style and children's language learning. *Topics in Language Disorders,* 4 (4), 15–23.

Litowitz, B. (1977). Learning to make definitions. *Journal of Child Language,* 4, 289–304.

Lucariello, J., & Nelson, K. (1982, March). Situational variation in mother-child interaction. Paper presented at the Third International Conference on Infant Studies, Austin, TX.

Lund, N., & Duchan, J. (1983). *Assessing children's language in naturalistic contexts.* Englewood Cliffs, NJ: Prentice Hall.

Maxwell, S. E., and Wallach, G. P. (1984). The language-learning disabilities connection: Symptoms of early language disability change over time. In G. P. Wallach and K. G. Butler (Eds.) *Language learning disabilities in school-aged children* (pp. 15–34). Baltimore: William and Wilkens.

McGhee-Bidlack, B. (1991). The development of noun definitions. A metalinguistic analysis. *Journal of Child Language,* 18, 417–434.

McLean, J., & Snyder-McLean, L. K. (1978). *A transactional approach to early language training.* Columbus, OH: Merrill/Macmillan.

Menyuk, P. (1977). *Language and maturation.* Cambridge, MA: MIT Press.

Miller, J. F. (1981). *Assessing language production in children: Experimental procedures.* Baltimore: University Park Press.

Moerk, E. L. (1975). Verbal interactions between children and their mothers during the preschool years. *Development of Psychology,* 11, 788–794.

Nelson, N. W. (1993). *Childhood language disorders in context: Infancy through adolescence.* New York: Macmillan Publishing Company.

Nippold, M., Leonard, L., & Kail, R. (1984). Syntactic and conceptual factors in children's understanding of metaphors. *Journal of Speech and Hearing Research,* 27, 197–205.

Owens, R. (1988). *Language development and communications disorders in children* (2nd ed.). Columbus, OH: Merrill/Macmillan.

Owens, R. (1996). *Language development: An introduction* (3rd ed.). Needham, MA: Allyn & Bacon.

Prather, E. M., Hedrick, D. L., & Kern, A. (1972). Articulation development in children aged two to four years. *Journal of Speech and Hearing Disorders,* 37, 55–63.

Rees, N. (1978). Pragmatics of language. In R. Schiefelbusch (Ed.), *Bases of language intervention.* Baltimore: University Park Press.

Rees, N. (1980). The nature of language. In T. Hixon, L. Shriberg, & J. Saxman (Eds.), *Introduction to communication disorders* (pp. 2–41). Englewood Cliffs, NJ: Prentice Hall.

Schultz, T. R., & Pilon, R. (1973). Development of the ability to detect linguistic ambiguity. *Child Development,* 44, 728–733.

Shatz, M., & Gelman, R. (1973). The development of communication skills: Modifications in the speech of young children as a function of listeners. *Monographs of the Society on Research on Child Development,* 38, 55.

Snow, C. (1983). Literacy and language: Relationships during the preschool years. *Harvard Educational Review,* 53 (2), 165–189.

Tanz, C. (1980). *Studies in the acquisition of deictic terms.* Cambridge: Cambridge University Press.

Templin, M. C. (1957). *Certain language skills in children: Their development and interrelationships.* Minneapolis: University of Minnesota Press.

Thorndyke, R. (1976). Reading comprehension in 15 countries. In J. Merritt (Ed.) *New horizons in reading.* Newark, DE: International Reading Association.

Tiegerman-Farber, E. (1995). *Language and communication intervention in preschool children.* Needham Heights, MA: Allyn & Bacon.

Trantham, C., & Pedersen, J. (1976). *Normal language development.* Baltimore: Williams & Wilkins.

Tough, J. (1977). *The development of meaning.* New York: Halstead Press.

Tyack, D., & Gottsleben, R. (1986). Acquisition of complex sentences. *Language, Speech, and Hearing Services in Schools, 17* (3), 160–175.

van Kleeck, A. (1995). Learning about print before learning to read. In Katherine Butler (Ed.), *Best practices II: The classroom as an intervention con-*

text (pp. 3–23). Gaithersburg, MD: Aspen Publishing Co.

Warden, D. (1976). The influence of context on children's use of identifying expressions and references. *British Journal of Psychology, 67,* 101–112.

Weiner, P. S. (1985). The value of follow-up studies. *Topics in Language Disorders,* 6 (3), 60–70.

Wiig, E. H., Gilbert, M. D., & Christian, S. H. (1978). Developmental sequences in the perception and interpretation of lexical and syntactic ambiguities. *Perceptual and Motor Skills, 46,* 959–969.

Wotten, J., Merkin, S., Hood, L., & Bloom, L. (1979). *Wh- questions; linguistic evidence, the sequence of acquisition.* Paper presented to the Society for Research in Child Development, San Francisco.

Chapter 5

Language Development: The School-Age Years

DEENA K. BERNSTEIN
Lehman College
City University of New York

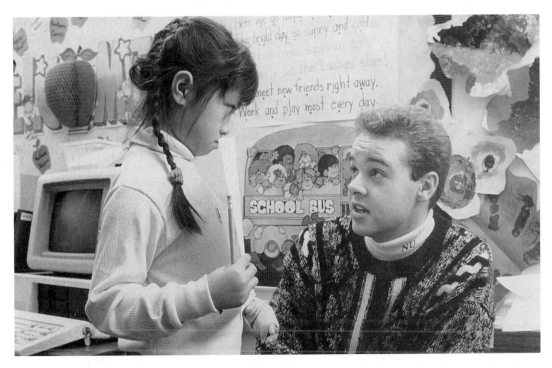

Until recently, it was assumed by many linguists that a child's language development was nearly complete by the time she entered school. However, recent research (Menyuk, 1983; Owens, 1996) tends to indicate that the school-age years are a very creative period for language development. These years are characterized by growth in all aspects of language: form, content, and use. However, the development of semantics and pragmatics seems to be the most prevalent. During this period, the child not only masters new forms but also learns to use these forms as well as existing structures to communicate more effectively She learns to clarify messages and to monitor communication that indicates the success or failure of her communicative efforts. She expands the range of her communicative functions as she learns to use language in the classroom. in this environment, the child must negotiate her turn by seeking recognition from the teacher and responding in a highly specific and precise manner to the teacher's questions. During the school-age years, the child also develops metalinguistic skills that enable her to think and talk about language. Metalinguistic skills help her master two important language-related skills that will have great impact on her life: reading and writing.

Learning to read and write requires the child to build on her oral language skills and communicate in a new mode: the visual one. This chapter includes aspects of language that develop during the school years. (A more detailed account of school-age language development can be found in Owens, 1996.) It is important for the reader to keep in mind that (a) *the later stages of language development cannot be separated from the earlier ones; language growth is a slow, gradual process;* and (b) *phonological morphological syntactic, semantic, and pragmatic acquisition in spoken language is related to the acquisition of written language.* Increasing knowledge of these later acquisitions is vital to our understanding of older children with language learning disabilities who exhibit deficits in reading and writing (Beck & Juel, 1995; Catts, 1991; 1996; Greene, 1996; Henry, 1993; Rubin, Patterson, & Kantor, 1991; Wallach, 1984).

Later Syntactic Development: An Overview

In the realm of morphology and syntax, school-age language development consists of simultaneous expansion of existing forms and acquisition of new ones. The child continues to expand her sentences by elaborating noun phrases and verb phrases. She expands her understanding and use of conjoined sentences with the addition of *therefore, although,* and *unless,* which are used to join clauses (Menyuk, 1969). Correct interpretation of these words usually does not emerge until age 7, and consistent correct comprehension may not occur until age 10 or 11 (Emerson, 1979). The child's use of embedding expands with her comprehension of more syntactically complex embedded sentences; her understanding will depend on the place and type of embedding used. (Embeddings may occur in the center of the sentence or at its end; the two clauses of the embedded sentence may share the same subject or object—called **parallel embedding**—or they may not—called **non-parallel embedding.**) The comprehension of embedded sentences progresses from the easiest to the most difficult, reflecting the child's cognitive development. Table 5-1 outlines the order in which various types of embedded sentences are acquired.

TABLE 5-1   Development Sequence of Embedded Sentence Comprehension

Type	Example
Parallel Center Embedding—same subject (*girl*) serves both clauses	The girl who bought the dress went to the party.
Parallel Ending Embedding—same object (*gift*) serves both clauses	He gave me a gift that I don't like.
Nonparallel Ending Embedding—the object of the main clause (*boy*) is the subject of the embedded clause	She hit the boy who ran away.
Nonparallel Central Embedding—the subject of the main clause (*cat*) is the object of the embedded clause	The cat that was chased by the dog ran up a tree.

Adapted from Abrahamsen & Rigrodsky (1984), Lahey (1974), and Owens (1996).

Several morphological structures also emerge during the early school-age years. By school age, 6-year-olds are just beginning to produce gerunds (Menyuk, 1969). **Gerunds** are verbs to which -*ing* has been added to produce a form that fulfills a noun function. (For example, *to fish* becomes *fishing;* "Fishing is fun.") Between 6 and 7 years of age, children also acquire the derivational morphemes, which change verbs into nouns; for example, -*er* (*catcher*), -*man* (*fireman*), and -*ist* (*cyclist*) (Carrow, 1973). Last, the adverbial -*ly* is understood and produced after the age of 7.

By the end of the second grade, children comprehend irregular noun and verb agreement ("The fish are eating," "The sheep is sleeping"), the implicit negative ("Find the one that is *neither* red *nor* blue"), and several verb tenses, such as the past participle (*had eaten*) and the perfect (*has been eating*).

Although children 5 to 7 years of age are able to use most elements of the noun and verb phrase, they frequently omit them. Even at age 7, they will omit some elements (articles) while expanding others, such as double negatives, redundantly. In addition, children of school age may still have difficulty with some prepositions, verb tensing, and plurals (Menyuk, 1969). And they are just beginning to learn to use reflexive pronouns (*myself, himself, herself*) and to use pronouns across sentences. (The use of pronouns anaphorically is discussed in Chapter 4.)

During the preschool years, reversible passive sentences ("The boy was hit by the ball") are difficult for children to understand and produce because the passive sentence violates the child's strategy of seeking "who did what to whom" from the word order. Children do not begin to abandon this strategy until after 6 years of age, at which time their comprehension of passive sentences begins to improve (Bridges, 1980). As for passive sentence formulation, only about 80 percent of 7½- to 8-year-olds produce full passive sentences (Baldie, 1976). The development of passive sentence understanding and production continues through age 9, and researchers have reported that some passive forms do not appear until children are 11 years of age (Horgan, 1978).

Other linguistic forms are acquired during the school-age years. The ability to distinguish between mass and count nouns and their quantifiers grows slowly (Gathercole, 1985).

Mass nouns refer to nonindividual substances that are homogeneous, such as *water, sand,* and *money.* **Count nouns** refer to heterogeneous individual objects such as a *glass, toy,* or *house.* Mass nouns take different quantifying modifiers (*much* and *little*) than those (*many* and *few*) taken by count nouns. By early elementary school the child has learned most of the correct noun forms, so that words like *monies* and *mens* are rare. *Many* then appears with plural count nouns, as in *many houses. Much* is usually learned by late elementary school, although the adolescent still makes many errors. Early on the child discovers a way around the quantifier question by using *lots of* with both types of nouns (Owens, 1996).

Summary

During the school-age years, the child adds new morphological and syntactic structures to her linguistic repertoire and expands and refines existing forms. These developments enable her to express increasingly more complex relationships and to use language more creatively.

In the next section I will discuss semantic development during the school-age years. The focus will be on two aspects of meaning: vocabulary growth and the development of nonliteral meaning.

Semantic Development

Vocabulary

During the school-age years, the child increases the size of her vocabulary and the specificity of her word definition (Crais, 1990). Gradually she acquires an abstract knowledge of meaning that is independent of particular contexts or individual interpretations. But adding lexical items is only a portion of the change that occurs in a child's vocabulary growth. Meaning increases in two directions: horizontal and vertical (McNeil, 1970). **Horizontal meaning** is the child's addition to a single definition features that are common to the adult definition. **Vertical meaning** involves bringing together all the definitions of a single word. Both horizontal and vertical growth occur during the school years. Between the ages of 7 and 11, the child makes significant increases in the comprehension of words that represent spatial, temporal, familial, and logical relationships. In addition, the child acquires the meaning of many words that have multiple meanings (Menyuk, 1971, Owens, 1996).

Differences between the abilities of older and younger school-age children become evident when defining words. Whereas preschoolers define words narrowly in terms of their sentence meaning, children in the middle-school years can abstract and synthesize meaning to form new definitions. During the school years, children also move from defining words according to individual experiences to defining words with more socially shared meanings (Litowitz, 1977). In addition, their definitions move from single words to sentences that express complex relationships, a shift that occurs at about the second grade (Wehren, DeLisi, & Arnold, 1981). Similar shifts in definition content occur throughout the grade-school years. In high school, adolescents' definitions are abstract and/or represent a concept of function modified by perceptual attributes. The definitions of upper-high-school children (as well as of adults) tend to be descriptive, having concrete terms of references to specific instances used to modify a concept, and contain synonyms, explanations, and categorizations. (Johnson & Anglin, 1995).

Vocabulary knowledge is highly correlated with general linguistic competence and academic aptitude. Acquiring a broad vocabulary will allow the child not only to understand and express more complex ideas with great facility but also to achieve a higher degree of competency in reading and writing.

The Development of Nonliteral Meaning

Nonliteral meaning adds richness and depth to language by communicating indirectly what would otherwise be communicated directly. Consider the meaning in the metaphor "Her eyes were ice" or in the proverb "The early bird catches the worm." Metaphors, proverbs, and jokes are examples of **nonliteral language**—language that doesn't mean what it says. The understanding and use of nonliteral meaning depend on the ability to disregard literal interpretation and to rely on nonreferential, abstract, general meaning. Current research that focuses on the development of nonliteral meaning—specifically, on the understanding and use of metaphoric language, idioms, proverbs, and humor—is discussed in the following section.

Metaphoric Language.   Studies dealing with children's comprehension and use of nonliteral language have focused on **metaphors,** which use a likeness to stand for a word, a referent, or an idea ("He has a heart of stone"). When metaphoric language is marked by the connectives *as* or *like*, it is called a **simile** ("It is as light as air").

The basic ability to comprehend nonliteral language emerges early and continues to develop with time (Bernstein, 1987; Nippold, 1985, 1991; Nippold, Leonard, & Kail, 1984). in the development process (Winner, Rosentiel, & Gardner, 1976), young children understand cross-sensory metaphors ("Her perfume was bright as sunshine") better than psychological-physical metaphors ("The prison guard was a hard rock"). In addition, similarity metaphors, in which objects are compared on the basis of shared features ("The stars are a thousand eyes"), are comprehended better than proportional metaphors, in which three objects are mentioned and a fourth must be inferred to complete a proportion ("My head is like an apple without a core"). Performance on each of the more difficult metaphoric types increases with age. Billow (1975) suggested that the precise use and understanding of metaphors are related to the cognitive abilities attained in adolescence. At this stage, children are able to understand that figurative language is based on a variety of links between domains.

Idioms.   Figurative, nonliteral expressions that express complex ideas in colorful and concise ways are called idioms. Included in different idiomatic types are semantically based idioms that can be assigned to various categories (foods—*sour grapes,* animals—*dark horse,* colors—*in the red*). Idiom comprehension is a skill that develops slowly and improves throughout childhood, adolescence, and into the adult years (Nippold, 1988, 1991; Nippold & Taylor, 1995, Nippold & Martin, 1989, Nippold & Taylor, 1995). Although preschoolers comprehend the nonliteral meaning of some idioms, their literal interpretation predominates during early childhood. As children are exposed to and encounter a larger number of idioms in various contexts, they tend to give idioms a more nonliteral interpretation.

Proverbs.   Another form of nonliteral language, **proverbs** are more abstract than metaphors. In a proverb, the domain that is the topic is never mentioned. Wise sayings such as "Don't put all your eggs in one basket" or "A stitch in time saves nine" mean something more general and abstract than their literal meaning. The real topic is never named. Billow (1975) found that preadolescents are generally unable to interpret proverbs and that it is not until adolescence that proverbs are understood.

Humor.   We often infer information about children's semantic knowledge (or lack of knowledge) from the riddles and jokes they understand and tell (Bernstein, 1986). The source of humor in riddles and jokes is largely semantically based. It depends on understanding words that sound the same but are spelled differently (*bear, bare*) or words that sound the same and are spelled the same way but have more than one meaning (*glasses, nail*). The comprehension of humor often depends on perceiving the incongruity among the meanings of homonyms or multiple-meaning words.

Fowles and Glanz (1977) found that before age 6, children tell jokes in a confused manner and show no evidence of riddle structure. Between 6 and 9 years of age, children understand the frame of riddles but not their meaning. When telling riddles, 6- to 9-year-olds delete or add portions to the riddle, making it informative rather than puzzling. When asked to explain jokes and riddles, 6- to 9-year-olds tend to be quite literal. They may identify something in the joke or riddle as funny but do not recognize that the riddle's language is contributing to its humor. Note the explanation of a riddle given by a child in Fowles and Glanz's study (1977):

Question: How do you keep fish from smelling?

Answer: Cut off their noses.

Child's Explanation: It's funny because I don't think fish really have noses.

After 9 years of age, children tell riddles using the appropriate structure. Their explanation of jokes and riddles focuses on the attributes of language that contribute to the humor rather than on the nonlinguistic situation.

Jokes, another form of humor, require suspending the usual literal meaning to appreciate the unexpected. The comprehension of jokes often depends on an incongruity or a sudden shift in perspective.

Researchers have identified different joke types (Lund & Duchan, 1983) as well as an order in which they are acquired (Shultz & Horibe, 1974). Before age 6, children understand only nonlinguistic, pie-in-the-face jokes. Between 6 and 9 years of age, children become sensitive to jokes that are based on the phonological structure of a word or a group of words within the utterance (Lund & Duchan, 1983).

Man: What is this?

Waiter: It's bean soup.

Man: I don't care what it's been. What is it now?

Between 9 and 12 years of age, children begin to develop an appreciation of humor that depends on a dual interpretation of a lexical item (multiple-meaning word).

Question: What is black, white, and red (read) all over?

Answer: A newspaper.

After 12 years of age, children appreciate humor that involves alternative deep structure of the same surface structure.

Question: What animal can jump higher than a house?

Answer: Any animal. Houses can't jump.

Although research in this area is relatively new (Bernstein, 1986), current investigations are beginning to shed light on children's development of various types of nonliteral meanings.

Summary

In this section, current trends in the study of children's later semantic development were presented. I examined children's development of vocabulary and their understanding and use of nonliteral meaning as evidenced by their comprehension and use of figurative language and humor. (These areas of semantic development are assessed during a language evaluation and may be targeted for remediation if found deficient. For a discussion of se7mantic assessment, see Chapter 7.)

The next section traces the expansion of school-age children's use of language in social contexts. The focus will be on pragmatic development; that is, the increased social use of language and the development of discourse skills.

Pragmatic Development

The most important area of linguistic growth during the school-age years is in language use, or pragmatics. Throughout the school years children increase their range of communication functions and learn how to become good conversational partners, how to make indirect requests, and how to process the language of the classroom.

Two processes enable the child to become a more effective communicator: neo-egocentrism and decentration. **Neo-egocentrism** is the ability to take the perspective of another person. (This ability has also been called presuppositional ability.) In general, as a communication task becomes more difficult, the child is less able to take a speaker's perspective. As the child advances cognitively and socially and gains greater facility with language structure, she can concentrate more effectively on her audience. Being able to shift perspective enables her to consider what the listener knows (and needs to know) when she constructs a message. This ability is refined during the school years. Being neo-egocentric also allows the child greater facility in the use of deictic terms. You will recall that the understanding and use of these terms depend on the nonlinguistic context—the perspective of the speaker and the listener. The acquisition of deictic terms begins in the preschool period and advances during the school years.

Decentration is the ability to consider several aspects of a problem simultaneously. This cognitive achievement allows the child to move from one-dimensional descriptions of objects and events to coordinated, multi-attributional ones. The child recognizes that there are many dimensions that can be used to describe an object or an event and adjusts her messages accordingly (Owens, 1996). Whereas a younger child's descriptions are more personal and do not consider the information that must be available to the listener, a school-age child's messages are more accurate because the child considers the listener's perspective and provides more extensive information. Thus, the school years bring the development of new and more effective communication strategies. By the time children reach Piaget's concrete operational stage, they perceive the needs of their listeners and make undifferentiated adaptations in their communication to satisfy those needs. In settling peer disputes, children give reasons for disagreements involving their own feelings and beliefs about an event or an action. In the stage of formal operations, children adapt to their listeners' needs in a differentiated manner by negotiating, justifying, and stating reasons for their positions. Table 5-2 summarizes the different communication strategies used by children in Piaget's preoperational, concrete, and formal operational stages.

Expansion of Communicative Functions

In addition to the wide variety of communicative functions that preschoolers use, the changing world of the school-age child requires her to use language in a wider variety of social contexts. The child's social-emotional and cognitive skills enable her to expand her repertoire of language use. White (1975) maintained that the school-age child displays the following communicative abilities and talents:

1. To gain and hold adults' attention in a socially acceptable manner
2. To direct and follow peers
3. To use others, when appropriate, as resources for assistance for information
4. To express affection, hostility, and anger, when appropriate
5. To express pride in herself and her accomplishments
6. To role-play
7. To compete with peers in storytelling

Narratives

By the time children are in school, they exhibit a storytelling talent; that is, they can communicate information through coherent and cohesive units called **narratives.** As toddlers, children are exposed to narratives, or stories, in picture books and on television. They begin to relate stories early in the preschool years. By first grade, demands are placed on them to relate narratives: participating in show-and-tell, relating vacation activities or holiday experiences, or retelling a story previously heard. These are activities common to all first- and second-grade children and later appear in the form of written assignments. "My Summer Vacation," "How I Spent the Holidays," or a synopsis of a book are frequently assigned topics for speeches and compositions.

Narratives are a form of discourse. They contain sentences and statements that are logically connected to reflect causal and temporal relationships. They also contain principles

TABLE 5-2   **Communication Strategy Development: An Overview**

Cognitive Stage	Strategy	Examples
Preoperational (ages 2–7)		
Early	Self-oriented perception Nonadaptation to listener	CONTEXT: Jim and John in sandbox. John wants to play with the pail and shovel. Jim is playing with it. JOHN: Gimme pail and shovel.
Late	Perception of listener Nonadaptation to listener	CONTEXT: Sue and Jean are in the yard. Sue has been riding the bike for 5 minutes. JEAN: Now *I* want to ride the bike!
Concrete (ages 7–11)	Perception of listener Undifferentiated adaptation to listener	CONTEXT: Bill and Sam are on the playground. BILL: Please, pretty please, can I try your baseball glove? CONTEXT: Linda borrowed Stacy's pen. LINDA: I'm sorry I broke your pen.
Formal (ages 11–14)	Perception of listener Differentiated adaptation to listener needs	CONTEXT: Jason and Peter are on the playground. JASON: If you'll let me try your mitt, I'll let you try my head-to-head football game. (Jason takes the game out of his pocket.) CONTEXT: Lisa has returned from school. Her mother is upset. LISA: I know you're upset, but the English teacher assigned a composition about El Salvador for tomorrow, and I stopped off at the library to get some books to do the research.

and structure that give them cohesiveness. One perspective on the nature and structure of narratives is seen in the work of Stein (1978). Stein and Glenn (1979) suggested that stories are combined according to various categories, or units, and rules. Category definitions and rules of the story grammar model, as outlined by Johnston (1982), are shown in Table 5-3.

According to Stein and Glenn (1979), stories have an internal structure, and competent storytellers structure their information in a form that guarantees the full understanding of the story. They sequence and organize events in time and space so that the consequential nature of the story is ensured.

When children hear stories in which the information sequences (as shown in Table 5-3) are inverted (for example, they are told the consequence unit before the initiating event), they remember them less well than if the story is told to them in the order given by the model. If children are given individual narrative statements and asked to make up a story, the sequence of their stories correlates highly with the sequence predicted by the story

TABLE 5-3   Story Grammar Model

STORY = SETTING UNIT + EPISODE STRUCTURE

SETTING UNIT—introduction of main characters, protagonist, context of time and place

EPISODE STRUCTURE—initiating event + internal response + plan + attempt + consequences + reaction unit

Initiating Event—action or occurrence that influences the main characters

Internal Response—characters' motivations, thoughts, and feelings about the initiating event

Plan Unit—protagonist's intended action or verbal responses to the initiating event

Attempt Unit—protagonist's actions in pursuit of the goal

Consequence Unit—outcome of the attempt; success or failure of the protagonist

Reaction Unit—protagonist's response to the outcome

Based on Stein (1978). Adapted from "Narratives: A New Look at Communication Problems in Older Language Disordered Children" by J. Johnston, 1982, *Language, Speech and Hearing Services in Schools, 13,* pp. 144–155. Copyright 1982 by the American Speech-Language-Hearing Association. Reprinted by permission.

grammar model. Also, when asked to retell a story, children are most likely to include the setting unit, initiating event, and the consequence unit.

Although children use the schematic knowledge of story grammars to understand stories and to formulate narratives, there are developmental differences between the abilities of younger and older children to formulate these narratives. The following characteristics are more likely to be found in the stories of 10-year-olds:

1. Greater detail in the setting information
2. More complex episode structure
3. More concern with motivations, thoughts, and feelings of the character
4. Less extraneous detail in general; greater detail in the internal response unit
5. Greater information regarding changes in time and place
6. Fewer unresolved problems
7. Greater adherence to the story grammar model (Clancy, 1979; Crais & Lorch, 1994; Keman, 1977; Owens, 1996; Stein & Glenn, 1979).

Crais and Lorch (1994) identified other features characteristic of the narratives of school age children. These include:

1. Embedding of one episode into another
2. Including multiple episodes in a narrative
3. The referencing of emotional states
4. Producing double meanings and mystery stories
5. Attitude statements and story evaluations

The older adolescent storyteller not only utilizes the above abilities but also uses argumentation and dramatization, and includes asides and morals in their narratives (Larson & McKinley, 1995).

Conversation

As noted in the previous chapter, the preschool child is not very adept at repairing her messages when she has not been understood. During the school-age years, the child learns to clarify her conversation with a variety of strategies (Konefal & Folks, 1984). Rather than repeating a message verbatim, as most 3- to 5-year-olds do, a 6-year-old will elaborate some elements in her repetition, enabling her to provide more information to the listener. The 9-year-old not only elaborates her repetition but also seems capable of addressing the perceived source of communication breakdown. She provides additional input for her listener by clarifying her messages, repairs her conversation by defining her terms, provides background context, and monitors her own communication. Last, she is sensitive to cues that indicate the failure of her communicative attempt and can talk about the process of conversational repair (Brinton, Fujiki, Loeb, & Winkler, 1986, Crais & Lorch, 1994; Hulit & Howard, 1993). Much of the control of conversation during the young school-age years is exercised by adults who ask children many questions. First graders' responses to adults' questions are usually brief, simple, and appropriate, whereas school-age children's responses to peer questions tend to be more complex, more elaborate, and of a great variety (Mischler, 1976).

During the school-age years, approximately 60 percent of children's peer interactions are effective. Effectiveness is measured by the clarity and structural completeness of the message sent, the relevance to the situation, the form of the utterance, and the requirement for and maintenance of attention (Mueller, 1972). When they talk to their peers, 8-year-olds speak differently than when addressing infants or adults. When speaking with infants, school-age children tend to reduce the length and complexity of their utterances, appearing to understand that very young children require a different form of interaction. Among adults, school-age children vary their codes for parents and for those outside the family. In general, parents are usually the recipients of demands, whining, and short (less conversational) narrative (Owens, 1996). It is not surprising that parents are often shocked when their child, who talks to them with language that is less than polite and informative, is described by other adults as charming, entertaining, and interesting.

During the older school age years, conversation becomes more demanding for adolescents. It is an important medium for them for social interaction. During conversation, they add information during their turn and also can "shade" from one topic to another (Larson & McKinley, 1995).

During this period, the adolescent can make transitions between formal and informal language, relying more on formal registers with not only adults, but their peers as well (unless particularly close to the peer). Modification of the verb phrase is key in switching between informal and formal codes (e.g., "Pass me my pen" as opposed to "would you pass me my pen"); a skill that the adolescent masters. Lastly, conversation directed to peers by adolescents usually involves more expressed feelings than conversation directed toward adults (Larson & McKinley, 1995).

Topic Maintenance

Almost from the time the child begins to speak, she is able to discuss topics briefly. However, the 3-year-old can sustain a topic of conversation only 20 percent of the time. Topic maintenance in preschoolers usually occurs only when the previous utterance of the child's partner was a topic-sharing response to one of the child's prior utterances (Bloom, Rocissano, & Hood, 1976). In other words, in the preschool years children change conversational topics very rapidly. However, the school-age child can not only introduce, close, or switch a conversational topic but, more importantly, can sustain it through several turns. These skills develop gradually through elementary school and contrast sharply with the preschooler's performance. in general, the proportion of introduced topics maintained in subsequent turns increases with age. The greatest change occurs during the years from late elementary school to adulthood (Brinton & Fujiki, 1984, Nelson, 1993). A related decrease in the number of different topics introduced or reintroduced occurs during this same period. Thus, the school years bring a growing adherence to the concept of conversational relevance and topic maintenance. Although an 8-year-old can sustain a topic through a number of conversational turns, her topics tend to be concrete. Discussions involving abstract topics usually are not sustained until age 11 (Owens, 1996).

Indirect Requests

Another dimension of pragmatic development that occurs during the school-age years is the ability to use indirect requests. The development of indirect requests is particularly noteworthy because it represents the child's growing awareness of both socially appropriate requests and the communication context (Hulit & Howard, 1993).

All of us are aware of indirect requests such as "It's awfully hot in here." This directive is an indirect request for lowering the heat or opening a window, for example. Indirect requests are first produced in the preschool years; the proportion of their occurrence to direct requests increases between the ages of 3 and 5 (Garvey, 1977). This proportion does not change markedly between ages 5 and 6 (Levin & Rubin, 1982). In general, the 5-year-old gets what she wants by asking for it *directly*. By age 7, however, she gains greater facility with indirect forms (Garvey, 1975; Grimm, 1975). Flexibility in the use of indirect requests continues to increase with age; for example, Ervin-Tripp (1980) found that the proportion of hints ("That sweater would go so nicely with my new skirt") increases from childhood through adulthood.

Language in the Classroom

The language of the classroom, where children are expected to do most of their formal learning, differs from that used in informal social interactions. In the classroom, children are expected to process the language of the teacher and the language of the textbooks. As grade level increases, so does the complexity of the language that the students are expected to process (Nelson, 1986; see also Chapter 9). Children with language abilities commensurate with the linguistic demands of the classroom do well in school. However, children who have linguistic deficits have difficulty with those same linguistic demands and feel both emotional and social repercussions (Gerber, 1981; Nelson, 1985, 1993).

The language of the classroom differs in several ways from the language spoken at home. Children of preschool age receive their major linguistic input from caretakers and can rely on the familiarity of the home context to help them understand what is expected of them. Because language at home depends heavily on context, children can act appropriately by following familiar routines, even if they understand only a little of what is presented to them linguistically. In addition, interactions between children and caretakers during the preschool years is dyadic; if children misunderstand the language directed to them, their caretakers repair the message. In school (and as children advance through the grades), however, teachers use long sentences, more complex syntactic structures, and more rapid speaking rates (Cuda & Nelson, 1976; Nelson, 1986, 1993). They provide very little nonverbal support for their linguistic messages. Lastly, the group communication of the classroom context allows less opportunity for conversational repairs to be made when communication breakdowns occur. Thus, language in the classroom is highly **decontextualized.** That is, there are few contextual cues that the child can rely on to better understand classroom language. Because of the increased linguistic demands of the classroom, children with language learning deficits often cannot benefit maximally from classroom instruction. The consultative role of speech-language pathologists in relation to classroom teachers who instruct these children is discussed more fully in Chapter 9.

Summary

As the child gains greater facility with the form and content of language, she is able to concentrate more on language use. As her communicative functions increase, she is able to participate more fully in conversation and she learns to process the language of the classroom. In the next section, I will focus on children's abilities to think about language independently of their comprehension and production ability.

The Development of Metalinguistic Abilities

During the preschool period, children view language primarily as a means of communication. They do not focus on the manner in which language is conveyed (Van Kleeck, 1982). During the school-age years, the child begins to reflect on language as a decontextualized object. This ability, called **metalinguistic ability,** enables the child to think and talk about language; that is, to treat language as an object of analysis and to use language to talk about language. The development of metalinguistic abilities is most obvious during middle childhood, between about 5 and 8 years of age.

Van Kleeck (1984) identified three important aspects of metalinguistic development: (a) recognizing that language is an arbitrary conventional code, (b) recognizing that language is a system of units and rules for combining those units, and (c) recognizing that language is used for communication. These three aspects involve awareness of all of the components of the linguistic system—phonological, morphological, syntactic, semantic, and pragmatic.

Understanding that language is an arbitrary conventional code includes understanding that words are arbitrary labels, separate from the objects or events they represent. Young children do not recognize the arbitrary nature of language; thus, they tend to treat words as though they were part of their referents. For example, a 4-year-old might say that the word *jet* is a big word because jets are big and that *ant* is a short word because ants are short. In contrast, a 7-year-old is likely to say that the word *jet* is a small word because it doesn't have many letters. Evidence of the arbitrary nature of language can also be seen in children's ability to recognize ambiguity, that is, that words and sentences can have more than one meaning. An example of detecting ambiguity would be recognizing that the sentence "The duck is ready to eat" could mean either (a) the duck (that is in the field) is ready to eat some grass or (b) the duck (which has been cooked) is ready to be served for dinner. Another metalinguistic skill that depends on the awareness that language is an arbitrary code is the ability to understand that different sentence forms can convey the same meaning. This ability is called **recognizing synonymy.** An example of recognizing synonymy would be realizing that the following sentences describe the same event: "The girl chased the boy," "The boy was chased by the girl," and "It was the girl who chased the boy." Children are not able to either detect ambiguity or recognize synonymy until the early to middle elementary school years (Tunmer, Pratt, & Herriman, 1984).

The awareness that language is a system of units is demonstrated by children's ability to break down larger linguistic units into smaller parts. This ability allows the child to divide the sentence "The dog chased the cat" into five words.

It also enables the child to "break down" the word *cat* into three phonemes. The ability to segment words into their component sounds is a result of the child's phonological awareness. Phonological awareness is also evident in the preschool child's ability to rhyme, and the school-age child's ability to group words together based on their common sounds (e.g.,/pen/ and /pot/ both begin with /p/), reverse phonemes (e.g., the child's game Pig Latin), and delete phonemes (e.g., /tin/ without the /t/ is in/) (Wallach & Butler, 1994; Owens, 1996).

You will recall (see previous chapter) that some areas of phonological awareness can be developed in preschool children. Home factors such as time spent on word play, nursery or Dr. Suess rhymes, and general exposure to story books appears to contribute to phonological awareness. In a 15-month longitudinal study of British children, Maclean, Bryant, and Bradley (1987) found a strong relationship between children's early knowledge of rhyme and the later development of philological awareness. In addition, phonological awareness predicted early reading ability.

Last, there is considerable evidence that indicates that deficits in phonological awareness and phonological processing are implicated in reading disabilities (Catts, 1996; Torgensen, Wagner, & Rashotte, 1994).

Also emerging during the early school years is children's ability to recognize that linguistic rules must be used to combine units (Owens, 1996; Ryan & Ledger, 1984). This ability is illustrated by children's awareness of the grammatical acceptability of sentences, for example, judging that the utterance "The cat chasing the dog" is ungrammatical. The child could make it acceptable either by adding an auxiliary verb (*is* or *was*) or by changing the progressive form to the third person singular (*chases*) or the past tense (*chased*).

Although children use language to communicate even in the earliest stages of language development, their awareness of the communicative nature of language does not develop until later. Preschool-age children demonstrate some awareness of the social rules for language use (Bates, 1976), but it is not until the early elementary school years that children can judge the adequacy and appropriateness of their messages—what constitutes good communication. Table 5-4 outlines the metalinguistic abilities that develop during the school-age years. Note that these abilities involve understanding of all the components of language—form, content, and use.

TABLE 5-4 Metalinguistic Abilities of School-Age Children

I. Recognizing that language is an arbitrary conventional code
  A. Understanding and using multiple-meaning words
  B. Understanding and using figurative language
  C. Using different sentence forms to express the same meaning
  D. Detecting ambiguous sentences and explaining their ambiguity
II. Recognizing language as a system of units and rules for combining those units
  A. Segmenting words into phonemes and sentences into words
  B. Judging grammatically
  C. Correcting ungrammatical sentences
  D. Applying appropriate inflections to new words
III. Recognizing that language is used for communication
  A. Judging utterances as appropriate for a specific listener or setting
  B. Awareness of the politeness of various request form

Metalinguistic abilities emerge about the same time children are learning to read. It has been suggested that metalinguistic awareness and reading development are related (Blackman & James, 1985; Catts, 1996; Saywitz & Cherry-Wilkinson, 1982; Tanmer & Bowey, 1984; Van Kleeck, 1995).

Research has also shown that some language-disordered children demonstrate deficits in metalinguistic abilities (Kamhi & Koenig, 1986; Van Kleeck, 1995; Wallach & Butler, 1994), and that metalinguistic and language processing deficits underlie reading disabilities (Brady & Shankweiler, 1991; Catts, 1996; Catts & Kamhi, 1987; Fletcher et al., 1994; Vellutino, Scanlon, Small, & Tanzman, 1991). Silliman and James (Chapter 7) suggest that speech-language pathologists need to assess metalinguistic abilities in school-age children suspected of having a language disorder or a reading disability.

Learning to Read

Preliteracy

In the previous chapter, I introduced the concept of emergent literacy and preliteracy preparation. As noted, for most children, the introduction to written language is a gradual process that begins in infancy with the child's first baby book and is augmented by parents and caretakers who read storybooks or recite the alphabet. These activities give the child tools to develop models of reading and writing. Slowly the child becomes aware that books are full of words that tell stories (Sulzby, 1981) and that words are made up of letters (written by people). Narratives and stories help children learn that language can be used in a more decontextualized manner—that is, language can describe events outside the context of their own lives (Heath, 1982) and can create make-believe tales (Rubin & Wolf, 1979; Wolf & Dickinson, 1993). Chomsky (1972) examined a range of factors that contribute to early success in reading. She found that the single largest factor in the child's achievement of reading skills begins at home.

Certain kinds of TV programs can also encourage preliteracy skills in children (Lesser, 1974). Lesser found that *Sesame Street* and *The Electric Company* (no longer produced) had an impact on very specific aspects of early reading, such as alphabet learning and recognizing words that rhyme.

Familiarity with nursery rhymes also appears to be correlated with better reading skills (Bryant, Bradley, MacLean, & Crossland, 1989). Nursery rhymes help children become sensitive to rhymes and phonemes and provide experience with language play, a building block for metalinguistic skills.

It appears that both the home and a child's preschool experiences have an impact on literacy acquisition (Van Kleeck, 1995; Wolf & Dickinson, 1993). The existing research also tends to indicate that the earlier the exposure to print, the better the early reader will be.

Linguistic Bases of Reading

Reading is a complex process that is not totally understood by development and education professionals. However, it is believed that reading is the synthesis of a network of perceptual and cognitive acts along a continuum from word recognition and decoding skills to comprehension and integration. Skilled readers draw conclusions and inferences from what they have read. The following sections describe the linguistic bases of reading by examining the reading process and outlining reading development. This information should provide guidance to speech-language pathologists and special educators on the role of language in reading and reading disabilities. A detailed analysis of these issues is beyond the scope of this chapter; interested readers are urged to refer to Owens (1996), Wolf and Dickinson (1993), Chall (1983), Vellutino (1977, 1979; Vellutino et al., 1991; and Catts, 1996). Because speech-language pathologists target linguistic structures in their therapy with language learning disabled as well as reading disabled children (see Chapter 11), their understanding of the links between oral language, reading, and reading problems is crucial (Catts & Kamhi, 1987; Rees, 1974; Stark, 1975; Catts, 1996; Greene, 1996; Moats & Lyon, 1996). For many years, reading was considered primarily a visually based, perceptual activity. Thus, children with reading disorders were believed to have visual problems, and remediation focused on correcting this deficit. During the 1960s and 1970s, however, researchers challenged this assumption and replaced it with an entirely new viewpoint (Kavanagh & Mattingly, 1972; Liberman, Shankweiler, Liberman, Fowler, & Fischer, 1977). They stated that reading was language-based (Vellutino, 1977, 1979; Catts, 1996) and that vision's role in reading was limited. Liberman (1973) stated that reading was parasitic on language, and Mattingly (1972) wrote:

> *Reading is seen not as a parallel activity in the visual mode to speech perception in the auditory mode.* . . . Reading . . . is a *deliberately acquired,* language based skill, dependent upon the speaker-hearer's awareness of certain aspects of primary linguistic activity. (p. 145) (emphasis added)

The impact of this view on reading instruction in general, and on the diagnosis and remediation of children with reading disabilities in particular, cannot be overemphasized.

Children with reading impairment, whom neurologists had long suspected of language dysfunction (Denckla, 1972), began to be perceived by the educational community as exhibiting a broad variety of disorders. At the root of most of those disorders were language problems; visual disturbances caused only one small group (Mattis, French, & Rapin, 1975). Although work remains to be done in classifying reading disorders, the emphasis on the relationship between language and reading has dramatically changed clinical and diagnostic work in this area (Catts, 1996; Catts & Kamhi, 1987; Dickinson et al., 1993; Greene, 1996; Vellutino et al., 1991).

Models of Reading

Since the early 1970s, various theoretical models of reading have been proposed, including many from the cognitive sciences that attempt to describe the underlying process of reading. It is beyond the scope of this chapter to detail these reading models. However, it is important to point out that these models largely share the assumption that reading is a complex, language-based, componential process that requires automaticity for rapid processing to function. Theoretical positions that attempt to explain the processes involved in reading follow two major approaches. They are termed the bottom-up approach and the top-down approach, and they describe the extremes of a theoretical continuum. Most professionals, however, believe that an intermediate approach—the interactive approach—more appropriately describes the reading process.

The Bottom-Up Approach.   Theories that subscribe to the **bottom-up approach** conclude that "reading is the translation of written elements into language" (Perfetti, 1984, p. 41). Bottom-up theories emphasize lower level perceptual and phonemic processes and their influence on higher cognitive functioning. According to this view, knowledge of the perceptual features of letters and of their correspondence to sounds aids word recognition and decoding. Bottom-up theories propose that the processing of textual material is the same as the processing of oral language, except for breaking the grapheme code (Owens, 1996).

Bottom-up theory assumes that the child must learn to decode print into language. That is, the child must be able to divide each word into phonemic elements—and also learn the alphabetical letters (graphemes) that correspond to these phonemes. Only when this process is automatic can the child give sufficient attention to the meaning of the text. If the child gains automaticity processing at the visual and auditory levels, the other stages of processing will be more easily acquired. According to the bottom-up theory, each word acts like a switchboard that activates the visual, auditory, and semantic features of that word. If the reader has enough information from these features, the information is automatically presented to the other parts of the system for processing. In sum, the bottom-up theory of reading emphasizes that lower level processes (e.g., perceptual and phonological stages) critically influence all further stages of processing.

Top-Down Approach.   In contrast to the bottom-up theories, theories that subscribe to the **top-down approach** emphasize the cognitive task of deriving meaning from print. This approach has been termed the problem-solving approach (Owens, 1996). Higher cognitive functions, such as concepts, inferences, and levels of meaning, influence the processing of lower order information. The reader generates hypotheses about the written material based on her world knowledge, the content of the material in the text, and the syntactic structures used. Sampling of the reading confirms or disconfirms the hypotheses.

The top-down model views reading as a "psycholinguistic guessing game" (Goodman, 1976) in which the reader uses her knowledge of language as well as her conceptual knowledge to aid her in recognizing words sequentially (Bransford & Johnson, 1972; Smith, 1971).

Interactive Approach.   The **interactive approach** to explaining the reading process incorporates portions of both bottom-up and top-down models (Rumelhart, 1977; Stanovich, 1980). According to this view, top-down and bottom-up processes provide information to the reader simultaneously, at various levels of analysis. This information is then synthesized. The processes are interactive, and relative reliance on each varies with the skills of the reader and the material that is being read. It has been proposed that by third or fourth grade, children rely on a bottom-up strategy when reading isolated words and a top-down strategy when reading text. Context supports the more rapid, top-down processes; when such support is lacking, the slower, bottom-up processes are used.

Although variations on bottom-up and top-down models of reading abound, all researchers agree that learning to read requires the integration of multiple sensory, perceptual, linguistic, and conceptual processing strategies. The importance of higher level language processing in constructing the meaning of text can be appreciated when we consider the strategies used by mature readers. These are discussed more fully in Chapters 7 and 11.

Reading Development

Five stages of reading development have been identified (Chall, 1983). At the prereading stage (prior to age 6), the child learns to recognize and discriminate between the letters of the alphabet. At this stage, most children are able to scan print, identify letters, recognize their name in print, and read a few memorized words such as those seen on common signs (*stop, exit*).

In stage one of reading development (through approximately the second grade), the child concentrates on decoding single words in simple stories. Meaningful words in context are read faster than random words (Doehring, 1976). At this stage, the child relies heavily on the visual configuration of a word in order to recognize it (Torrey, 1979). She pays particular attention to the first letter of the word and the word length while ignoring the order of the letters. Next, the child learns letter-sound correspondence rules, recognizes their importance, and is able to sound out novel words by using the phonetic approach. In addition, the child learns that the text provides messages and does more than just describe pictures (Ferreiro & Teberosky, 1982). Thus, first grade oral readers begin to use the text to analyze unknown words. Whenever they read a word incorrectly, it is because they have substituted a word that makes sense in the context for a word they do not know. Whereas poor readers in the first two grades tend to make wild guesses when analyzing unknown words (Biemiller, 1970), good readers try to use contextual clues to figure them out.

By stage two (approximately the third and fourth grades) the child's ability to analyze unknown words by using orthographic patterns and contextual inferences is firmly established. At stage three (from the fourth to the eighth grade) the emphasis in reading shifts from decoding skills to comprehension. During this stage the child's scanning rate continues to increase and her ability to answer complex questions based on textual material is tested in the classroom. By secondary school—stage four—lower level skills are firmly established. The adolescent must use higher level skills, such as inference and the recognition of the author's viewpoint, to aid reading comprehension.

Not all children follow the same progression in reading development. Individual differences abound, because children have different cognitive styles that influence the manner in which they approach learning to read.

Learning to Write

As in reading, children progress through various stages when learning to write. Writing development begins with children's drawing and scribbling, as they struggle to create forms that resemble letters. Although at this stage the child may pretend to write, she usually does not know letter names, nor does she know that print represents spoken words (Sulzby, 1981).

Next, the child learns to write her name and "well-learned words" such as *stop*. These familiar words help the child understand that different letters represent different sounds. With the emergence of the following stage, **inventive spelling,** the child tries to impose regularity on her writing system by matching sounds and letters (Read, 1981). The sound the child hears is matched to the letter, and her writing reflects this match. Initially, the child represents the entire word with the first letter and pays little attention to the other letters of the word. For example, *DRLM* or *DBC* might represent *Daddy*. This is similar to the initial stage of reading, in which the child pays attention to only the first letter. Next, the child will represent syllables, often without vowels. For example, *girl* might be written as *GRL* or *boy* as *BY.* In the final stage of inventive spelling, called **phonemic spelling,** the child is aware of the alphabet and the correspondence of graphemes to phonemes. Words such as *cat, it,* and *me* are spelled correctly, but words such as *knife, night,* or *soup* are not. The formal instruction of school brings mastery of the conventional spelling system.

Writing, however, involves much more than spelling. Like preschool speakers, preschool writers are often oblivious to the needs of the reader. The 6-year-old pays little attention to format, spacing, spelling, and punctuation when producing a written piece of work. In addition, better developed aspects of a child's writing will often deteriorate when new ones are introduced; for example, spelling and sentence structure deteriorate when a child changes from print to script. Writing on a difficult topic can also result in spelling, handwriting, and sentence structure deterioration.

By the middle-school years, the length and diversity of children's written productions increase. With the demands for lengthier writing that middle school imposes come increasing cognitive demands for cohesion and organization of ideas. In early writing, the child uses drawings to highlight important parts and to help her organize her text; in later writing, she must recall the order and sequence of events to formulate a cohesive text.

A shift in the child's writing from an egocentric focus to a concern for reader reaction occurs in the third or fourth grade. Writers at this stage can revise and proofread their work (Bartlett, 1982; Graves, 1979) because of their knowledge of syntactic rules. The third and fourth school years bring a decrease in the use of incomplete written sentences, an increase in the use of complex clauses and phrases, and a variety of sentence types (deVilliers & deVilliers, 1978). By the end of elementary school, the complexity of children's written language surpasses that of their spoken language (Gundloch, 1981).

Summary

Once children have gained a working knowledge of spoken language, most of them adapt to the new mode of written language (reading and writing) with relative ease. The underlying linguistic relationships between spoken and written language make success in this mode possible. In addition to the child's linguistic knowledge, emerging metalinguistic abilities enable her to decontextualize language and use her knowledge to understand language in another mode.

Summary

By kindergarten, the child has acquired much of the mature language user's form (Bloom, 1975). Development continues, however, and the child adds new forms and gains new skills in transmitting messages. Her vocabulary increases, and she learns to be a more effective communicator. Through the formal instruction of school, the child learns a new mode of language—reading and writing, essential skills in a literate society.

For children with language disorders, the school years pose special problems. Their needs must be met by a variety of specialists who assess their skills (see Chapter 7) and integrate programming (see Chapter 9) so that they can fully benefit from classroom instruction.

Study Questions

1. Outline the syntactic achievements of the school-age years.
2. Discuss the development of figurative language in school-age children.
3. Describe the changes that take place in school-age children's conversational abilities.
4. What are metalinguistic abilities? How are they related to the development of reading?
5. Briefly describe the bottom-up and top-down theories of reading.

References

Abrahamsen, E., & Rigrodsky, S. (1984). Comprehension of complex sentences in children at three levels of cognitive development. *Journal of Psycholinguistic Research, 13,* 333–350.

Baldie, B. (1976). The acquisition of the passive voice. *Journal of Child Language, 3,* 331–348.

Bartlett, C. (1982). Learning to write: Some cognitive and linguistic components. In R. Shuy (Ed.), *Lin-*

guistics and literary series (No. 2). Washington, DC: Center of Applied Linguistics.

Bates, E. (1976). *Language and context: The acquisition of pragmatics.* New York: Academic Press.

Beck, I., & Jeul, C. (1995). The role of decoding in learning to read. *American Educator,* 19, (2) 8–13.

Berko Gleason, J. (1993). The development of language. New York: Macmillan.

Bernstein, D. K. (1986). The development of humor: Implications for assessment and intervention. *Topics in Language Disorders,* 4, 65–73.

Bernstein, D. K. (1987). Figurative language: Assessment strategies and implications for intervention. *Folia Phoniatrica,* 39, 130–144.

Biemiller, A. (1970). The development of the use of graphic and contextual information as children learn to read. *Reading Research Quarterly,* 6, 75–96.

Billow, R. (1975). A cognitive developmental study of metaphor comprehension. *Developmental Psychology,* 11, 415–423.

Blackman, B., & James, S. (1985). Metalinguistic abilities and reading achievement in first grade children. In J. Niles & R. Lalid (Eds.), *Issues in literacy: A research perspective.* Thirty-fourth Yearbook of the National Reading Conference.

Bloom, L. (1975). Language development. In F. Horowitz (Ed.), *Review of child development research* (No. 4). Chicago: University of Chicago Press.

Bloom, L., Rocissano, L., & Hood, L. (1976). Adult-child discourse: Developmental interactions between information processing and linguistic interaction. *Cognitive Psychology,* 8, 521–552.

Brady, S., & Shankweiler, D. (Eds.). (1991). Phonological processes in literacy. Hillsdale, NJ: Lawrence Erlbaum.

Bransford, J., & Johnson, M. (1972). Contextual prerequisites for understanding: Some investigations of comprehension and recall. *Journal of Verbal Learning and Verbal Behavior,* 11, 717–726.

Bridges, A. (1980). SVD comprehension strategies reconsidered: The evidence of individual patterns of response. *Journal of Child Language,* 7, 89–104.

Brinton, B., & Fujiki, M. (1984). Development of topic manipulation skills in discourse. *Journal of Speech and Hearing Research,* 27, 350–358.

Brinton, B., & Fujiki, M., Loeb, D., & Winkler, E. (1986). Development of conversational repair strategies in response to request for clarification. *Journal of Speech and Hearing Research,* 39, 75–82.

Bryant, P., Bradley, L., MacLean, M., & Crossland, J. (1989). Nursery rhymes, phonological skills and reading. *Journal of Child Language,* 16, 407–428.

Carrow, E. (1973). *Test of Auditory Comprehension of Language.* Austin, TX: Urban Research Group.

Catts, H. (1991). Early identification of reading disabilities. *Topics in Language Disorders,* 12 (l), 1–17.

Catts, H. (1996). Defining dyslexia as a developmental language disorder: An expanded view. *Topics in Language Disorders,* 16 (2), 14–25.

Catts, H., & Kamhi, A. (1987). The linguistic basis of reading disorders: Implications for the speech-language pathologist. *Language, Speech and Hearing Services in Schools,* 17, 329–342.

Chall, J. (1983). *Stages of reading development.* New York: McGraw-Hill.

Chomsky, C. (1972). Write now, read later. *Childhood Education,* 47, 296–299.

Clancy, P. (1979). The development of narrative discourse in Japanese. *Papers and Reports in Child Language Development # 17* (pp. 41–48). Stanford, CA: Stanford University, Department of Linguistics.

Crais, E. (1990). World knowledge to word knowledge. *Topics in Language Disorders,* 10 (3), 45–63.

Crais, E. R., & Lorch, N. (1994). Oral narratives in school age children. *Topics in Language Disorders,* 14 (3), 13–28.

Cuda, R. A., & Nelson, N. (1976, November). *Analysis of teacher speaking rate, syntactic complexity, and hesitation phenomena as a function of grade level.* Paper presented at the Annual Convention of the American Speech-Language-Hearing Association, Houston, TX.

Denckla, M. B. (1972). Color naming defects in dyslexic boys. *Cortex,* 8, 164–176.

deVilliers, J., & deVilliers, P. (1978). *Language acquisition.* Cambridge: Harvard University Press.

Dickinson, D., Wolf, M., Stotsky, S. (1993). Words move: The interwoven development of oral and written language. In J. Berko Gleason (Ed.), *The development of language* (3rd ed.) (pp. 225–257). Columbus, OH: Merrill/Macmillan.

Doehring, D. (1976). Acquisition of rapid reading responses. *Monographs of the Society of Research in Child Development,* 41(2).

Emerson, H. (1979). Children's comprehension of "because" in reversible and nonreversible sentences. *Journal of Child Language, 6,* 279–300.

Ervin-Tripp, S. (1980). Lecture. University of Minnesota. May 14, 1980.

Ferreiro, E., & Teberosky, A. (1982). *Literacy before schooling.* Exeter, NH: Heinemann.

Fletcher, J., Shaywitz, S., Shankweiler, D., Katz, L., Liberman, I., Stuebing, K., Francis, D., Fowler, A., & Shaywitz, B. (1994). Cognitive profiles of reading disabilities: Comparison of discrepancy and low achievement definitions. *Journal of Educational Psychology,* (86), 6–23.

Fowles, B., & Glanz, M. E. (1977). Competence and a talent in verbal riddle comprehension. *Journal of Child Language, 4,* 433–452.

Garvey, C. (1975). Requests and responses in children's speech. *Journal of Child Language, 2,* 41–63.

Garvey, C. (1977). The contingent query: A dependent act of communication. In M. Lewis & L. Rosenblum (Eds.), *Interaction, conversation, and the development of language.* New York: Wiley

Gathercole, V. (1985). "Me has too much hard questions": The acquisition of the linguistic mass-count distinction in much and many. *Journal of Child Language, 12,* 395–415.

Gerber, A. (1981). Problems in the processing and use of language in education. In A. Gerber & D. N. Bryen (Eds.), *Language and learning disabilities.* Baltimore: University Park Press.

Goodman, K. (1976). Behind the eye: What happens in reading. In H. Singer & R. Ruddell (Eds.), *Theoretical models and processes of reading* (2nd ed.). Newark, DE: International Reading Association.

Graves, D. (1979). What children show us about revision. *Journal of Language Arts, 56,* 312–319.

Greene, J. (1996). Psycholinguistic assessment: The clinical base for identification of dyslexia. *Topics in Language Disorders, 16* (2), 45–72.

Grimm, H. (1975, September). *Analysis of short-term dialogues in 5–7 year olds: Encoding of intentions and modifications of speech acts as a function of negative feedback loops.* Paper presented at the Third International Child Language Symposium, London.

Gundloch, R. (1981). On the nature and development of children's writing. In C. Frederiksen & J. Dominic (Eds.), *Writing: The nature, development and teaching of written communication* (Vol. 2). Hillsdale, NJ: Lawrence Erlbaum Associates.

Heath, S. B. (1982). Toward an ethnohistory of writing in American education. In M. F. Whiteman (Ed.), *Writing: The nature, development and teaching of written composition* (Vol. 1). Hillsdale, NJ: Lawrence Erlbaum Associates.

Henry, M. (1993). Morphological structure: Latin and Greek roots and affixes as upper grade code strategies. *Reading and Writing: An Interdisciplinary Journal* (5), 227–41.

Horgan, D. (1978). The development of the full passive. *Journal of Child Language, 5,* 65–80.

Hulit, L. M., & Howard, M. R. (1993). Born to talk: An introduction to speech and language development. New York: Macmillan.

Johnson, C. J., & Anglin, J. M. (1995). Qualitative development in the content and form of children's definitions. *Journal of Speech and Hearing Research,* (38), 612–625.

Johnston, J. (1982). Narratives: A new look at communication problems in older language disordered children. *Language, Speech and Hearing Services in Schools, 13,* 144–155.

Kamhi, A., & Catts, H. (1986). Toward an understanding of developmental language and reading disorders. *Journal of Speech and Hearing Disorders, 51,* 337–348.

Kamhi, A., & Koenig, L. (1985). Metalinguistic awareness in language disordered children. *Language, Speech and Hearing Services in Schools, 16,* 199–210.

Kavanagh, J., & Mattingly, I. G. (1972). *Language by ear and by eye.* Cambridge: MIT Press.

Kernan, K. (1977). Semantic and expressive elaboration on children's narratives. In S. Ervin-Tripp & C. Mitchell Kernan (Eds.), *Child discourse* (pp. 91–103). New York: Academic Press.

Konefal, J., & Folks, J. (1984). Linguistic analysis of children's conversational repairs. *Journal of Psycholinguistic Research, 13,* 1–11.

Lahey, M. (1974). The role of prosody and syntactic markers in children's comprehension of spoken sentences. *Journal of Speech and Hearing Research, 17,* 656–668.

Larsen, V. L., and McKinley, N. (1995). Language disorders in older students, preadolescents and adolescents. Eau Claire, WI: Thinking Publication.

Lesser, G. (1974). *Children and television.* New York: Random House.

Levin, E., & Rubin, K. (1982). Getting others to do what you want them to: The development of children's requestive strategies. In K. Nelson (Ed.), *Children's language* (Vol. 4). New York: Gardner Press.

Liberman, I., Shankweiler, D., Liberman, A., Fowler, C., & Fischer, F. (1977). Phonetic segmentation and receding in the beginning reader. In A. Reber & D. Scarborough (Eds.), *Towards a psychology of reading.* Hillsdale, NJ: Lawrence Erlbaum.

Liberman, I. Y. (1973). Segmentation of the spoken word and reading acquisition. *Bulletin of the Orton Society, 23,* 65–77.

Litowitz, B. (1977). Learning to make definitions. *Journal of Child Language, 4,* 289–304.

Lund, N., & Duchan, J. (1983). *Assessing children's language in naturalistic contexts.* Englewood Cliffs, NJ: Prentice Hall.

Maclean, M., Bryant, P., & Bradley, L. (1987). Rhymes, nursery rhymes, and reading in early childhood. Special issue, Children's reading and the development of phonological awareness. *Merrill-Palmer Quarterly, 33* (3), 255–281.

Mattingly, J. G. (1972). Reading the linguistic process and linguistic awareness. In J. F. Kavanagh & J. G. Mattingly (Eds.), *Language by ear and by eye.* Cambridge: MIT Press.

Mattis, S., French, J., & Rapin, I. (1975). Dyslexia in children and young adults: Three independent neuropsychological syndromes. *Developmental Medicine and Child Neurology, 17,* 150–163.

McNeil, D. (1970). *The acquisition of language: The study of developmental psycho-linguistics.* New York: Harper & Row.

Menyuk, P. (1969). *Sentences children use.* Cambridge: MIT Press.

Menyuk, P. (1971). *The acquisition and development of language.* Englewood Cliffs, NJ: Prentice Hall.

Menyuk, P. (1983). Language development and reading. In C. Prutting & T. Gallagher (Eds.), *Pragmatic assessments and intervention issues in language.* San Diego: College-Hill Press.

Mishler, E. (1976). Studies in dialogue and discourse: 3—Utterance structure and utterance function in interrogative sequences. *Journal of Psycholinguistic Research, 5,* 88–99.

Moats, L., & Lyon, G. R. (1996). Wanted: Teachers with knowledge of language. *Topics in Language Disorders, 16* (2), 73–86.

Mueller, E. (1972). The maintenance of verbal exchanges. *Child Development, 43,* 930–938.

Nelson, N. W (1985). Teacher talk and children listening—Fostering a better match. In C. Simon (Ed.), *Communication skills and classroom success: Assessment of language-learning disabled children.* San Diego: College-Hill Press.

Nelson, N. W (1986). Individual processing in classroom settings. *Topics in Language Disorders, 6,* 13–27.

Nelson, N. W. (1993). Childhood language disorders in contexts: infancy through adolescence. New York: Macmillan Publishing Co.

Nippold, M. (1985). Comprehension of figurative language. *Topics in Language Disorders, 3,* 1–20.

Nippold, M. (1988). Figurative language. In M. A. Nippold (Ed.), *Later language development: Ages nine through nineteen* (pp. 179–210). Austin, TX: Pro-Ed.

Nippold, M. (1991). Evaluating and enhancing idiom comprehension. *Language, Speech and Hearing Services in Schools, 22* (3), 100–105.

Nippold, M., Leonard, L., & Kail, R. (1984). Syntactic and conceptual factors in children's understanding of metaphors. *Journal of Speech and Hearing Research, 27,* 197–205.

Nippold, M., & Martin, S. T. (1989). Idiom interpretation in isolation versus context: A developmental study with adolescents. *Journal of Speech and Hearing Research, 32,* 59–66.

Nippold, M. A., & Taylor, C. L. (1995). Idiom understanding in youth: Further examination of familiarity and transparency. *Journal of Speech and Hearing Research, 2,* 426–443.

Owens, R. (1996). *Language development: An introduction* (3rd ed.). Columbus, OH: Merril/Macmillan.

Perfetti, C. (1984). Reading acquisition and beyond: Decoding includes cognition. *American Journal of Education, 93,* 40–60.

Read, C. (1981). Writing is not the inverse of reading for young children. In C. Frederiksen & J. Dominic (Eds.), *Writing: The nature, development, and teaching of written communication.* Hillsdale, NJ: Lawrence Erlbaum Associates.

Rees, N. (1974). The speech pathologist and the reading process. *ASHA, 16,* 225–258.

Rubin, H., Patterson, P., & Kantor, M. (1991). Morphological development and writing ability in children and adults. *Language, Speech and Hearing Services in the Schools, 22* (4), 228–236.

Rubin, S., & Wolf, D. (1979). The development of maybe: The evolution of social roles into narrative roles. *New Directions for Child Development, 6,* 15–28.

Rumelhart, D. (1977). Toward an interactive model of reading. In S. Dornic (Ed.), *Attention and performance* (Vol. I). Hillsdale, NJ: Lawrence Erlbaum Associates.

Ryan, E., & Ledger, G. (1984). Learning to attend to sentence structure: Links between metalinguistic development and reading. In J. Downing & R. Valtin (Eds.), *Language awareness and learning to read.* New York: Springer-Verlag.

Saywitz, K., & Cherry-Wilkinson, L. (1982). Age related differences in metalinguistic awareness. In S. Kuczaj (Ed.), *Language development: Vol. 1. Language, thought and culture.* Hillsdale, NJ: Lawrence Erlbaum Associates.

Shultz, T. R., & Horibe, F (1974). The development of the appreciation of verbal jokes. *Developmental Psychology, 10,* 13–20.

Smith, F. (1971). *Understanding reading: A psycholinguistic analysis of reading and learning to read.* New York: Holt, Rinehart & Winston.

Stanovich, K. (1980). Toward an interactive-compensatory model of individual differences in the development of reading fluency. *Reading Research Quarterly, 16,* 32–71.

Stark, J. (1975). Reading failure, A language based problem. *ASHA, 17,* 832–834.

Stein, N. (1978). *How children understand stories: A developmental analysis* (Tech. Rep. No. 69). Urbana-Champaign: University of Illinois, Center for the Study of Reading.

Stein, N., & Glenn, C. (1979). An analysis of story comprehension in elementary school children. in R. Freedle (Ed.), *New directions in discourse processing.* Norwood, NJ: Ablex.

Sulzby, E. (1981). *Kindergarteners begin to read their own compositions.* Final report to the Research Foundation of the National Council of Teachers of English.

Torgensen, J., Wagner, R., & Rachotte, C. (1994). Longitudinal studies of phonological processing and reading. *Journal of Learning Disabilities, 27,* 276–286.

Torrey, J. (1979). Reading that comes naturally: The early reader. In T. Waller & G. Machinnon (Eds.), *Reading research: Advances in theory and practice.* New York: Academic Press.

Tunmer, W., & Bowey, J. (1984). Metalinguistic awareness and reading. In W. Tunmer, C. Pratt, & M. Herriman (Eds.), *Metalinguistic awareness in children: Theory, research and implications.* New York: Springer-Verlag.

Tunmer, W., Pratt, C., & Herriman, M. (Eds.). (1984). *Metalinguistic awareness in children: Theory, research and implications.* New York: Springer-Verlag.

Van Kleeck, A. (1982). The emergence of linguistic awareness: A cognitive framework. *Merrill-Palmer Quarterly, 28,* 237–265.

Van Kleeck, A. (1984). Metalinguistic skills: Cutting across spoken and written language and problem solving abilities. In G. Wallach & K. Butler (Eds.), *Language learning disabilities in school age children* (pp. 129–153). Baltimore: Williams & Wilkins.

Van Kleeck, A. (1995). Learning about print before learning to read. In K. Butler (Ed.), *Best practices II. The classroom as an interaction context* (pp. 3–23). Gaithersburg, MD: Aspen Publishing Co.

Vellutino, F. R. (1977). Alternative conceptualizations of dyslexia: Evidence in support of a verbal-deficit hypothesis. *Harvard Educational Review, 47,* 334–354.

Vellutino, F. R. (1979). *Dyslexia: Theory and research.* Cambridge: MIT Press.

Vellutino, F., Scanlon, D., Small, S., & Tanzman, M. (1991). The linguistic bases of reading disability: Converting written to oral language. *Text, 11,* 99–133.

Wallach, G. (1984). Who shall be called "learning disabled": Some new directions. In G. Wallach & K. Butler (Eds.), *Language learning disabilities in school age children.* Baltimore: Williams & Wilkins.

Wallach, G., & Butler, K. (1994). Language learning disabilities in school age children and adolescents. New York: Macmillan Publishing Co.

Wehren, A., DeLisi, R., & Arnold, M. (1981). The development of noun definition. *Journal of Child Language, 8,* 165–175.

White, B. (1975). Critical influences in the origins of competence. *Merrill-Palmer Quarterly,* 22, 243–266.

Winner, E., Rosentiel, A., & Gardner, H. (1976). The development of metaphoric understanding. *Developmental Psychology,* 12, 189–297.

Wolf, M., & Dickinson, D. (1993). From oral to written language: Transitions in the school years. In J. B. Gleason (Ed.), *The development of language.* Columbus, OH: Merrill/Macmillan.

P a r t **II**

Language Assessment and Intervention

Chapter 6
*Early Communication Assessment
and Intervention: An Interactive Process*

Chapter 7
Assessing Children with Language Disorders

Chapter 8
*Planning Language Intervention
for Young Children*

Chapter 9
Language Intervention in School Settings

Chapter 10
*Language and Communication Disorders in
Culturally and Linguistically Diverse Children*

Early Communication Assessment and Intervention: An Interactive Process

NANCY B. ROBINSON
University of Hawaii at Manoa

MICHAEL P. ROBB
University of Connecticut at Storrs

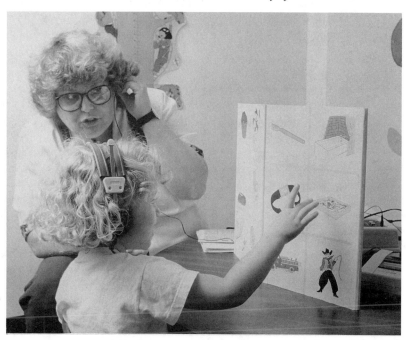

The term *infant,* typically used to describe the child from birth to 12 months of age, was originally a Latin term meaning "one unable to speak." This literal definition implies the absence of speech and expressive language, but that is not to say the infant is without capacities that significantly preconfigure spoken language (Kent & Hodge, 1991). Several investigators have documented nonverbal behavior in very young infants that is clearly communicative, signaling physiological states and interactive preferences (Barnard, 1978; Brazelton & Als, 1979). Studies of early communicative signaling and social interaction patterns of young infants have shown strong predictive relationships to language emerging between 12 and 18 months of age (Bates, Benigni, Bretherton, Camaioni, & Volterra, 1979; Bates, Bretherton, & Snyder, 1988; Snow, 1979). Kopp and Kaler (1989) referred to infancy as the foundation period of our species. Growing support for the continuity of early prelinguistic, communicative behaviors with emergent verbal language adds further importance to the task that confronts the speech-language pathologist (SLP) involved in early language assessment.

The goal of this chapter is to introduce to the student a foundation of behaviors that describe the infant's developing language and communication system. These behaviors provide a framework with which to assess and intervene with infants at risk for communicative disorders. The chapter is divided into four parts, beginning with policy guidelines for SLPs involved in early intervention, followed by an overview and description of the populations of infants and toddlers most at risk for language/communication delays. The third section includes a proposed model for early communication assessment and intervention planning. In the fourth section, the assessment model is applied to three children representing early, middle, and later periods of infancy. Throughout the chapter, we present recommended processes and practices for early language and communication assessment and intervention that are consistent with the position of the American Speech-Language-Hearing Association (ASHA) and regulations for Public Law 99-457. Of special importance is the involvement of the family at each step of the assessment and intervention process.

Policy Guidelines for the SLP in Early Intervention

The involvement and role of the SLP in early intervention is changing rapidly. With the 1986 passage of PL 99-457, the urgency to provide early intervention services for infants and toddlers with special needs pushed this population to the forefront in federal and state policy and program development. The role of the SLP in serving infants and toddlers and their families is described by ASHA (1989):

> *Families and their infants and toddlers (birth–36 months) who are at-risk or have developmental disabilities present a broad spectrum of needs that the appropriately certified and/or licensed speech-language pathologist is uniquely qualified to address. These include delays and disabilities in communication, language, and speech, as well as oral-motor and feeding behaviors. Speech-language pathologists, and independent practitioners, assume various roles in addressing these needs of families and their infants. (p. 116)*

This ASHA position statement describes possible roles of SLPs in early intervention to include (a) screening and identification; (b) assessment and evaluation; (c) design, planning, direct delivery, and monitoring of treatment programs; (d) case management; and (e) consultation with, and referral to, agencies and other professionals. The intention is SLP is expected to assume these multiple and changing roles within a community-based, family-centered program, as part of an early intervention team. Although brief in content, the position statement embodies considerable thought and broad implications about the way we interact with families and their infants at risk for communicative disorders (Catlett, 1991).

Children at Risk for Communication/Language Delays

When genetic heritage and prenatal life are favorable, the infant's roots are securely anchored and normal development should occur (Kopp, 1990; Kopp & Kaler, 1989). Unfavorable genetic or prenatal factors set the stage for vulnerabilities, that is, the child becomes "at risk" for developmental delays. Since the inception of PL 99-457, attention has been directed toward identifying and intervening with the at-risk infant. There are two basic forms of risk: biological and environmental. Biological risks stem from genetic conditions as well as from exposure to harmful nonsocial environmental factors (e.g., viral infections, drug use). Environmental risk generally refers to adverse rearing conditions (e.g., maternal depression, abuse, environmental toxins).

Following is a list that describes biological and environmental factors that place infants at risk for communicative disorders. The list is not meant to be all-inclusive. Many other sources have reviewed well-known biological risks that can be identified early in life, such as Down syndrome, cerebral palsy, cleft lip and palate, and so on. The reader is referred to Hanson (1983a) for an overview of established biological risk conditions. The present review highlights recent information regarding risk factors that are increasingly identified among newborn infants. The risk factors range from minor to significant involvement.

Biological Risks

Illegal Substances.   When considering the perinatal effects of illegal or illicit substances, the basic tenants of maternal-fetal physiology and pharmacology apply (Dattel, 1990). Illicit drugs tend to be of low molecular weight, passing freely between the mother and child within minutes after ingestion. Because of the rapid transfer across the placental barrier, the drug concentration received by the fetus is usually 50 percent to 100 percent of maternal levels. Unfortunately, incidence and prevalence data are difficult to establish. The substance being abused is often illegal; thus, parental disclosure of drug use is rare. In addition, identifying and isolating a specific drug used by a parent is problematic because of the mixture with other over-the-counter drugs (e.g., caffeine, alcohol). Chasnoff (1987) reported that the percentage of newborns exposed to drugs has quadrupled within the past ten years.

Cocaine.   The increased use of cocaine in the United States has changed the classic picture of the drug addict. Thousands of women from middle and upper socioeconomic groups are addicted to this so-called drug of the 1980s. Reportedly, as of 1989, more than 11 percent of babies born each year in the United States have been exposed to cocaine (Chasnoff, 1987). It is still the most commonly abused illicit substance in pregnancy. There is no difference between cocaine and "crack" cocaine. Crack is created by mixing the cocaine with water and bicarbonate soda to form a hard substance. The substance allows for the cocaine to vaporize. The vaporized cocaine produces a rapid "high" when inhaled. The effects of cocaine on the central nervous system include increased respiratory and heart rates, restlessness, and excitement. Developmental outcomes of infants exposed to cocaine include shorter body length, smaller head circumference, and lower birthweight than infants delivered to drug-free women. Associated behavioral outcomes include tremulousness and muscle rigidity. Cocaine babies often will not suck, swallow, or feed well. They do not interact freely with caregivers and are difficult to console. Their APGAR scores are less than 7 at 1 minute and 5 minutes, and they tend to perform poorly on other neonatal assessment scales.

Ice.   If cocaine is referred to as the drug of the 1980s, then crystal methamphetamine hydrochloride, or "ice," is the drug of the 1990s. The overall stimulant effect is similar to cocaine. However, the effects of ice persist for hours, whereas cocaine's effects may last less than 60 minutes. As with crack cocaine, ice is usually inhaled so as to create a volatile vaporization in the lungs. It is not a new drug—in fact, its abuse has been documented in the United States and abroad (e.g., in Japan and Sweden) for more than 30 years. The persistence of ice in the body greatly enhances the medical problems associated with the drug. For example, because of longer exposure, children born of ice users have greater developmental problems than cocaine babies. The hazardous effects to the user include acute toxicity; cardiovascular problems; seizures; psychiatric, social, and law enforcement problems; and, of course, death. Developmental outcomes of ice are largely unknown at this time, although users are often sleep and nourishment deprived. They also experience periods of psychosis and depression.

Marijuana.   The use of marijuana is on the rise. In 1985, approximately 31 percent of American women in their late teens and early 20s reported that they had used marijuana within the past year. The finding of such widespread use during the prime reproductive years raises important questions about the effects of marijuana used during pregnancy on fetal growth and development (Zuckerman, Frank, Hingson, Amaro, & Levenson, 1989). The main psychoactive ingredient of marijuana is delta-9-tetrahydro cannabinol. Marijuana used during pregnancy is associated with a variety of adverse outcomes, including prematurity, low birthweight, decreased maternal weight gain, complications of pregnancy, difficult labor, congenital abnormalities, increased chance of stillbirth and perinatal mortality, poor neonatal assessment scores, and limited verbal and memory abilities (Fried & Watkinson, 1990).

Commonly Used Teratogens.   Whether, or to what extent, pregnant women should abstain from drinking alcohol, smoking, or drinking caffeinated beverages is a subject that has been debated for years. It's been only in recent years that researchers have pinpointed the dangers of these practices. Alcohol, nicotine, and caffeine are indeed teratogens, drugs or substances capable of interfering with the development of a fetus.

Alcohol.   Alcohol is the most widely used, and abused, drug in the United States. A 1988 national household survey by the National Institute on Drug Abuse revealed that 3 of every 5 women of childbearing age currently consume alcoholic beverages (ASHA, 1991). Historically, children have been exposed to mothers' consumption of alcohol since people began to drink. Jones and Smith (1973, 1974) were the first to describe fetal alcohol syndrome (FAS), resulting from excessive prenatal exposure to alcohol. FAS is a pattern of altered tissue and organ development that involves cardiovascular problems, craniofacial abnormalities (e.g., cleft lip and/or palate), and limb defects accompanied by prenatal growth deficiency and developmental delay (Gerber, 1990). FAS is a leading cause of birth defects characterized by mental retardation. It is still unknown how much alcohol is necessary to produce the symptoms of FAS. The syndrome appears in 1.9 per 1000 live births (Abel & Sokol, 1986). Children with FAS are usually born small (below the 10th percentile for size) and remain small throughout postnatal development. Reported communication problems include delayed language and problems with speech articulation, fluency, and swallowing (ASHA, 1991; Sparks, 1984).

Nicotine.   Approximately 30 percent of women smoke during pregnancy (Gerber, 1990). Smoking during pregnancy—specifically, the ingestion of nicotine—is the most common cause of low birthweight and accounts for at least 20 percent of all low birthweight infants born in the United States. Approximately 90 percent of the nicotine inhaled is absorbed into the mother's body (Dattel, 1990). Documented effects of nicotine ingestion upon the infant include long-term impairment of neurological and intellectual development. In addition, potential consequences of smoking during pregnancy include infant respiratory distress, sudden infant death syndrome (SIDS), and increased risk of in utero placenta complications and in utero growth retardation.

Caffeine.   Caffeine is a substance commonly used during pregnancy. At least 80 percent of pregnant women ingest caffeine in some form (e.g., in coffee, cola) daily (Dattel, 1990). As with other chemicals, caffeine freely crosses the placenta from mother to child. However, because caffeine is broken down much more slowly than some other substances, its potential influence upon the developing child is greater. No confirmed studies show the direct influence of caffeine upon the developmental outcome of infants. Animal studies have shown an increase in birth defects and a decrease in fetal weight.

Other Health Risks.   Two medical conditions currently being examined for their role in affecting communication outcomes are the commonplace middle ear infection and infection with the virus that causes acquired immunodeficiency syndrome (AIDS).

Otitis Media.   The rapid and short onset of signs and symptoms of inflammation in the middle ear is termed acute otitis media (Bluestone, 1990). Acute otitis media occurs in almost every child at some time during the first years of life. Many infants experience multiple episodes of acute otitis media; some spend months, with fluid discharge (or effusion) in both ears (Bauer & Mosher, 1990; Teele, Klein, Chase, Menyuk, & Rosner, 1990). Considerable data show that conductive hearing loss can accompany otitis media with effusion (OME), although the extent of loss varies from child to child. Thus, impaired hearing occurs, to some extent, in most children at the time when language and other skills are being acquired. Robb et al. (1993) evaluated the dramatic effects OME can have in delaying an infant's phonetic development. Further, Teele et al. (1990) reported that children who experienced OME during the first three years of life were subsequently found to have lower scores on tests of cognitive ability and on follow-up speech and language tests at 7 years of age.

HIV.   Although in the United States AIDS was initially described in young homosexual men in the early 1980s, the epidemic of human immunodeficiency virus (HIV) infection has since come to encompass large numbers of heterosexuals, intravenous drug abusers, persons with hemophilia, and other recipients of contaminated blood products (Diamond & Cohen, 1989). Of women in the United States infected with HIV, a large number are intravenous drug users or sexual partners of intravenous drug users (Cohen, 1990). Most infants with HIV infection contracted the virus by perinatal exposure. The first reports of pediatric AIDS were in 1983. Central nervous system involvement is prominent in children with HIV infection. Estimates of the prevalence of central nervous system dysfunction in children with HIV infection range from 73 percent to 93 percent (Hopkins, Grosz, & Lieberman, 1990). To date, we know little of the communicative outcomes resulting from HIV infection and the subsequent contraction of AIDS.

Environmental Risks

Socioeconomic Status.   The offspring of families who are economically stressed have been found to be at developmental risk. Low socioeconomic (SES) appears to be predictive of lower mental development scores, impoverished language development, placement in special classes, and school failure (Bryant & Ramey, 1987). Low SES is also a significant predictor of childhood psychopathology during the school years (Rutter, Yule, Quinton, Rowlands, Yule, & Berger, 1975). Risk factors associated with low SES include infant prematurity, adolescent parenthood, single parenthood, and parental psychiatric disorder (Lyons-Ruth, Connell, & Grunebaum, 1990). Other investigators have shown that such risk factors are correlated with one another so that poor child outcomes multiply with successive additional risk. In other words, children in multirisk families represent the most serious developmentally impaired group (Rutter, 1979).

Maternal Influences.   Maternal anxiety is regulated by the sympathetic division of the autonomic nervous system. As such, anxiety can produce a variety of psychological changes, including changes in heart rate, the constriction of blood vessels, and decreases in gastrointestinal motility. Generally, the greater the anxiety, the more severe the response. Environmental factors that the mother may exhibit include depression, social isolation, and low IQ. Lyons-Ruth et al. (1990) have studied maternal depression and subsequent effect on infant development. The results indicate that these children generally exhibit poor cognitive abilities when compared to children of nondepressed mothers.

Lead.   Around the beginning of the 1900s, it was recognized that women employed in the lead trades often gave birth to infants who were small, weak, and neurologically damaged (American Academy of Pediatrics, 1987). Lead had crossed the placental barrier, resulting in retarded intrauterine growth and postnatal failure to thrive. Excess levels of environmental lead are still found in houses where lead-based paints were used, exhaust of leaded gasoline, hazardous waste, and in glazes and decorative paint used on dishware. Children are also exposed to lead in soil and water. Noted outcomes of lead exposure include mental retardation and language learning disabilities.

TABLE 6-1   Selected Risk Factors Related to Adverse Developmental Outcomes

Risk Factor	Possible Outcome
Biological risks	
Cocaine/crack	Low birthweight, shorter body length, smaller head circumference, tremulousness
Methamphetamines, "ice"	Cognitive, social, behavioral differences
Marijuana	Prematurity, low birthweight, congenital abnormalities
Alcohol	Low birthweight, shorter length, fetal alcohol syndrome
Smoking/nicotine	Neurological impairment, respiratory distress
Caffeine	Possible decrease in fetal weight and birth defects
Otitis media	Conductive hearing loss, delayed phonetic development
HIV infection	Central nervous system disorder, death
Environmental influences	
Socioeconomic status	Low mental development, psychopathology
Maternal influences (e.g., stress)	Low mental development
Lead	Mental retardation
Nutrition	Low mental development, learning disorders

Nutrition and Diet.   The infant's intake of nutrition is vital to his developmental outcome. Before 1980, no federal laws regulated the composition of infant food formulas (Wing, 1990). From 1971 to 1979, between 26,000 and 150,000 babies were fed chloride-deficient formulas. Most infant formulas were based primarily on soybeans. These soy-based infant formulas were lacking in chloride, an essential element for facilitating rapid brain cell growth and nerve myelinization during the first year of life (Finberg, 1980). Recent articles have suggested that children born in the United States in the 1970s who were fed a chloride-deficient formula in infancy may now have expressive language or learning disorders (Roy, 1984; Wing, 1990).

This section addressed several prevalent risk factors described in recent studies of infants and toddlers born in the United States. Table 6-1 summarizes the foregoing discussion, identifying risk factors and predicted developmental outcomes related to each risk factor. The reader should keep in mind that a single risk factor alone cannot clearly predict a specific outcome, given the mediating effects of the infant's own resiliency and the caregiving environment.

Communication Assessment Model for Infants (CAMI)

We now turn to assessment and intervention planning for very young children with identified risk factors that could be associated with adverse communicative and language development outcomes. Communication assessment typically encompasses three broad phases:

screening, diagnosis, and ongoing evaluation (Ensher, 1989). Moreover, assessment (as distinguished from testing) involves the use of several measures and techniques that should serve at four major purposes: (a) to identify those in need of intervention, (b) to determine goals, (c) to monitor developmental progress, and (d) to evaluate the effectiveness of intervention.

Sparks (1989) advised that assessments be serial and that they address the infant, the primary caregivers, and their interactions. Types of infant assessment tools that evaluate early communication and language include screening tools, in-depth assessments, and neonatal behavioral assessments. To integrate environmental and biological influences with early communication and language development, the SLP needs a conceptual framework.

The two most commonly applied models of assessment are developmental models and naturalistic models. Developmental models rely almost exclusively on age-expected or normative criteria. The tests are age-expected behaviors. There are a number of commercially available assessments and instruments adhering to a developmental model. Some of these instruments are listed in Table 6-2. Far fewer assessment instruments are based on a naturalistic model. Naturalistic assessment involves viewing the infant's communication skills in commonly occurring settings and contexts such as play and daily routines (Crais, 1995). Wetherby and Prizant (1992) have voiced dissatisfaction with many of the available developmental instruments because of their limited scope and difficulty in thoroughly evaluating preverbal communication behaviors.

Given the rapid sequence and complexity of developmental processes in the first year of life, we agree with Wetherby and Prizant (1992) that developmental assessment models are perhaps too static in their examination of the infancy period. Naturalistic models tend to allow much-needed flexibility, which is particularly important when confronted with children with special needs. On the other hand, a naturalistic approach may not provide the milestone information necessary to evaluate the child's communication abilities compared to his same-age peers. We propose a conceptual model of assessment that provides an organizational framework for the SLP. The proposed model is, in essence, a combination of developmental and naturalistic models and therefore, provides more dynamic approach to early communication assessment. The model allows the clinician to move easily between assessment and intervention phases in working with families and infants and toddlers with language/communication delays.

We have applied more general guidelines found in early intervention literature (i.e., Bailey, 1988; McGonigel, Kaufmann, & Johnson, 1991) to early communication and language assessment in the form of the Communication Assessment Model for Infants (CAMI). The conceptual model combines six components, or strands, of the assessment process that are recommended in best practice and policy guidelines for early intervention. The six strands of the CAMI are: (a) family preferences, (b) developmental processes, (c) individual differences, (d) communicative contexts, (e) early intervention teams, and (f) intervention strategies. Together, these strands provide the clinician with a structural plan from which to proceed with observations, data gathering, interviews with family members, and specific test procedures required for comprehensive assessment and intervention planning.

As shown in Figure 6-1, the CAMI establishes a blueprint for the clinician to plan initial assessment questions and potential assessment tools for individual children and fami-

TABLE 6-2   **Popular Instruments Used in the Evaluation and Assessment of Infants**

Instrument	Authors
Preschool Language Scale-3	Zimmerman, Steiner, & Pond (1992)
Infant-Toddler Language Scale	Rossetti (1990)
Receptive-Expressive-Emergent Language Scale-Revised	Bzoch & League (1991)
Birth to Three Developmental Scales	Bangs & Dodson (1986)
MacArthur Communicative Development Inventories	Fenson et al. (1993)
Sequenced Inventory of Communicative Development-Revised	Hendrick, Prather, & Tober (1984)
Early Language Milestone Scale	Coplan (1993)
Assessing Linguistic Behavior	Olswang et al. (1987)
Neonatal Behavioral Assessment Scale	Brazelton (1973)
Communication and Symbolic Behavior Scales	Wetherby & Prizant (1993)
Mother/Infant Communication Screening	Raack (1989)
Parent-Child Interaction Assessment	Comfort & Farran (1994)

Adapted from Crais (1995).

lies. The family preferences strand is always the beginning point, as the information gathered and shared at this level will drive the subsequent assessment and intervention activities. Each strand is distinct, yet interdependent, and each has a direct bearing on intervention strategies. Implicit in the CAMI is the flexibility for the SLP to conduct brief assessments of the infant's current status and to immediately implement or demonstrate intervention to support further communication/language development.

Strand 1: Family Preferences

The field of early intervention is rapidly changing, as professionals move from direct intervention with children to a supportive and collaborative role with family members. In many ways, early intervention services are changing in concert with the cost-effective reorganization of the health-care industry. According to Cochrane, Farley, and Wilhelm (1990), "The field of early intervention is evolving from discipline-specific, child-centered services, to a family-oriented context within which professionals from many disciplines address the educational, medical, psychological, and therapeutic needs of handicapped infants and their families" (p. 373). Cochrane et al., among other leading voices in the field, have called for empowerment models that place families in key decision-making and goal-setting positions for their young children with disabilities. To meet these new challenges, pro-

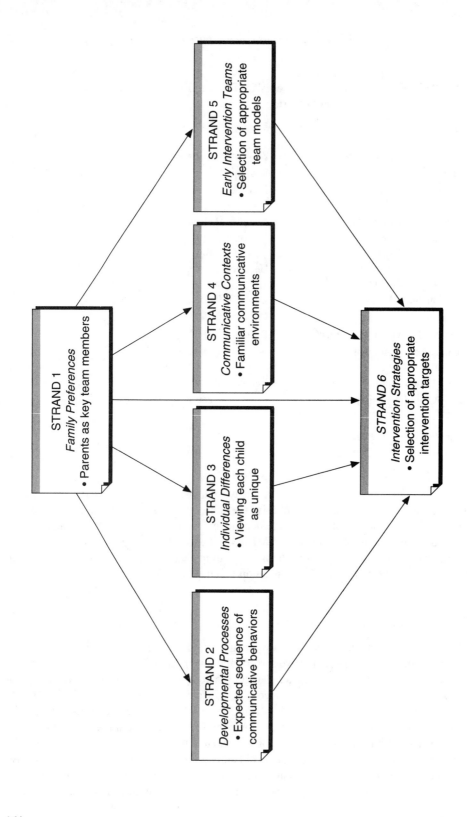

FIGURE 6-1 **Six strands of the Communication Assessment Model for Infants.**

fessionals must acquire competency-based training in family support skills. Such training should include communication with families, case management, interdisciplinary teaming, family intervention, and family-centered values and ethics.

The unique characteristics of families in the United States today call for SLPs to cultivate highly developed sensitivity to cultural and individual strengths and preferences (Turnbull & Turnbull, 1990; Hanson, Lynch & Wayman, 1990). Diverse cultural groups have differing views that range from seeing the child with a disability as a "good luck omen" to viewing the disability as a more shameful event, caused by wrong-doing in previous generations. Direct questioning by the professional may be aversive to families from some cultures, and the subject of disability within the family must be approached very gradually. In Hawaii, for example, a "talk story" format of interaction is preferred with some time allowed for small talk and relationship building before moving to the central focus, the developmental status of the child. In addition to the need for sensitivity to parents' preferred cultural styles of interaction, professionals also need to be attuned to individual styles of families made up of single parents, extended family caregivers, foster families, working parents, as well as teenage parents.

The importance of sensitivity to individual family preferences is clearly important in early communication and language assessment. Because the initial contact with families begins the assessment/intervention process, the success of that first meeting has implications for the continuing parent-professional relationship and, ultimately, intervention outcomes for the child (Gradel, Thompson, & Sheehan, 1981). During the initial family contact, the SLP needs to acknowledge that family members play a key role in the assessment/intervention team. The information gathered during the initial meetings helps the SLP determine the degree of responsibility that individual parents desire in the assessment process; their primary concerns about the child; strengths identified in parent-child interactions; and appropriate assessment tools to match parents' stated strengths, concerns, and needs for information and support.

Strand 2: Developmental Processes

The term *development* implies a high degree of continuity and stability in behavior change within and between children across time (Dunst & Rheingrover, 1982). Development for each child takes place at a relatively consistent rate, a pace established and maintained from birth to adolescence. Some children develop more slowly than their peers and others more quickly, although the *sequences* followed by both are usually the same. The sequence of behaviors expressed by the child are assumed to be orderly and lawful. For practically all children, for example, sitting upright precedes standing, and smiling precedes talking.

The approach used most often to evaluate the development of a child is to organize the child's changing behavior as a function of stage intervals occurring at a specific chronological age. A **stage model of development** is a description of measurable aspects of behavioral development (Brainerd, 1978). In the typical stage model of development, shown in Figure 6-2, the sequence of development is based on one behavior serving as the antecedent for the next behavior. The antecedent must occur in order for the ensuing behavior to develop. For the most part, a stage model of development is conceptually similar to the previously described developmental assessment model.

There are at least two primary drawbacks to using a stage model for evaluating a young child. First, an important characteristic of stage models is that the particular stages are assumed to occur in an invariant sequence, yet, the determination of stages seems to be quite arbitrary, because stage models are constantly revised. For example, a group of researchers in 1950 may have identified three stages in a child's development of walking; whereas 20 years later another group of researchers may have identified five stages. Thus, the more we learn about development, seemingly the more stages we require (Kent, 1982). The second drawback relates to ascribing an age expectancy to each stage. Chronological age often misrepresents readiness skills and expectant behavior. To post norms based on age is often a matter of convenience and practicality, and deviations should be weighed accordingly, because early- and late-maturing children do not display similar characteristics at the same chronological age. Thus, although a developmental assessment instrument may be useful as a gauge to which normal behaviour can be compared, caution is warranted. One needs to be careful not to adhere too closely to specific age-expected requirements. That is not to say, however, that stages are not important in infant assessment protocols. Stage models play an important role in guiding the SLP to be on the lookout for expected behaviors.

We believe that a more appropriate approach to describing a child's ongoing development is through the use of a process model. A **process model of development** allows for overlaps of behavior, as well as for the individual differences displayed by infants (Kent, 1982). For the most part, a process model of development is conceptually similar to previously discussed naturalistic models. Although the advantages of applying a process model to early communication seems clear, there are surprisingly few instruments commercially available that adhere to such a philosophy. Examples of such tools are the Mother/Infant Communication Screening (Raack, 1989), and the Communication and Symbolic Behavior Scales (Wetherby & Prizant, 1993).

Vocal Stages and Processes.   A child's early vocal development is usually described with respect to a stage model of development. Several versions of this model have been published, but they differ somewhat in the number of stages recognized, the particular characteristics of each stage, and the age period covered. However, most models recognize

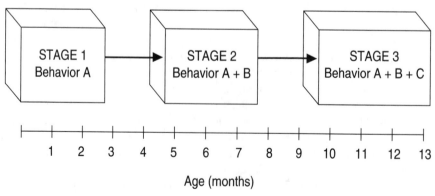

FIGURE 6-2   **Stage model of behavioral development.**

approximately five major stages, referenced according to chronological age (refer to Figure 6-3). These include

1. *Reflexive and cry vocalizations.* Usually thought to occur during the first month of life.
2. *Cooing or gooing.* The basic syllable shapes (V, CV) and consonants /k/ and /g/ are identified between ages 2 and 3 months.
3. *Reduplicated or canonical babbling.* The same CV syllable shape is produced in repetitive strings and occurs by 6 months of age.
4. *Variegated or nonreduplicated babbling.* The variety of sounds and syllable strings produced increases markedly by 8 months of age.
5. *Single-word production.* Occurs around 12 months of age.

Stages of development serve as a useful *general* framework for organizing early vocalization behaviors (Proctor, 1989). However, because stages are descriptive and somewhat impressionistic, they can become obsolete and their inadequacies more obvious (Shatz, 1983). For example, recent research (Mitchell & Kent, 1990; Smith, Brown-Sweeney, & Stoel-Gammon, 1989) suggests that because reduplicated and variegated babbling were found to co-occur, they are not separate stages of vocal development. Futhermore, the notion of a discrete single-word stage has been criticized due to the apparent mixture of identifiable word forms, as well as nonword (e.g., jargon) forms (Rob, Bauer, & Tyler, 1994). A guideline when using the stage model is to allow for overlap or individual differences from one child to the next.

Gestural Stages and Processes. Stages of gestural development appear to follow a sequence similar to that found in vocal development, as the infant moves from early reflexive activity to intentional control over planned sequences of behavior. Gestural communication

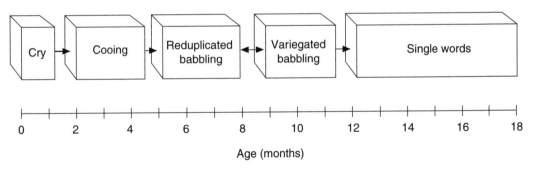

FIGURE 6-3   Schematic representation of a traditional stage model of vocalization development. The various stage assignments, according to chronological age, are based on the work of Holmgren et al. (1986), Koopmans van-Beinum and van der Stelt (1986), Oller (1980), Proctor (1989), and Stark (1980). The two-way arrow between reduplicated and variegated babbling stages indicates co-occurring behaviors.

proceeds from the infant's first year of life and continues well beyond the emergence of verbal language. Individual differences occur and are expected in the specific gestures used. Furthermore, there seems to be a direct relationship between motor development and the infant's ability to use precise gesturing toward caregivers.

The earliest gestures are found during the the first month of life when the neonate displays engagement and disengagement cues, signaling readiness to interact or to "take a break" from interaction. Brazelton (1973) has described both subtle and potent forms of engagement and disengagement cues of young infants that let caregivers know how to adjust and respond during daily care and play routines. Engagement cues are those that convey to caregivers that the infant welcomes interaction; these nonverbal behaviors include facial brightening, eye widening, smiling, open hands, smooth movements of extremities, head turning toward the caregiver, and reaching toward the caregiver (Barnard, 1978). Disengagement cues are signals that the infant is ready for a break from interaction; these behaviors include whimpering, hiccoughs, increased rate of sucking, frowns, yawning, leg kicking, and immobility. Sensitive and trained caregivers who respond to engagement cues by interacting with the infant and to disengagement cues by giving the baby a break from interaction can assist their newborns to express their own communicative behaviors.

During the second month of life, the infant displays increasing mastery over discrete facial expressions and movements of arms, legs, and fingers, to express pleasure, anticipation, hunger, and readiness to play. As infants become accustomed to daily caregiving routines, they display to caregivers a range of gestural responses, including lifting legs in diapering routines, grasping adult's hands or facial parts, whole body orientation toward the parent, and exploring mother's clothing during feeding.

An infant's reciprocal imitation of facial and hand gestures begin to emerge by 6 months of age (Moore & Meltzoff, 1978). For example, an infant will attempt to restart games such as patty-cake and peek-a-boo by reaching toward the adult's hands or the cloth hiding the adult's face. By 9 months of age, gestures play a key role in the emergence of verbal language, particularly during the period of intentional communication. Transitions from nonintentional to intentional communication are aided by a range of vocal, gestural, and gaze patterns that differ across individual children. Common patterns are found, however, in the sequence of increased refinement and range of meanings expressed. Infants typically display intentional gesturing during use of protoimperatives (i.e., preverbal requests), as reported by Bates et al. (1979). The essence of the display of intentional communication is the repeated and increasingly ritualized means of signaling adults (see Table 6-3). As discussed in earlier chapters, in the case of protoimperatives the child desires a specific item or action from the adult. Protodeclaratives are intentional communication sequences that indicate the child's desire to gain adult attention related to a specific object or environmental event (Bates, Bretherton, Snyder, Shore, & Volterra, 1980; Bates et al., 1979; Halliday, 1979; Harding & Golinkoff, 1979; Snyder, Bates, & Bretherton, 1981). Gestural sequences observed in protodeclarative sequences of behavior include showing and giving.

Protoimperative and protodeclarative sequences are observed before systematic use of pointing in communication. With the development of intentional forms of communication comes the development of **reference,** which is the ability to differentiate one entity from many and to note its presence (Owens, 1992). Reference coincides with the age period of approximately 11 months. Bates et al. (1979) have taken the position that showing and giv-

TABLE 6-3   Sequence of Intentional Communication Behavior in Protoimperatives at 9 Months of Age

Communicative Behavior	Example
1. Gaze alternation	Mother and cookie are not in same line of vision. The child looks back and forth from the cookie to the adult—indicating that he expects adult intervention.
2. Repair of failed message	If initial signalling (gaze and/or gesture) fails to result in adult action, child repeats and expands signaling (reaching toward object, looking back at adult, vocalizing loudly).
3. Ritualization of previously instrumental gestures	True reaching toward the object becomes abbreviated grasping motion, and vocalization for the cookie may become insistent "mmmm" sound.

Adapted from Bates, Camaioni, & Volterra (1975).

ing gestures are precursors to pointing, as the child learns how to conduct referential communication acts. Bates has termed the gestures observed during the intentional period and their rapid ritualization the **gesture complex.** The role of the gesture complex in establishing reference has been found to be strongly correlated with the subsequent emergence of verbal naming.

Social Interaction Stages and Processes.   Caregiver-child social routines are important in the development of prelinguistic and early linguistic communication. During the first months of infancy, children take a responsive role in interactions with caregivers; toward the end of the first year, they gain more intentional control. The growth-fostering aspect of social interaction with caregivers is often referred to as social scaffolding, providing a context for the development of social, emotional, psychological, and cognitive development (Brazelton & Als, 1979; Brazelton, Koslowski, & Main, 1974; Bruner, 1983). Through daily caregiving routines, games, and other interactions with caregivers, infants have repeated opportunities to experience the effect of their actions upon caregivers and the home environment. The role of the caregiver is a supportive and structural responsibility. The caregiver's ability to make adjustments in timing, verbal stimulation, presentation of objects, changing positions in space, and introducing a variety of activities and experiences contributes to the infant's growing world of referents.

Social interactions develop over the first year of life, expanding from early face-to-face interactions with caregivers to intentional and referential communication in less specific environmental contexts (Goldberg, 1977). Key elements in this developmental process include the dyad, infant's state control, mutuality, reciprocity, synchronicity, and turn-taking. The **dyad** refers to the interactive pair, including the infant and caregiver. Mother-infant dyads are observed most often, but sibling-infant, father-infant, relative-infant, and babysitter-infant are all viable caregiving dyads that may play an important role in fostering the infant's communication development. **Infant state control** refers to the neonate's mastery over smooth movement from sleep to wake states. Brazelton and Als (1979) described progressive states, including deep sleep, drowsiness, quiet alert, and crying. Neonates repeatedly cycle through these states during the first month of life, demonstrating increased physiological and neurological maturity. The quiet alert state is the optimal state for the infant to interact with caregivers. As the infant matures in state regulation, longer periods of the quiet alert state are observed. Other terms applied to parent-infant communication include **mutuality, reciprocity, synchronicity,** and **turn-taking.** These terms, defined in Table 6-4, refer to qualities of interaction between caregivers and infants that are considered to enhance communication development with young infants over the first year of life.

The supporting role of caregivers is significant because it provides multiple opportunities for infants to practice and refine the vocal, gestural, and social communication behaviors. For the SLP and other early intervention professionals, understanding the developmental processes underlying prelinguistic and early linguistic communication is critical to providing appropriate services.

Strand 3: Individual Differences

The third strand of the CAMI involves the notion of individual differences. The possibility that children may follow different paths or strategies in language acquisition was noticed as early as the 1960s, when the prevailing emphasis in the field was on universal aspects of development (c.f. Vihman & Greenlee, 1987). Since then, there have been numerous accounts of variation across subjects in the acquisition of syntax and single-word vocabulary

TABLE 6-4   Social Scaffolding Qualities in Caregiver-Infant Interaction

Quality	Definition
Mutuality	Both partners in the interactive dyad are aware and attentive to each other, accepting any contribution to the interaction made by the other partner (Brazelton, Koslowski, & Main, 1974).
Reciprocity	Adaptive modifications are made within the dyad by both partners in response to communicative behavior of the other partner. Reciprocity can be observed in repair strategies by both the mother and child that serve to continue, or to "repair" the interaction. Infants learn to repair interactions through repeated signalling to re-engage caregivers (Brazelton, Koslowski, & Main, 1974).
Synchronicity	Building on sensitivity and awareness of the other partner, synchronous dyads include mutuality and reciprocal interaction. Mutual sensitivity to the emotional and attention state of the other partner is coupled with continuous adjustments in timing and intensity of stimulation (Clark & Siefer, 1983).
Turn-Taking	A turn is defined as any single communicative act, verbal or nonverbal, that is directed toward another person. Turn-taking is considered one of the primary social interaction skills learned in infancy. Parents initially take more turns, but infants later take a more active role in social games and routines. Turns between parents and infants become more balanced as each partner learns to respond contingently to the other (Kaye & Charney, 1981).

(Nelson, 1973; Peters, 1977); pragmatic development (Bates et al., 1979); and phonological development (Stoel-Gammon & Cooper, 1984; Vihman & Greenlee, 1987). However, individual differences in language acquisition are not limited to vocal/verbal forms of communication. Concomitant aspects of communication development also vary considerably from child to child. Among these aspects are intentional acts (Bates et al., 1988; Harding & Golinkoff, 1979), turn-taking (Mahoney & Powell, 1984), and gesturing (Bates, Thal, Whitesall, Fenson, & Oakes, 1989; Thal & Bates, 1988).

Given the complexities of communication development and varied opportunities for learning, variability in rate of learning is to be expected (Muma, 1986). In general, we can conclude that children exhibit a high degree of variability in the individual competence each brings to communication development. For the SLP, accepting that a child displays individual differences helps in recognizing the uniqueness of a child's development, specifically the approach he takes to acquire language. The differing rates and styles of language development increasingly found among normally developing infants support the need to approach developmental assessment of infants and toddlers with language/communication delays with caution. The CAMI acknowledges these differences and incorporates them into the assessment paradigm.

Strand 4: Communicative Contexts

Language development occurs within familiar contexts. Developmentally, children go through a gradual process of decontextualization, in which utterances are no longer bound to limited contexts. Snyder et al. (1981) have described the process of decontextualization in relation to a child's acquisition of first words and early word combinations. Young children first exhibit utterances that are bound to specific contexts, such as saying "Daddy go" only when Daddy is walking out the front door at home. Later, the same child may generalize such utterances to other people, in other locations, and possibly in picture contexts (i.e., decontextualization). When assessing infants, clinicians need to be aware that familiar routines at home may be the only contexts that elicit vocalizations and communicative intent. Situational variables, such as degree of structure (low/high), environment (familiar/unfamiliar), persons (familiar/unfamiliar), age of communicative partner (adult/ peer/younger child), and communicative function (request, comment, showing off, greeting, etc.) influence the communicative and linguistic performance of young children.

For children with language/communication delays, the relationship between familiar context and communicative behavior takes on additional significance. Kennedy, Sheridan, Radlinshi, and Beeghly (1991) recently studied the relationships between play behavior and subsequent language development in a small sample of children with developmental delays. Using Nicolich's (1977) symbolic play scale, play behavior and early language skills were compared for six children ranging in age from 2 years 9 months to 3 years 4 months. Although relationships between language comprehension, expression, and symbolic play schemes were similar to those found in normally developing children of similar language development skills, wide fluctuations in play and language behavior were found. Observed differences in language skills demonstrate that children with language/communication delays may be more sensitive to context, structure of assessment situation, and the demands placed upon them.

Strand 5: Early Intervention Teams

The next strand of the CAMI involves selecting an appropriate early intervention team. Three types of team models are identified in the literature and in practice: the multidisciplinary, interdisciplinary, and transdisciplinary models (Campbell, 1987; McConnick & Goldman, 1978). Although among the models clear differences exist in the patterns of interactions with families and in the delivery of early intervention services, early intervention professionals actually use variations and combinations of all three team models. The three models can be outlined as follows:

- *Multidisciplinary model*—professionals from multiple disciplines work independently to provide services to an individual child and family. For example, in the case of a speech and language delay related to a child born with cleft lip and/or palate, the child's parents may see multiple medical specialists, an audiologist, SLP, genetic counselor, hospital social worker, and other professionals over the course of many months, in relatively separate interactions. Parents and children are involved in a number of different assessments and interventions, as each professional interacts individually with the family.
- *Interdisciplinary model*—involves a greater degree of interaction among disciplines and more coordinated service delivery with families and young children. For example, in an interdisciplinary model, parents of an infant with health and developmental needs related to prenatal drug exposure and positive HIV status may interact with medical, social work, public health nursing, speech-language pathology, physical therapy, occupational therapy, and psychology professionals. Rather than interact with families individually throughout the identification, assessment, and intervention process, professionals meet together to discuss findings of individual assessment and, most often, to synthesize individual findings into a single report intended to be comprehensive to family members. Similar to the multidisciplinary model, interdisciplinary services are provided through professionals interacting individually with families and children.
- *Transdisciplinary model*—requires a great deal more communication between team members, as coordinated interactions with families and children with disabilities are the primary goal of this model. Transdisciplinary approaches move beyond single-discipline interactions with families at all levels of identification, assessment, and intervention with young children and their caregivers. For example, a child with early communication and language delays related to combined biological and environmental risks, such as a very low birthweight infant born to a teenage mother, may have maximum contact with the SLP and minimal contact with other related disciplines. In this case, the SLP relies on the input and consultative roles of professionals from other disciplines, such as the physical therapist (PT), the occupational therapist (OT), the social worker, and others, to provide comprehensive services with the young mother, infant, and other family members involved.

The transdisciplinary model is often considered the preferred model for increasing communication and collaboration among disciplines and for maintaining continuity in services to families (Hanson, 1983b). However, individual family and child needs, as well as the particular needs of the program (e.g., staffing, location, etc.), may necessitate the use of multidisciplinary and interdisciplinary models at times. For example, children who are identified at birth to have been exposed to drugs in utero require confidentiality to prevent possible stigma and further isolation for them and their caregivers. A multidisciplinary model may be required to identify these children; however, a transdisciplinary model may best serve them when planning intervention. Because the transdisciplinary model calls for a primary care provider to maintain sole contact with the parent and child during the intervention process, the intervention should be more confidential and meaningful to family members. Keep in mind that the ultimate goal is to improve the health and developmental outcome for the child.

Collaborative Team Models.   The three types of team models described above apply to interactions of team members *within* teams, or intrateam processes. Also critical to the coordination of services for families and young children are the interactions *across* teams, or interteam processes. Professionals in early intervention services are increasingly urged to develop collaboration across disciplines and service systems, in order to create more effective transitions and services with families. For example, families with high-risk newborns born prematurely are faced with interactions with a hospital team, a home-health care team, and possibly an early intervention team. Interactions with each of these teams are made in very rapid succession, often within one–two months after the birth of the child. The importance of coordination and collaboration across teams has emerged as an element of best practice in providing family-centered care that is responsive to the needs of families for linkages in information and support from one team of providers to the next. Collaborative models of team workers are described by Wyly, Allen, Pfalzer, and Wilson (1996) within the context of the neonatal intensive care unit for cooperation and transitions to early intervention services in home and community settings. The need for cooperation and communication between health care teams is outlined by Wyly et al. with the following key components:

- Establishing partnership with family members at the outset
- High-risk infant interventions
- Transition information and support to early intervention services
- Continuity of care from hospital, home, center-based services
- Communication between hospital, home, and center-based team members

Collaboration between teams requires that a **care coordinator** be appointed from the initial contact with family members and the identification of potential risk factors such as low birthweight, developmental delay, other biological or environmental risk factors. The care coordinator often serves in the role of the primary partner with family members to assist them in negotiating the early assessments, medical interventions, developmental support for the infant, parent education, referral, and development of short- and long-term goals related with the care of the child. While many challenges remain to achieve collaboration in service with families and young children with disabilities, increased awareness and cooperation across teams can improve the family's experience toward "seamless" or continuous services that are cohesive and coordinated.

Strand 6: Intervention Strategies

The last strand of the CAMI involves selection of intervention strategies for infants and toddlers. The selection of these strategies is guided by assessment information and individual characteristics of children and families. As the clinician moves through the assessment process, beginning with identification of family concerns, intervention goals may become evident. For example, a parent may identify increased vocalization and "talking" as intervention targets. Keeping this intervention target in mind, information regarding developmental processes, individual differences, communicative contexts, and roles of team members will allow the SLP and parent to refine the initial target and develop collaborative goals. At each stage in the assessment process, linkages to intervention can be developed. The interaction goals are then based on a synthesis of shared information, between parents, the SLP, and other team members.

Bailey (1988) outlined a process of developing collaborative goals and objectives for early intervention personnel and families. An **intervention goal** is a long-term statement that includes an outcome statement for a given time frame (e.g., 6 months to 1 year). **Intervention objectives** are specific, short-term goals that include (a) the precise behaviors to be accomplished, (b) a description context for the behaviors expected of the individual, and (c) specific criteria to evaluate the attainment of the objective. This chapter briefly addresses the development of intervention goals and objectives; the reader is referred to Bailey for a more complete discussion. However, the CAMI, as discussed and applied in the following sections, provides a context for the SLP to integrate findings from differing perspectives with family members as key decision makers throughout the entire process. These procedures are consistent with guidelines for developing the Individualized Family Service Plan (IFSP), as required in federal legislation and policy. Detailed guidelines for the IFSP process are found in McGonigel et al. (1991).

Selection of goals and objectives will greatly influence the types of communication intervention strategies selected. As the student will discover in the case studies presented later in this chapter, individual child characteristics, family preferences, and professional findings influence the selection of intervention approaches. Two primary types of intervention approaches are used in practice and described in the literature: naturalistic and direct (McCormick, Loeb, & Schiefelbusch, in press). Differing theory and principles underlie the two types of intervention. Naturalistic approaches are based on a developmental/ cognitive/social model, and direct approaches are based on a behavioral model incorporating reinforcement principles. Each approach and some examples are briefly described.

Naturalistic Communication Intervention.   Naturalistic approaches to language and communication are based on the assumptions that (a) young children learn to communicate using speech and language in variety of daily routines and activities with caregivers; and (b) intervention is best conducted within the context of familiar environments. Based on the work of Hart and Risely (1975), naturalistic approaches to language intervention have their basis in "incidental teaching" techniques that relied primarily on a time-delay procedure (withholding desired items briefly) in order to elicit further communicative attempts with children with developmental delays. Since that time, the many forms and procedures of naturalistic approaches to intervention to support young children with language delays have more commonly been referred to a "mileu approaches." Other terms that are used to refer to similar methods of embedding language intervention withing naturally occurring activities and routines include (a) transactional teaching (McLean & Snyder-McLean, 1978); (b) pragmatic intervention (Duchan, 1986); (c) child-oriented teaching (Fey, 1986); (d) interactive modeling (Wilcox, Kouri, & Caswell, 1991); (e) social partnership (MacDonald & Carroll, 1992); and (f) enhanced mileu teaching (Kaiser & Hester, 1995). A more complete review of the past development of naturalistic/mileu intervention approaches was provided by Warren and Gazdag (1990), who defined several common elements, including incidental teaching, social routines, turn-taking, and environmental arrangement.

Incidental Teaching. The concept and application of incidental teaching has remained central to the application of naturalistic interventions, as SLPs, parents, and other members of the team are required to become skilled in observation and identification of "teachable moments" with young children. For example, an infant who is reaching toward her bottle provides caregivers the opportunity to hold the bottle momentarily and comment, "Yes, that's Ana's milk!" thus engaging the baby's attention and providing a verbal label for her behavior. The importance of joint attention between caregiver and child and responsiveness to the child's focus of attention are stressed in naturalistic intervention as the key starting points.

Social Routines and Daily Activities. Bruner (1983) identified the importance of familiar names and social routines such as peek-a-boo due to their defined structure, repetition, and opportunities for young children to experience anticipation, response, initiation, and conclusion. The adult's use of naturally occurring games, interactions, and routines as teaching opportunities with the child was described as "scaffolding" by Bruner. The application of naturalistic or milieu approaches are by nature embedded within daily routines and familiar activities for young children. In application, authors range from carefully planned environments and activities to naturally occurring events; agreement is stated that young children demonstrate increased generalization of language and communication behaviors when familiar routines are used for the context of intervention such as play, mealtimes, bath, and so on (Kaiser & Hester, 1995). Norris and Hoffman (1990) have described specific steps that caregivers can structure and respond to child communication through selection of toys, expansion of child behavior, and natural consequences.

Turn-taking. The notion of "balanced" turns between adult and child were incorporated into conversational forms of language intervention by MacDonald and Gillette (1985) and Mahoney and Powell (1984). Turn-taking interventions are planned primarily as play sessions between the parent and child with the focus on achieving a balanced turn ratio between partners. MacDonald and Carroll (1992) have more recently proposed a social partnership model that is designed to support parents to learn that communication "develops even from the (child's) simplest actions and sounds." Parents are encouraged to respond to any child behavior that might be communicative, treating each child behavior as one conversational "turn." The effects of the social partnership model are reported to increase levels of child imitation, vocalization, and communicative turn-taking in the context of interaction with parents.

Environmental Arrangement.   The arrangement of activities and the play environment has received increased attention in naturalistic methods of language intervention. The structuring of the environment and the role of the adult to mediate the environment are considered key to the implementation of naturalistic intervention methods. Included in the arrangement of the environment is the selection of appropriate toys for the child, arrangement of materials to promote requests and initiated communication behaviors from the child, and the role of the adult to employ environmental modifications in communication. Rather than assuming the role of an observer, naturalistic approaches require active monitoring and utilization of multiple opportunities to extend communication with the child.

The application of naturalistic intervention approaches was originally demonstrated within the context of early language development in preschool children with developmental delays (Halle, Baer, & Spradlin, 1981). In recent years, increased applications of naturalistic methodology are reported with infants and toddlers in stages of prelinguistic communication and emergent language development (Norris & Hoffman, 1990; McDonald & Carroll, 1992; Yoder, Warren, Kyoungram, & Gazdag, 1994). Yoder et al. described the application of a **modified milieu** approach combined with **linguistic mapping** to teach intentional requesting with young children with Down syndrome. Intervention techniques were implemented in a play setting while adults employed time-delay, joint-attention, and environmental arrangement to elicit requesting behaviors with young children. In addition, linguistic mapping was employed as adults verbally labeled the child's actions and focus of attention. As children increased **intentional requesting** (nonverbal gestures to signal requesting), Yoder et al. found that adults also increased verbal labeling (mapping) of the child's actions. The effect of increased child communicative behavior on increased adult responsiveness was described as a **transactional effect.** As children increased in their intentional communication behaviors, adults increased responsive communication toward the children.

In a similar approach, MacDonald and Carroll (1992) have extended earlier work to support verbal language between children and caregivers to intervention with infants and toddlers. The ECO model has specific applications to children with communication disorders and families in daily routines. The context of play interactions are recommended for assessment and intervention processes with young children and family members. In the ECO approach to intervention, parents are supported to learn that communication "develops even more from the (child's) simplest actions and sounds" and to respond to any child behavior that might be construed as communication. Similar to findings in the work by Yoder et al., MacDonald and Carroll have reported that parents demonstrated qualitative changes in communication behavior directed toward their children that included actions and words that are more closely matched to the child's play.

Through the increased modification and demonstration of naturalistic intervention approaches to communication and language intervention with young children, researchers have demonstrated positive effects for the **parent-child dyad** and the reciprocal communication between child and caregiver, rather than a single focus on the increase in child behavior that was reported in earlier research.

Direct Communication Intervention.   **Direct intervention** models are based on learning principles, as defined in behavioral psychology. Applications of direct intervention strategies are often incorporated in naturalistic settings but, as opposed to naturalistic methods, are highly structured. Direct intervention principles are discussed thoroughly by

McCormick and Schiefelbusch (1990), and the reader is referred to that source for a detailed overview of modeling, reinforcement, shaping, chaining, fading, and prompting-cueing strategies. The beginning SLP often feels more comfortable pursuing direct intervention over naturalistic techniques because of the highly structured nature of direct intervention. However, direct intervention approaches are not easily applied with infants and toddlers who have communication and language delays; play-based and naturalistic methods are better aligned with the attention, focus, and behaviors of this age group. However, direct intervention approaches have been successful in developing contingency awareness in infants and toddlers with severe disabilities (Dunst, Cushing, & Vance, 1985).

Applications of the CAMI: Three Case Examples

Example 1: Early Infancy

The CAMI allows for assessment of children across several periods of development. The first case focuses on the period of early infancy. Early infancy is characterized by basic physiological responses to the external world and development of primary relationships with caregivers.

> *Kwan was born 3 months prematurely, weighing only 949 grams, placing her within the very low birthweight range. Her condition at birth was such that she required breathing assistance with a respirator and feeding with a gavage tube. She remained in the hospital three months, going home at her term gestational age of 9 months. Her weight at discharge was improved, at nearly 1500 grams. At the time of discharge, Kwan was medically stable, having overcome irregular breathing patterns. She was discharged with a gastrostomy tube for feeding. Kwan's mother, a 20-year-old single parent, cared for her with the help of her own mother and sister in the home that the three adults share. Kwan's mother and her family originally immigrated to a large urban area on the U.S. mainland from Taiwan 10 years ago. Kwan's mother and grandmother were referred to the early intervention program through the public health nurse, and a home visit was scheduled for an assessment. Kwan's mother expressed concern because her baby did not seem to make many movements or vocal sounds (except prolonged crying every day between 6:00 and 9:00 p.m.). Kwan's mother reported that she had difficulty handling Kwan, as she cried often and stiffened when picked up out of her crib.*

Family Preferences. Because Kwan's mother is young and offers only a small amount of information about her daughter's early development, it may be tempting to assume that her limited knowledge in some way contributes to Kwan's fussiness and slow development. However, the characteristics that Kwan brings to the caregiving interaction are significant and contribute to her mother's reported frustration. Further questioning about the primary concerns for Kwan's development reveal that her mother is a very concerned and knowledgeable caregiver for her daughter. With the help of Kwan's grandmother, Kwan's mother has spent many hours watching her daughter in the hospital and learning how to feed and care for her. The grandmother carries on most of the home chores so that Kwan and her mother can be together. Further, the grandmother and Kwan's mother have different concerns about the baby and these must be incorporated in the assessment plan. Kwan's mother sincerely wants to learn skills to better handle and soothe her daughter, and the grandmother feels the baby would grow better with formula fed through a bottle rather than a gastrostomy tube. The concerns of each of these key people in Kwan's caregiving will guide the continuing assessment and intervention process. As the clinician observes and gathers further information about Kwan's early development, Kwan's family members can be encouraged to participate actively, as primary informers about Kwan's interactive cues and feeding behaviors at home.

Developmental Processes.   Based on information gathered from the brief report provided by Kwan's mother and grandmother, certain questions emerge regarding Kwan's development thus far in her early life. Knowing her multiple biological and potential environmental risks at birth, assessment of Kwan's physiological, sensory, and motor development are needed. The following questions can now be formulated to systematically determine her developmental status and relationships to her communication development:

1. To what extent does Kwan respond to voices and familiar sounds in her environment, now that she has been home for approximately one month?
2. How does Kwan respond to familiar faces in her environment?
3. What are Kwan's sleep and waking patterns? How does she make transitions through waking and sleep states?
4. What are Kwan's overall muscle tone and movement patterns when she is placed in prone, supine, and feeding positions?
5. What primitive reflexes are observed in Kwan's repertoire at this time?
6. When Kwan is placed in close proximity to her caregivers, what social responses (e.g., brightened gaze, smile, open mouth, arm thrust, foot movement, or other generalized response to caregivers) are observed?
7. What is Kwan's regular intake of formula/breastmilk at each feeding? How steady is her weight gain?

As these questions indicate, the focus of assessment at this point is to gather further information about critical developmental processes that are typically observed in infants at one month of age. Communication development is clearly not the only concern for this child. With Kwan's early and very low birthweight history, a number of developmental processes are affected. Developmental measurement tools available to assist the clinician include the Minnesota Infant Development Inventory, a subtest of the Minnesota Child Development Inventory (MCDI) (Ireton & Thwing, 1974) and the Hawaii Early Learning Profile (HELP) (Furuno, O'Reilly, Inatsuka, Hosaka, Allman, & Zeisloft-Falboy, 1986). Both of these tools can be administered through parent report and supplemented with direct observation. Although only limited items on both instruments assess developmental processes in very young infants, these instruments allow for flexibility in administration and strongly encourage parent report.

Individual Differences.   With information regarding the developmental status of Kwan's communication behavior, we gather a more complete picture of Kwan's individual communication patterns.

Kwan's mother reported that her daughter is beginning to recognize familiar peo-ple when she is awake, generally after a feeding and in her swing. Kwan's mother is not sure if her own voice or face are more effective in getting Kwan to gaze in her direction. When observed at home, Kwan did not localize to sounds readily but exhibited a "whole-body" response when her mother said her name. Her mother reported that Kwan's waking from sleep in the midmorning is more gradual than other times. At other times, Kwan has difficulty waking, sleeping on-and-off throughout the day, fussing and quickly developing an agitated cry before her mother can get to the room to pick her daughter out of bed. According to the mother, preparation of the gastrostomy tube, formula, and attaching the tube takes more time than Kwan is willing to wait. Her intake of formula is quite good, as the entire 4 ounces are absorbed rapidly through the tube. Kwan does show some re-flexive sucking activity near the beginning of feeding, and her family wants to be-gin bottle feeding. Observations of Kwan's muscle tone and motor development showed low muscle tone and weak startle reflexes in response to loud sounds.

Further report by Kwan's mother and grandmother and direct observation will provide a daily record of sleeping, feeding, and waking times so that we can mutually understand the best times to play with Kwan and support her responsive interactions with her family. Two different types of assessment tools are now helpful, the Nursing Child Assessment Sleep/Activity Manual (NCASA) (Barnard, 1978) and the Bayley Scales of Infant Development (BSID) (Bayley, 1969). The first instrument, the NCASA, is part of a series developed to provide understanding of caregiver and child interactions in a variety of activities; administration requires extensive training within an approved Nursing Child Assessment Satellite Training (NCAST) course (Barnard, 1978). However, the NCASA offers a very clear method for the parent to assess sleep, wake, activity behaviors, and feeding patterns in the lives of their very young infants. The BSID, on the other hand, is a standardized test with limited reliability for use with young infants. However, the early items on the BSID lend themselves to further exploration of Kwan's gaze, reach, and preferred motor positions and can be interpreted to highlight individual differences and strengths. From what we know about her individual preferences thus far, Kwan requires support to adjust to environmental stimulation throughout the day. For example, her intense crying periods in the evening may be a result of increasing stimulation throughout the day that result in potent disengagement cues including body arching, hands at sides, and inconsolable crying.

Communicative Contexts.   The contexts in which Kwan shows communicative behavior can be determined through her daily caregiving routines. The individual engagement and disengagement behaviors that she displays are intimately tied to the context of the caregiving environment. Two additional NCAST scales, the Feeding Scale and the Infant Behavior Assessment Record (IBAR) (Barnard, 1978), help the clinician and caregiver determine the specific contexts that will reveal the most about Kwan's early behavioral signals (i.e., communicative behavior). Although the use of these scales requires rather extensive training, the specific information about individual infants can be extremely helpful to caregivers. Guidelines for assessment of parent-child interaction are also provided by Comfort and Farran (1994). The IBAR is based on concepts developed by T. Berry Brazelton, looking at neurological and behavioral maturation of the newborn. The IBAR offers the practitioner a brief assessment guide of alerting, visual responsiveness, auditory response, habituation, cuddliness, and consolability. Each of these behavior areas is related to state regulation, and use of the IBAR provides more specific information about optimal responses when the infant is awake and offers a potential source to develop support strategies for the infant to interact.

Early Intervention Teams.   Kwan's family has experienced intervention services provided by a number of health care professionals and will receive weekly follow-up from the public health nurse in their community. With a baby who is medically at risk, such as a very low birthweight baby, multiple contacts with a range of health care and social service professionals are unavoidable. Thus, a multidisciplinary team approach is needed to support Kwan and her family. To minimize the fragmentation the family may experience, a primary care coordinator, or case manager, is recommended. At the hospital level, this person may be the primary care nurse assigned to Kwan's mother or perhaps the SLP or other professional responsible for early assessment and parent education in the neonatal intensive care unit. After the family goes home, the public health nurse often becomes the case manager. At the point when Kwan's family contacts an early intervention program, they have made transitions between several different service systems and related professionals.

The SLP can build a parent-professional partnership with Kwan's family by taking a key role in coordinating recommendations from other disciplines that impact Kwan's intervention plan. Based on the assessment information gathered thus far, it is clear that concerns about Kwan's motor development, feeding, general health, hearing, vision, and communication will involve at least the following disciplines: speech-language pathology, audiology, physical therapy, occupational therapy, nursing, nutrition, pediatrics, and early intervention specialists. In this case, the SLP is the obvious professional to coordinate contacts and recommended interventions with Kwan's family, due to the central nature of her families' concern about Kwan's limited interactions. The team model that most applies in this situation is a combination of transdisciplinary and interdisciplinary approaches, as individual disciplines will continue to have direct involvement with Kwan's family.

Intervention Strategies.   Three primary areas of concern were voiced by Kwan's primary caregivers at the outset of the assessment process: soothing her when crying, feeding with a bottle, and a general lack of noncry vocalization. As the SLP and other team members contribute to the assessment process, these areas of concern can be elaborated and refined as collaborative goals for Kwan's early communication intervention program. Based on the information gathered, at least three possible goals can be generated for Kwan: (a) develop alternative techniques for Kwan's mother to soothe her daughter, (b) increase Kwan's tolerance for oral feeding, and (c) increase social interaction times between Kwan and her family members. Several researchers in the area of neonatal and high-risk infant development provide effective strategies to enhance the self-regulation and tolerance of external stimuli of even the most vulnerable infants. Several of these strategies are given in Table 6-5. The underlying principle for all the approaches is to continually monitor infant engagement and disengagement cues, adjusting caregiver behaviors in direct response to infant cues. Adjustments of caregiver behavior may include simply taking a break in the interaction, allowing the infant to brace her feet against the caregiver's hand, or providing a small toy for the infant to grasp. Of course, individual infants vary in their response to specific techniques and strategies; the parent and SLP must discover the appropriate techniques through trial and error. Table 6-5 also provides more extensive guidelines that may be applied and modified for individual infants.

TABLE 6-5   Communication Intervention Goals, Strategies, and Models for Kwan

Intervention Goal	Intervention Strategy	Intervention Model
Develop alternative techniques for Kwan's mother to soothe her daughter.	Demonstrate holding, wrapping, and soothing techniques with Kwan and her mother.	Swaddling, self-regulation, and slow movements (Cole, 1996).
Increase Kwan's tolerance for oral feeding.	Provide pacifier or nipple on bottle to increase oral tolerance; gradually increase amounts of formula by mouth.	Consult physician and OT regarding feeding techniques and plan for increasing oral feeding (Ahman, 1986).
Increase social interaction times between Kwan and her family members.	Encourage Kwan's mother and grandmother to respond to vocal, visual, and gestural behaviors during Kwan's awake/alert times.	Support parent-child interaction (Hanson & Krentz, 1986; McCollum & Yates, 1994).

Example 2: Middle Infancy

In middle infancy, the child becomes a more active participant in the world around him. He or she sleeps less, sits upright, and vocalizes often. The following referral applies the CAMI to a child in middle infancy:

> *Lucy was referred at the age of 7 months for an evaluation of her general developmental status, particularly in communication, as her mother reported that "Lucy's muscles are weak and do not allow her to make sounds like my other children." Lucy's mother reported that her pregnancy was normal but that Lucy was born in a "breech" position and was diagnosed as having cerebral palsy shortly after birth. Lucy's mother reported that an earlier developmental assessment of Lucy performed at 3 months of age indicated that her cerebral palsy is considered "spastic hemiplegia" affecting the right side of her body. Reportedly, Lucy is able to sit upright with support. However, she appears to have difficulty tracking objects visually. Her mother said that she is most worried now that Lucy makes only a few vocal sounds, including crying and some vowel sounds.*

Family Preferences.   Lucy is the youngest of four siblings. She comes from an extended family consisting of her mother and siblings, her grandmother, and an aunt and uncle, who all reside in the same home. Lucy's mother works outside the home, so Lucy is cared for at home by her aunt and older siblings. Lucy's siblings and her aunt are important to include in the assessment process because of their roles as primary caregivers. Each of Lucy's family members has information about her personality, daily communicative behavior, feeding, fussiness, and overall development. Because Lucy has multiple caregivers, the SLP has a unique opportunity to develop teamwork with these key family members. Placing Lucy's family members in the role of primary informants is most important. Use of parent/caregiver interview tools with family members is a helpful strategy to build collaborative teamwork from the first contact between the SLP, the family and child, and other early intervention personnel.

Developmental Processes.   Information provided thus far by Lucy's mother indicated generalized developmental delays in the areas of gross and fine motor, feeding, communication, and visual development. The following questions can be formulated to gather critical information for understanding and planning intervention to support Lucy's progress in developmental and functional skills:

1. What is Lucy's pattern for digesting liquid and solid foods? What are her likes and dislikes of liquid and solid foods?
2. What is Lucy's general muscle tone? Does she attempt (and accomplish) any mobility on her own?
3. What is the exact nature of Lucy's vocalizations? In what contexts is she most likely to vocalize?
4. What early social and gestural communications are reported when Lucy interacts with caregivers?
5. In what positions is Lucy most comfortable and observed to vocalize?
6. What degree of physical support is needed to help Lucy maintain sitting or other upright postures?
7. What is Lucy's range of visual response to her caregivers and objects in her environment?

As discussed, Lucy's extended family plays a critical role in her daily development. Gathering developmental information through informant report will empower family members to identify Lucy's strengths and needs, rather than being "told" of these by professionals. Further exploration of Lucy's development may best begin with her family through a structured interview process, using developmental stages as guidelines for discussion. Several instruments are available for this purpose. The Vineland Scale of Adaptive Behavior (VSAB) (Sparrow, Balla, & Ciccetti, 1984) is a comprehensive evaluation of the major domains of development through a parent interview format. As a standardized instrument, the VSAB provides a normative score; however, such a score may not be relevant to the needs of Lucy's family. Other tools appropriate at this stage of the assessment process include the HELP developmental checklist (Furuno et al., 1986) and the MCDI (Ireton & Thwing, 1974).

Individual Differences.   Having gathered critical information covering the preceding developmental areas, we can begin to identify the specific characteristics of Lucy's individual prelinguistic communication patterns. We gain the following information through careful observation and parental information:

Results of developmental assessment based on parent report and clinical observations showed that Lucy's oral mechanism is somewhat tactilely defensive, showing low tolerance for solid foods. She can sit upright with support, however, she has yet to walk on "all fours." She shows interest toward objects presented directly in her line of vision and will reach for those objects. On the other hand, when objects are presented away from Lucy's midline, she is less responsive, probably due to her motoric and visual limitations. She demonstrates differentiated cries for hunger, discomfort, and pain. Aside from crying and other reflexive vocalizations (e.g., burping, sneezing), she occasionally laughs, and she is just beginning to make some vocal sounds, including a "grunting" /h/ sound and an "aah" /ah/ sound. She is particularly vocal when lying on her back during diaper changes. She is also generally more attentive toward familiar family members than to strangers.

This information leads to the hypothesis that Lucy's primary strength is her overall interest in the environment. She is responsive to familiar people and will reach toward objects. Her primary weaknesses are in the areas of motor and visual development. These weaknesses may prevent Lucy from gaining everyday experiences in the environment that nondisabled children take for granted. Her present oral motor abilities also suggest that normal speech sound development may be impaired.

Additional questions can now be generated for further assessments. Continued assessment should probably focus on Lucy's strengths, as well as further define the range of her motoric and visual limitations. Continuing assessment will focus around the following questions:

1. What events occur regularly throughout Lucy's day? What gestural/vocal behaviors does she display during these routines?
2. How does Lucy demonstrate her attentiveness toward familiar people?
3. What are the specific food items that Lucy can/cannot tolerate?
4. What are Lucy's imitation skills, both gesturally and vocally?
5. What specific items/events will Lucy attend most/least to?
6. What specific vowellike and consonantlike sounds can Lucy produce?

Assessment instruments that will address these specific questions include the Early Language Milestone (ELM) Scale (Coplan, 1993) and the Rossetti Infant-Toddler Language Scale (ITLS) (Rossetti, 1990). The ELM scale uses parent report, incidental observation, and direct testing to evaluate expressive, receptive, and visual development (in monthly intervals) across the first three years of life. With respect to Lucy, the assessment of her visual development is particularly important. Coplan and Gleason (1990) have demonstrated that the ELM scale is valid for both normal and at-risk populations.

Similar to the ELM scale, the ITLS (Rossetti, 1990) is designed to assess children between the ages of birth to 3 years. The ITLS uses both parent report (and interview) and actual testing of children's social interaction, pragmatics, gestural development, play behavior, language comprehension, and language expression. For Lucy, developmental ages obtained on both the ELM and ITLS measures may not be as critical as the degree of effort and attention she displays on the test items.

Communicative Contexts.   What are the contexts in which Lucy appears to communicate? Lucy's prelinguistic behavior appears to be tied to three different contexts. The first context is one of the family in general. Lucy is most attentive when interacting with familiar people. Such a context should be stressed as being an important one, with familiar members playing the role as primary interactive partners. A second context appears to be tied to a daily routine—diaper changing. Recurring situations such as these should be identified. Such daily routines provide opportunities for Lucy to communicate with her caregivers and for her caregivers to communicate in return, stressing turn-taking, vocalization expansion, and vocal and gestural imitation. The third context, and perhaps the most important, is directly related to Lucy's motoric visual limitations. Specifically, she responds to items and activities presented at her midline. This important context will serve as the foundation for presenting new information to Lucy.

Early Intervention Teams.   Events at birth contributing to cerebral palsy are seldom so site-specific that they bring about only one kind of clinical problem. As already noted, Lucy is demonstrating feeding, motor, and visual impairments, in addition to a delay in communication development. Other problems found to be associated with cerebral palsy include hearing impairment, mental retardation, and seizure activity. Because the problems associated with cerebral palsy are numerous and complex, intervention involves the integrated efforts of many professionals. Rather than schedule separate evaluations for Lucy's family to see these various professionals, the SLP may wish to utilize these persons as consultants while maintaining direct contact with the child and family herself. This approach represents a transdisciplinary model and limits the number of personnel that must initially be involved in the child assessment and family conferencing steps.

Intervention Strategies.   Infants born with special needs and their caregivers require specialized professional support in the early months so that both parent and child can adjust to the communicative styles and behaviors of the other (Richard, 1986). A child with motor development involvement related to cerebral palsy from birth may have severely limited movement and gestural capabilities, requiring family members to extensively adapt and augment their infant's communicative efforts. The specific areas that need to be strengthened and supported for Lucy's prelinguistic and emerging communication skills with her caregivers include (a) fuller use of gaze patterns to maintain interaction with caregivers, (b) gradual introduction of thicker textures in feeding, and (c) the discovery on Lucy's part that her communicative behaviors have an effect on her family members. The intervention goals, strategies, and suggested models found in Table 6-6 are based on Lucy's developmental needs as well as her reported and observed preferences. Her family members all demonstrate active involvement with Lucy; their preferences for certain intervention strategies will determine what priority is placed on the goals outlined.

Example 3: Transitions to Toddlerhood

The conclusion of the infancy period and the beginning of toddlerhood is characterized by the emergence of recognizable language. The following referral begins our application of

TABLE 6-6   **Communication Intervention Strategies for Lucy (Age 7 Months)**

Intervention Goal	Intervention Strategy	Intervention Model
Increase chewing of solid foods.	Include small bites of soft foods and thick liquids.	Have OT/PT team member provide feeding program.
Increase eye gaze and tracking of objects and people.	Introduce colorful, movable objects to visual midline and periphery.	
Develop skills to reach/touch/ activate switches.	Introduce musical/sound making toys (at visual midline) that require switch attention.	Uses language intervention organizational framework (Messick, Anketell, & Chapman, 1987).
Increase gestural/facial expression.	Identify daily routines (e.g., diaper changes) that provide opportunities for face-to-face contact.	
Increase vocalization.	Identify daily routines that elicit frequent vocalization from Lucy and encourage her to vocally imitate.	Milieu teaching and linguistic mapping (Yoder et al., 1994).
Increase conversational behavior.	Identify daily routines that elicit vocalizations from Lucy and encourage her to "take turns."	Social partnership model (MacDonald & Carroll, 1992).

recent findings in studies of emerging language to assessment and intervention planning during the period of toddlerhood:

> *Josh, age 19 months, was referred for an evaluation of his communication skills, based on his parents' report that he is not yet talking. Josh's mother provided the following information: His birth history is reported to be normal, although he was diagnosed to have Down syndrome at birth. His health history is characterized by a "number of ear infections," that "never seem to clear up." His mother stated that "aside from the infections," his health has been "good." Josh's mother also reported that he cannot yet stand on his own, although he can stand with support. He still drinks fluids from a bottle and is not yet able to tolerate solid foods. Josh communicates with his parents using "only a few sounds," and "lots of gesturing," including gestures for "bye-bye" and "eat." When compared to her older child, Josh's mother said, "Josh is not doing much."*

Family Preferences.   Josh's family consists of his mother, father, and older brother, age 5. His mother coordinates most of the medical and developmental activities with her children, as his father works full time. However, Josh's father is very much involved in the care of his children and keeps well informed about the special needs of his youngest son. Both parents are very much concerned that they do "everything possible to help Josh." Based on the comments made about Josh's development, particularly his communication development, the SLP may gather that his parents' perception of Josh's strengths are limited. This initial impression that Josh's parents may not perceive his prelinguistic and early linguistic behaviors as strengths may alert the SLP that his parents require support and careful guidance to identify every means of communication that Josh exhibits.

Developmental Processes.   Having considered the background information, a number of questions can be generated regarding developmental processes present in Josh's communicative behavior. Note that the areas addressed in the preceding description provided by Josh's mother include possible concerns about hearing, motor development, oral-motor development, cognitive development, social, and vocal development.

1. Does Josh appear to respond to voices and sounds in his environment?
2. What is Josh's overall muscle tone and body posture in a variety of positions?
3. What are Josh's sucking, swallowing, and chewing patterns?
4. Does Josh demonstrate interest in toys? What types of actions are performed?
5. How does Josh respond when family members begin to play with him? Does he begin favorite games with them?
6. What vocal sounds does Josh make? What changes are reported in recent months?
7. What is the total number of different gestures that Josh produces?

Based on the areas of concern for Josh, several developmental assessment tools may be appropriate to gather initial information with his parents. Several of the tools provide extensive developmental information—the selection will ultimately rest on the clinician's judgment about appropriateness for Josh and his family. Possible tools include the HELP (Furuno et al., 1986), VSAB (Sparrow et al., 1984), MCDI (Ireton & Thwing, 1974), and the Sequenced Inventory of Communication Development (SICD) (Hedrick, Prather, & Tobin, 1984). At this point in the assessment, general developmental information is needed. Parent-report measures such as the MCDI may be most informative to Josh's parents about developmental skills he demonstrates. Of the other tools listed, the HELP is a nonstandardized developmental scale; the VSAB is a standardized developmental interview scale; and the SICD is a standardized early assessment that also includes several parent-report items for children under 20 months of age. There are several advantages to using a tool such as the MCDI for initial assessment and intervention planning with Josh's parents. Recall that Josh's mother reported she does not perceive him to be doing much communicating for his age. Through completion of the MCDI, with professional support, Josh's parents may be able to identify his specific developmental skills and provide the clinician with data for further assessment and initial intervention strategies. In addition, recent studies report a strong correlation between the MCDI and other developmental assessments, including the BSID (Bayley, 1969) and more recently the SICD. Tomblin, Shonrock, and Hardy (1989) examined the predictive relationship of the MCDI Expressive and Comprehension-Conceptual scales with the SICD Receptive and Expressive scales and found moderate to strong correlations between the two assessment tools. Interestingly, the MCDI Comprehension-Conceptual scales were most strongly correlated to the SICD Expressive scales, a finding that indicates that parents may report both expressive and comprehension information on the MCDI Comprehension-Conceptual scale.

Individual Differences.   With specific developmental information, we will learn more of the developmental bases for Josh's delay in language and begin to identify his individual communication patterns. We gain the following information through careful observation and parental information:

> *Results of developmental assessment based on parent report and clinical observations showed that Josh responds to many environmental sounds and voices of family members. He appears to understand a number of words that refer to names of family members, to familiar items including his bottle, blanket, teddy bear, and inflated ball with noise makers inside, and to some daily activities including eating, bathtime, and story time. He enjoys sitting in either parent's lap at bedtime to read stories, although he only looks at the pictures fleetingly. Recently, he has begun to pat the pages of the books. Further observation of his body posture showed that Josh pulls to stand on furniture with his back curved and stomach out. He drops to the floor in sitting and generally sits with legs widespread, with his center of balance on his lower back. Feeding patterns were described as "messy" by his mother, with frequent drooling. Observation of chewing skills showed some vertical munching of soft crackers and forward tongue thrusting when attempting to swallow sips of milk from a small plastic tumbler. Interactions with others were generally described as visual and sometimes vocal responses. Josh's parents thought he tended to use gaze patterns to get attention, followed by pointing when he really wants his bottle. Vocal sounds were described primarily as vowels. He was found to use gestures to indicate "up," "bye-bye," "eat," and "no."*

This information leads to the hypothesis that Josh's strengths lie in his social responsiveness to members of his family and his understanding of familiar events and daily routines. Concerns about motor development and apparently hypotonic patterns (low muscle tone) involve both large and small for body movement and control in space as well as feeding skills and preferences. Consultation with other disciplines, including the physical therapist and occupational therapist, is supported by these observations. Additional questions can now be generated for further assessment, as the first steps of supporting parents to become the primary informants about their own child are accomplished. From this point, Josh's parents and the SLP can continue to work together, even setting initial assessment goals for the IFSP. Continued assessment can now focus specifically on Josh's individual strengths and developmental patterns in the areas of responsiveness to the home environment, social routines, word comprehension, and use of combined vocalizations and gestures. Continued assessment will focus around the following questions:

1. Which environmental sounds are most likely to get a response from Josh? How does he respond?
2. Does Josh respond to particular voices more than others? What type of physical, vocal, or other reactions are noted?

3. What differences are found in Josh's responses when his parents name and point to particular toys and familiar objects versus just naming the same items?
4. How does Josh respond to familiar routines when his parents mention "It's bath time, Josh," and so on?
5. Does Josh move toward favorite objects on the floor and attempt to bring them to family members to start games or other interactions?
6. Does Josh offer objects to family members during any games or daily routines?
7. Does Josh enjoy particular pictures and books more than others in his bedtime story routine?
8. In what positions and with what degree of physical support is Josh most likely to point to and/or reach for objects he wants?
9. To what extent is Josh able to imitate fine motor "gestural" movements of the hands and arms?

These questions require more specific information about Josh's individual communicative behaviors. Particularly useful at this point are structured parent-report measures that help parents catalog more specific understanding of gestural, vocal, and verbal communication and language. Parent-report measures are beneficial because (a) parents can provide data that is more representative of typical infant behavior, (b) parents report what the child knows more accurately than clinical observations that merely sample linguistic use, (c) they are a cost-effective means of identification and assessment, (d) they define further directions for intervention, and (e) they are an evaluation tool that monitors generalized changes in communication and language related to early intervention (Dale, 1991). Recently developed tools include the MacArthur Communicative Development Inventories (CDI) (Fenson et al., 1993) and the Language Development Survey (LDS) (Rescorla, 1989).

The CDI provides two scales, the CDI/Infants and the CDI/Toddlers, to assess preverbal development related to emerging language including nonverbal gestures, games and routines, actions with objects, imitation of actions, use of early language forms, and the degree of decontextualization present in the young child's language. Dale, Bates, Reznick, and Morisset (1989) and Dale (1991) reported significant correlations between the CDI/Toddlers and the BSID (Bayley, 1969). Miller, Sedey, and Miolo (1995) recently reported strong predictive correlation between CDI vocabulary scores and MLU. Rescorla (1989) conducted multiple studies of the LDS and reported repeatedly high correlations of the LDS with the BSID, the Preschool Language Scale (PLS) (Zimmerman, Steiner, & Pond, 1992), and the Reynell Expressive and Receptive Language Scales (Reynell, 1985). The LDS was found to be a reliable predictor of language delay with children at 2 years of age. Although each tool is somewhat different in content and in level of communication and language assessed, all have common elements, in particular a focus on current and newly emerging communication and language behaviors.

Communicative Contexts.   What are the contexts in which Josh appears to communicate? We know from the work of Bruner (1983), Snow and Ratner (1984), and Snyder, Bates, and Bretherton (1981) that familiar routines and games are the natural contexts for the expansion and elaboration of early communication forms. We also have learned about the important process of gradual decontextualization in early language. In Josh's case, verbal language has not yet fully emerged, so we might anticipate that his communication behavior is likely to occur in familiar, daily routines with familiar caregivers. Suggested methods to identify communicative contexts include ecological inventories (Richard, 1986), assessment of play sessions (Kennedy et al., 1991; Nicolich, 1977), and direct observations of caregivers and infants.

Early Intervention Teams.   Throughout the foregoing discussion of the assessment and initial intervention process for Josh, there are several points of linkage that must made with other professionals. Appropriate team members for the completion of Josh's assessment include the audiologist, pediatrician, nurse practitioner, physical therapist, occupational therapist, social worker, and possibly other professionals. The manner of referral and utilization of other disciplines in the assessment process with Josh and his family can be guided by current understanding of best practice in early intervention and, ultimately, the preferences of Josh's parents.

As mentioned earlier, the assessment/intervention process can be streamlined for families if the number of contacts with different professionals for different purposes can be minimized. This approach represents a transdisciplinary model. The core early intervention team—typically the SLP, occupational therapist, and physical therapist—have the unique opportunity to consult with one another through case review and observation. Additional referrals to other specialists, such as the pediatrician and audiologist, might also be necessary. However, these visits can be discussed with family members before and following the event to maximize the information provided.

Intervention Strategies.   Although Josh's assessment process has been presented as a linear series of steps leading up to intervention, in actuality the process is not linear. Intervention may begin at any point in the process—whenever a problem has been identified and Josh's parents and the clinician agree to address it. Some of these points in our discussion include reports by Josh's mother of her concern about his use of only a few sounds, frequent ear infections, and general pattern of responding rather than initiating games with his family. Further development of family goals around each of these concerns for Josh will provide opportunities for the clinician to assist the parents. Recommended strategies for each of these concerns are displayed in Table 6-7. General principles to support Josh and his family include enhancing daily routines rather than creating "teaching" situations; expanding play interactions with Josh; identifying functional communication through Josh's use of gestures, vocalizations, and emerging word patterns; and taking a preventative approach to upper respiratory infections.

Summary

The purpose of this chapter was to provide students of speech-language pathology with an overview of normal communication development during the period of infancy and early toddlerhood. As part of this overview, biological and environmental factors that contribute

TABLE 6-7   Communication Intervention Strategies for Josh (Age 19 Months)

Intervention Goal	Intervention Strategy	Intervention Model
Monitor general health and ear infections.	Consult with pediatrician on regular basis.	Have Josh undergo periodic audiological testing. Use prevention approach for chronic otitis media (Northern, 1981).
Increase vocalization repertoire in daily routines and games with family members, especially older brother.	Select favorite routine, such as reading books at night, and pause often to give opportunities for, Josh to vocalize before turning pages. Imitate and expand his sounds ("aa . . . ba . . .," "aa . . . da . . .," "aa . . . ma . . .".	Use conversational teaching (MacDonald, 1985; Mahoney & Powell, 1984; MacDonald & Carroll, 1992). Scaffolding structured intervention (Norris & Hoffman, 1990).
Increase vocal and gestural initiation in games and functional communication.	Before daily activities such as eating, bath time, going in the car, etc. Josh's parents and/or brother should pause and wait for Josh to gesture or vocalize to eat, turn on the bath water, or get picked up to go out to the car.	Enhanced milieu teaching (Kaiser & Hester, 1995). Group intervention (Wilcox, Kouri, & Caswell, 1991).
Increase Josh's social communication with other children and adults.	Involve Josh in playgroup.	

to placing the infant at risk for normal communication development were presented. Following a review of normal and at-risk development, a model of infant communication assessment, the CAMI, was presented and applied to three individual cases. The CAMI integrates six strands in the assessment process: family preferences, developmental processes, individual differences, communicative contexts, early intervention teams, and intervention strategies. We believe that using a broad framework such as the CAMI and placing family members in the role of key personnel is an appropriate approach to evaluating and treating children during infancy and early toddlerhood.

Study Questions

1. Explain the differences between environmental and biological risk factors. Provide examples of each.
2. What is a stage model of development? What are the advantages and disadvantages of using a stage model to evaluate a child?
3. Explain the differences between the multidisciplinary, interdisciplinary, and transdisciplinary team models.
4. Explain the six strands of the CAMI model.
5. List some of the commonly used communication assessment instruments for infants.

References

Abel, E., & Sokol, R. (1986). Fetal alcohol syndrome is now the leading cause of mental retardation. *Lancet, 2,* 1222–1224.

Ahman, E. (1986). *Home care for the high risk infant.* Rockville, MD: Aspen.

American Academy of Pediatrics. (1987). Statement of childhood lead poisoning. *Pediatrics, 79,* 458–459.

ASHA. (1989). Issues in determining eligibility for language intervention. *ASHA,* March, 113–118.

ASHA. (1991). Let's talk: Fetal alcohol syndrome. *ASHA,* August, 53–54.

Bailey, D. B. (1988). Considerations in developing family goals. In D. Bailey & R. Simeonsson (Eds.), *Family assessment in early intervention,* Columbus, OH: Merrill/Macmillan.

Bangs, T., & Dodson, S. (1986). *Birth to Three Developmental Scales.* Allen, TX: DLM Teaching Resources.

Barnard, K. (1978) *Nursing Child Assessment Satellite Training.* Seattle: University of Washington Press.

Bates, E., Benigni, L., Bretherton, I., Camaioni, L., & Volterra, V. (1979). *The emergence of symbols: Cognition and communication in infancy.* New York: Academic Press.

Bates, E., Bretherton, I., & Snyder, L. (1988). *From first words to grammar: Individual differences and dissociable mechanisms.* New York: Cambridge University Press.

Bates, E., Bretherton, I., & Snyder, L., Shore, C., & Volterra, V. (1980). Vocal and gestural symbols at 13 months. *Merrill-Palmer Quarterly, 26,* 408–423.

Bates, E., Camaioni, L., & Volterra, V (1975). The acquisition of performatives prior to speech. *Merrill-Palmer Quarterly, 21,* 205–226.

Bates, E., Thal, D., Whitesall, K., Fenson, L., & Oakes, L. (1989). Integrating language and gesture in infancy. *Developmental Psychology, 25,* 197–206.

Bauer, H., & Mosher, G. (1990). Ohio infants at risk for communicative disorders. *Journal of the Ohio Speech and Hearing Association, 5,* 43–45.

Bayley, N. (1969). *The Bayley Scales of Infant Development.* Atlanta: Psychological Corp.

Bluestone, C. (1990). *Update on otitis media: 1990.* Unpublished manuscript, University of Pittsburgh School of Medicine, Pittsburgh.

Brainerd, C. (1978). The stage question in cognitive-developmental theory. *The Behavioral and Brain Sciences, 1,* 173–182.

Brazelton, T. (1973). *Neonatal Behavioral Assessment Scale.* Philadelphia: Lippincott.

Brazelton, T. B., & Als, H. (1979). Four early states in the development of mother-infant interaction. *The Psychoanalytic Study of the Child, 34,* 349–369.

Brazelton, T. B., Koslowski, B., & Main, M. (1974). The origins of reciprocity: The early mother-infant interaction. In M. Lewis & L. A. Rosenblum (Eds.), *The effect of an infant on its caregiver* (pp. 49–76). New York: Wiley.

Bricker, D., & Carlson, L. (1980, May). *The relationship of object and prelinguistic social-communication schemes to the acquisition of early linguistic skills in developmentally delayed infants.* Paper presented at Conference on Handicapped and At-Risk Infants: Research and Applications, Monterey, CA.

Bruner, J. (1983). *Child's talk: Learning to use language.* New York: Norton.

Bryant, D., & Ramey, C. (1987). An analysis of the effectiveness of early intervention programs for environmentally at-risk children. In M. Guralnick & F. Bennett (Eds.), *The effectiveness of early intervention for at-risk and handicapped children.* New York: Academic Press.

Bzoch, K., & League, R. (1991). *Receptive-Expressive-Emergent-Language Test* (REEL-2). Los Angeles: Western Psychological Services.

Campbell, P. (1987). The integrated programming team: An approach for coordinating professionals of various disciplines in programs for students with severe handicaps. *Journal of the Association for Persons with Severe Handicaps, 12,* 107–116.

Catlett, C. (1991). ASHKs early intervention projects. *ASHA.* April, 50–51.

Chasnoff, I. (1987). Parental effects of cocaine. *Contemporary Ob/Gyn, 26,* 1–8.

Clark, F. N., & Siefer, R. (1983). Facilitation of mother-infant communication. *Infant Mental Health Journal, 4.*

Cochrane, C. G., Farley, B. G., & Wilhelm, I. J. (1990). Preparation of physical therapists to work with handicapped infants and their families: Current status. *Physical Therapy, 70,* 372–380.

Cohen, H. (1990). Case management and care coordination for children with HIV infection. In P. Kozlowski, D. Snider, P. Vietze, & H. Wisniewski (Eds.), *Brain in pediatric AIDS*. Basel, Switzerland: Karger.

Cole, J. G. (1996). Intervention strategies for infants with prenatal drug exposure. *Infants and Young Children, 8*, 35–39.

Comfort, M., & Farran, D. C. (1994). Parent-child interaction assessment in family-centered intervention. *Infants and Young Children, 6*, 33–45.

Coplan, J. (1987). *Early Language Milestone Scale.* Tulsa, OK: Modern Educational Corporation.

Coplan, J. (1993). *Early Language Milestone Scale* (2nd Ed.). Austin, TX: Pro-Ed.

Coplan, J., & Gleason, J. (1990). Quantifying language development from birth to 3 years using the Early Language Milestone Scale. *Pediatrics, 86*, 963, 971.

Crais, E. (1995). Expanding the repertoire of tools and techniques for assessing the communication skills of infants and toddlers. *American Journal of Speech-Language Pathology, 4*, 47–59.

Dale, P. S. (1991). The validity of a parent report measures of vocabulary and syntax at 24 months. *Journal of Speech and Hearing Research, 34*, 565–571.

Dale, P. S., Bates, E., Reznick, S., & Morisset, C. (1989). The validity of a parent report instrument of child language at twenty months. *Journal of Child Language, 16*, 239–250.

Dattel, B. (1990). Substance abuse in pregnancy. *Summaries in Perinatology, 14*, 179–187.

Diamond, G., & Cohen, H. (1989). *HIV infection in children: Medical and neurological aspects.* Technical report on developmental disabilities and HIV infection. American Association of University Affiliated Programs.

Donahue, M. L., & Pearl, R. (1995) Conversational interactions of mothers and their preschool children who have been preterm. *Journal of Speech and Hearing Research, 38*, 1117–1125.

Drash, P. W., & Tudor, R. M. (1990). Language and cognitive development: A systematic behavioral program and technology for increasing the language and cognitive skills of developmentally disabled and at-risk preschool children. *Programs in Behavior Modification, 26*, 173–220.

Duchan, J. (1986). Special education for the nonhandicapped: How to interact with those who are different. In P. Knochhlock (Ed.), *Book on special education*. New York: Wiley.

Dunst, C., Cushing, P. J., & Vance, S. D. (1985). Response-contingent learning in profoundly handicapped infants: A social system perspective. *Analysis and Intervention in Developmental Disabilities, 5*, 33–47.

Dunst, C., & Rheingrover, R. (1982). Discontinuity and instability in early development: Implications for assessment. In J. Neisworth (Ed.), *Assessment in special education*. Rockville, MD: Aspen.

Ensher, G. (1989). Newborns at risk. *Topics in Language Disorders, 10*, 80–90.

Fenson, L., Dale, P., Reznick, S., Thal, D., Bates, E., Hartung, J., Pethick, S., & Reilly, J. (1993). *MacArthur Communicative Development Inventories*. San Diego: Singular Publishing.

Fey, M. (1986). *Language Intervention with young children.* San Diego: College-Hill Press.

Finberg, L. (1980). One milk for all—not ever likely and certainly not yet. *The Journal of Pediatrics, 96*, 240–241.

Frankenburg, W. K., Dodds, J., & Fandal, A. (1975). *Denver Developmental Screening Test.* Denver: LADOCA Project and Publishing Foundation.

Fried, P., & Watkinson, B. (1990). 36- and 48-month neurobehavioral follow-up of children prenatally exposed to marijuana, cigarettes, and alcohol. *Developmental and Behavioral Pediatrics, 11*, 49–58.

Furuno, S., O'Reilly, K., Inatsuka, T., Hosaka, C., Allman, T., & Zeisloft-Falboy, B. (1986). *Hawaii Early Learning Profile*. Palo Alto, CA: Vort Corp.

Gerber, S. (1990). *Prevention: The etiology of communicative disorders in children.* Englewood Cliffs, NJ: Prentice Hall.

Goldberg, S. (1977). Social competence in infancy: A model of parent-infant interaction. *Merrill-Palmer Quarterly, 23*, 163–177.

Gradel, K., Thompson, M. S., & Sheehan, R. (1981). Parental and professional agreement in early childhood assessment. *Topics in Early Childhood Special Education, 1*, 31–39.

Halle, J. W. Baer, D., & Spradlin, J. E. (1981). Teacher's generalized use of delay as a stimulus control procedure to increase language use in handicapped children. *Journal of Applied Behavior Analysis, 14*, 389–411.

Halliday, M. (1979). One child's protolanguage. In M. Bullowa (Ed.), *Before speech* (pp. 171–190). New York: Cambridge University Press.

Hanson, M. (Ed.). (1983a). *Atypical infant.* Baltimore: University Park Press.

Hanson, M. (1983b). Social development. In M. Hanson (Ed.), *Atypical infant.* Baltimore: University Park Press.

Hanson, M. J., & Krentz, M. S. (1986). *Supporting parent-child interactions: A guide for early intervention program personnel.* San Francisco: San Francisco State University, Integrated Special Infant Services Program Department of Special Education.

Hanson, M. J., Lynch, E. W., & Wayman, K. (1990). Honoring the cultural diversity of the family when gathering data. *Topics in Early Childhood Special Education,* 10, 112–131.

Harding, C., & Golinkoff, R. (1979). The origins of intentional vocalizations in prelinguistic infants. *Child Development,* 50, 33–40.

Hart, B., & Risely, T. (1975). Incidental teaching of language in the preschool. *Journal of Applied Behavioral Analysis,* 8, 411–420.

Hedrick, D., Prather, E., & Tobin, A. (1984). *Sequenced Inventory of Communication Development* (Revised). Los Angeles: Western Psychological Services.

Holmgren, K., Lindblom, B., Aurelius, G., Jaling, B., & Zetterstrom, R. (1980). On the phonetics of infant vocalization. In B. Lindblom & R. Zetterstrom (Eds.), *Precursors of early speech.* New York: Stockton.

Hopkins, K., Grosz, J., & Lieberman, A. (1990). *Working with families and caregivers of children with HIV infection and developmental disability.* Technical report on developmental disabilities and HIV infection. American Association of University Affiliated Programs.

Ireton, H., & Thwing, E. (1974). *Manual for the Minnesota Child Development Inventory.* Minneapolis: Behavior Science Systems.

Jones, K., & Smith, D. (1973). Fetal alcohol syndrome is now the leading cause of mental retardation. *Lancet,* 2, 1222–1224.

Jones, K., & Smith, D. (1974). Outcomes in offspring of chronic alcoholic women. *Lancet,* 3, 1076–1078.

Kaiser, A. B. & Hester, P. P. (1995). Generalized effects of enhanced milieu teaching. *Journal of Speech and Hearing Research,* 37, 1320–1340.

Kaye, K., & Charney, R. (1981). Conversational asymmetry between mothers and children. *Journal of Child Language,* 8, 35–49.

Kennedy, M. D., Sheridan, M. K., Radlinshi, S. H., & Beeghly, M. (1991). Play-language relationships in young children with developmental delays: Implications for assessment. *Journal of Speech and Hearing Research,* 34, 112–122.

Kent, R. (1982, June). *Structure and function times three.* Paper presented at the Symposium on Research in Child Language Disorders, Madison, WI.

Kent, R., & Hodge, M. (1991). The biogenesis of speech: Continuity and process in early speech and language development. In J. Miller (Ed.), *Research on child language disorders.* Austin, TX: Pro-Ed.

Koopmans-van Beinum, F., & van der Stelt, J. (1986). Early stages in the development of speech movements. In B. Lindblom & R. Zetterstrom (Eds.), *Precursors of early speech.* New York: Stockton Press.

Kopp, C. (1990). Risk in infancy: Appraising the research. *Merrill-Palmer Quarterly,* 36, 117–139.

Kopp, C., & Kaler, S. (1989). Risk in infancy. *American Psychologist,* 44, 224–230.

Lyons-Ruth, K., Connell, D., & Grunebaum, H. (1990). Infants at social risk: Maternal depression and family support services as mediators of infant development and security of attachment. *Child Development,* 61, 85–98.

MacDonald, J. (1985) Language through conversation. In S. Warren and A. Rogers-Warren (Eds.), *Teaching functional language.* Austin, TX: Pro-Ed.

MacDonald, J. & Carroll, J. Y. (1992) A social partnership model for assessing early communication development: An intervention model for preconversational children. *Language, Speech and Hearing Services in Schools,* 23, 113–124.

MacDonald, J., & Gillette, Y. (1985). *Social play: A program for developing a social play habit for communication development.* Columbus, OH: O.S.U. Research Foundation.

Mahoney, G., & Powell, A. (1984). *The transactional intervention program, preliminary teacher's guide.* Unpublished manuscript. School of Education, University of Michigan, Ann Arbor.

McCollum, J. A., & Yates, T. J. (1994). Dyad as focus, triad as means: A family-centered approach to supporting parent-child interactions. *Infants and Young Children.* 6, 54–63.

McCormick, L., & Goldman, R. (1978). The transdisciplinary model: Implications for service delivery and personnel preparation for the severely and profoundly handicapped. *AAESPH Review,* 4, 152–161.

McCormick, L., Loeb, D., & Schiefelbusch, R. (in press). *Early language intervention: An introduction* (3rd Ed.). Columbus, OH: Merrill/Macmillan.

McGonigel, M., Kaufmann, R., & Johnson, B. (1991). *Guidelines and recommended practices for the individualized family service plan.* Bethesda, MD: Association for the Care of Children's Health.

McLean, J., & Snyder-McLean, L. (1978). *A transactional approach to early language training.* Columbus, OH: Merrill/Macmillan.

Messick, C., Anketell, M., & Chapman, K. (1987). *Language intervention with 0–5 population: An organization framework.* Paper presented at the American Speech-Language-Hearing Association Convention.

Miller, J. P., Sedey, A. L., & Miolo, G. (1995). Validity of parent report measures of vocabulary development for children with Down syndrome. *Journal of Speech and Hearing Research,* 38, 1037–1044.

Mitchell, P., & Kent, R. (1990). Phonetic variation in multisyllabic babbling. *Journal of Child Language,* 17, 247–266.

Montagu, M. (1968). Constitutional prenatal factors in infant and child health. In M. Haimowitz & N. Haimowitz (Eds.), *Human development: Selected readings* (2nd Ed.). New York: T. Crowell Co.

Moore, M. K., & Meltzoff, A. N. (1978). Object permanence, imitation, and language development: Toward a neo-Piagetian perspective. In R. D. Minifie and L. L. Lloyd, *Communicative and cognitive abilities—Early behavioral assessment.* Baltimore: University Park Press.

Muma, J. (1986). *Language acquisition: A functionalistic perspective.* Austin, TX: Pro-Ed.

Nelson, K. (1973). Structure and strategy in learning to talk. *Monographs of the Society for Research in Child Development,* 38 (No. 149).

Nicolich, L. (1977). Beyond sensorimotor intelligence: Assessment of symbolic maturity through analysis of pretend play. *Merrill-Palmer Quarterly,* 23, 89–99.

Norris, J. A., & Hoffman, P. (1990). Language intervention within naturalistic environments. *Language, Speech, and Hearing Services in the Schools,* 21, 72–84.

Northern, J. (1981). *Hearing disorders.* Boston: Little, Brown.

Oller, D. K. (1980). The emergence of the sounds of speech in infancy. In G. Yeni-Komshian, J. Kavanagh, & C. Ferguson (Eds.), *Child phonology* (Vol. 1, pp. 93–112). New York: Academic Press.

Olswang, L., Stoel-Gammon, C. Coggins, T., & Carpenter, R. (1987). *Assessing linguistic behavior.* Seattle: University of Washington Press.

Owens, R. (1992). Language development: An introduction (3rd ed.). Columbus, OH: Merrill/Macmillan.

Peters, A. (1977). Language learning strategies: Does the whole equal the sum of the parts? *Language,* 53, 560–573.

Proctor, A. (1989). Stages of normal vocal development in infancy: A protocol for assessment. *Topics in Language Disorders,* 10, 26–42.

Raack, C. (1989). *Mother/Infant Communication Screening.* Schaumburg, IL: Community Therapy Services.

Ratner, N., & Bruner, J. S. (1977). Games, social exchange and the acquisition of language. *Journal of Child Language,* 5, 391–401.

Rescorla, L. (1989). The Language Development Survey. *Journal of Speech and Hearing Disorders,* 54, 587–599.

Reynell, J. (1985). *Reynell Developmental Language Scales.* Los Angeles: Webster Psychological Corp.

Rice, M., Buhr, J., & Nemeth, M. (1990). Fast-mapping word-learning abilities of language-delayed preschoolers. *Journal of Speech and Hearing,* 55, 33–42.

Richard, N. (1986). Interaction between mothers and infants with Down syndrome: Infant characteristics. *TECSE,* 6, 54–71.

Robb, M., Bauer, H., & Tyler, A. (1994). A quantitative analysis of the single-word stage. *First Language,* 14, 37–48.

Robb, M., Psak, J., & Pang-Ching, G. (1993). Chronic otitis media and early speech development: a case study. *International Journal of Pediatric Otorhinolaryngology,* 26, 117–127.

Rossetti, L. (1990). *The Rossetti Infant-Toddler Language Scale.* Moline, IL: Lingua Systems.

Roug, L., & Landberg, L. (1989). Phonetic development in early infancy: A study of four Swedish children during the first eighteen months of life. *Journal of Child Language,* 16, 19–40.

Roy, S. (1984). The chloride depletion syndrome. In L. Barnes (Ed.), *Advances in Pediatrics,* 31.

Rutter, M. (1979). Protective factors in children's response to stress and disadvantage. In M. Kent and T. Rolf (Eds.), *Social competence in children.* Hanover, NH: University Press of New England.

Rutter, M., Yule, B., Quinton, D., Rowlands, O., Yule, W., & Berger, M. (1975). Attainment and adjustment in two geographical areas: III. Some factors accounting for area differences. *British Journal of Psychiatry,* 126, 520–533.

Shatz, M. (1983). On transition, continuity and coupling: An alternative approach to communicative development. In R. Golinkoff (Ed.), *The transition from prelinguistic to linguistic communication.* Hillsdale, NJ: Erlbaum.

Smith, B., Brown-Sweeney, S., & Stoel-Gammon, C. (1989). A quantitative analysis of reduplicated and variegated babbling. *First Language,* 9, 175–190.

Snow, C. (1979). The role of social interaction and the development of communicative ability. In A. Collins (Ed.), *Children's language and communication.* Hillsdale, NJ: Erlbaum.

Snow, C., & Ratner, N. (1984, November). *Talking to children: Therapy is also social interaction.* Paper presented at the Annual American Speech-Language-Hearing Association Convention, San Francisco.

Snyder, L., Bates, E., & Bretherton, I. (1981). Content and context in early lexical development. *Journal of Child Language,* 8, 565–582.

Sparks, S. (1984). *Birth defects and speech-language disorders.* San Diego: College-Hill Press.

Sparks, S. (1989). Assessment and intervention with at-risk infants and toddlers: Guidelines for the speech-language pathologist. *Topics in Language Disorders,* 10, 43–56.

Sparrow, S., Balla, D., & Ciccetti, D. (1984). *Vineland Adaptive Behavior Scales.* Minneapolis: American Guidance.

Stark, R. (1980). Stages of speech development in the first year of life. In G. Komishan, J. Kavanagh, & C. Ferguson (Eds.), *Child phonology* (Vol. 1). New York: Academic Press.

Stoel-Gammon, C., & Cooper, J. (1984). Patterns of early lexical and phonological development. *Journal of Child Language,* 11, 247–271.

Sweeney, J. (1985). Neonates at developmental risk. In D. A. Umphred (Ed.), *Neurological rehabilitation.* St. Louis: Mosby.

Teele, D., Klein, J., Chase, C., Menyuk, P., & Rosner, B. (1990). Otitis media in infancy and intellectual ability, school achievement, speech and language at age 7 years. *Journal of Infectious Diseases,* 162, 685–694.

Thal, D., & Bates, E. (1988). Language and gesture in late-talkers. *Journal of Speech and Hearing Research,* 31, 115–123.

Tomblin, J. B., Shonrock, C. M., & Hardy, J. C. (1989). The concurrent validity of the Minnesota Child Development Inventory as a measure of young children's language development. *Journal of Speech and Hearing Disorders,* 54, 101–105.

Turnbull, A., & Turnbull, H. (1990). *Families, professionals, and exceptionality: A special partnership* (2nd Ed.). Columbus, OH: Merrill/Macmillan.

Vihman, M., & Greenlee, M. (1987). Individual differences in phonological development: Ages one and three years. *Journal of Speech and Hearing Research,* 30, 503–521.

Warren, S. R. & Gazdag, G. (1990). Facilitating early language development with milieu intervention procedures. *Journal of Early Intervention,* 14, 62–86.

Warren, S., & Kaiser, A. (1986). Incidental language teaching: A critical review. *Journal of Speech and Hearing Disorders,* 51, 291–299.

Wetherby, A., & Prizant, B. (1992). Profiling young children's communicative competence. In S. Warren & J. Reichle (Eds.), *Causes and effects in communication and language intervention* (pp. 217–253). Baltimore: Brookes Publishing.

Wetherby, A., & Prizant, B. (1993). *Communication and Symbolic Behavior Scales.* Chicago: Riverside.

Wilcox, M. J., Kouri, T. A., & Caswell, S. B. (1991). Early language intervention: A comparison of classroom and individual treatment. *American Journal of Speech-Language Pathology,* 1, 49–61.

Wing, C. (1990). Defective infant formulas and expressive language delay: A case study. *Language, Speech and Hearing Services in Schools,* 21, 22–27.

Wulz, S., Meyers, S., Klein, M., Hall, M., & Waldo, L. (1982). Unobtrusive training: A home-centered model for communication training. *Journal of the Association for the Severely Handicapped, 7,* 36–48.

Wyly, M., Allen, J., Pfalzer, S. M., & Wilson, J. R. (1996). Providing a seamless service system from hospital to home: The NICU Training Project. *Infants and Young Children, 8,* 77–84.

Yoder, P., Warren, S., Kyoungram, K., & Gazdag, G. E. (1994). Facilitating prelinguistic communication skills in young children with developmental delay II: Systematic replication and extension. *Journal of Speech and Hearing Research, 37,* 841–851.

Zimmerman, I., Steiner, V., & Pond, R. (1992). *Preschool Language Scale-3.* San Antonio: Psychological Corporation.

Zuckerman, B., Frank, D., Hingson, R, Amaro, H., & Levenson, S. (1989). Effects of maternal marijuana and cocaine use on fetal growth. *New England Journal of Medicine, 320,* 762–768.

Chapter *7*

Assessing Children with Language Disorders

ELAINE R. SILLIMAN
University of South Florida

SHARON JAMES
University of Wisconsin

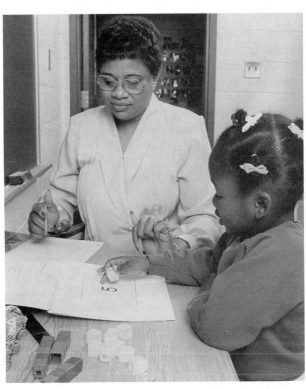

As speech-language pathologists, we are responsible for identifying school-age children with language disorders and for designing and implementing effective intervention programs for them in a variety of settings. Because we now understand that oral language and literacy learning are interconnected, our responsibilities have expanded in two important ways: the inclusion of language and literacy learning as components of assessment and the development of approaches that recognize language intervention as "an integral part of the child's classroom life" (Naremore, Densmore, & Harman, 1995, p. 50). To fulfill these multiple responsibilities, we must obtain accurate and comprehensive information about a child's language and language-related abilities in both the oral and print domains, interpret that information, and use it to make decisions about the need for and focus of intervention. Thus, assessing a child's language and communication behaviors is a very important aspect of meeting our professional responsibilities.

The task of assessing children's language abilities would be relatively simple if language were easily quantified, like height or weight. However, language is not a unitary dimension that can be measured with a yardstick or scales. It is multidimensional, complex, and dynamic; it involves many interrelated processes and abilities; and it changes from situation to situation depending on why we are talking, who we are talking with, and what we are talking about. As Miller (1981) points out, the elusive nature of language makes it very difficult to measure and quantify. The task is complicated further in the range and variety of behaviors exhibited by individual children with language disorders. Every child that you evaluate will have a unique pattern of language abilities and problems in how language is used. In fact, individual differences will be the rule, not the exception. For example, one child may have an adequate vocabulary and good social communication skills but may have severe problems in using grammatical morphemes appropriate to the syntactic structures being expressed. Another child may be able to produce easily a variety of grammatically acceptable sentences but may use many nonspecific terms, like *that one, it,* and *the thing,* because she has trouble rapidly retrieving the appropriate words for objects, people, and events in particular situations. One of the challenges in assessment is to reveal and describe the unique pattern of language behaviors for each child with a suspected or known language impairment.

Another complicating variable in assessment is that, today, we are dealing with an increasingly diverse population that reflects a rich fabric of cultural and linguistic differences. Being able to differentiate sociocultural variability in language use from uses of language that result from an impaired system requires comprehensive knowledge of other cultures and their patterns of language and communication (Westby, 1995). We can meet the many challenges of the assessment task if we: (1) have an open and curious mind; (2) develop keen observational skills; (3) maintain a current disciplinary and interdisciplinary knowledge base about language theory and research; and (4) understand how different conceptual frameworks about language and literacy learning lead to different questions and focuses for both assessment and intervention (Vigil & van Kleeck, 1996). The task of assessing children's language and communication is not only our professional responsibility, it is also one of the most creative and exciting facets of our work.

Special appreciation for their valuable assistance in preparation of certain materials for this chapter is extended to Carolyn Ford, Department of Communication Sciences and Disorders, University of South Florida, and Mary Kepich, Nicole Nystrom, Kim Taczak, and Deborah VanDam, graduate students in the Department of Communication Sciences and Disorders.

This chapter is designed to introduce the nature and scope of the assessment task in school-age children rather than to provide all of the information necessary for carrying out an in-depth language assessment. The following major questions will be explored:

1. Why do we assess a child's language and communication abilities?
2. What aspects of the child's functioning will we assess?
3. How will we assess those aspects?
4. How will we interpret and use the results of our assessments?

Although this chapter focuses on assessing children's language and communicative behaviors, there are other aspects of development that need to be considered in evaluating a child. It is crucial to remember that a child's communicative functioning involves not only language knowledge and skills but also cognitive and social knowledge. The development of early cognitive and social-communicative behaviors is discussed in Chapters 2 and 3. In addition, Chapter 6 discusses the principles of assessing these behaviors in infants and toddlers.

We also may be concerned with a child's physical status, motor abilities, and socioemotional development. In regard to socioemotional development, being a competent communicator is intertwined with our self-esteem; thus our abilities as a communicator affect the development of our personal identity, and, in turn, significantly influence how others judge our competence (Fujiki & Brinton, 1994). For example, it is estimated that between 50 to 70 percent of school-age children in special education because of emotional or behavioral problems may have undiagnosed language impairments (Hummel & Prizant, 1993). We also will need to be concerned with those situations in which the child spends a good deal of time, such as the classroom, or interacting with peers or family at home. We will not need to obtain information in all of the areas just mentioned, but it is important to remember that children's language and communicative performances can never be separated from the context in which children are being asked to perform. Also, our choice of particular assessment procedures will always depend first on why we want to assess a particular child; thus we will need to be prepared to assess whatever areas are relevant for a particular child in relation to the questions being asked.

Models and Purposes of Assessment

Models of Assessment

An assessment model can be thought of as a blueprint or a set of assumptions that guide the scientific or clinical questions asked about the functioning of a child's communication system and how this functioning will be interpreted. Models tend to derive from different conceptual frameworks of what language learning is and how it works. Different models are not necessarily always compatible with each other (Chapman, 1991).

Deficit Models

Lund and Duchan (1993) illustrate this point about the incompatibility of assessment models. When we ask a deficit question such as, "What is the deficit and how severe is it?" we are asking a question typically associated with normative/deviance models of assessment. These models tend to define normal versus atypical in terms of the degree of deviance from a statistical mean (Peterson & Marquardt, 1994). This type of statistical definition derives from the average performance of large groups of individuals, what is called a norming sample, and is associated with one general kind of assessment tool: standardized measures of language performance.

Deficit models often have a *discrete-point* perspective on language assessment (Damico, 1991; Shulman, Katz, & Sherman, 1995). In this perspective, language proficiency is viewed as its own system relatively uninfluenced by other systems, such as cognition, memory, or emotional factors. Moreover, the language system itself is considered as consisting of separate components, such as sound structure, syntax, or meaning, which implies that each can be assessed independently of the other (Damico, 1991). The purpose of assessment, therefore, is directed to identifying the specific components of the language system that are missing or incomplete, for example, the speech sounds or syntactic structures that the child does not produce. Often the information obtained is not useful for intervention purposes, although it may be used for determining whether a child is eligible for speech and language services in the school setting.

Etiological Models

On the other hand, when we ask an assessment question, like "What is causing the problem?" we are asking an etiological question. Etiological models are common to medically based assessment approaches. As a result, these models are oriented to differentiating one set of symptom clusters from another in order to arrive at a category of diagnosis, e.g., that an individual's set of "symptoms" is more consistent with a specific language impairment than with mental retardation. Etiological models are also concerned with factors that may cause, contribute to, or maintain a language impairment (Nation & Aram, 1991), a very important issue for the prevention and treatment of language impairment. Many etiological models share a discrete-point perspective about language similar to deficit models.

Developmental Models

A third kind of assessment question more directly addresses the connection between assessment and intervention (Lund & Duchan, 1993): "What plan should we design to help this child?" Developmental models most often see this question as the important purpose of assessment.

Because of this concern, developmental models of assessment tend to share in common a *holistic* or *synergistic* perspective on language and communication (Damico, 1991). That is, "Language exists only as an integrated whole and that communication is *highly* influenced by context, cognitive ability, experience, and learning potential" (Shulman et al., 1995, pp. 53–54). In this view, language components are seen as an integrated system whose components interact with each other and with other cognitive and socioemotional systems. As a result, developmental models are oriented to discovering and describing patterns of regularity in an individual child's language performance, using normal aspects of development as a reference. Knowing what a child cannot do (a "deficit" view) must be balanced with learning about a child's potential (an "ability" view), what the child is capable of doing more proficiently in particular situations, including the circumstances that might promote a higher level of competence.

Developmental models do not reject etiological models of assessment (although they may find normative deviance models more incompatible). The major issue concerns the extent to which causal information illuminates how best to meet individual children's needs. For example, even if we know that a child's language impairment may be related to maternal drug use during pregnancy, that information alone provides little guidance for the best language intervention.

A final point is that the model(s) selected for understanding communicative behaviors and their disruption should represent a valid conceptual framework about the development of language (Lund & Duchan, 1993). These same models influence clinical and educational practices. Approaches based on discrete point models often emphasize the language system as consisting of splinter skills, which can result in learning disconnected from functional communication. In contrast, approaches grounded to more holistic perspectives value integrating the real communicative processes of listening, speaking, reading, and writing across the curriculum as strategies for learning how to learn. Again, these significant differences in assessment and intervention models mean that, as speech-language pathologists, we must continuously assess and reassess our clinical practices in light of changing scientific knowledge about children with language impairment and how their needs can be met best.

Purposes of Assessment

The purposes for assessment influence the nature of the information to be obtained, the methods used to obtain the information, and how that information will be interpreted. There are a variety of purposes associated with the assessment of children's language and communicative behaviors.

1. Identifying children with language disorders
2. Designing appropriate language intervention programs
3. Monitoring changes resulting from intervention, including the ongoing appropriateness of intervention goals and the effectiveness of procedures

Identification

States are required under the Individuals with Disabilities Education Act (IDEA, PL 101-476), the federal law and regulations governing the education of children with disabilities, to identify children who might need special services because of delays in developing basic oral language skills (Nelson, 1993). This step usually involves some kind of **screening** procedure, usually the administration of a standardized measure, to decide if a child's learning of language may be sufficiently different to warrant a full assessment. Those children who perform below a given acceptable level for their age or grade level are recommended for more comprehensive evaluations. Within many school districts, the speech-language pathologist is responsible for conducting these brief evaluations of the oral language abilities of all kindergarten children served by that district. A major issue in the selection of screening instruments, whether they are standardized instruments or informal methods, are their psychometric acceptability (Paul, 1995). This topic will be discussed shortly.

As the academic and social demands of schooling increase, some older school-age children may also be referred for screening by teachers or parent because these children are encountering difficulties with effectively using language for learning. Teachers and parents have numerous opportunities to observe how a child's language behaviors are used for a variety of communicative purposes in many different situations; therefore, these adults are often in a position to detect subtle indications of a language learning problem that might be missed in a brief screening procedure when a child is younger or that may not have been tapped by that procedure. For example, because language disabilities change over time and may look different depending on the nature of cognitive and social demands, some students may not experience serious academic problems until they enter middle school (Bashir & Strominger, 1996; Ehren, 1994). At this level, the curriculum demands the application of more complex cognitive and linguistic strategies for comprehending a wide variety of different contents in oral and print domains and expressing what one knows in both domains.

Regardless of how or when a child with a potential language problem is located, the second step in identification is to determine whether the child actually has a language impairment. Might we expect this child to continue developing normally in either basic language learning or the use of language to learn or may some intervention be required to facilitate further development? To answer this critical question, we must understand what atypical language learning is and be able to obtain valid information about the child's linguistic and communicative behaviors, interpreting these findings in relation to normal developmental expectations for the child's age. We also want to know what areas of language functioning are involved and the situations that influence variability in performance.

This kind of decision making is complicated by four issues. First, apparent difficulties can exist in language and communication despite the lack of documented evidence for a known neurobiological etiology or etiologies; however, there is some correlational evidence, based on family studies, that certain patterns of language impairment may be inherited (Crago & Gopnik, 1994; Gilger, 1995; Lahey & Edwards, 1995; Tomblin, 1989). Second, the difference between a language delay and a language disorder is unclear (Kahmi, 1996). Initial language development may not be slow or delayed, but protracted (Locke, 1994). In other words, a late start means that normal "windows of opportunity" for language learning may not be available unless young children are challenged to use their existing linguistic and communicative resources, for example, through early language intervention. Third, in determining eligibility for intervention services, children with atypical language learning are expected to show normal intellectual potential based on nonverbal test performance; but studies consistently show, to the contrary, that nonverbal abilities are also affected in many children (Kamhi, 1996; Parnell, 1995). For example, as a group, children with atypical language learning have problems in so-called nonlanguage areas, such as the complexity of their symbolic play, manipulating visual imagery, and the efficiency of their problem solving. Johnston (1994) suggests, "A portion of this disability must reflect the role of language in higher level problem solving. . . . Another portion of the cognitive disability is nonverbal and can be presumed to be responsible for inefficient learning in many domains, including language" (p. 114). A very real question, therefore, is whether impairment is specific to language for all children or whether, for some, more general information processing limitations are responsible for the profiles found. Only continuing study will verify whether the concept of specific language impairment as traditionally defined is a clear diagnostic category (Aram, Morris, & Hall, 1993).

The fourth complicating issues deals with the fact that a language impairment is a persistent, chronic condition. Children do not "catch up" in the sense of being in phase with children of their own age or grade level. However, it is important to remember that individual profiles will change over time as the child matures and new strategies are learned for managing interpersonal and intrapersonal activities. The **interpersonal** domain refers to the social relations that we create and sustain with others through communication. These social relations also define our conversational roles in any situation (Beaumont, 1995; Brinton & Fujiki, 1989; Rees & Gerber, 1992). For example, think of how your own discourse style changes when you interact with your professor about a project you must complete versus interacting with a friend that you have known for many years. The **intrapersonal** domain, in contrast, concerns those cognitive and affective processes that regulate our abilities to think, communicate, and experience emotion in everything that is heard, said, read, and written. Children and adolescents with language impairment may have less appropriate discourse options available for establishing acceptance and status at home, school, and in the community (Black & Logan, 1995; Brinton & Fujiki, 1994; Rees & Gerber, 1992). As a result, they are faced with rejection, which can then seriously affect socioemotional development (Hummel & Prizant, 1993). This may mean that many develop a form of self-esteem in which their view of themselves is centered in less competence as a learner and as a communicator. To cope with feelings of incompetence, some children may learn to "keep a low profile" (the so-called quiet child), while others may present an aggressive profile (the child who acts out) for interacting with others (Donahue, 1994).

Designing Appropriate Language Intervention

Once a child is identified as demonstrating a language impairment, we will be concerned with the second purpose of language assessment: designing an appropriate language program. To meet this purpose, we need a detailed description of the child's understanding and use of all components of language—phonology, semantics, syntax, and discourse—and the interactions of these components across multiple situations, including their applications to literacy learning. We can think of human communication as multilayered, with the components embedded within each other to create an integrated system.

Least Restrictive Environment.   IDEA requires that every effort be made to keep a child in the least restrictive environment (LRE). The appropriate education and related services necessary for that child to achieve satisfactorily must be determined. Once that decision has been made, then the LRE for service delivery is decided on a case-by-case basis. All efforts must be demonstrated to keep the child in the general education classroom. It is important to remember that IDEA prohibits decision making about the LRE based on a student's category of disability (Bateman, 1995). Because a child has a language impairment does not mean that the child must be placed in a classroom for children with language impairment.

The responsibility to maintain a child in the LRE means that the kind of in-depth information needed for appropriate identification and intervention in the LRE requires multiple observations of the child's communication system. This means that we must collaborate with teachers and parents to plan observations. We need to observe the child systematically in the classroom in a variety of activities involving the teacher and peers and, if possible at home. Information should be obtained on the child's typical functioning and on optimal functioning. Learning to be a systematic observer, therefore, requires far more than just looking. Instead, it requires understanding the purposes for assessment, which then should guide the selection of the appropriate observational tools (Silliman & Wilkinson, 1991). The ways in which observational information is obtained should allow questions about the child to be addressed at a level of detail sufficient to draw valid conclusions. It is important to keep in mind that assessment and intervention are not two distinct activities. The authenticity of assessment depends on the degree to which it is linked to learning about what the child is capable of in real communicative contexts, given the support to be successful. All good intervention involves ongoing assessment.

Monitoring Progress

The third major purpose of language assessment is to monitor changes resulting from intervention. The integration of communication goals and procedures with the curriculum should be a priority. The same process for monitoring progress is followed regardless of whether the child is in the general education or special education education setting. We will be observing and recording the child's language and communicative behaviors so that we can modify our intervention goals and strategies as needed. This type of ongoing monitoring is the heart of authentic assessments where assessment and intervention are integrated.

For example, if the child is not making progress toward one of the goals initially established, we need to analyze carefully what conditions may be hindering progress. Perhaps what the child is being asked to do is too hard and the child is experiencing failure as a result. Or it may be that the child has insufficient background knowledge to engage in particular communicative activities effectively; or that more explicit written organization of information needs to be provided, such as charts or other organizers, for the child to hang onto less familiar concepts. This kind of continual analysis should lead us to modify approaches for teaching the target behaviors, to know what works for a particular child and what does not work effectively to support the child's needs.

We also will be concerned with whether the child can apply increasingly on his or her own new language and communicative behaviors to new social situations. For example, if the child has been focusing on initiating topics using more variety of linguistic forms in various classroom activities, can the child now apply what has been learned to buying lunch in the school cafeteria, where she must ask what choices are available? Or if the child has been learning new word meanings in a unit on farming, can he use some of these new meanings in a creative way to write a short sentence for a book that the class is making? Questions to ask would include, What kind of support to succeed does the child need from the teacher or speech-language pathologist? Might the child first need the teacher or speech-language pathologist to model explicitly in different situations the strategies for arriving at the desired target behavior? With some practice in role playing and other more natural situations, can the teacher or speech-language pathologist then become a coach or mentor as the kind of support for the child to be successful in a new situation? With repeated experience, can the child now accomplish this activity more independently? The ultimate test of the ability to generalize, as well as a test of the effectiveness of any language intervention program, is whether the child can now use new behaviors for functional communicative purposes *with minimal aid and assistance from others.* To assess the scope of generalization, we must observe the child in a number of different communicative situations. This issue is discussed in more detail in Chapter 9.

Components of Assessment

After determining the major purposes for the language assessment, we need to consider what we are going to assess. Because language and communication assessment with school-age children should be concerned with a child's knowledge and use of language in relation to the demands of schooling, we will focus on aspects of metalinguistic and meta-cognitive development. Both are critical for literacy learning, including higher-order thinking and more literate uses of oral language. Being able to understand, remember, and express oneself in more conscious or explicit ways crosses over the domains of listening, speaking, reading, and writing (Baker & Brown, 1984). Literacy is more than learning to read and write. Rather, literate communication in either the spoken or print domains involves flexible new ways of thinking (Wallach & Butler, 1994). Literacy is a linguistic lifeline to learning novel information about the real and imagined worlds of ourselves and others (Hewitt & Duchan, 1995; Wallach, 1990). Although not discussed further here, we also need to remember that language expression in both the oral and print realms depends on a child's motor abilities; therefore, we may need to consider this area as a component of assessment.

Also, we sometimes find ourselves responsible for assessing some children who are preverbal, who have not yet begun to comprehend or produce language consistently for social communicative purposes. In these cases, we do need to focus on cognitive, social, and communicative precursors to the development of language. Chapter 6 is devoted to assessing preverbal children.

Knowledge and Uses of Language: What to Assess

The development of literacy foundations begins at birth and is interrelated with the developing richness of a child's oral language system (van Kleeck, 1990). Table 7-1 outlines the interactive nature of language components as they function in expert readers (Pressley & McCormick, 1995).

Knowledge consists of two forms. Both types comprise long-term memory, our "storehouse" of what we know. One form is *declarative knowledge,* our factual knowledge about the world, including our knowledge of language form (phonology, morphology, and syntax) and language content (semantics). The other type is *procedural knowledge.* The knowledge in our storehouse is of little value unless we can access and use it in ways appropriate to the specific communicative context. Thus, procedural knowledge guides our selection of strategies for *comprehension,* making sense of what others say or write, and for *expression,* making ourselves understood to others either orally or in print.

The brain is a highly complex information processing mechanism. At the same time, the brain is also a limited capacity processing system (Lahey & Bloom, 1994). Only so much can be attended to at any one time depending on how task complexity is interpreted. Two types of information processing, or *levels of analysis,* occur simultaneously in both

TABLE 7-1   **Interactive Language Components in Reading: Declarative and Procedural Knowledge Necessary for Various Levels of Analysis**

Level of Analysis	Declarative Knowledge	Procedural Knowledge
Metacognitive-level analysis	What to monitor; self-awareness	Strategies for comprehension monitoring and taking corrective actions
Schema-level analysis	General world knowledge obtained from life experiences	Strategies for predicting what will happen next and for identifying the general idea of what is to be read
Discourse-level analysis	Superstructures of information organization; patterns of organization; types of relationships between ideas; linguistic signals for patterns and relationships	Strategies for identifying superstructures, patterns, and relationships in written information
Semantic-syntactic-level analysis	Syntactic rules of English; lexical and relational meanings	Strategies for accessing word meanings, using syntactic cues to identify unknown words, and predicting what will come next in a sentence
Word identification analysis	Basic sight vocabulary; spelling patterns, including morphophonological markers	Strategies for word identification using spelling patterns, including morphophonological markers
Phonological analysis	English phonological structure; letter-sound relationships	Strategies for phonemic segmentation and manipulation
Letter recognition analysis	Lines and shapes used in English orthography; alphabetic recognition	Strategies for recognizing unknown letters

Adapted from: C. Westby (in press). Working in the zone of proximal development. In E. R. Silliman, L. C. Wilkinson, & L. P. Hoffman (Eds.), *Children's journeys through school: Assessing and building competence in language and literacy learning.* San Diego: Singular.

Based on: R. J. Marzano, P. A. Hagerty, S. W. Valencia, & P. P. DiSteano (1987). *Reading diagnosis and instruction: Theory into practice.* Englewood Cliffs, NJ: Prentice-Hall.

reading and listening: *bottom-up* and *top-down.* These information processing resources are synergistic and function in parallel to produce the behaviors we call language and communication in spoken and written mediums.

Bottom-Up Processes
Expert readers are able to utilize bottom-up processes automatically, rapidly, and accurately to recognize words in reading and produce them in spelling (Ehri, 1991). These bottom-up processes are analytic because they are directed to how parts make up the whole. They in-

clude the recognition of graphemic (alphabetic) and phonological (sound structure) information, as well as spelling patterns and their associated meanings at the word level.

Most importantly, these bottom-up processes are thought to be phonologically driven (Kamhi, 1989). Because phonemes are abstract categories (unlike syllables, phonemes have no acoustic correlates in the speech stream), correspondences must be inferred between phonemic structure and their alphabetic counterparts. Also, words are phonological structures; they consist of phonemes: "If we have perceived or produced a word, whether in speech or in reading, we have in fact engaged a phonological structure" (Liberman & Shankweiler, 1991, p. 5). Thus, our mental lexicon, where individual vocabulary meanings are stored, is part of declarative knowledge and consists of both lexical and phonological information. Also, automatic word recognition in reading is facilitated when a rich network of word meanings exists in the mental lexicon (Pressley & McCormick, 1995).

Top-Down Processes

At the same time that bottom-up processes are figuring out the parts, top-down processes are working to make sense of the parts as an integrated whole. This sense making is the core of comprehension, which is an active, constructive process involving inferencing. Semantic-syntactic processing of linguistic cues supports the ability to anticipate "What comes next?" and "Does it make sense?" in the particular discourse context.

At the level of discourse processing, we activate knowledge of different text patterns for organizing information. These superstructures are a basic part of comprehension because they help to cue whether information is organized as narrative discourse, a chronologically based type of organization that focuses on what people are doing and feeling, or is arranged as expository discourse. In expository text, information is not organized chronologically, but instead has a variety of structures depending on their function, such as description, enumeration, comparison/contrast, cause/effect explanation, or problem/solution (Westby, 1994; Westby & Rouse, 1993). Moreover, as shown in Table 7-2, expository structures, unlike narratives, are more focused on logical connections between objects and ideas. The linguistic forms of expository discourse also differ from narrative texts (Scott, 1995). Another issue is that efficient processing at both the semantic-syntactic and discourse levels requires sufficient working (short-term) memory to hold in mind in an active state what was read, or said, as new information comes in. This new material then must be rapidly integrated with existing information in order to construct an interpretation (Kamhi, 1989; Lahey & Bloom, 1994; Pressley & McCormick, 1995; Sternberg, 1987).

Comprehension involves more than understanding the phonological structures, word meanings, syntax, and discourse structure of one's language. Consider the following text:

> *When Ulysses S. Grant and Robert E. Lee met in the parlor of a modest house at Appomattox Courthouse, Virginia on April 9, 1865, to work out the terms for the surrender of Lee's Army in Northern Virginia, a great chapter in American life came to a close, and a great new chapter began. (Hirsch, 1987, in Wallach & Butler, 1994, p. 4)*

To understand this stretch of discourse, readers must bring their real world knowledge of American history to interpretation. This kind of declarative knowledge allows us to access

TABLE 7-2 Types of Expository Structures, Their Functions, and Linguistic Cues

Text Pattern	Text Function	Key Words
Description	The text tells what something is	is called, can be defined as, is, can be interpreted as, refers to, is a procedure for, is someone who, means
Collection/ enumeration	The text gives a list of things that are related to the topic	an example is, for instance, another, next, finally, such as, to illustrate
Sequence/ procedure	The text tells what happened or how to do something or make something	first, next, then, second, third, follow-ing this step, finally, subsequently, from here . . . to, eventually, before, after
Comparison/ contrast	The text shows how two Things are the same or	different, same, alike, similar, although, however, on the other hand, contrasted with, compared to, rather than, but, yet, still, instead of
Cause/effect explanation	The text gives reasons for why something happened	because, since, reasons, then, therefore, for this reason, results, effects, consequently, so, in order to, thus, depends on, influences, is a function of, produces, leads to, affects, hence
Problem/ solution	The text states a problem and offers solutions to the problem	a problem is, a solution is

From: C. E. Westby & G. R. Rouse (1993). Facilitating text comprehension in college students: The professor's role. In L. Clark (Ed.), *Faculty and student challenges in facing cultural-linguistic diversity*. Springfield, IL: Thomas.

appropriate strategies for drawing inferences. In this case, our schema knowledge of histor-ical events allows to make connections between information presented in the text and our previous knowledge of the American Civil War. Schema knowledge is an organizational structure that has three interrelated functions: (1) to predict in specific social contexts what content might plausibly occur; (2) to support recall of information from long-term memory (Naremore et al., 1995); and (3) to transform "old schemas to fit new experiences" (Duchan, 1995, p. 88). When schema knowledge for particular events is familiar and elab-orated, comprehension is enhanced. In contrast, when schemas are less familiar and less well-developed, then processing resources will be stretched. For example, children with language impairment might not be able to attend to both the content and linguistic demands of particular discourse activities when the topic elicits less familiar schemas. As a result of this resource competition, the coherence of their comprehension is affected.

The metacognitive level of processing functions to keep us on track in sense making. Metacognition refers to the ability to think more intentionally about our own thinking, to monitor and self-direct it when information must be actively organized and applied for par-ticular purposes (Baker & Brown, 1984; Brown & Palincsar, 1987; Pressley & McCormick, 1995). It allows us to: (1) be aware of whether our predictions are verified, for example, that the names Ulysses S. Grant and Robert E. Lee in this discourse context do refer to the Civil War; (2) know the purpose for reading this passage (perhaps to compare and explain how the surrender changed the course of our country's destiny); (3) change our style of reading consistent with the purpose (we cannot skim, but must use strategies to process content at a deeper level); and (4) know when to apply different strategies when we fail to make connections (such as rereading, taking notes to organize the main points, or looking up unfamiliar words in the dictionary).

Oral Language and Written Language: Two Issues

Structurally Different Systems.   Depending on what they are being asked to do, children with language impairment may experience breakdowns with various bottom-up processes, top-down processes, or both in either oral or print activities. Two qualifications must be mentioned, however. First, the exact causal relationships between oral and print mediums are unknown. Are they structurally different systems or do they overlap in terms of their communicative functions?

Speech and print differ structurally (Kamhi & Catts, 1989; Liberman & Shankweiler, 1991). The speech stream is continuous and unsegmented; we do not hear "boundaries" between phonemes. In contrast, print is discrete, not continuous; letters are separated from one another by clear visual boundaries. Moreover, children are not formally instructed in how to talk, but breaking the alphabetic code to engage interactively with print does require explicit instruction for most children (Adams, 1990), typically through using phonics approaches.

Functionally Similar Systems.   When the speech-print issue is examined from a functional perspective, one position is that, like oral language, written language is also discourse and roles in this discourse overlap with oral language. Both share the same communicative processes.. The role as a speaker or author is to be understood for a specific purpose by a real or hypothetical audience, while the role of a listener or reader is to understand another's intentions.

Another overlap involves linguistic complexity. Oral and written language are both structurally complex but the type of linguistic complexity may differ. Consider these two examples of the same message (Halliday, 1987, p. 62):

More Spoken: Whenever I'd visited there before I'd end up feeling that other people might get hurt if I tried to do anything more.

More Written: Every previous visit had left me with a sense of the risk to others in further attempts at action on my part.

In the spoken example, syntactic structures meet the real-time constraints of speaking. As a listener, we must engage in rapid temporal processing. What is said is here and gone. To met these limitations, oral language may have evolved as a linear code characterized by strings of clauses, which may be the primary units of spoken language for preliterate children rather than the sentence (Halliday, 1987; Scott, 1995). In the spoken example, meaning develops through the use of four successive clauses, which are linked by connectives (*whenever, that, if*). We "hang onto" these successive clauses and keep them active in working memory as a strategy for processing and integrating what still will be said.

The written example shows that complexity is produced through a hierarchical code (Halliday, 1987). Here, syntactic structures meet the demands of a visual/spatial processing system, which is less bound to time. This one clause sentence is characterized by more lexical density and embedding through the use of a complex noun phrase strategy (use of pre- and post-modification structures). Scott (1995) proposes that the final form any sentence takes depends on the interactions among four factors: (1) the audience; (2) the discourse context; (3) the mode of communication (whether spoken or written); and (4) the type of discourse being produced (narrative or expository); thus, a major part of later syntactic development may be "learning to apply *discourse-motivated syntactic options*" (Scott, 1995, p. 109) that are consistent with the purposes and meanings being expressed. Table 7-3 shows some of these syntactic options in writing development.

Another point concerns the developmental sequences of oral and written language. Wallach and Butler (1994) observe that the older view of oral-print relationships presented an oral language-to-written-language developmental sequence. Proficiency in oral language was a precursor for proficiency in written language. This "one-way" concept, also reflected in intervention approaches, is contradicted by new research in emergent literacy that clearly documents a reciprocal relationship. Children learn about the forms and functions of print before they learn to read and write. In other words, emergent literacy influences their oral language development further, which, in turn, influences proficiency with written language.

The second qualification pertains to children with disruptions in their learning of both the oral and print systems. Despite the fact that spoken and written language problems are strongly linked, the specific causal relationships remain indirect (Kamhi, 1989). For example, it is unclear how specific patterns of difficulty with phonological processing relate to reading comprehension problems later on or how semantic-syntactic processing is associated with specific patterns of reading or writing problems (Snyder & Downey, 1991). What is known is that children learn about print before they learn to apply reading and writing as tools of discovery for new language learning. Our focuses of assessment needs to be directed to these areas to determine what a child can do and where breakdowns may be occurring.

Emergent Literacy: Learning to Read and Write

Most of the research on emergent literacy is based on children's language socialization experiences grounded in the values of the dominant, or mainstream, culture. This is the school-oriented culture, where parent-child interactions provide repeated experiences that are similar to classroom interactions (Heath, 1982). It is well documented that many children from this cultural orientation learn a good deal about print before they ever learn to read and write (Morrow, 1993; van Kleeck, 1990, 1995; van Kleeck & Schuele, 1987).

The traditional one-way view of literacy is that it is an activity begun when children begin formal schooling because children must be "ready" to learn to read and write (Terrell, 1994). Emergent literacy, in contrast, is a newer perspective. It refers to the knowledge children acquire about relationships among oral language, reading, and writing before entering school (Morrow & Smith, 1990). Learning to read and write is not a matter of readiness but

TABLE 7-3   Structures Cited as Markers of Grammatical Development in Writing

Complex noun phrases (NP)

Postmodification of head noun via prepositional phrases and nonfinite clauses:

a boy named Yanis . . .
a little girl with braids running down the road . . .
a plant in the desert by the oasis . . .

Postmodification of head nouns via relative clauses, particularly nouns used as grammatical subjects:

The first dance I ever went to was . . .
The fisherman who came to his rescue convinced the others . . .

Complex NPs used as grammatical subjects

Appositives

Mrs. Smith, my first grade teacher, . . .
Desert creatures, such as scorpions, . . .

Nonrestrictive relative clauses

Harold, whose army had just marched across England, was . . .

Adverbial fronting

Every Sunday we have waffles for breakfast.
In the early evening you can always see him.
When it finally rains, the plants bloom.

Adverbial fronting with subject/verb inversion

There stood a little tiger cub . . .
On the other side of the mountain was a small cabin.

Nonfinite adverbial clauses

Hoping to catch him, she hurried.
They are on their own *after hatching.*

Verb phrase expansion via tense, aspect, and modal auxiliaries

Could have been talked into . . .
Will not be coming.

Coordinated NPs, predicates, and series constructions

Animals found in the desert such as badgers, snakes, lizards . . .
Many mice and other rodents will be . . .

From: C. M. Scott (1995). Syntax for school age children: A discourse perspective. In M. E. Fey, J. Windsor, & S. F. Warren (Eds.), *Language intervention: Preschool through the elementary years* (p. 113). Baltimore: Paul H. Brookes.

is integrated with and naturally embedded in the many routine social interactions with literate adults encountered from infancy onwards (Heath, 1982; Stallman & Pearson, 1990). One powerful example of how young children are socialized into a literate orientation before they learn to read is the book reading routine. The schemas that young children acquire over time about how to construct increasingly complex meanings from dialogues centered on book reading events influence how they ultimately learn to talk about meaning and the features of print (Heath, 1982, 1983; van Kleeck, 1995; van Kleeck & Schuele, 1987).

Metalinguistic Awareness

As just noted, children first acquire language for everyday social communication. The next phase, which overlaps with first language acquisition, is the progressive acquisition of metalinguistic ability.

Metalinguistic knowledge, or language awareness, is another aspect of metacognition. But, unlike metacognition, which is concerned with the self-regulation of thinking, metalinguistic awareness involves the ability to think in more intentional ways about the nature and properties of language forms and meanings apart from their everyday uses for social communication (van Kleeck, 1994). For example, it is one thing for a child to use word meanings and syntactic constructions as the means to accomplish social communicative goals. But it is another level of development for a child to know in a more explicit way that *boat* is a word (a formal lexical unit) and *tiv* is not a word (van Kleeck, 1994, p. 66) or to be able to segment *boat* into its phonemic elements. To focus on meaning as an arbitrary conventional code requires knowing more consciously that words and their meanings are not in a direct relationship; rather the relationship is indirect. A *boat* can become a *tiv* if we could agree as a linguistic community on the name change. Similarly, understanding that words can have both literal and figurative (nonconventional) meanings is the basis of vocabulary richness. Being able to manipulate figurative language is the foundation of metaphor, humor, satire, and poetic uses of language.

Dominant culture children also come to understand that language is a structured system consisting of "a finite set of elements . . . that are combined in systematic ways" (van Kleeck, 1994, p. 75). These finite elements include words, which are composed of phonemes. The ability to approach printed words as a formal unit of language is the heart of word recognition or decoding, the result of bottom-up processing. Children must apply appropriate strategies for analyzing words into their phonemic units or to synthesize phonemic units into a whole word. This ability to segment and manipulate is an essential aspect of more fully developed *phonological awareness.* More than two decades of research show that performance on phonological awareness tasks in kindergarten and first grade is strongly predictive of success with learning to read as defined by word recognition (Adams, 1990; Ball, 1993; Blachman, 1994a, 1994b; Kamhi & Catts, 1989; Mann, 1993,1994; Swank & Catts, 1994). However, again, the exact nature of this connection remains elusive. Is the relationship causal? This would mean good phonological awareness directly influences good word recognition (Blachman, 1994a). Or is the relationship reciprocal? Early interactions with the functions and forms of print trigger phonological awareness before formal instruction begins, which then supports further phonological awareness (van Kleeck, 1994; van Kleeck & Schuele, 1987).

In a similar vein, significant difficulties with phonological awareness tasks are characteristic of many children who, potentially, might have a language impairment or a learning disability. The position taken, consistent with current views, is that developmental dyslexia (a reading disability) is a developmental language impairment whose patterns of difficulty evolve throughout the lifespan (Catts, 1991a, 1996; Kamhi, 1992). These changing patterns, found in Table 7-4, may have a variety of causes and represent a continuum of severity (Spear-Swerling & Sternberg, 1994).

TABLE 7-4 Changing Profiles of Language Impairment Related to Difficulties with Phonological Processing

PRESCHOOL YEARS

➤ Oral language delay apparent, including slower vocabulary growth and less rapid retrieval of words in discourse where is less contextual support for topic development (Catts et al., 1994; Nippold, 1992).

➤ Less sensitive awareness of phonological structure in terms of reduced sensitivity to rhyming, alliteration, and nonsense sequences (Fey, Catts, & Larrivee, 1995; Catts, 1991a, b; 1993).

ELEMENTARY YEARS

➤ Significant problems with phonological processing, such as use of segmentation strategies to analyze phonemic structure; ease, accuracy, and speed of word recognition in reading and spelling are affected due to reduced insight that phonemic and alphabetic segments correspond in a systematic way (Ehri, 1989a, b; Catts, 1989a; Kamhi, 1989).

➤ If severe-to-profound expressive phonological impairment is present (unintelligible speech production) combined with problems in phonological awareness, spelling may also contain high levels of phonological deviations (Clarke-Klein & Hodson, 1995).

➤ Slower in adding new word meanings to vocabulary, expanding and elaborating existing word meanings into multiple meanings, including figurative meanings, and speed of word retrieval (Catts et al., 1994; McGregor & Leonard, 1995; Milosky, 1994; Snyder & Godley, 1992; Wolf & Siegel, 1992).

➤ Comprehension problems emerge in oral and print domains because of less flexible top-down strategies for interpreting semantic-syntactic cues, utilizing discourse-level information structures, and accessing appropriate schemas for inferring purpose and meaning (Catts, 1996; Snyder & Downey, 1991; Spear-Swerling & Sternberg, 1994)

LATER SCHOOL YEARS

➤ Persistent problems with manipulating phonological segments, including ease in oral production of complex words (Catts, 1989b; Hodson, 1994); reading comprehension, writing, and spelling may continue to be effortful and less strategy-based (Pressley, Brown, El-Dinary, & Afflerbach, 1995; Scott, 1989, 1994, 1995).

➤ May develop compensatory strategies for facilitating word recognition, such as using sentence context, but are then diverting processing resources that could be allocated to comprehension (Snyder & Downey, 1991; Spear-Swerling & Sternberg, 1994).

YOUNG ADULTHOOD

➤ Patterns of difficulty become more selective, for example, problem writing and spelling may be most prominent (Bashir & Scavuzzo, 1992)

The Phonological System and Phonological Awareness

The basic phonological system is predicated on the existence of a phonological code that allows speech to be produced. This basic system is first used in a primarily automatic way to formulate and execute speech.

Phonemes are the smallest relevant sound units in any language. They are considered relevant because they signal meaning differences among words; when you change a phoneme, you create a different word. For example, the words *bat, fat, cat, mat,* and *sat* differ

TABLE 7-5   **Phonological Awareness: A Developmental Continuum—
From Holistic to Analytic Processing**

1. *Emerging Segmental Awareness* *(Recognition)*

➤   Age level: Nursery/kindergarten

➤   Transitory attention to speech segments for activities only requiring minimal levels of explicit analysis

➤   Examples:

 ∽ Knows how to hold books and how print is organized on a page

 ∽ Variably understands that sentences can be segmented into words and words can be segmented in syllables

 ∽ Engages in spontaneous sound play and production of rhyme and alliteration; comments on or attracts attention to pronunciations

 ∽ Spontaneously produces invented spellings (in situations where writing encouraged)

 ∽ Prefers highly familiar or predictable sound sequences (e.g., nursery rhymes or songs such as the "Alphabet Song"); may have rote recall of alphabet, but minimal recognition of letter names, shapes, and sounds

2. *Simple Segmental Awareness* *(Detection/Emerging Comparison)*

A. Rhyme *(attention to rime)*

➤   Age level: Nursery/kindergarten

➤   Increasing sensitivity to parts smaller than the syllable in activities that are low in explicit analysis and use highly predictable sound structures

➤   Examples:

 ∽ Produces rhymes on demand

 ∽ Produces rhymes to nonsense words (e.g., tiv-miv)

 ∽ Identifies initial sounds (onsets) that may be learned by example (e.g., *"L is for Lauren"*), but ability to identify initial sounds does not mean child can independently produce own example (Chaney, 1992)

 ∽ Categorizes by rhyme (*odd one out*)—Which word in a three or four word series does NOT rhyme? (e.g., *hen-men-sun-pen*)

 ∽ Judges rhymes—Which word rhymes with *hill: heel or pill*?

B. Alliteration *(attention to onset)*

➤   Age level: Kindergarten–Grade 1 for more advanced activities

➤   Task demands require isolating first phoneme of each word

 ∽ Produces words on demand that begin with a specific phoneme (e.g., Tell me words that start with "L.")

 ∽ Categorizes by *similarity* of initial phoneme (e.g., grouping pictures according to shared phoneme—*hen-hat-hill* (unclear if "odd one out" activity, a rime focus, is more or less difficult than a focus on onset [Blachman, 1991a; Treiman, 1993])

 ∽ Makes judgments based on comparison: Which word begins with a sound that is different from other words: *rat, roll, ring, pop. . .nut, sun, sing, sort?*

C. Phoneme synthesis *(blending)*

➤   Age level: Late kindergarten–Grade 1

2. *Simple Segmental Awareness (<u>Detection/Emerging Comparison</u>)* continued

➤ A transitional phase from holistic to analytical; requires more explicit analysis because emphasizes segmental (phonemic) properties of words

➤ Most likely, influenced by beginning experiences in learning to read

➤ Example:

ʞ**Blending task:** Using a puppet "who has trouble with words," child "fixes" the words (synthesizes parts into a whole; e.g. "My name is /P/ eter.")

A complexity order followed in presentation (Blachman, 1991a, 1994a): Single phoneme segmented first [/p/ eter; /r/at]; then *3-phoneme words* with *continuant sounds* in initial position [/s/ /u/ /n/]; then *stop sounds* in initial position [/p/ /a/ /s/]

D. Phoneme analysis (*segmentation*)

➤ Age level: Grade 1+

➤ Strong correlation with word recognition

➤ Influenced by learning to read and write

➤ Example:

ʞ**Segmentation task** (Blachman, 1991a): We are going to play a tapping game (demonstrate). Now I'll say a word, then you say it and tap out the sounds in the word: *dinner, apple, shoe, cheese, boat, hamburger,* etc."

3. *Complex Phonological Awareness (<u>Manipulation of Phonemic Segments</u>)*

➤ Age level: Grade 3–4

➤ Requires skill in explicit analysis

➤ Strongly influenced by learning to read and write, not direct instruction in phonological awareness (Blachman, 1991a)

➤ Example:

ʞ**Phoneme deletion task** (Swank & Catts, 1994)—Child shown picture of cow and a boy's head, asked to "say cowboy,"and then asked to say it again "but without the cow"; task continues using words without pictorial support, e.g., <u>Su</u>nday, <u>s</u>now, <u>sp</u>ring

a. By end of Grade 1, can delete initial phonemes in one, two, and three phoneme items; by Grade 3, should be able to do more complex phoneme manipulations (Blachman, 1991a, p. 62)

b. Ease and accuracy of phoneme deletion requires availability of spelling strategies (Ball, 1993)

ʞ**Invented spellings task** (uses nonsense words to assess complex knowledge of phoneme-grapheme relationships) (Vellutino, et al., 1994): Child compares the correct number of phonemes versus correct number of graphemes in the nonsense word, e.g., *nad (3 phonemes/3 graphemes), moke (3 phonemes/4 graphemes), perven (5 phonemes/6 graphemes), lemble (5 phonemes/6 graphemes)*

Involves "name encoding ability" or memory strategies for nonsense words; appears to be a task that consistently discriminates between good and poor readers in their alphabet mapping ability (Vellutino et al., 1994, p. 313)

Based on: Adams, 1990; Ball, 1993; Blachman, 1991a, 1994a; Catts, 1991a, b; Chaney, 1992; Swank & Catts, 1994; Treiman, 1993; van Kleeck, 1990, 1995; van Kleeck & Schuele, 1987; Vellutino, Scanlon, & Tanzman, 1994.

only in the first sound, and yet they all mean something different because /b/, /f/, /k/, /m/, and /s/ are different phonemes in English. Important aspects of assessing children's phonological systems include: (1) obtaining an inventory of the phonemes they produce correctly and incorrectly relative to age expectations; (2) exploring the sound contexts in which accurate and inaccurate production occurs, e.g., /k/ may be produced accurately in *cake,* but in, saying *car,* /t/ is substituted for /k/; and (3) analyzing the child's inaccurate productions for phonological processes that are being used longer than the age expectations for their use. Most children achieve adult speech production by age 7 years (Hodson, 1994).

There is a difference, however, between the automatic, or holistic, use of phonemic structure to produce intelligible speech and the ability to analyze parts of that structure for a new purpose, to recognize and spell printed words. This requires that the child shift from a holistic orientation to an analytical orientation towards sound segments, a development that it is not all-or-none, but gradual, beginning in very early childhood. The task confronting the child is made all the more difficult because nothing exists in alphabetic information that signals to the child the specific linguistic units that print symbolizes (Blachman, 1994a). A developmental continuum for phonological awareness (Ball, 1993) is shown in Table 7-5.

Word Recognition.   In the early grades, problems with word recognition account for the most variation in reading ability (Swank & Catts, 1994). Phonological awareness influences the gradual ability to recognize printed words in more controlled and automatic ways. Because young children, and older children with language impairment, have more limited processing capacities, they are less able to focus their resources in a more controlled way on language as an arbitrary code (meaning) *and* language as systematic (form).

Prior to age 6 to 7 years, children can attend separately to either the form or meaning aspects of language, but are less likely to be able to attend to both simultaneously and integrate them (van Kleeck, 1995). From an instructional or intervention perspective, this may mean, as van Kleeck (1995) points out, that for many children their emergent literacy foundations may not be consolidated sufficiently for them to be successful with particular approaches for learning to read and write. For example, the phonics approach strongly emphasize sound-symbol relationships, which are at the high end of simple segmental awareness. A first grade child whose level of phonological awareness is still within the emerging segmental awareness end of the continuum will be at a serious disadvantage (Blachman, 1994a). This child may need to be challenged by more natural experiences with onset-rime activities (Adams, 1990). Onset-rime is a linguistic unit intermediate between the syllable and the phoneme (Bradley, 1992; Treiman, 1993). This unit underlies both rhyming (rime) and alliteration (onset). For example, the onset in the word *split* is a subunit consisting of consonantal information, *spl-,* and the rime subunit begins with the vowel and remaining consonant(s), *-it.*

Comprehension.   The ultimate goal of reading is comprehension. In middle school and high school, problems with reading comprehension explain most of the variation in reading ability (Swank & Catts, 1994). A history of struggle with word recognition can result in less enjoyment of reading as a tool of learning and less motivation to read, with the result that effective strategies for reading comprehension are never well integrated (Spear-Swerling & Sternberg, 1994). Unless the connection between phonological awareness and word recognition is appreciated, the child may be identified as learning disabled without an appropriate understanding of the real underlying issue.

A final point concerns the child who may have a "speech problem." Although the data are conflicting (Hodson, 1994), evidence suggests that, as a group, children whose sole problem is less accurate production of certain phonemes but whose speech is *intelligible* do not encounter problems in learning to read, write, and spell (Catts, 1991b, 1993; Catts, Hu, Larrivee, & Swank, 1994). In contrast, severe-to-profound intelligibility problems, referred to as an expressive phonological disorder (Hodson, 1994), may be reflective of underlying disruptions in the representation and use of the phonological code and may affect proficiency in word recognition for spelling (Clark-Klein & Hodson, 1995). On the other hand, many children who have significant problems along the developmental continuum of phonological awareness do not have any disruptions in their basic phonological system as used for speech production.

Critical Literacy: Reading and Writing as Tools for Learning

Literacy extends far beyond understanding or expressing words on the printed page. The broader view of literacy is critical literacy, the use of literacy to problem solve, "the ability to reflect, to objectify, and to analyze what is read (and written)" (Westby, 1995, p. 51). As shown in Table 7-6, the demands of schooling begin to change around third grade. The curriculum shifts from learning to read and write to using reading and writing as tools for problem solving. Moreover, beginning around fourth grade, most new vocabulary is acquired through reading and writing, with vocabulary learning increasing rapidly in the school-age years (Anglin, 1993; Nippold, 1995). One explanation for this rapid new learning is that children start to encounter more uncommon words in written texts that they may not use in their everyday oral communication (Snow, 1994).

The language learning problems of some children may not become apparent until the third or fourth grade, particularly those who do not have phonological processing difficulties, but who may have more top-down limitations. They may be able to "get by" in the lower primary grades when learning is highly teacher-directed and children are not encouraged to talk and write creatively (Kushinoff & Creaghead, 1994). Consider just these two examples of text demands, one expository and the other narrative, at the upper primary level.

> *Reading to learn about factual or technical information (expository discourse— description structure) (see Table 7-2)*
>
> *All matter is made of tiny bits of material called* **molecules** *(mol' kulz). The largest molecules are so small that a million of them could fit along a line one inch long! (Kushinoff & Creaghead, 1994, p. 51)*

> *Reading to learn from literature about people and their cultures (narrative discourse)*

TABLE 7-6 Reading and Writing Skills for Problem Solving Demanded in and after Grade 3

<u>Reading</u>

- Deal with a variety of discourse genres and styles of print
- Identify organizational structures of these genres
- Recognize and benefit from varying organizing structures and devices used in curricular materials
- Apply new vocabulary learned from reading experience
- Comprehend material not controlled for grammatical complexity
- Extract main idea from details and summarize information
- Ask questions of text during reading
- Comprehend questions to be answered
- Draw inferences and make predictions
- Evaluate facts, accuracy of information, opinions/different viewpoints
- Use print as supplement to obtain information from visual formats (maps, charts, graphs, pictures, mathematical computations, etc.)

<u>Writing</u>

- Use a variety of discourse genres and styles
- Use different structures to begin organizing writing
- Organize information for clarity and cohesion; begin to use writing for self-directed learning (note taking, summarizing, outlining)
- Use increasingly complex and varied vocabulary
- Use increasingly complex and varied grammatical forms, more accurate spelling, punctuation, and paragraphing
- Recognize errors and edit
- Answer test questions accurately and in appropriate form
- Use print to clarify visual information on maps, graphs, charts, pictures, and so on.

Adapted from: B. E. Kuvshinoff & N. E. Creaghead (1994). Literacy in elementary school: Getting started. In D. N. Ripich & N. A. Creaghead (Eds.), *School discourse problems (second edition).* San Diego: Singular, pp. 45–46.

> *Ch'idzigyaak sat quietly as if trying to make up her confused mind. A small feeling of hope sparked in the blackness of her being as she listened to her friend's strong words. She felt the cold stinging her cheeks where her tears had fallen, and she listened to the silence that The People left behind. She knew that what her friend said was true, that within this calm, cold land waited a certain death if they did nothing for themselves. (Wallis, 1993, pp. 17–18.)*

Each reading requires a problem-solving orientation as guided by metacognitive and metalinguistic knowledge. The purposes of each reading differ, as do their discourse structures and choices of vocabulary and syntactic structures. A good assessment plan includes these areas as needed for individual children.

Semantic Knowledge and Awareness

The Lexicon.   "Words are the stuff of language" (Snyder & Godley, 1992, p. 10), but the meanings of word and concept are not so easy to define. In assessing children's knowledge of the semantic component, we are concerned with word meaning, both literal and nonliteral, because words represent concepts. There are two kinds of word meaning that comprise our semantic networks: *lexical meaning,* the word meanings we recognize, and *relational meaning*, the semantic connections between word meanings within and across sentences.

As discussed earlier, words are phonological structures. This also means that information about "modulators of meaning" (Brown, 1973) are stored as part of word knowledge. These modulators, another component of language form, make up our understanding of *morphology,* nouns, pronouns, main verbs, and adjectives that have their own meanings (*lexical morphemes*) and the inflectional endings that carry subtle information about time, number, possession, and so on (*grammatical morphemes*). The distinction between lexical and grammatical morphemes is best illustrated by "telegraphic messages." A family member in a rush might leave the following message on your answering machine: "Arrive 2:00 p.m. Saturday American flight 436. Expect you there." Lexical morphemes make understanding of this message possible. If you expand these telegraphic sentences, you can see that several grammatical morphemes are absent: "I *will* arrive *at* 2:00 p.m. *on* Saturday *on* American's flight 436. I *will* expect you *to be* there." In practice, it is not always easy to differentiate lexical from grammatical morphemes (Nelson, 1993). However, our mental lexicons store this *morphophonological* information in long term memory.

Other critically important information is encoded in the lexicon. This includes information about the social and linguistic contexts of word use, the syntactic frames within which words can appear, and how individual word meanings are related to each other within those syntactic frames (Snow, 1994). For example, the writer of the sentence "All matter is made of tiny bits of material called **molecules**" formulated this sentence based on: (1) the purpose to be accomplished (define **molecule**); (2) inferences about the audience to read it (elementary school children); (3) knowledge of syntactic constraints on the selection of lexical meanings (in this linguistic context, **matter** refers to a substance and is a noun, not a verb, which then affects clause choices, including use of grammatical morphemes); and (4) how meanings can be related through choosing particular cohesive devices, such as lexical cohesion (**matter-bits-material-molecules** all share similar referents in this linguistic context). Cohesive devices were defined in Table 4-9.

Learning New Words.   We learn new words in two ways (Nippold, 1988). One method is direct instruction where teachers or parents define or label words; the other method is indirect. We infer new meanings based on the contexts of their use. Like research on emergent literacy, most of what is known about children's vocabulary learning is based on studies with children and their families in the dominant culture (for an exception, see the longitudinal study of Hart & Risley, 1995). Estimates are that children from the dominant culture comprehend more than 14,000 different word meanings by age 6 years and over 80,000 by high school graduation (Crais, 1992; Nippold, 1988a). School promotes a *literate lexicon,* the use of words that are more common to the language of textbooks, oral lectures, and formal writing (Nippold, 1993).

Estimates of vocabulary knowledge depend on how we define the meaning of "knowing a word." There is a distinction between a child's *recognition vocabulary,* understanding words because they have been previously learned and stored in the mental lexicon, and *rate of word learning.* With the latter, word meaning is not previously familiar, but is potentially knowable because the meaning can be inferred on the spot when the situation requires it (Anglin, 1993). One important strategy for problem solving the meaning of less-familiar words may involve applying procedural knowledge of morphology, such as a derivational strategy. Consider whether the following sets of words come from (are derived) from one another (Anglin, 1993):

1. Bash/Bashful
2. Cat/Kitten
3. Teach/Teacher

In the bash/bashful example, the words are phonetically similar (share similarity in the form of pronunciation), but are semantically unrelated. The cat/kitten pair is semantically related, but phonetically dissimilar. With teach/teacher, they are related phonetically, semantically, and morphologically because of the *-er* inflectional marker (suffix). Younger elementary age children, in judging whether two words are related, use either semantic similarity (cat/kitten), which would lead to a correct judgment, or phonetic similarity (bash/bashful), for example, "sounding-out the word," which might not lead to a correct outcome. The ability to apply derivational strategies for new word meanings based on the comparison and evaluation of semantic, phonetic, and morphological similarities is gradually acquired throughout the school years (Anglin, 1993; Windsor, 1994). Relatively advanced metalinguistic ability is required for effective use of morphologically based problem solving in new word learning across the oral, reading, and spelling domains (Ehri, 1989a, b, 1991; Hoffman, 1990). The ability to apply these strategies effectively is most likely facilitated through extensive experience with reading, writing, and spelling as tools for learning more about language (Lewis & Windsor, 1996).

Thus two paradoxes are created in acquiring a literate lexicon for many children with a language impairment and other children at risk for school failure (Snow, 1994). The first dilemma stems from consistent research findings. Children with atypical language learning have smaller oral recognition vocabularies, often described as a "poor vocabulary." Most critically, their persistent problems with automatic word recognition in reading may be related more to the speed, ease, and accuracy of new word learning than it is to problems of explicit phonemic analysis (Blachman, 1994b; Catts, 1993; Catts et al., 1994; Gathercole, 1993; Nippold, 1992). Speed, ease, and accuracy of new word learning, in turn, are related to the ability to use the phonological code for the *storage and rapid retrieval of information* (Vellutino et al., 1994) (remember that words are phonological structures). When word meaning is insufficiently integrated into a flexible semantic network of relational meanings in the mental lexicon, then children will have significant difficulties in reading or spelling many unfamiliar words. The dilemma arises because the most effective way to expand vocabulary knowledge for a literate lexicon is to acquire new word meanings "on-the-spot" in the actual context of reading the very expository and narrative texts in which these new words are encountered (Blachowicz, 1994; Snow, 1994). More-successful experiences with reading and writing lead to enriched vocabularies; less successful experiences result in vocabularies inadequate for effective communication.

The second paradox stems from another consistent pattern of findings for some children and adolescents in their oral language use. Persistent problems remain with many of the grammatical morphemes when the linguistic context requires their use (Leonard, 1994; Rice, 1994). An example is verb agreement, as in "He walk" (for a present tense situation) and "He walk" (for a past tense situation) (Crago & Gopnik, 1994, p. 47). These variations are unrelated to normal dialect variations, such as African-American English. Whether these variations in atypical use of grammatical morphology reflect lexical learning differences or other difficulties associated with mastering aspects of syntax is unknown. However, chronic problems with certain grammatical morphemes may: (1) affect new word learning, particularly the use of more advanced derivational morphology strategies in both reading and spelling, and (2) contribute to the increasing selectivity of patterns of language impairment with increasing age (see Table 7-4).

The Type Token Ratio (TTR) is one method commonly used to assess a children's scope of lexical development when a naturalistic sample of their language is obtained. This measure is a ratio and examines the number of different words that occur in relation to the total number of words produced. TTRs below .50 are a general guideline to indicate a low level of vocabulary diversity often associated with a language impairment. However, the TTR has been criticized on the grounds that insufficient information exists on normal variation in vocabulary diversity, among other concerns, which then compromises the use of the TTR for diagnostic purposes (Watkins, Kelly, Habers, & Hollis, 1995).

Learning Multiple Meanings: Figurative Language.   Another aspect of semantic knowledge important to assess in school-age children is their understanding and use of multiple meanings, specifically, nonliteral meaning. Whether word meaning is literal or nonliteral (nonconventional) is a matter of degree, not an absolute (Milosky, 1994). Figurative language is integral to routine discourse because it is the basis of linguistic creativity, from "figures of speech," like metaphors, to idioms ("You put your foot in it"), to irony (Nippold, 1993; Nippold & Taylor, 1995; Milosky, 1994; see also Chapter 5). In the classroom, figurative expressions are a common device for "making a point" (e.g., "Let's not put the cart before the horse"). In written texts, figurative language is often the basis for analogies and for inferring relationships about others' feelings and attitudes.

To illustrate, the excerpt on Ch'idzigyaak, a Native American character living in the arctic region of Alaska, is organized around the use of metaphors. A child may know (recognize) the word *black* but not fully understand the metaphorical meanings of "*blackness* of her being." A semantic similarity strategy will be insufficient to derive meaning, as will a morphological strategy for compounding (i.e., black/blackness). Even the sentence context may be of little assistance in inferring the meaning unless the child knows that what is being compared is a category violation: the literal meaning of black is transformed into a new meaning to convey a character's perspective on her feelings (Milosky, 1994).

Much of figurative language learning, which extends well into adolescence, is inferential. Interpretation depends on social and cultural knowledge and well-developed vocabulary learning (Nippold, 1988b, 1993; Milosky, 1994). It is an area not well studied in children with language impairment (e.g., Nippold & Fey, 1983; Nippold & Taylor, 1995; Seidenberg & Bernstein, 1986). However, there is little clinical question that these children and adolescents encounter significant problems with different kinds of figurative meanings. The result is that teachers and other adults often refer to them as "concrete." Also, these same children may be locked out of the worlds of fiction and autobiography, where we "enter the mental universe of other beings, a universe fabricated by language alone" (Hewitt & Duchan, 1995, p. 14).

Syntactic Knowledge and Awareness

The term *grammar* actually subsumes several levels of language form, its phonology, syntax, and morphology, which was referred to in the previous section. For the purposes of our discussion here, we will focus on the relationships between early and later developing syntax as they affect the learning of critical literacy skills. Two points are pertinent. First, because the communication system functions as an integrated whole, syntax cannot be easily separated from meaning and discourse. Second, most of what we know about syntactic development comes from research during the preschool years. There is less information about syntactic development during the school-age years, the syntactic proficiencies of children and adolescents with language impairments, and how particular patterns of syntactic difficulties in the oral domain are linked to specific patterns of difficulties in literacy learning (Scott, 1995; Scott & Stokes, 1995; Snyder & Downey, 1991).

As shown in Table 7-7, starting around age 18 to 24 months and continuing throughout the preschool years, children acquire a basic knowledge of English word order, which includes three aspects of syntax: (1) clause structure; (2) noun phrases (NP) and verb phases (VP) within clauses; and (3) rules for forming different types of constructions, such as negatives and questions. Syntactic rules for English word order express relational meaning in terms of who (subject) is doing what (action) to whom (object) (Lahey, 1988).

Basic Structures as High-Frequency Structures

Basic knowledge refers to the fact that young children gradually acquire a set of syntactic structures that they use with more frequency compared to other structures. However, a typical pattern is that these high-frequency structures "are used with a restricted range of meaning and intention as well as structural flexibility" (Scott, 1988a, p. 50).

The basic unit of early syntax is the clause. All clauses contain a subject and a verb phrase, although the subject may be omitted in imperative sentences (e.g., *See the doggie*). In other words, a main clause always contains a verb or verb phrase and the type of clause—intransitive, transitive, or equative—depends on the nature of the verb. Intransitive clauses contain action verbs (*see, look, do*) or state verbs (*sleep, go, think*) that cannot take an object, but intransitive clauses may contain one or more adverbials, which are adverbs or prepositional phrases. Transitive clauses contain action verbs (*run, walk, drink, move*) or state verbs (*eat, take, open*) that can take a direct object. In addition, transitive clauses may contain indirect objects and adverbials. Equative clauses contain a copula, or linking verb. Cop-

TABLE 7-7   Basic High-Frequency Clause Structures Acquired during the Preschool Years

Clause Type	Verb	Optional Elements (±)	Structure
Intransitive	Cannot take direct object	Adverbials (adverbs or prepositional phrases)	Subject + Verb ± Adverbial, e.g., The dog barked, The dog barked *loudly,* The dog barked *at the man,* The dog barked *loudly at the man every day*
Transitive	Takes direct object	Indirect object and/or adverbials	Subject + Verb ± Direct Object ± Adverbial, e.g., The girl ate the candy, The lady gave *her* the candy, The girl ate the candy *quickly,* The lady gave *her* the candy *on the bus*
Equative	Copula and complement (noun phrase with a noun and/or article, adjective, preposition)	Adverbials	Subject + BE + Complement ± Adverbial, e.g., He is *the boss,* The dog looks *big,* They are *in the house,* They are *in the big house today*

ulas are forms of the verb *be* (am, is, are, was, were) that are used as the main verb in a clause. They link the clause subject to some additional element that relates to the subject and is referred to as the **complement.** Other verbs, such as *seem, become, feel,* and *look,* may function as linking verbs and receive a complement. Complements can be nouns, adjectives (both of which comprise noun phrases), or adverbials.

Developmental complexity of basic clause structure is typically assessed by **mean length of utterance** (MLU), a measure of structural complexity based on the average number of morphemes that a child produces per utterance in a sample of language (Brown, 1973). For example, the utterance *Dog run* contains two morphemes (dog and run), while *Dogs walked in the street* has seven morphemes (the plural marker for dog counting as two, the past tense form for walk counting as two, and the noun phrase *in the street* counting as three morphemes). Increases in early utterance length are due to two major developments: expansions of noun phrases containing more modifiers and verb phrases containing more auxiliaries and adverbials, and emergence of the grammatical morphemes (Owens, 1996). MLU, rather than age, is the preferred measure for assessing the length and complexity of sentences because there is significant variability in rate of acquisition among children.

Beginning around 24 months, and continuing through adolescence, children begin to acquire syntactic devices for advancing the complexity and flexibility of expression. They expand noun phrase information through coordination and combine and condense clausal information through subordination as seen in Table 7-8. Thus, in developing high-frequency structures, the child can use a linear code that is best designed to meet the temporal processing demands of face-to-face communication (Halliday, 1987; Scott, 1995).

TABLE 7-8 **Producing Interclausal Structures: High Frequency Syntactic Devices for Coordination and Subordination**

Clause Type	Example	Emerging Complexity
Coordination		
1. Additive (simultaneous) and temporal (sequential) conjoining of events (Lahey, 1988)		• Well-developed by age 2½ years; remains most common connective throughout childhood particularly in narrative discourse and with the subject repeated (Scott, 1988a; Lahey, 1988)
a. Sentential *and* with same verb in both clauses	I walk here *and* I walk there (simultaneous order of events)	
b. Sentential *and* with different verbs in both clauses	He got the Halloween mask *and then* he put it on (sequential order of events)	
c. Phrasal (co-referential) *and* where subject of second clause deleted	He got the Halloween mask *and* put it on (sequential order of events)	
2. Causal, adversative, comparative (see also adverbial clauses)	I'm gonna wet my hair *and* get it tangled up (causal)	• *Because, so, but, like* uncommon before late preschool years (Lahey, 1988); all occur less frequently than *and* in oral narratives through adolescence (Scott, 1988a)
	My hair got tangled *because* I wet it (causal)	
	I wanted to wet my hair *so* it would get tangled (casual), *but* I didn't do it (adversative)	
	I wanted to get my hair wet *like* mommy (comparative)	
Subordination		
1. Nominal clauses (infinitive as complement in object position)	He's trying *to make a sandwich*	• Earliest subordination form to emerge (27 to 30 months) (Tyack & Gottsleben, 1986; Wells, 1985); object position frequent because is easiest way to mark new information for listener (Scott, 1988b)
2. *That*-clauses as object (relative clause)	And the end is *[that]* My-My and Rosie went west (unmarked for *that,* but is coreferential with the main clause *And the end is*) (Romaine, 1984, p. 85)	• Emerge about age 4 years, but not found frequently (Tyack & Gottsleben, 1986); but cross-linguistic data from Scotland show marked and unmarked *that* still preferred over *wh-* from ages 6 to 10 years (Romaine, 1984)
	There's lots of people *that* got hurt (*that* preferred to *who* to mark interclausal relations)	
	Do you think *that* I can go?	

Clause Type	Example	Emerging Complexity
3. *Wh*-clauses as object (relative clause)	Do you know *what* I know? I can't guess *what* you know She's somebody *who* I don't know Can you tell me *where* you left the keys?	• Emerge about age 4 years (Wells, 1985), but is much variability in frequency of use throughout childhood (Romaine, 1984); relative clauses occur less frequently than nominal and adverbial clauses (Scott, 1988a, b)
4. Adverbial clauses	I want to go *because* I do (reason) You can go *when* I do (time)	• *Because* and *when* most frequent of preschool children's adverbial clauses in everyday and narrative discourse (Scott, 1988a)

Literate Uses of Syntax: Learning about Low Frequency Structures

As children progress through school, their immersion in reading and writing and the many aspects of the curriculum increasingly forces them to analyze the language structures found in books and in classroom discussions. School tasks also require syntactic awareness: "Being able to talk about language, pull its units apart and put them back together, compare and contrast words, (and) reorganize paragraphs and topic sentences." (Wallach & Butler, 1994, p. 8). Syntactic awareness, like phonological and semantic awareness, is another aspect of metalinguistic ability also intertwined with metacognitive abilities. It involves being able to think, talk, and write about grammatical structures in explicit ways.

Syntactic Awareness in the Oral Domain.   Think about the kinds of grammatical problem solving that certain tasks demand, including many formal measures for assessing whether a language impairment exists (all examples are from Ricciardelli, 1993):

1. Say the sentence exactly as I say it: **Dad at home is.**
2. I will say everything with a mistake in it and you fix up what I say: **Bananas not are blue.**
3. I am going to say something that might sound silly. You have to tell me if it's the right or wrong way, not if it's funny: **They are drinking apples.**

The first example is a repetition task. Successful performance requires that the child *be able to separate* meaning from its structure of expression through applying metacogitive strategies (Ricciardelli, 1993). The child must refocus attention in a more conscious away from the meaning of the sentence to the word order that intentionally violates normal word order.

The second example does require correction of word order violations and a high degree of metalinguistic analysis. The child must be able to *evaluate* the specific nature of the violations and know the strategies for correction.

In the third example, the child must be able to *compare and contrast* underlying syntactic rules for grammaticality while simultaneously *analyzing meaningfulness* (Are they drinking a glass of apples? Are they apples to drink? Or does neither interpretation make sense?). This task requires application of both metacognitive and metalinguistic strategies (Ricciardelli, 1993). Children must have a flexible command of syntactic and semantic regularities to judge sentence acceptability on linguistic grounds alone. Younger children and many older children with language impairment might evaluate a sentence as "The men wait for the bus" to be unacceptable because they are using their social (schema) knowledge, not their linguistic knowledge, as the source of judgment (children wait for buses, not men) (van Kleeck, 1994).

Syntactic Awareness and Literate Language Use.   Table 7-9 presents excerpts from successive drafts of a script for a student-produced television news show as written by Jackie, a 16-year-old with a language impairment, initially identified at age 4 years. The script is a type of expository discourse (a collection of items related to the overall theme), but also combines elements of narrative in the writing style because the intent is to "say" the script as part of video filming). Thus, Jackie's understanding of the task purpose, her knowledge of the audience, and the mode of communication influence her choice of structures, many of which are still high-frequency structures.

Scott (1995) reviews evidence that written discourse experiences influence the development of syntactic awareness more than oral discourse experiences. Meaningful writing

---

TABLE 7-9   Excerpts from Jackie's First and Final Drafts of Her Television News Show Script (all spellings, punctuations, and spacings retained)

First draft

Benton High School has received new books in library some examples are: Chicago Fire Disneyland: inside story, Suicide. They are very interesting books to read. You can go down to the library and check it out.......

In woodshop Chad is making bows and varnish them. They are making cups and varnish them, making shelves, and making a wooden or metal tool boxes, and making clocks, a key rack. Also, making a maple spoon, a step stool, and wood ducks.........

Final typed version (typed in uppercase)

BENTON HIGH SCHOOL HAS RECEIVED MANY NEW BOOK IN THE LIBRARY THIS YEAR. SOME OF THE BOOKS INCLUDE: THE CHICAGO FIRE; DISNEYLAND: THE INSIDE STORY; AND SUICIDE. THEY ARE VERY INTERESTING BOOKS TO READ. YOU CAN GO DOWN TO THE LIBRARY AND CHECK THEM OUT.......

I RECENTLY HAD THE OPPORTUNITY TO INTERVIEW CHAD C ABOUT HIS WOODSHOP CLASS. IN WOODSHOP, CHAD IS MAKING BOWS AND VARNISHING THEM. THEY ARE MAKING CUPS, SHELVES, CLOCKS, KEY RACKS AND THEY ARE VARNISHING THEM. THEY MAY ALSO MAKE WOODEN OR METAL TOOL BOXES.....

From: Silliman, Wilkinson, & Hoffman, 1994, p. 121.

experiences with a wide variety of narrative and expository texts serve as the basis by which children, even those with language impairment, may work out the grammatical features of a "sentence." To state this another way, oral discourse experiences are less effective in teaching children, like Jackie, about syntactic units because the primary unit of spoken language, as we have seen, are clauselike units linked together via coordinates and simple subordinates. Also, much of everyday speaking is less planned. Writing, on the other hand, is a process that requires more planning. Notice how Jackie's drafts show evidence of more self-directed planning from the first to final drafts. As a result of this need to plan more explicitly, writing pushes children to attend to such syntactic units as the sentence because written language is more consistent with a hierarchical code (Scott, 1995). These written experiences begin to influence new ways of using spoken language. Children learn how to "talk like books" and "write like books" (Silliman & Wallach, 1991, in Wallach & Butler, 1994, p. 9). They have begun to master more literate language use in the oral domain. Children with language impairment, like Jackie, tend to "write like talk" even as adolescents, regardless of whether this more oral style is appropriate or not for the intended communicative purpose. They have less flexible syntactic options available to talk and write like books. This analysis makes the strongest possible case for the integration of reading *and* writing into oral discourse activities for children with language impairment, even during the preschool years.

Contrasted with spoken language, the syntactic structures of writing, particularly for expository texts, are low frequency. Sentence length is increased through the use more complex of noun phrase constructions and expansions of verb phrases through modal and use of the passive voice (see Table 7-3). Jackie shows some evidence of reaching toward more length of expression via verb phrase expansion, even in her first draft (e.g., "Benton High School *has received* new books in library").

Moreover, by age 10 years, for dominant-culture children, written language becomes more subordinated than spoken language (Scott, 1998b; 1994), as assessed by the terminable unit (T-unit), a measure for assessing clause density. Syntactic devices responsible for increasing clause density include adverbial clauses with nonfinite verbs (**Having seen the house,** she decided not to buy it.) and nominal clauses in subject position (**What bothered President Lincoln** was the long duration of the war) (Scott, 1988b; Scott & Stokes, 1995). Jackie's drafts show less evidence for selection of low frequency structures that advance information complexity through increased subordination (Nippold, 1993).

Narrative Discourse: From Oral to Literate Uses

As top-down processes, schema and discourse level knowledge are central to understanding, remembering, and being understood (see Table 7-1). Both are important aspects of our declarative knowledge stored in long-term memory that allow us to know how to behave in real time interactions. Declarative knowledge is our conceptual knowledge of situations that represents our autobiographical memory, our personal experiences about events and actions organized into superstructures called macrostructures (van Dijk, 1987).

A **macrostructure** frames the big picture, or overall topic, of discourse, and guides the general plan for comprehension or production.. **Topic sharing** is a collaboration where conversational partners (whether speakers and listeners or readers and writers) jointly attend to a particular aspect of the discourse. Topic construction requires that thematic continuity be maintained in order for participants to have a shared frame of understanding. Moreover, as part of this general plan, we must be aware of what **discourse strategies** to select, whether spoken or written, that will be appropriate to maintain topic coherence during the interactions in which we are engaging. These include strategies for introducing a topic as a focus of discussion, producing utterances related to that focus in order to maintain thematic continuity and contribute new information, and shifting to a new topic focus while still keeping shared understanding (Brinton & Fujiki, 1989; Mentis, 1994). For example, if we know that we want to share experience about a specific event that happened to us at work during the day, we first must have an existing organizational structure for events in long-term memory into which this event can be compared. We must then know what kind of discourse organization or plan will best communicate this event so that our audience can interpret our intention and meanings. The likelihood is that we will utilize a narrative organization and discourse strategies most consistent with the specific topic of narration to implement the plan.

Most importantly, macrostructures allow us to engage in **inferencing** so that, each time we encounter new experiences or information, we can use existing schemas or form new ones as the way to make sense of the situation without having to figure it out all over again. Inferencing allows comprehension and production to be active and "constructive" processes. Real understanding or expression is always gradual, takes place moment to moment as it is happening (on-line), often makes use of incomplete information, requires information from other top-down and bottom-up processes as well as from the communicative context, and is governed by the goals we are trying to accomplish (Pressley & McCormick, 1995; van Dijk, 1987).

The Relevance of Narratives in Assessment

There are many different kinds of discourse superstructures. Our focus for assessment will be narrative discourse for four reasons. First, the narrative genre is map or plan for making sense of human experience (Heath, 1986). Narratives are a universal way of communicating memories about how people think, feel, and act through reference to a series of events and actions (Bruner, 1990; Hicks, 1991). Every culture in the world uses narration for a variety of overlapping functions (Westby, 1994): to share experience, teach others, plan one's thinking about events, and entertain others. In other words, narratives are a kind of social problem solving (Stein, 1983). Although there is much cross-cultural variation in how narratives are organized and communicated, narratives share in common predictable patterns of organization and certain types of prosodic, semantic, and syntactic devices that are used for creating dramatic tension.

Second, narratives are among the earliest oral discourse forms that children understand and produce because they are an integral part of routine social interaction with adults and peers (Westby, 1994). Third, the ability to understand and produce a variety of narratives is closely linked with school success and further social development (Gillam, McFadden, & van Kleeck, 1995; Heath, 1986; McCabe & Rollins, 1994; Paul & Smith, 1993), although the specific connections remain unclear. The school curriculum at both the primary and secondary levels assumes increasing proficiency with a variety of narrative genres (Scott, 1988c). Both emergent and critical literacy require learning to enjoy, and to be challenged by, the processes of interpreting others' meanings through reading good literature, creating personal meanings for oneself (e.g., through diary or journal writing), and creating a rich variety of public meanings to share with others through writing.

Finally, many aspects of spoken and written narrative development, their analysis, assessment, and intervention strategies have been extensively studied over the past 15 years in children with language impairments or learning disabilities (Crais & Chapman, 1987; Feagans & Short, 1984; Garnett, 1986; Gillam & Johnston, 1992; Graybeal, 1981; Griffith, Ripich, & Dastoli, 1986; Gutierrez-Clellan & Quinn, 1993; Hedberg & Stoel-Gammon, 1986; Hogan & Strong, 1994; Johnson, 1995; Liles, 1987; 1993; Liles & Purcell, 1987; Liles, Duffy, Merritt, & Purcell, 1995; MacLachlan & Chapman, 1988; McCabe & Rollins, 1994; Merritt & Liles, 1987, 1989; Milosky, 1987; Miranda, McCabe, & Bliss, 1994; Montague, Maddux, & Dereshiwsky, 1990; Paul & Smith, 1993; Roth, 1986; Roth & Spekman, 1986; Scott, 1988c; Silliman, 1989; Sleight & Prinz, 1995; Strong & Shaver, 1991; Westby, 1984, 1985, 1989, 1994; Westby, Van Dongen, & Maggert, 1989; Wilkinson, Silliman, Nitzberg, & Aurilio, 1993). Wide variations exist in the methods employed in these studies, which makes comparisons difficult. However, studies show consistent patterns of developmental difficulties in this unique kind of social problem solving. A significant implication from this body of research is that "Problems in spoken and written narration might reflect an underlying difficulty with using narration in the service of thought, a basic problem that could have a profound impact on numerous aspects of academic achievement and social acceptance" (Gillam et al., 1995, pp. 146–147).

Types of Narratives

There are four narratives genres associated with the dominant culture (Duchan, 1995; Heath, 1986): (1) **accounts,** which are descriptions of events that children spontaneously share, e.g., "You know what happened to me? (followed by an account)"; (2) **recounts,** typical of school-based narratives, that occur when children are asked to retell a real or fictionalized event to an adult already familiar with the event, such as retelling a story just heard; (3) **eventcasts,** where children provide a running commentary about what is happening or will happen (e.g., while playing, "I'm gonna feed the little bear first cause she's sad and then I'm gonna put her to bed and tell her a story about the three little pigs"); and (4) **stories** that children create. Children's stories differ from accounts in two important ways (Heath, 1986). First, stories represent fictionalized knowledge of events, the actors in events, and outcomes that do not have to exist outside of the child's imagination and, second, for the story to be worth telling, the expectation is that the audience will play a central role in story interpretation. (For a discussion of cultural variations in these narrative genres, see Westby, 1994.) A narrative assessment should include samples of these different types.

Further, regardless of the genre, a good narrative, whether real or imagined, is more than its structure. Rather, a good story is always involving. In addition to the telling of a series of events and actions, dramatic focus is placed on characters' internal conditions, such as their emotional, attitudinal, or mental states.

Narrative Structures

The Temporal-Causal Narrative.   In Western cultures, mature narrative organizations have a linear macrostructure that is consistent with the telling of events and actions. This linear structure helps to cue information retrieval from long-term memory because it consists of story episodes in which there is an anticipated order for the unfolding of the theme. We typically refer to this temporal order of events as a three-part structure consisting of a beginning, middle, and end.

Narratives are more than a temporal sequence of events, however. In reality, narratives consist of temporal-causal chains of events. An inherent part of narrative knowledge are the **categories** of information that narrative propositions represent and the **relationships** created that connect the categories. These causal events are linked in a predictable order through characters' intentions (motivations), their actions, and how these motivations and actions affect the outcomes. Think of the narrative plot as an interwoven fabric consisting of many layered threads. How the patterns of regularity are described is the result of the method of analysis applied for understanding the fabric's construction. Shown in Table 7-10, one such tool is a "story grammar," a type of episode analysis. Story grammar is a method for revealing how narrative structure and its theme (plot) are layered in terms of its categories and relationships between categories.

It is important to note that not all categories need be present for the definition of an episode. For example, setting information is not part of the episode structure, but to be an episode, as a minimum, three categories must be present: an initiating event, an action, and an outcome. Also, stories must consist of more than one episode. In the excerpt from *Melvin, the Skinny Mouse* (Stein & Glenn, 1979), both initiating events (#1 and #2) serve to create a "problem" for Melvin, which needs to be resolved according to some kind of plan or strategy. The setting and initiating event information guides the reader or listener to access schema knowledge that is applied to predicting what might happen next. Melvin's reactions to the to initiating events (#4) and his plan to reach his goal (#5) should then serve

TABLE 7-10   Story Grammar: First Episode of *Melvin, the Skinny Mouse*

1. Once upon a time there was a skinny little mouse named Melvin who lived in a big red barn (Category—*setting information;* cues orientation to the story's time, place, and characters)
2. One day, Melvin found a box of Rice Krispies underneath a stack of hay (Category—*initiating event*)
3. Then he saw a small hole in the side of the box (Category—*second initiating event*)
4. Melvin knew how good the cereal tasted and wanted to eat just a little bit of cereal. (Category—*reaction or internal state;* represents how character feels as result of initiating events)
5. He decided to get some sugar first so he could sweeten his cereal (Category—*reaction;* also an internal state, but represents a plan or strategy to reach a goal)
6. Then Melvin slipped through the hole in the box and quickly filled his cereal bowl (Category—*action;* states what character actually does to begin reaching his goal)
7. Soon Melvin had eaten every bit of the Rice Krispies and become very fat (Category—*outcome;* success of failure of the actions taken)
8. Melvin knew he had eaten too much and felt very sad (Category—*reaction,* resolution that represents characters' feelings or thoughts as result of initiating events, actions, and outcomes)

Adapted from: Stein & Glenn, 1979, p. 61.

to verify earlier prediction, while guiding a new set of predictions about the next series of events. We need to note, however, that Melvin's plan must be inferred from what was read thus far. As we discover Melvin's strategies for implementing his plan (#6), the outcomes of his actions (#7), and his reaction to his plan (#8), the reader at this point has sufficient information to know what happened and what might happen next (in the next episode). Our predictions are confirmed through the causal relationships between Melvin's motivation, his plan, and the actions he took to problem solve. In other words, thematic relationships are established through temporal-causal chains. These same relationships also allow the reader to infer there may be a moral to this story.

Development of Basic Narrative Structure.   Development of a basic temporal-causal structure follows a sequence (Applebee, 1978) (for a full discussion, see Hedberg & Westby, 1993, and McCabe & Rollins, 1994). Samples of two narrative retellings from wordless video stories are shown in Table 7-11.

Children's earliest narratives are heaps, a mere listing of events that do not have an organization. The syntax of heaps may be repetitive (Hedberg & Westby, 1993, p. 67), for example, in telling a story about animals: "Lookee. There monkey. Monkey. They're all lost. There's doggy.... There's duck. See duck." The next phase is the leap-frog narrative, typical of 4-year old narration (McCabe & Rollins, 1994). Here, at least two past events are present and there may be a causal sequence to those events, but there is not a clear order to when events occur. The narrator jumps around in time; however, the presence of a sequence is the first evidence for the centering of a main idea, which may be repeated: "Mommy in park. Baby in park. Swing in park" (Hedberg & Westby, 1993, p. 69).

By ages 5–6 years, children's narratives have a sequencing of events in a focused chain, a chronological order that parallels the real world, although their actual ordering of ideas (propositions) may not mirror the order of events (McCabe & Rollins, 1994). But events do lead from one another in a more natural way, although the relationship between events may be more temporal than causal, for example (Hedberg & Westby, 1993, p. 81): (the child is describing a picture sequence) "They going on a picnic and have a home. They going on a picnic, packing a basket way. They leave to go on a picnic." Bill's narrative, in this instance, has elements of a focused chain, where event relations are primarily temporal and the ending is not predictable from the beginning (see Table 7-11).

By age 8 years, the true narrative macrostructure exists. Telling a story now involves, as well, a clearly evaluated high point, or dramatic point of the story (McCabe & Rollins, 1994, p. 50): (child is telling about a fight with her brother, including the day he got into trouble and he went into her room) "... and tore all my pictures down that I painted and he tore them up. And he broke one of my best, my very best doll, my Raggedy Ann, she was my favorite [story continues to the end]." Other aspects of a mature narrative organization include more coherence in topic continuity, such as (Miranda et al., 1994): (1) the clear centering of narrative propositions in a discourse theme; (2) sufficient presentation of new information so that the listener understands the story; and (3) use of cohesive ties to connect propositions semantically in a more explicit way and appropriate use of pragmatic links that contextualize the story (e.g., marking its beginning, end, and changes in topic focus). Bobbie's narrative meets most of the criteria for a true narrative, including one that is thematically coherent although there is not a distinctly evaluated high point.

TABLE 7-11   Narrative Retellings (Recounts) of Two Wordless Video Stories about Max the Mouse

• "Bobbie" age 8 years with normal language development, and "Bill" age 7 years 7 months, who has a language impairment (both children were told that the purpose of video watching was to determine whether "other kids" might like the video). (Note: Numbers refer to Terminable-units [T-units].) Bobbie retells "Friend," a story in which Max the mouse, while looking at the stars, sees an alien land. The alien then wants some carrots, which Max provides, but the alien eats the carrot leaves, not the carrot. At the end the picture fades to show the whole world. (CD refers to the adult eliciting the retelling.)

CD: OK, Bobbie, now that you saw the video, tell me everything that happened in the story

Bobbie: **1.** First Max was eating his meal

                         2. And then he went outside to look at some stars

                         3. And then a space alien came down from the sky and got out of his spaceship

                         4. And, well, he met Max

                         5. And he wanted to find some carrots

                         6. And Max said he knew where some carrots were

                         7. So—um—he went to go get a whole bunch of carrots

                         8. And so Max ate the carrot, the root of the carrot

                         9. And then the alien ate the leaves

                         10.* So they started sharing when Max—um—they'd take a carrot out

                         11. And Max would eat the carrot and give the leaves to the alien

                         12. And the alien would eat the leaves and give the carrot to Max

                         13. And that's how it ended

• Bill retells "Sandwich," where Max decides to make a sandwich and continues to add so many ingredients that, finally, the sandwich is bigger than his mouth. The result is that Max cannot fit the sandwich into his mouth until he makes a strenuous effort to do so. (MK refers to the adult eliciting the narrative.)

MK: Tell me about Max the Mouse cartoon we just saw

Bill: **1.** He was trying to make a sandwich

                         2. And his sandwich, he put too much

                         3. And he put stuff on it

                         4. And it wasn't enough

                         5. And he put some more

                         6. And it wasn't enough

                         7. He put some more

                         8. And it wasn't enough

                         9. And he put some more

                        10. And it wasn't enough

                        11. He try to eat it

                        12. But he couldn't

                        13. So he took one breath ate it

*Indicates a revision of structure; the T-unit is actually... *they'd take a carrot out*

From: Society for Visual Education, 1989.

Narrative Development of Children with Language Impairment.   As mentioned earlier, significant variations exist across studies in their methodologies. Given this important qualification, the evidence suggests that school-age children with language impairment or a learning disability eventually develop a basic narrative macrostructure, at least in terms of event sequencing and simple causal chains. However, this basic structure may be insufficiently elaborated or flexible to meet literacy learning needs. Studies investigating both story recall (recounts) and story generation find that children with language impairment order events in appropriate chronological sequences, recall plausible information, but do not recall as much detail as children without language impairments. Also, they may have more problems with inferences that require the integration of information (Crais & Chapman, 1987). For example, Bill's narrative appears to indicate that he "missed the point;" however, when guided to be more specific about why Max could not eat the whole sandwich, he was able to state that it was because "He put too much stuff on it," but he could not go beyond that.

A number of studies also show that another prominent difficulty relates to the understanding of planning. This involves shifting mental perspectives in order to infer characters' psychological states as the motivation for actions. This means that many children with language impairment do not always understand internal states as the basis for planning (Roth & Spekman, 1986; Westby, 1994).

Moreover, compared to chronological age peers, they evidence more problems with local management of narrative discourse, referred to as the **microstructure.** During production, particularly when asked to "make up a story" on their own, they are less effectively able to manage the on-line production demands for the moment-to-moment selection of cohesive devices and syntactic devices that would make their references clearer and knit the episodes of the plot together (Liles et al., 1995).

In terms of syntactic complexity, children with language impairment, like Bill, tend to use more high-frequency syntactic structures, such as more coordinates rather than subordinates, as a linear strategy for adding new information in their spoken versus written narratives (Gillam & Johnston, 1992; Scott, 1988a). Even though Bobbie and Bill have a comparable number of T-units, Bobbie's clausal density and other nonclausal forms are more complex than Bill's. Two qualifications merit mention. First, by virtue of its focus on people, events and actions, narrative discourse, whether spoken or written, does not lend itself to the use of low-frequency structures compared to expository discourse (Scott, 1995). Second, the nature of children's educational experiences influences the complexity of sentence production in both spoken and written narratives (Gillam et al., 1995), a factor that may be operating for both Bobbie and Bill.

Summary

As we have seen, children with language impairments are continuously confronted by language learning challenges that are the bases for emergent and critical literacy. Furthermore the nature of the problems that result from meeting new or different challenges will change over time. Finally, children with language impairment will demonstrate various pattern as a function of the particular academic, social, and communicative challenges they must solve. Within individual children, these patterns may not mutually be exclusive (Brinton &

Fujiki, 1989; Gillam et al., 1995; McTear & Conti-Ramsden, 1992; Mentis, 1994; Scott, 1995). They may have inadequate or less elaborated conceptual or procedural knowledge (a schema-level breakdown); problems in being able to inference, which affects their ability to take the perspective of the listener or writer into account (also a breakdown at the cognitive or schema level); difficulty with easily or efficiently organizing information (a discourse level breakdown); limited flexibility in the linguistic strategies they have available to use in real time (a breakdown at the semantic-syntactic levels); or limitations in easily manipulating the phonological code for new purposes, such as word recognition (a breakdown at the phonological level).

General Plan for Assessment

The communicative system always functions as an integrated system. Decision making about an assessment plan for a school-age child or adolescent should consider three criteria (Damico, 1993; Duchan, 1995; Shulman et al., 1995). Assessment should be **authentic** to the extent that we want to observe how children actually use their systems in real communicative interactions. Assessment should also be **functional** in evaluating how the components interact to produce appropriate and effective communication. For example, if we focus only on the form component, such as syntax or expressive phonology, our interpretations of performance may be in biased because "Learning syntax and phonology does not necessarily make a child an adept conversationalist. Any of us who have ever learned a second language in the classroom, doing well on all the grammar tests, and then tried to converse in the language with native speakers will know this" (Naremore et al., 1995, p. 66). Finally, assessment has to be **descriptive** of what children can do, the difficulties they encounter, and variations in the situations that facilitate, or cause stress for, more effective communication (Lahey & Bloom, 1994). This means that we must learn to become systematic observers of the communicative contexts in which children must function since observing is always more than just looking or listening (Silliman & Wilkinson, 1994b; Silliman, Wilkinson, & Hoffman, in press).

Specific evaluation formats (the specific behaviors to be assessed and the procedures to be used) will vary, depending on the purpose of assessment and the characteristics and age of the particular child to be assessed, e.g., the child's estimated level of functioning and sensory or motor abilities (Miller, 1981). We need to think in terms of a flexible assessment plan, one that will allow adapting the format to different goals, different children, and the different communicative contexts of the curriculum and other social interactions that interface with the individual's communicative and linguistic abilities (Nelson, 1994; see also Chapter 9). There are some general principles of assessment, however, that transcend the type of assessment.

Purposes of Assessment

Children are typically referred for a language assessment because of some concern that the child's performance is not meeting expectations and assistance may be indicated. This is the eligibility question, whether a child's performance sufficiently differs from some standard that special education services are necessary. As discussed earlier (pp. 199–201), our models of assessment matter. The eligibility question has traditionally been asked as "Does the child have a deficit and how severe is it?" not as "What plan could we design to help this child?" The deficit question does not address whether a child might benefit from an intervention program.

The single most important aspect of a plan is developing clear purposes for assessment, the **"why"** of assessment. A good assessment, one that meets reasonable standards of reliability and validity, should address answerable questions about a child. One implication is that we should be able to define target behaviors clearly with examples at phonological, semantic, syntactic, discourse, and schema levels so that others can consistently recognize the specific behaviors when they see or hear them in real communicative contexts. Remember, "The first law of diagnostics is: Describe the behavior. If you cannot describe it, you do not understand it; or, you cannot expect to understand the behavior if you cannot describe it" (Peterson & Marquardt, 1994, p. 2). There should be a clear sequence of the evidence obtained, from the questions asked about specific behaviors, the procedures used to address these questions, and the conclusions reached (Silliman & Wilkinson, 1991).

Often, answerable questions may only emerge from the collection and interpretation of preliminary information from a variety of sources. These sources can include: (1) written reports of previous evaluations, including medical and audiological evaluations that might document possible causes; (2) interviews with the child's parents, teachers, and other significant individuals who make up that child's world; (3) an open-ended interview of the child, an important way to determine how that child understands his or her problems and needs (Reid & Button, 1995); and (4) a general observation of the classroom communicative context to ascertain how the classroom is organized for learning across the day. Nelson (1994) suggests that these initial steps should assist in identifying zones of significance for the particular child. Zones of significance are authentic communicative contexts that two or more individuals identify as being of primary concern, either emotionally, socially, or academically, which should then assist in developing a set of answerable questions.

Focus of Assessment

The specific purposes for assessment should then guide decision making about the **"what"** of assessment, the communicative contexts in which assessment will take place and the content of assessment. For example, in what kinds of activities will assessment occur, such as observing the child during small-group versus large group activities or assessing the child in a separate room as a formal "evaluation activity"? Will assessment involve different conversational partners, such as teachers, peers, siblings or other family members, and the speech-language pathologist? Or will the child's only conversational partner be the speech-language pathologist? What kinds of discourse genres will be incorporated into assessment, such as creating narrative or expository genres, participating in question-answer sequences in lessons, or others? Will be the medium for assessment be focused on the spoken or written domains or a combination of both? Again, the decision made about the specific reason for assessment will steer selection about where the assessment questions will be directed.

The second aspect of what to assess concerns the specific areas discussed in the previous section to be evaluated. The particular areas of linguistic and communicative functioning chosen should be derived from addressing the purposes and focuses of assessment.

Methods of Assessment

The next step in building an evaluation plan is concerned with "**how**" to obtain information to answer the questions being asked. This aspect of the plan also has two subcomponents: selection of assessment methods and the analysis and interpretation of the information gathered. We will need to select assessment procedures that can provide the relevant information and are appropriate for the child's current level of knowledge and abilities. Flexibility in planning is also required since particular assessment procedures may not turn out to be appropriate; thus, alternative procedures should be part of planning.

Once assessment activities are completed, we will need to analyze the child's patterns of responses. In many cases, we must think about the kinds of analysis that we might want to do. For example, if our answerable question concerns the types of topic management strategies that a child displays in two different classroom events with the teacher versus peers as conversational partners, then we must know about the development of children's strategies for topic initiation and maintenance and the methods available to analyze these strategies. On the other hand, if we give a standardized test, then we must be equally knowledgeable about how test construction influences options for analyzing performance.

Specific interpretation of results will depend, to a large extent, on the purpose of assessment. To illustrate, what do the results tell us about variations in the child's use of topic management strategies in different communicative contexts? Are these variations consistent with expectations for the child's age or developmental level? Or are these variations indicative of problems with maintaining thematic continuity when, for example, there is less physical support available for the discourse referents, such as pictures or objects.

Traditional approaches to assessment are typically directed to revealing the child's current level of performance. Often the current level may only show that child's lower level of competence, what the child does when expected to perform independently. Based on our assessment purpose, we can also develop further questions about specific aspects of behavior, either to clarify the results or to provide a more comprehensive view of the child's **learning potential,** what the child's upper level of competence may be when provided with a challenging task and given the necessary support to succeed. Assessment directed to children's ongoing learning potentials are clearly interconnected with the development of interventions that might meet that child's unique needs.

Recommendations from Assessment

Finally, we can make recommendations based on the assessment results. In the best of all possible worlds in the school setting, assessment will be a team effort. Recommendations for particular kinds of intervention in educational and communicative areas should be integrated and linked to the child's authentic and functional needs in the classroom. They should be need-focused and not placement-focused. If the child's educational and communicative needs can be met with appropriate support for both the child and teacher in the general education classroom, then that type of recommendation is best for that child.

Summary

This general plan for assessment allows considerable flexibility. The types of questions asked in each area can be adapted to varying levels of preliminary information, to individual children, and to different purposes. The particular procedures chosen can be adapted to the type of information needed, the characteristics and age of the individual child, and the communicative contexts in which that child is expected to function. Analyses and interpretations of the results can be adjusted to the specific purposes of assessment. In addition, the plan provides a framework for linking assessment with intervention or instruction as a means for continuing evaluation of a child's learning potential regardless of the educational setting.

Methods of Assessment

A thorough description of a child's current language and communication abilities, as well as potential abilities, requires obtaining information from a variety of sources. As the general assessment plan indicates, the two major sources of information are others who have contact with the child and direct observation of the child's performance. The information collected must meet basic standards for validity. In this case, validity is defined as having sufficient and representative information logically connected in relevant ways to the purposes of evaluation.

Obtaining Information from Parents, Other Adults, and the Child

Parents or Primary Caregivers

Usually the adults who can give the most information about a child's past and current behaviors are the child's parents or other primary caregivers. The family must know how valuable their information is so that their answers will be as accurate and complete as possible.

One common method of obtaining information from parents as a way to narrow the zones of significance (Nelson, 1994) is for them to fill out a questionnaire on the child's developmental history and current language functioning before the scheduled evaluation. Questionnaires can cause unintentional obstacles for those parents whose level of functional literacy may be inadequate or whose sociocultural beliefs are that family information is not to be shared with strangers (Heath, 1983; Terrell & Terrell, 1993).

A second method commonly used is to interview the parents or caregiver, which usually takes place in the professional setting. It may also be helpful to observe the parent and child, or other siblings, interacting. A combination of all three methods—a questionnaire, an interview, and the direct observation of parent-child interaction—provides the most complete and useful information about the child's past and present language functioning and gives some insight into the parent-child relationship.

Interviewing skills take time and experience to acquire. We must define the purpose of the interview, since we want to obtain the most critical information without causing feelings of unnecessary stress in those being interviewed, know the types of information to be obtained, and the method for recording information in a reliable way, for example, the use of audio or video recordings (Haynes, Pindzola, & Emerick, 1992; Nation & Aram, 1991). Most important for skill acquisition in interviewing is to understand the interview as a discourse process. It is a collaboration for the purpose of problem solving about a possible communication problem (Nation & Aram, 1991). How this collaboration is organized as a dialogue becomes critical. For example, if our purpose is to discover the family's perspective, then our ways of asking for information will determine whether or not the information accurately reflects the parent's interpretation. Compare the following two questions and think of the possible responses that might be obtained from each one: (1) "Why do you think Bill doesn't talk well to strangers?" and (2) "Give me some examples of when Bill doesn't talk well with strangers." In the first example, an explanation for the behavior is being requested, which the parent may not know, while in the second example, the parent's schema knowledge of personal experience is being evoked (Westby, 1990). The second type of question is more likely to keep communication open.

Other Adults and the Child

In addition to the perspectives of the child's parents, we will want to obtain the perspectives of other professionals, such as an audiologist, physician, psychologist, classroom teacher, and other educational specialists who may know the child. This information can be obtained by written reports, interviewing the individual, following the same principles for interviewing just mentioned, or requesting that checklists be completed that focus on aspects of the child's classroom functioning. If possible to videotape a classroom activity, the teacher can then be asked to view the video and stop it whenever the child is doing something that is interpreted as significant (Mehan, Hertweck, & Meihls, 1986).

For any kind of learning to be meaningful, children must have an investment in their own learning. It is increasingly recognized that children and adolescents must actively participate in planning their own communication and related educational goals (Larson, McKinley, & Boley, 1993; Reid & Button, 1995; Silliman & Wilkinson, 1991; Silliman, Wilkinson, & Hoffman, 1994). The child interview can also help to validate how the child interprets the world of classroom discourse by using an alternate interview format designed for this specific purpose (Morine-Dershimer, 1985).

Direct Observations of Children's Performance

The major source of information about a child's linguistic and communicative knowledge derives from direct observation. These observations will serve as the basis for the decisions about the need for and the nature of language intervention integrated with instructional modifications. Therefore, it is crucial that the samples of behavior obtained be as representative as possible of the child's current abilities, potential abilities, and problems with language and literacy learning. The issue of representativeness must be a major consideration in choosing assessment approaches and instruments. Representative samples are those obtained from multiple communicative contexts. We want to learn about a child's demonstration of comprehension and production strategies that are (1) **typical** of everyday use and (2) more characteristic of **optimal** use when supported to be a more effective communicator (Silliman & Wilkinson, 1991). Samples should be representative of a child's lower level of competence (typical use), as well as indicative of an upper level of competence when the child is given appropriate aid and assistance to be successful (optimal use).

Procedures for structuring observations of the child's communication system can be divided into two basic categories: standardized and nonstandardized. Because of the computer revolution, a brief discussion will be included for the role of microcomputer analysis in assessment.

Standardized Tests of Language

Table 7-12 contains 30 standardized tests used to assess current levels of language abilities in school-age children and adolescents. The list is not exhaustive; rather, it shows some of the more recent and commonly used language tests.

Standardized language tests, including screening tests, are psychometric creations rooted in concepts of statistical probability. They provide a uniform set of instructions and content to elicit behaviors and a specific set of standards for scoring and interpreting these behaviors. They also consist of contrived tasks whose correspondences to authentic and functional communication activities are often tenuous. A major assumption underlying all standardized tests is that children's performance is homogeneous; that is, regardless of individual differences, we can expect similar patterns of performance from all children. As summarized in Table 7-13, standardized tests vary along eight dimensions. The degree of variation along these dimensions significantly affects the reliability and validity of any single measure.

Reliability, a subcomponent of validity, concerns the confidence we can have that any score obtained on a single test performance predicts that child's true score if the test were given repeatedly (Salvia & Ysseldyke, 1991). Measurement error is a significant issue that can never be eliminated, only minimized, and is a major reason accounting for why two different test batteries will not consistently identify the same children as having a language impairment (Cole, 1995). Validity refers to the evidence that a test is measuring what it claims to be measuring. A test can be reliable, but invalid. Because of these factors, speech-language pathologists must be educated consumers of a particular test's construction to know whether it meets basic psychometric standards for adequacy. This kind of analysis also applies to screening tests (Paul, 1995). A test should always be accompanied by a manual that contains sufficient technical information about the eight dimensions so that an educated decision can be made about whether or not that test should be selected. Some of these issues in test selection are reviewed next.

Conceptual Framework and Purposes.   In examining the conceptual frameworks and purposes of the 30 tests, a reader will find wide variation in the extent to which a developmental model of language learning is present. For example, many vocabulary measures simply assess changes over a given age span in the amount of vocabulary recognition or production without linking test premises to any model of natural word learning. Another point is that approximately one-third of the measures in common use, as listed in Table 7-12, are more than 15 years old, meaning that their norms do not meet standards of adequacy. Finally, although many of these measures may be predictive of academic achievement, specific connections are lacking between the content of these measures and essential aspects of emergent or critical literacy for individual children.

Focus Targeted.   Most of the tests shown are broadly focused on various aspects of the syntactic and semantic domains. A number of these focuses are actually metalinguistic and metacognitive, although test titles would lead the reader to believe that the measure is ac-

TABLE 7-12 Selected Language Tests by Type of Score, Components Assessed, and Age Range

Name and Author	Type of Score			Comprehension					Production					Ages
	Standard	Age Equivalent	Percentile	SYN*	SEM*	PHO*	PRG*	DIS*	SYN*	SEM*	PHO*	PRG*	DIS*	
Adolescent Language Screening Test (Morgan & Guilford,1984) Modern Ed. Corp.		X	X	X	X				X	X	X	X	X	11–17
Analysis of the Language of Learning (Blodgett & Cooper, 1987) Linguisystems	X	X	X		X				X	X	X			11–17
Carrow Elicited Language Inventory (Carrow-Woolfolk,1974) Learning Concepts		X	X						X	X				3:0–7:11
**Clinical Evaluation of Language Fundamentals—Third Edition (Semel, Wiig, & Secord, 1995) Psych. Corp.	X	X	X	X	X			X	X	X				6–21
**Comprehensive Receptive & Expressive Vocabulary Test (Wallace & Hammill, 1994) Pro-Ed	X	X	X						X	X				4–17
Detroit Test of Learning Aptitude—3 (Hammill, 1991) Pro-Ed	X	X	X	X	X									6–17
Developmental Sentence Analysis (Lee, 1974) Northwestern Univ. Press		X	X						X	X		X		1:6–6:6
Expressive One-Word Vocabulary Test- Revised (Gardner, 1983) Academic Therapy	X	X	X							X				2:0–11:11
Expressive One-Word Upper Extension (Gardner, 1983) Academic Therapy			X							X				12:0–15:11
Peabody Picture Vocabulary Test - Revised (Dunn & Dunn, 1981) AGS	X	X	X		X									2:3–18:5
Receptive One-Word Picture Vocabulary Test (Gardner, 1985) Academic Therapy	X	X	X		X									2:0–11:11

Test										Age
Structured Photographic Expressive Language Test II (Werner & Kresheck, 1983) Janelle Pub.		X								4:0–9:5
Test for Auditory Comprehension of Language–Revised (Carrow-Woolfolk, 1987)	X	X	X	X						3:0–9:11
Test of Adolescent/Adult Word Finding (German, 1990) Riverside	X	X	X					X		3:0–9:11
**Test of Adolescent and Adult Language—Third Edition (Hammill et al., 1994) Pro-Ed	X	X	X	X		X		X		12:0–24:11
Test of Awareness of Language Segments (Sawyer, 1987) Pro-Ed					X					4:7–7
Test of Early Language Development—2 (Hresko, Reid, & Hammill, 1981) Pro-Ed.	X	X	X	X		X		X		3:0–7:11
Test of Language Competence—Expanded (Wiig & Secord, 1989) Psych. Corp.	X	X	X	X		X				9–adult
Test of Language Development-2 Primary (Hammill & Newcomer, 1988) Pro-Ed	X	X	X	X		X		X		2–7:11
**Test of Pragmatic Language (Phelps-Terasaki & Phelps-Gunn, 1992) Pro-Ed	X	X				X			X	5–13
Test of Pragmatic Skills—Revised (Shulman, 1986) Commun. Skill Builders		X							X	3:0–8:11
Test of Word Finding (German, 1987) Riverside	X	X	X					X		7–11
Test of Word Finding in Discourse (German, 1991) DLM	X	X						X		6:6–12:11
Test of Word Knowledge (Wiig & Secord, 1992) Psych. Corp.	X	X	X					X		5–17
Token Test for Children (DiSimoni, 1978) Pro-Ed.		X	X							3:0–12:6

Continued

TABLE 7-12 *Continued*

Test	Type of Score			Comprehension					Production					Ages
Name and Author	Standard	Age Equivalent	Percentile	SYN*	SEM*	PHO*	PRG*	DIS*	SYN*	SEM*	PHO*	PRG*	DIS*	
Utah Test of Language Development—3 (Mecham, 1989) Comm. Research Assoc.	X		X		X					X				3–9
Wiig Criterion Referenced Inventory of Language, (Wiig, 1990) Psych. Corp.	Criterion	referenced	score						X	X		X		4:0–13:0
Woodcock Language Proficiency Battery (Woodcock, 1991) Psych. Corp.		X	X		X	X			X	X				2–95
The WORD Test—Revised (Elementary)(Huisingh et al., 1989) Linguisystems	X	X	X							X				7:0–11:0
The WORD Test—Adolescents (Zackman et al., 1989) Linguisystems	X	X	X							X				12:0–17:11

*Key: SYN—Syntax, PHO—Phonology, DIS—Discourse, SEM—Semantics, PRG—Pragmatics

**Contains subtest(s) assessing limited aspect of reading and writing

tually assessing basic syntactic or semantic development. Another issue is that tests or subtests of syntactic knowledge in adolescents vary considerably in their sentence length, clause density, types of structures, variety of structures, processing requirements, and formats of administration (Scott & Stokes, 1995). This type of variability makes it difficult to draw conclusions about how well a child utilizes syntactic options in the service of real communication in either the spoken or written mediums. However, an increasing number of measures are designed to focus specifically on more developmentally advanced phonological awareness (for a review, see Catts, 1996).

There are few measures of discourse comprehension or production. When available, measures are more often designed to assess different focuses of pragmatic comprehension or production. Pragmatics is part of the discourse system and deals with the functions of individual utterances and their appropriateness in natural communication situations. These kinds of individual speech acts always have multiple functions, which are almost infinite in number. For example, "Can you pass the salt?" has a question form but, in reality, is a request to take action. Depending on how it is said, it may also communicate anger, humor, or a neutral affect. When contrived situations are used to assess "pragmatic responses," we may fail to obtain accurate information about a child's understanding of an utterances that actually convey many communicative functions.

Methods for Quantifying Performance.   When a child's score is compared to the average scores for all of the age groups in the standardization sample, an age-equivalent score is obtained. For example, an 8-year-old might score closest to the average score for 5 years 6 months. It might be convenient to say that this 8-year-old is performing like a child at 5 years 6 months but it is statistically improper to draw this conclusion. Age equivalent scores have been criticized as an inappropriate basis for comparing performance (Bain & Dollaghan, 1991; Haynes et al., 1992; Lahey, 1990; Lawrence, 1992; McCauley & Swisher, 1984a, b; Peterson & Marquardt, 1994; Salvia & Ysseldyke, 1991). First, the term *age equivalent* means average performance, not identical performance for children of that age. To achieve the same age equivalent as a child 5 years 6 months old does not mean that the same items were missed or that the same strategies were used to answer the items. Second, age equivalent comparisons ignore the wide variability existing among children in the ages at which different language behaviors emerge (Lahey, 1990). This means that the average 5-year, 6-month-old child does not exist; rather this hypothetical child is a composite (an average) of all 5-year, 6-month-old children in the normative sample, assuming a normal distribution. Third, because age equivalents are based on standardization samples that have different standard deviations at different ages, the same age equivalent on separate tests is not based on the same value of standard deviations. Since these kinds of scores are easily misinterpreted, the strong recommendation is to avoid selecting tests that offer only age equivalent scores (Haynes et al., 1992; Salvia & Ysseldyke, 1991).

More preferred comparisons of performance involve scores of relative standing. These include percentile ranks and standard scores. Percentiles are typically ordinal scales derived by arranging all of the scores obtained from the sample age group and computing the percentage of children at and below each score. The 50th percentile corresponds to the median and is the score that divides the group into equal halves. A child scoring at or below the 10th percentile performed more poorly than 90 percent of the particular standardization group.

TABLE 7-13 **Eight Dimensions of Variation for Standardized Tests, Their Key Features, and the Kinds of Criteria Applied for Assessing Psychometric Adequacy of Particular Dimensions**

Dimension	Key Features	Criteria for Adequacy
1. Conceptual framework and purposes	• Conceptual basis reflects era in which test developed • Different models of assessment describe similar communication problems differently • When using a test, are "buying" into a specific view of what these behaviors are (Lund & Duchan, 1993) • Test purposes should clearly derive from its framework (Lund & Duchan, 1993)	• Affects construct validity (internal validity or adequacy of test's theoretical premises)
2. Focus targeted	• Global test titles often mislead as to the actual focus • Real focus can only be determined from careful analysis of the kinds of behaviors included	• Affects content validity (degree to which test items reflect specific behaviors being measured)
3. Range of difficulty	• Must demonstrate sufficient sampling of items related to focus • Range of item selection and difficulty sufficient so that test is neither too easy nor too hard (Meitus & Weinberg, 1983)	• Affects content validity
4. Depth of assessment	• More global the focus, the less are opportunities present for in depth analysis of any aspect • Wider the age range covered, less likely that tasks are appropriate for specific ages (Meitus & Weinberg, 1983)	• Affects construct validity

5. Methods for quantifying performance	• Different kinds and combinations of mathematical units may be used to compare performance
	• Different units often derive from different scales of measurement
	• Most common units (scores):
	  1. age-equivalent score
	  2. percentile rank
	  3. standard score
		1. Unacceptable: No scores reported or raw scores reported only as age or metal age equivalents
		2. Acceptable: Scores reported as percentile ranks; requires least assumptions about relative standing in a group
		3. Good: Scores reported as standard scores; cut-off scores based on discriminant analysis (Plante & Vance, 1995)

Dimension	Key Features	Criteria for Adequacy
6. Nature of standardization procedures	• Adequacy of test norms depends on: 1. Sample representativeness 2. Total number included and distribution of subtotals within age levels or diagnostic categories 3. Relevance of norms for test purposes, e.g., if test is diagnostic, has the special population been included in the sample?	1. Unacceptable: Sample characteristics unstated; normative sample size unstated; norms 15+ years old 2. Acceptable: Sample characteristics better correspond to specified population; total sample 750+ with 75+ in each age interval; norms 7–14 years old 3. Good: Total sample 1000+ with 100+ in each age interval; norms 6 years old or less
7. Nature of reliability data	• Measurement error always present; uncertainty invariably exists about reliability of individuals' true scores (Wiig & Secord, 1991, p. 9)	1. Unacceptable: Reliability coefficients unreported or below .80 at most ages 2. Acceptable: Coefficients at .80+ for most ages spanning no more than three years each 3. Good: Coefficients at .90+ for two or more age intervals covering no more than three years each
	• Standard error of measurement (SEM) important to apply to scores	
	• Other reliability evidence also includes: 1. Test-retest reliability 2. Interrater reliability 3. Split-half reliability	• Reliability coefficients for diagnostic tests should be at least .90 and .80 for screening tests (Salvia & Ysseldyke, 1991)
8. Nature of validity data	• Evidence of external validity includes: 1. Content validity 2. Criterion-related validity 3. Discriminative validity	1. Unacceptable: Unreported 2. Acceptable to Good: Extent to which direction of results match predictions for the test, e.g., age, abilities, item discrimination, predicts over time, etc.

From: Hammill, Brown, & Bryant, 1992; Salvia & Ysseldyke, 1991.

A caution is in order, however. The distance between points on an ordinal scale is not constant. Thus, small differences in ranks at the high or low end of the scale, for example the difference between the 10th and 8th percentiles or the 90th and 92nd percentile, often reflect large differences in scores (McCauley & Swisher, 1984a). Thus, "it is important to look at the total distribution and variation in scores and not simply at the child's score" (Siegel & Broen, 1976, p. 90) when using percentile ranks to interpret a child's performance.

The most sophisticated comparison of relative standing and one found in two-thirds of the measures on Table 7-12 is the standard score. This type of score, based on a ratio scale, is derived by assigning an arbitrary number to the mean score and a constant value to the standard deviation. For example, on one type of standard score scale, the arbitrary number for the mean is 50 and the standard deviation value is always a constant 10. A child who obtains a standard score of 30 would fall 2 standard deviations below the mean and, therefore, might be suspected of having a language impairment. Another advantage of standard scores is that performance from different tests can be compared for the same child. Recall that age equivalent scores and percentiles are based on ordinal scales that do not have constant values in terms of standard deviations; therefore, we cannot make compare the performance of the same child across different tests.

Nature of Standardization Procedures.   A significant issue for standardized measures that have a diagnostic purpose is that populations with disabilities are often excluded from the normative sample. This produces a truncated sample, which seriously impacts on the ability to describe individual differences in performance (McFadden, 1996). It also introduces sampling bias because: "Even the most deviant scores contained in the normative sample represent normal performance . . . Thus, it may be harder to tell just how different a score needs to be before it reflects the possible presence of (an) impairment" (McCauley & Swisher, 1984a, p. 36). Many of the tests in Table 7-12 did not include children with language impairment in the norming sample.

The truncated sample problem has a major influence on how individual measures define cut-off points for "impairment." Diagnostic and screening tests must met accuracy in classifying who is and is not language impaired. Many test manuals fail to offer adequate statistical information for how their cut-off scores are derived (Plante & Vance, 1995). This leads speech-language pathologists to apply arbitrary cut-off scores, which is not a valid method for decision making about accuracy. As a result, children may be misdiagnosed as having a language impairment, a major concern for all children, but specially those who may represent cultural or linguistic differences.

All of these problems contribute to the reliability and validity of standardized tests for the identification of a language impairment. Generally, standardized tests are best approached as global measures most useful for screening whether or not a child's communication system may be age appropriate. However, they rarely provide the kind of comprehensive in depth information required for planning an intervention program.

However, when used to complement the results of nonstandardized assessment, standardized measures may have an important supportive function in the identification of a language impairment. As described in the components of assessment, there appears to be a cluster of behaviors that distinguish atypical language functioning from normal language functioning (Lahey, 1995). Selective subtests that tap into known metacognitive and metalinguistic processing difficulties characteristic of language impairment can be used as supplemental tools to confirm or disconfirm the results of nonstandardized assessment. Depending on a child's age and developmental level, examples might include the: *Test of Awareness of Language Segments* (Sawyer, 1987) for aspects of phonological awareness; *Test of Word Knowledge (TOWK)* (Wiig & Secord, 1990), which assesses selective relational knowledge of antonyms, synonyms, definitions, and figurative language (see also, Nippold, 1995); *Test of Word Finding (TWF)* (German, 1986), *Test of Adolescent/Adult*

Word Finding Skills (TAWF) (German, 1990), or the rapid, automatic naming subtest of the *Clinical Evaluation of Language Fundamentals-3 (CELF-3)* (Semel, Wiig, & Secord, 1995), all of which assess the speed or accuracy of word retrieval; the speaking and listening grammar subtests of the *Test of Adolescent and Adult Language-3 (TOAL-3)* (Hammill, Brown, Larsen, & Wiederholt, 1994, which assess a limited range of low frequency syntactic structures (Scott & Stokes, 1995); and selective subtests of the *Test of Language Competence-Expanded (TLC)* (Wiig & Secord, 1989) and the *CELF-3* (Semel et al., 1995), such as the listening to paragraphs subtest, where the application of various comprehension strategies are required to draw inferences. We need to remember that, even with this more circumscribed use of standardized tests or their subtests, standards of psychometric adequacy must still be met.

Nonstandardized Language Assessment Procedures

Table 7-14 outlines the areas of oral and written discourse development that can be assessed through nonstandardized procedures. These kinds of procedures are not synonymous with informal or unstructured observations. Nonstandardized procedures differ from standardized procedures or tests in that they do not have a standard set of events or instructions that must be adhered to, nor do they have well-established standards or norms for interpretation. Instead, they are descriptive, grounded to conceptual frameworks and related research about language and communication development and its disruption. Unlike many standardized assessments, nonstandardized approaches have sufficient external validity to be used in assessing various aspects of language and communication (Miller, 1981).

Nonstandardized assessments can include relatively unstructured observations, as well as structured observations, in authentic and contrived settings. They also consist of a wide variety of observational tools for collecting and analyzing information. One of the primary assets of nonstandardized procedures is that they are flexible and can be adapted to fit the needs, characteristics, and age of the child being evaluated. Because assessors are not locked into a particular method for obtaining information, variations in a child's patterns of performance can be explored by varying the **activity structures** for participation. All human activity, including any kind of learning, is collaborative because it is constructed through the medium of dynamic social interactions with others (Palincsar, Parecki, & McPhail, 1995). Activity structures consist of the unfolding events in which children and adults participate (Rogoff, 1995), including the assessment event. Whether these activities are located in a classroom or a separate room for "testing," this social organization of involvement with others determines the roles children assume, their expectations for how to perform, the verbal and nonverbal strategies they select to maintain self-esteem, and how the components of language and discourse are used to accomplish communication goals. When we refer to the need to obtain multiple samples from multiple contexts, we are actually referring to obtaining an integrated portrait of a child's participation along a continuum of activity structures that have differing degrees of contextual support for them to display communicative competence.

Nonstandardized procedures can be categorized according to this continuum of support within activity structures. The continuum extends from the naturalistic sampling of discourse contexts, such as a reading activity in the classroom, to more restricted discourse

TABLE 7-14   Areas of Oral and Written Discourse to Be Assessed

I. *Phonological Knowledge and Awareness*
   A. Emerging awareness
   B. Simple awareness
   C. Complex awareness
II. *Lexical/Semantic Knowledge and Awareness*
   A. Knowledge of print functions
   B. Oral vocabulary estimates: literal word meaning
      1. Recognition vocabulary
      2. Explicit meanings (definitions)
   C. Speed, ease, and accuracy of learning new meanings
   D. Speed, ease, and accuracy of word retrieval in different situations and levels of demand
   E. Strategies for topic initiation and maintenance
      1. Within own speaking turns
      2. Across speaking turns
   F. Nonliteral word meaning: comprehension and production in meaningful contexts
      1. Perceptually based idioms and metaphors
      2. Psychologically based idioms and metaphors
   G. Nature of error patterns in oral reading and spelling
III. *Syntactic Knowledge and Awareness*
   A. Types and complexity of interclausal structures produced in different samples of oral and written discourse
      1. High-frequency structures
      2. Low-frequency structures
   B. Nature of error patterns unrelated to dialect differences
      1. Grammatical morphemes (spoken and written samples)
      2. Punctuation strategies to denote sentence as a unit (written samples)
IV. *Discourse/Schema Knowledge and Awareness*
   A. Coherence of oral and written discourse structures
      1. Narrative genres: Comprehension and production
         a. Accounts
         b. Recounts
         c. Stories
      2. Expository genres: comprehension and production
         a. Description
         b. Enumeration
         c. Procedural
         d. Comparison/contrast
         e. Cause/effect
         f. Problem-solution
   B. Inferencing strategies in oral and written discourse genres
      1. Predictive
      2. Organizational
      3. Monitoring/self-correction
      4. Summarization
      5. Intertextuality

contexts in which specific elicitation procedures are used with the intention to solicit particular language behaviors. Procedures that can be used along this continuum will be discussed.

Phonological Knowledge and Awareness

Naturalistic Discourse Sample.   Consider this classroom activity structure that we are observing in a special education classroom. The larger theme guiding this activity structure is learning about foods. A group of children—Jamie, Clayton, Leonard, and Alice—are engaged with their teacher in an emerging literacy activity that focuses on form. Our focus is Jamie, a 7-year-old female still struggling with precursors for word recognition. In this particular activity, the teacher writes on a chart rhymed words about food that the children are inventing (the original words rhymed, *munchy* and *crunchy,* are taken from the individual books that the children have written and illustrated). The question being asked about Jamie might be directed to her awareness of onset-rime, the first phase of simple phonological awareness (van Kleeck, 1995; see Table 7-15). Specifically, what happens when Jamie has to generate her own rhyming examples rapidly? (Numbers refer to speaking turns, T is teacher, C is Clayton, L is Leonard, and J is Jamie)

We learn from a written running record of this 35-minute activity that critical incidents occur (Wilkinson & Silliman, 1994). These incidents are critical because they are related specifically to the question being asked about Jamie. We then transcribe these incidents verbatim. For example, we discover from these **critical incident transcriptions,** when Jamie is given the example orally and can refer to their written forms on a chart, such as when asked, "What is the same about *munchy* and *crunchy?*" she has no difficulty in attending to the rime similarity. However, unlike the ease and accuracy demonstrated by her peers, when Jamie is asked to generate her own examples, she does not consistently attend to the rime component unless assisted to do so by her teacher and peers. She also needs the support of the chart as well. In finding such a pattern, we might conclude that Jamie is significantly behind expectations for her age in achieving the kind of phonologcal awareness necessary for learning to read through more explicit analysis of sound-letter correspondences. However, we also have some understanding of the kinds of contextual supports that assist Jamie to show what she might be capable of doing next.

Specific Elicitation Procedures.   Elicitation procedures are generally characteristic of activities that are intentionally designed either in whole or part to solicit specific behaviors from the child or adolescent being assessed. These kinds of activities are often referred to as more structured or contrived. If we wanted to probe Jamie's level of phonological awareness further, as we should, then we might want to present her with particular kinds of simple phonological awareness tasks that sample her ability to segment words into syllables, categorize by rime and onset, and, most critically, segment words into their phonemic units (Ball, 1993; Blachman, 1991, 1994; Swank & Catts, 1994).

One qualification is important about obtaining a representative sample. Often the conversational partner in an assessment situation is a clinician responsible for conducting the assessment in a diagnostic or therapy room within a school or clinic. This kind of evaluation

**TABLE 7-15   Example of a Critical Incident Transcription from a
Naturally Occurring Classroom Activity**

1	T:	(Holding up chart that has *munchy* and *crunchy* written on it) Who can think of another word that rhymes [with]
		[C and L overlap the teacher's speaking turn and each other's turn]
2a	C:	[munchy]
2b	L:	[crunchy]
3	T:	Well we have munchy/
		We have crunchy/ (Jamie raises both hands over her head, which lifts her shirt)
		Jamie, put your shirt down/
		Do you know another word that rhymes?/
		You can make up the word as long as it has those letters at the end/
		Munchy crunchy/
4	C:	Punchy/
5	T:	Punchy! Let's try punchy/
		(writes and spells each grapheme aloud) P-u-n-c-h-y/
		(addressing C) Did you make a rhyming word?/ (C nods yes)
		Good job, Clayton/
		Jamie, you try one/
		Munchy crunchy punchy. . . ./
5	J:	Juicy/
6	C:	Juncy/
7	T:	(looking at Jamie) Juicy has the same letters?/
8	J:	Junchy/
9	T:	Junchy?/
		How would I spell that to make it rhyme?/
		(The activity continues to evolve. Clayton spells *junchy* on his own and then Leonard offers *tunchy,* which he also spells without any assistance; the teacher then selects Jamie for another turn)
32	T:	Jamie, you make a rhyming word/ (holding the chart towards Jamie)
		Munchy crunchy punchy junchy tunchy/
		We're just making up words but they rhyme/
		How about if you put a "B" in the front/
		What would the word be?/
33	L:	Bunchy/ (Leonard responds before Jamie)
34	J:	Bunchy
35	T:	Bunchy/
		How would you spell bunchy?/
36	J:	B/ (looking at the chart on which the teacher is writing)
		U-N-C-H-Y
37	T:	Very good/

activity structure may have a number of potential constraints for collecting a representative sample that will effectively address the questions being asked. If interaction is structured primarily through question-answer sequences, where the clinician continually asks evaluative or known-answer questions (Silliman & Wilkinson, 1991), such as "What letter is this" or "What is the same about *munchy* and *crunchy?*" then the outcome might be a sample that reflects only a child's lower level of competence.

Lexical/Semantic Knowledge and Awareness

Again, how assessment of this aspect is approached depends on the questions being asked and the nature of the activity structures. Areas of concern about can include a basic question about emergent literacy, such as whether a child has knowledge of print functions, including awareness of the word as a lexical unit. Other questions may pertain to both emergent and critical literacy. These can include estimates of word meanings known, how easily new word meanings are acquired, the speed and accuracy of word retrieval, the linguistic strategies used to be to construct and maintain topics in oral and written discourse, and the understanding and use of nonliteral meaning. Remember that many children who find learning to read difficult may not have had sufficient experience with literacy events prior to school and do not understand that meaning is actively constructed as an interpretation of the words and sentences an author selects to convey a message.

Natural Discourse Samples. If the question relates to topic management strategies, then sufficient samples of participation on different topics must be obtained in order to transcribe for analysis. Similar to the critical incident transcription shown in Table 7-15, transcription consists of all participants in the event, not just the child of interest, and the overall sample must be long enough to include sufficient instances of the behaviors to be analyzed. A 30-minute sample of interaction is a minimum time period to meet these basic requirements (Lahey, 1988). The extent to which various topic components are effectively manipulated and supported can be analyzed through a topic coherence analysis, which addresses strategies used for maintaining the semantic continuity of topic sharing (Mentis, 1994; Mentis, Briggs-Whittaker, & Gramigna, 1995).

Estimates of lexical diversity, a measure of production vocabulary, can be obtained from these samples through computing a type-token ratio (TTR); however, as discussed earlier (p. 221), because of inadequate data on normal variation in lexical diversity, a type-token ratio below .50 needs to be interpreted cautiously (Watkins et al., 1995). To increase confidence, we would want to obtain type-token ratios from different kinds of activity structures, not just one, and compare them.

Word finding patterns can also be analyzed through discourse samples, using a system to classify types of word finding behaviors (German, 1987, 1994). An issue might be whether the child has an inherent word-finding problem, which might be difficult to prove or disapprove, or whether resource allocation demands in particular social situations better explain patterns of word finding (Snyder & Godley, 1992). For example, a child might demonstrate more word finding problems in particular kinds of instructional events that demand more metacognitive and metalinguistic processing than when engaging in peer interaction where spontaneous narrative accounts of recent shared experiences dominate.

If the discourse samples also contain a reading activity in which the child reads aloud, then patterns of errors can be analyzed. Errors need to be regarded, not as a wrong response, but as a child's attempt to "hit the mark." (Vigil & van Kleeck, 1996). Errors provide valuable information on the underlying processes that the child is attempting to apply to make sense of the "problem." One type of error analysis in oral reading is a miscue analysis (Goodman, Watson, & Burke, 1987). This approach emphasizes that, when meaning is not completely familiar, the reader draws on available resources in long-term memory, from phonological and graphemic levels to discourse and schema levels, to preserve meaning

(Nelson, 1993; Weaver, in press). Similar error analyses can be made of spelling inventions from samples of the child's writings (e.g., Ehri, 1989; Treiman, 1993). In general, the the the instructional approaches used strongly influence children's approaches to spelling (Graham, Harris, MacArthur, & Schwartz, 1991).

Specific Elicitation Procedures.   Emerging word awareness can be assessed using a specific protocol designed for this purpose (e.g., van Kleeck, 1994). The ability to define words, in contrast, requires the more advanced linguistic and metalinguistic ability to analyze word meaning explicitly in order to "talk about other words (Nippold, 1988a, p. 43). Word definition tasks are the staple of many standardized assessments. However, the nature of definitions change with development as children begin to reorganize their lexicon from meanings based on personal experience (e.g., *a long word is a snake*) to meanings that are semantically related. To be able to provide a definition, children must have linguistic knowledge of the superordinate category term combined with the ability to reflect on the category and its characteristics (Nippold, 1995). With second-grade and older children, depending on word familiarity, there is a general trend for definitions to proceed along a functional to formal continuum, for example, *a clock tells time* to *a clock kind of keeps time* to *a clock is a timepiece* (Nippold, 1988a, 1995).

Turning to the assessment of nonliteral meaning, there is general consensus that this area of difficulty for children with language impairment must be evaluated in meaningful contexts. All figurative language, including riddles and jokes, involves the resolution of linguistic ambiguity. The child cannot focus on the literal meaning of the individual words but must process at a more explicit level to infer the nonconventional or double meaning being conveyed in the particular communicative context (Milosky, 1994; Nippold, 1988b). To illustrate, the comprehension of perceptual metaphors, such as "A cloud is like a pillow," and the more difficult psychological metaphors, like "She lives in an ivory tower," are enhanced when presented in a short narrative context versus in isolation. An example of a context-based format is (Nippold, 1993): "Peter was bragging about all the fish he had caught. When he found out that his sister had caught more, it took the wind out of his sails. What does it mean to *take the wind out of someone's sails?*" (p. 25). Other elicitation formats for idiom and metaphor comprehension include sentence completion and multiple choice tasks (Milosky, 1994).

Syntactic Knowledge and Awareness

As academic demands require using reading and writing tools for critical literacy, children must be able to use their syntactic knowledge in a variety of new and creative ways. In real classroom activities, they must be able to "recognize paraphrases of what they have read . . . to infer the relationships between two different sentences with the same or almost the same meaning, to take true-false and multiple choice tests that require sophisticated sentence analysis strategies, and to find alternative structures for saying the same thing when revising their own written compositions" (Nelson, 1993, pp. 424–425). These new focuses for applying syntactic knowledge in more planned ways also demand more metalinguistic and metacognitive resources.

Natural Discourse Samples.   The same discourse samples obtained for assessing lexical/ semantic or discourse level proficiencies can be used to assess syntactic proficiencies, for example, to assess the type and complexity of interclausal structures produced in particular kinds of written discourse genres (see Table 7-9) or oral discourse genres (see Table 7-11). In school-age children and adolescents, production measures of syntactic diversity and complexity must take into account two dimensions: nonclausal structures that increase utterance length through elaboration and clausal structures that condense what is said through subordination. Because mean length of utterance (MLU) considers only utterance length, it is an inappropriate measure to use with children who are increasingly encoding complexity through subordination.

The narrative recounts of Bobbie and Bill in Table 7-11 are segmented by the terminable unit (T-unit) (Hunt, 1965), in which the clause functions as the basic unit for analysis. The T-unit is defined as "a main clause with all subordinate clauses or nonclausal structures attached to or embedded within. All main clauses that begin with coordinating conjunctions (*and, but, or*) initiate a new T-unit unless there is co-referential subject deletion in the second clause" (Scott, 1988b, p. 55). For example, Bobbie's sentence "First Max was eating his meal and then he went outside to look at some stars" is two T-units. In contrast, the sentence "And Max would eat the carrot and give the leaves to the alien" is one T-unit because of the subject deletion of *he* in the second clause.

A subordination index can also be determined as a measure of clause density from the T-unit analysis (Scott, 1998b, p. 92). For example, Bobbie's sample has 13 T-units and 19 clauses. When a clause has both a main and subordinate clause, then a value of at least 2 is assigned to that clausal structure (see T-unit #7, "And Max said *[that]* he knew *where* some carrots were," which has two subordinate clauses and a resulting value of 3). The subordination index of 1.46 is a ratio obtained by dividing the number of subordinate clauses (19) by the number of T-units (13) (19/13 = 1.46) This can also be interpreted as approximately 46 percent of Bobbie's utterances have a subordinate clause. Bill also has 13 T-units, but 15 clauses, both *to*-infinitives-as-objects. In contrast to Bobbie, Bill's subordination index is 1.15 (15/13 = 1.15) (about 15 percent of his utterances contain subordinate clauses).

Bobbie and Bill both used a similar linear strategy typically found in oral narrative discourse, that is, adding new information through coordination (*and, and then, and so*). As might be predicted, both used **high frequency structures.** However, in addition to the frequency of subordination devices, they also differ in their use of nonclausal structures, those that elaborate sentence length and provide explicit information. Bobbie has more noun phrase postmodifications via prepositional phrases ("he went outside to look at some stars," "he went to get a whole bunch of carrots") and, even, an appositive construction ("Max ate the carrot, the root of the carrot"). Bobbie also has more variety in verb relations, such as the use of modals (e.g., *would*). We would want to have more information on both children; however, if these patterns continue to be found across different activity structures, then one conclusion might be that Bill is considerably delayed in his development of high frequency structures that demonstrate syntactic diversity and clausal density. We would also have specific information on how to target intervention planning for him.

In deciding what kinds of syntactic structures to analyze, Scott (1988a) suggests that a top-down approach be used. Rather than analyzing every structure a child uses, which is more traditional and bottom-up, the purpose for assessment of syntactic structures should serve as a guide for selection. For example, if we are interested in an older child's use of **low-frequency structures,** then the assessor should look through the discourse samples, whether oral or written, for examples of emerging complexity in the specific categories that define low frequency structures. If, on the other hand, the intent is to examine error patterns, e.g., oral and written patterns in obligatory contexts for use of the grammatical morphemes, then that purpose would guide assessment. An obligatory context refers to those places in utterances where an adult speaker or writer of Standard American English (SAE) would use a grammatical morpheme. For example, in obligatory contexts it is unclear whether Bill, who is a SAE speaker, is misusing the morpheme for noun-verb agreement of the irregular verb **put** ("he put too much," "he put some more") or is using the verb as past tense, which would then be appropriate (but see "he try to eat it").

Specific Elicitation Procedures.   The major method of eliciting particular kinds of syntactic forms from a child involves providing a verbal frame designed to elicit specific responses. Frames can differ in the degree of structure.

The most highly contrived verbal frame for production results in an elicited imitation. The most common procedure is **sentence imitation,** a procedure frequently found in many of the standardized language tests listed in Table 7-12 as a measure of syntactic production. These kinds of tasks require that children suspend their understanding of real communicative intent to carry out the examiner's instructions ("Say what I say. Won't the girls play baseball?"). Also, repeating sentences verbatim is not part of natural language use. Instead, elicited imitation tasks often solicit metalinguistic analysis because they require that children deliberately attend to word order, suspending attention to meaning (Ricciardelli, 1993). Examples from language tests include the Recalling Sentences Subtest of the Clinical Evaluation of Language Fundamentals-3 (Semel et al., 1995) and the Speaking Grammar Subtest of the Test of Adolescent and Adult Language-3 (Hammill et al., 1994). The diagnostic rationale for sentence imitation is not clear, other than its' general role as a broad predictor of syntactic ability in natural discourse (Scott & Stokes, 1995). Because of their questionable value, sentence imitation tasks should be used with caution and never should be used as the only measure of a child's syntactic production.

A second type of verbal frame is **sentence completion.** This procedure, while contrived, allows more latitude in choice on the child's part. The assessor provides the first part of a sentence and the child completes it, for example, to elicit morphological endings for nonsense words (Berko, 1958) ("This is a wug. Now there are two of them. There are two _____"). The key to sentence completion tasks is to construct the first part of the sentence so that there are few possible correct responses for the fill-in. To illustrate, a sentence like "The sun came out and the dog _____" has a large number of possible responses that can be appropriate, whereas "The sun came out and the snowman _____" has only a few possible responses. Another kind of sentence completion format is somewhat less structured. It solicits production of more advanced adverbial conjuncts, such as moreover, consequently, furthermore, conversely, for example (Nippold, 1993, p. 23): "Father told Crystal that she had to complete all of her homework before she could go skating. Furthermore, _____." These clausal devices appear with increasing frequency in writing from early adolescence through young adulthood particularly in expository writing (Scott, 1995).

Many standardized tests also assess comprehension of a broad variety of syntactic structures. However, assessment of specific syntactic forms in school age children is less common. Miller and Paul (1995) use a variation of the verbal frame format to evaluate basic comprehension of adverbial conjuncts (*although, unless, until*) and adverbial clause types (*when, after, before, while, as*) in children, ages 6 to 12 years. For example, children are to comply appropriately with such directions as "Make a noise *while* I say 'Go'" and "Make a noise *until* I say 'Go'" (Miller & Paul, 1995, p. 162).

A final point is that these elicitation formats for production and comprehension generally do not ask children to discuss the strategies they use for arriving at a "response" nor do they necessarily require an error analysis (Scott & Stokes, 1995). These formats are directed to evaluating the accuracy of responses, not the underlying process. When the child does not perform accurately, we may be obtaining information only about that child's lower level of competence.

Discourse/Schema Knowledge and Awareness

More is known about narrative development in this population and its relationship to emergent and critical literacy skills than is known about the development of expository discourse; therefore, we will concentrate on narrative elicitation procedures. Because narrative development is so diverse, creative, and draws on a variety of cultural and schema knowledge for events, there are no standardized tests that directly assess narrative learning. Instead, many measures indirectly attempt to access children's understanding of oral narrative structure through simple picture description or writing a story on a preselected topic (Johnson, 1995), procedures that yield a limited amount of information if they are the only ones utilized. In a broader framework, methods of narrative elicitation can be categorized according to whether they primarily solicit comprehension or production schemas, the degree of structure imposed, and whether the medium for elicitation involves spoken or written discourse.

Elicitation Procedures: Spoken Discourse.   All elicitation procedures regardless of the medium create effects. In deciding whether to select more naturalistic or more contrived procedures, we have to keep in mind that, like any discourse participation, speakers and listeners in creating narrative activity structures have a purpose to achieve. The real question is whether the adult's or child's purpose is being fulfilled through narrative assessment, and, if it is the adult's purpose being realized, how the child interprets that purpose (Hedberg & Westby, 1993). Other considerations include the instructions that will be used to elicit narratives, whether the child (or listener) is familiar with the content, the complexity of themes and structure, and if and how adult probes will be employed to "keep the narrative going" (McCabe & Rollins, 1994).

Oral story retelling, or the recount, is the genre most often associated with **comprehension.** The reason for this association is that story recounts are often premised on **highly structured** procedures for elicitation. In showing picture sequence cards, having a child listen to an orally read story, reviewing together a wordless picture book, or, even having the child watch video cartoons or filmstrips, the assessor is providing the child with a preformulated schema for retelling. Children are furnished with information about a story's setting, it's characters, and the events that occur. In theory, giving this amount of schema structure for the recall of an event should better free up the child's linguistic resources to concentrate on the actual production of a retelling (Hedberg & Westby, 1993). In practice, careful examination may indicate that this is not the case. The two narrative excerpts from Bobbie and Bill shown in Table 7-11 and contrasted in the previous section were the result of highly structured elicitations. Because this type of narrative context is more controlled, children can be asked to recall story elements, as did Bobbie and Bill. The resulting recall may then be analyzed according to a story grammar or other methods, such as a dependency analysis (Miranda et al., 1994), and analyzed, as well for other components already discussed. Children can also be asked to answer literal questions about story details or inferential questions about thematic relationships (e.g., Crais & Chapman, 1987; Merritt & Liles, 1987, 1989).

Two other elicitation methods are directed more to narrative **production.** Because of this purpose, they have lesser degrees of structure imposed on the schemas and content that can be generated in contrast to story retelling, which is often based on fictional literary events. In a **partially structured** elicitation, the child must recognize a schema for a specific event that is incomplete, retrieve the event schema from long term memory, and use this schema to construct a narrative that is related in coherent ways to the elicitation. One type of elicitation procedure is the scenario, which provides a discourse frame to solicit reality-based narratives (McCabe & Rollins, 1994). An example would be (Miranda et al., 1994): "When I was about your age, I was smelling a flower and there was a bee on it and it stung me right on my nose. Did you ever get stung? [assuming the child says yes]. . . Tell me about it." Other kinds of partially structured elicitations appropriate for school-age children include; (Hedberg & Westby, 1993): (a) presenting pictures of a series of events, such as the occurrence of a hurricane and its effects where the focus might be physical causality; (b) presenting pictures depicting a theme, like homelessness, where the focus is on emotional events and their consequences, a psychological focus; and (c) using story starters or story stems. With a story starter, the child is given a specific beginning that also conveys information on the setting, characters, or possible theme of the story, which the child must then complete, for example: "Once a little girl (or boy) went into the woods where a lot of bees lived. . . ." A caution is in order. Hedberg and Westby (1993) warn that, if pictures are used as a medium for elicitation, then the picture should not literally tell the whole story. Since the narrative mode represents social problem solving, the point of elicitation with pictures is to determine how adequately children can infer the characters' planning and the resulting consequences when a partial schema is presented.

The second production method is an elicitation that is **unstructured.** In this situation the child spontaneously generates his or her event schema and content. If this contribution is volunteered, it is most consistent with the account genre. On the other hand, unstructured elicitations can also be solicited by asking the child to recall a general theme or experience, as is the situation that occurs when we ask a child to "Tell me a story" or "Tell me about a happy time." Recalling general schemas takes more cognitive and linguistic work than recalling a memory for a specific event (McCabe & Rollins, 1994); thus, the child may not produce as well-formed narratives as might be the likelihood when partially structured elicitations are used. The converse might also hold as well. If, with minimum assistance, children can consistently produce their own schemas and themes that present relatively well-organized macro-and-microstructures, then the probability is that they have a good concept of narration (Hedberg & Westby, 1993). Since not all children are equally eager to participate, some may need to begin with highly structured elicitations followed by partially structured before being asked to tell on their own without some degree of discourse support.

Elicitation Procedures: Written Discourse.   A major issue for all children and adolescents, but especially for those with impairments in language and literacy learning, is acquiring real comprehension strategies that will allow them to engage in critical literacy activities. In sum, real comprehension is always interpretative, not the literal recall of information (Pressley et al., 1995). Real comprehension leads to the discovery of intertextuality, the ability to "generate interconnections, or links, between (multiple) texts, which results in webs of meaning." (Palincsar et al., 1995, p. 506). Creating these webs of meaning is the heart of skillfulness with critical literacy.

Expert readers and writers are active constructors of their own understanding. They are able to predict information in written discourse based on activating their prior knowledge, know how to look for information relevant to the purposes for reading, have strategies available to monitor and enhance their understanding when confused, can interact with the author's perspective and overall meaning through comparing these aspects with existing schemas, and are able to evaluate that they have understand the main points (Pressley & McCormick, 1995; Pressley et al., 1995). Adolescents with language learning impairments (like Jackie, who was discussed earlier) may be able to recognize key vocabulary words, attend to isolated and literal pieces of information or, even infer an initial main idea (Blachowicz, 1994; Palincsar, Brown, & Campione, 1993). However, the information acquired does not get easily interconnected into networks of meaning. As a result, their interpretations remain unrevised and they tend not to apply information obtained from reading and writing in new ways. In other words, they do not know how to use knowledge acquired from reading and writing to build new interpretations about themselves, their own culture, and the culture of others (Palincsar et al., 1993).

Alternate assessment procedures can be designed to follow the constructive comprehension model. Assessment is linked with classroom instruction or a plan of intervention. The focus of evaluation becomes children's potential for narrative problem solving in real literacy events. The procedures are process oriented. They are designed to assist children and adolescents to predict, organize, monitor, clarify, and evaluate their understanding of fictional, and nonfictional, texts through collaborative participation in the reading of good literature and writing about what has been learned.

The first phase occurs prior to reading where the purpose is to activate and build children's content knowledge through applying general predictive processes (Blachowicz, 1994; Englert, Tarrant, Mirage, & Oxer, 1994). New vocabulary words are included but within the meaningful context of what they could mean in the story. Children are guided in examining what they know about a theme, as well as familiar and less familiar word meanings, as a way to establish the purposes for reading. For example, if the story to be read is about a young boy and his family who are homeless, children can brainstorm what they know about this topic, with the teacher guiding them to ask other questions about what they need to know about the topic and what words might help them in this search. The categories of information generated are then interconnected in a formal manner through the use of organizers, such as anticipation guides, contrast charts, semantic word maps, or many other types that are available. These organizers serve as an external anchor for children to hang onto their tentative understandings of how categories of information may relate to the overarching theme. Resources across grade levels for the selection of themes, literature, and organizers are available in Strong and North (1996) and Yopp and Yopp (1996).

During reading, the next phase, children apply strategies for enhancing their comprehension of themes and learning how to clarify any information gaps. Organizing activities assist them to critique and evaluate what they believe to be most important, including how certain word meanings or syntactic forms are used.

The post-reading phase, again using organizers, emphasizes the analysis and synthesis of what has been learned and the promotion of responses across texts through supporting intertexuality connections. The larger purpose is always to extend comprehension beyond what has been read in order to help children to bring new meaning to another text that they will read or write about. Carolyn, who has a language learning impairment and is in a self-contained special education classroom equivalent to Grades 3 and 4, provides a demonstration of this larger goal of comprehension as an ongoing problem-solving process (Palincsar et al., 1995). Carolyn has previously read a story about a unicorn who unselfishly gives up its horn to a sheep and then disappears. She now starts to predict on her own a similar theme for a story about two elephants, one of whom has pink ears: "I think the big elephant with pink ears isn't happy because her ears aren't gray, but they might be gray at the end of the story. I think the little one is gonna give him his ears, and the little one will disappear" (Palincsar et al., 1995, p. 506). In being challenged to go beyond her current level of competence, Carolyn has begun to show the first glimmers of intertextuality, a spark that will need constant nourishing to keep her on the pathway to critical literacy.

While an alternate assessment approach of this kind can be time consuming to implement, it best meets the three criteria for assessing communication as an integrated system. It is authentic because we are observing what a child is actually doing in meeting the cognitive, social, linguistic, and communicative goals of real language and literacy learning. It is also functional because we can evaluate how the components of the communicative system interact to produce behaviors meaningful to the child across a variety of activity structures. Finally, this type of alternate approach, in crafting a a supportive learning context, is descriptive of differences within individual children, what they can typically do versus what they are capable of when invited to reach beyond their current level of competence.

A Word about Computer Analysis in Assessment

Computerized assisted language analysis (CLA) in many respects is still in its infancy. Long and Masterson (1993) point out a major limitation. All CLA software programs base their analyses on particular models of language structure. Thus, like standardized tests, the data generated reflect the validity of the conceptual model underlying the software program and are subject to the same problems of measurement error based on the sampling procedures that produce the data.

Current software packages allow either a closed set or an open set analysis (Cochran & Masterson, 1995). A closed set program allows only predetermined words and functions to be entered into the data base, while an open set program accepts more semantic, syntactic, pragmatic, and phonological information for analysis. There are also differences in available programs on the ways that data can be coded to make them acceptable for analysis. Advantages of CLA include faster analysis of transcriptions, which are completed using a standard format, and more detailed analyses of particular language forms or other key measures, such as type-token ratios, which allow linguistic profiles to be produced. Moreover, software development for many of the analyses discussed in this chapter remains in the future because of the complexity involved in examining language as a multidimensional, synergistic system (Cochran & Masterson, 1995). Moreover, CLA does not yet "give the answers" because there is not consensus on the specific language behaviors that are diagnostically significant, much less how to assess them.

Finally, there are few computer-based versions of standardized language tests. While computer-administered versions have the same time saving advantages of CLA in scoring, they may not be equivalent to the standard version. Significant differences can exist in task complexity, formats, or response requirements, for example, in the computer based assessment of a standardized test of word knowledge (Wiig, Jones, & Wiig, 1996). Furthermore, computer-administered testing also requires that children have some degree of computer literacy and, depending on the program, a sufficient level of print literacy to take a computer-administered test (Wiig et al., 1996).

Using the Assessment

The purpose of assessment must be defined well since it determines the focus and content to be assessed, the choice of assessment approaches, and the methods of analysis. If the major purpose is to determine whether a child's comprehension and use of different language components is similar to his or her peers, then a standardized test would provide this general kind of information. However, this broad purpose is insufficient if we want to address how a child's language and literacy learning is or is not characteristic of a language impairment, much less what a plan of intervention might be. This is the real identification issue.

If the major purpose is to render an authentic, functional, and comprehensive description of the child's linguistic/communicative abilities and problems, then standardized tests are inappropriate to use as the basis for decision making. Instead, a variety of nonstandardized procedures are necessary to assess those categories of behaviors that distinguish atypical language learning from expected courses of development. Since it is not possible to assess all areas in equal depth, it becomes important to define first what aspects of functioning appear to be significant issues for the individual child in terms of academic, social, and communicative needs. This information should lead to the formation of answerable questions, which can then be addressed along a continuum of activity structures, from natural discourse samples to the design of specific elicitation procedures. Selected standardized tests or subtests that tap the characteristic processing difficulties of children with language impairment may be used as an additional source of information. To the greatest extent possible, we want to obtain an integrated profile that is representative of the child's current and potential levels of linguistic/communicative competence.

Interpretation of Assessment Results

The way in which assessment results are organized and interpreted depends on the purposes of assessment. If the purpose is to screen whether a child may have a language impairment, then interpretation is limited to the scoring system of the individual test. Generally, children's performance on a test will be compared to the norms to determine if they performed at the same level as their peers. For example, Bill, the 7½-year-old child who retold a narrative based on a wordless video story, was administered the *Peabody Picture Vocabulary Test-Revised (PPVT-R)* (Dunn & Dunn, 1981), a general measure of oral recognition vocabulary. He received a standard score of 85, which placed him within one standard deviation of the mean standard score of 100 (±15). We interpret this score to mean that Bill, compared to his peers, is within the normal range of oral vocabulary recognition as assessed by this measure. Thus, test scores may be helpful in deciding whether there might be a problem, but, in Bill's case, a test score can also provide misleading information. Ultimately the clinician must rely on professional knowledge and informed judgement to decide whether there is a problem and what the patterns of performance indicate.

When the purpose of assessment is to identify an individual child's patterns of performance indicative of strengths and problem areas, the concern is no longer one of comparing the child's performance with that of his or her peers. Thus, the organization and interpretation of results will be different. To return to Bill, an only child from a middle-class family, he was a "late talker," and was currently struggling with reading and writing in his first grade classroom. He also is becoming the "class clown." Based on information obtained from Bill's teacher and mother, nonstandardized assessment focused on his level of phonological awareness, using specific tasks designed for that purpose, his discourse/schema level knowledge and awareness, as elicited through narrative comprehension and production tasks, and the types and complexity of syntactic constructions that Bill used across a variety of narrative activities where themes varied from familiar to less familiar.

Bill's patterns of performance in phonological awareness activities showed that he was still in transition between emerging and simple phonological awareness, a possible reason for his significant difficulties with phonics instruction in his class. Using a *Dependency Analysis* (Miranda et al., 1994) to assess his developing concepts of narrative genres, patterns indicated that Bill seldom had difficulty with event sequencing, the ordering of events in an expected chronological order. But the analysis also showed the variability associated with Bill's understanding and production of narrative discourse.

One pattern found that the less planned was the narrative, the more difficulty he encountered in formulating specific experiences that were thematically coherent and linguistically cohesive. On the one hand, when narrative content was highly familiar and Bill did not have to expend cognitive and linguistic resources for schema recognition, the narratives produced were better formed. In contrast, when Bill had to engage in more "on-line" processing and production of schemas while figuring out what to say and how to say it to particular conversational partners, he provided evidence of significant difficulties in being able to attend to multiple dimensions simultaneously. His communicative system appeared to become more stressed when he engaged in discourse that was less planned. For example, one narrative was a spontaneous account of an event that involved Bill's obtaining a Halloween costume from a cousin. This narrative contained less detail, less adequate references, and less inclusion of the pragmatic devices that mark beginnings and endings and cohesive devices that glue meaning relationships together.

A T-unit analysis across these narratives found, that in using high frequency structures, Bill only had an average clause density of .15, indicating that he used subordination devices about 5 percent of the time. He primarily added new information through the use of coordination (*and, so, because*), as might be expected with narrative discourse, but the reduced amount of subordination clearly suggested this to be another problem area. When subordination occurred, it tended to be the *to*-infinitive, with some evidence for use of the *that*-relative clause with *that* deleted and the *what*-relative clause with pronouns. Nonclausal complexity was equally limited to the same reappearing structures. One possible conclusion is that Bill has achieved a syntactic repertoire of high frequency structures, but he tends to use these structures in less flexible and complex ways to achieve different communicative goals particularly when he has to attend to many interactional dimensions at once. We now have a better sense of why Bill is having academic and social difficulties.

This description of Bill illustrates the differences between the nature and interpretation of the information obtained from standardized and nonstandardized approaches. A rich interpretation of performance patterns made possible through nonstandardized assessments should lead to an understanding of the individual child and to the development of an intervention plan that will be authentic and functional for the child and the child's family and teachers.

Study Questions

1. How do different models of assessment influence the purposes for assessing children's language? In what ways do the three major purposes for assessment affect decisions made about the focus and methods of assessment? How do different methods of assessment influence the interpretation of assessment information?

2. Read this statement carefully: *"Literacy is more than learning to read and write."* Identify the interactive components of language that guided your recognition of the individual words and understanding of the whole statement. What kinds of declarative knowledge and procedural knowledge must you draw on for interpreting the statement's meaning? Describe some specific metacognitive and metalinguistic strategies that you applied to make sense of the statement.

3. What are some aspects of phonological, lexical/semantic, syntactic, and discourse knowledge and awareness associated with learning to read and write? Discuss specific areas that you would include in a comprehensive language evaluation directed to determining a child's development of skills in emergent literacy.

4. What aspects of phonological, lexical/semantic, and discourse knowledge and awareness seem related to the flexible use of reading and writing as tools for learning? Discuss specific areas you would examine in a comprehensive language evaluation of a child's abilities to manage critical literacy demands.

5. Compare differences in the kinds of information obtained from standardized tests contrasted with nonstandardized procedures, including alternate assessment approaches and computer-assisted language analyses. Justify the situation(s) in which you would recommend using standardized versus nonstandardized measures.

6. Compare and contrast the kinds of information obtained in using highly structured versus less structured elicitation procedures in syntactic and narrative discourse areas.

What is the diagnostic value in assessing the accuracy of responses only versus examining strategies the child may have used to produce and response? Why might the analysis of the child's error patterns be important for the purposes of assessment?

7. You are responsible for assessing a 9-year-old female in third grade who is suspected of having problems in "semantic and syntactic development." She is also having problems learning to read. Outline a specific plan of assessment oriented to description of the child's current level of competence. Your goal is to determine whether this child actually has a language impairment. Include in your plan: (a) the kinds of background information important to obtain and from whom; (b) the answerable question(s) you want to address; (c) the areas of linguistic/communicative functioning to be evaluated; (d) the activity structures for assessment; and (e) the procedures to be used. Be sure that the methods you choose, including any standardized tests, are age appropriate and will meet your assessment purposes. Justify the procedures you choose on these bases.

8. Assume the child you assessed above is found to be significantly below age expectations in her level of complex phonological awareness, the diversity and complexity of syntactic production of high-frequency structures in narrative discourse, and in the development of a basic narrative structure. However, she is within the normal age range for vocabulary recognition as assessed by a standardized measure, but her teacher reports that, in the classroom, she has a "limited vocabulary." Your goal is to maintain this child in the regular education class setting; thus, you are now concerned with determining this child's learning potential (her upper level of competence) when given support to be successful. Outline the additional information you would need to plan an intervention program that meets the child's specific needs and can be integrated with the academic and social requirements of the classroom. What procedures or instruments would you use to determine this child's learning potential?

References

Adams, M. J. (1990). *Beginning to read: Thinking and learning about print.* Cambridge, MA: MIT Press.

Anglin, J. M. (1993). Vocabulary development: A morphological analysis, with commentary by G. A. Miller & P. C. Wakefield and a reply by J. M. Anglin. *Monographs of the Society for Research in Child Development,* 58 (10, Serial No. 238).

Applebee, A. N. (1978). *The child's concept of a story.* Chicago: University of Chicago Press.

Aram, D. M., Morris, R., & Hall, N. E. (1993). Clinical and research congruence in identifying children with specific language impairment. *Journal of Speech and Hearing Research,* 36, 580–591.

Bain, B. A., & Dollaghan, C. A. (1991). Treatment efficacy: The notion of clinically significant change. *Language, Speech, and Hearing Services in Schools,* 22, 264–270.

Baker, L., & Brown, A. L. (1984). Metacognitive skills and reading. In P. D. Pearson (Ed.), *Handbook of reading research* (pp. 353–394). New York: Longman.

Ball, E. W. (1993). Assessing phoneme awareness. *Language, Speech, and Hearing Services in Schools,* 24, 130–139.

Bashir, A. S., & Scavuzzo, A. (1992). Children with language disorders: Natural history and academic success. *Journal of Learning Disabilities,* 25, 53–65.

Bashir, A. S., & Strominger, A. Z. (1996). Children with develomental language disorders: Outcomes, persistence, and change. In M. D. Smith & J. S. Damico (Eds.), *Childhood language disorders* (pp. 119–140). New York: Thieme.

Bateman, B. D. (1995). Who, how, and where: Special education issues in perpetuity. In J. M. Kaufman &

D. P. Hallahan (Eds.), *The illusion of full inclusion: A comprehensive critique of a special education bandwagon* (pp. 75–90). Austin, TX: Pro-Ed.

Beaumont, S. L. (1995). Adolescent girls' conversations with mothers and friends: A matter of style. *Discourse Processes, 20,* 109–132.

Berko, J. (1958). The child's learning of English morphology. *Word, 14,* 150–177.

Blachman, B. A. (1991). Early intervention for children's reading problems: Clinical applications of the research in phonological awareness. *Topics in Language Disorders, 12* (1), 51–65.

Blachman, B. A. (1994a). Early literacy acquisition: The role of phonological awareness. In G. P. Wallach & K. G. Butler (Eds.), *Language learning disabilities in school-age children and adolescents: Some principles and applications* (pp. 253–274). Boston: Allyn & Bacon.

Blachman, B. A. (1994b). What we have learned from longitudinal studies of phonological processing and reading, and some unanswered questions: A response to Torgesen, Wagner, and Rashotte. *Journal of Learning Disabilities, 27,* 287–291.

Blachowitz, C. L. (1994). Problem-solving strategies for academic success. In G. P. Wallach & K. G. Butler (Eds.), *Language learning disabilities in school-age children and adolescents: Some principles and applications* (pp. 304–322). Boston: Allyn & Bacon.

Black, B., & Logan, A. (1995). Links between communication patterns in mother-child, father-child, and child-peer interactions and children's social status. *Child Development, 66,* 255–271.

Bradley, L. (1992). Rhymes, rimes, and learning to read and spell. In C. A. Ferguson, L. Menn, & C. Stoel-Gammon (Eds.), *Phonological development: Models, research, implications* (pp. 553–562). Timonium, MD: York Press.

Brinton, B. B., & Fujiki, M. (1989). *Conversational management in language impaired children.* Rockville, MD: Aspen.

Brown, A. L., & Palincsar, A. S. (1987). Reciprocal teaching of comprehension strategies. In J. D. Day & J. G. Borkowski (Eds.), *Intelligence and exceptionality: New directions for theory, assessment, and instructional practice* (pp. 81–132). Norwood, NJ: Ablex.

Brown, R. (1973). *A first language: The early stages.* Cambridge, MA: Harvard University Press.

Bruner, J. (1990). *Acts of meaning.* Cambridge, MA: Harvard University Press.

Catts, H. W. (1989a). Phonological processing deficits and reading disabilities. In A. G. Kamhi & H. W. Catts (Eds.), *Reading disabilities: A developmental language perspective* (pp. 101–132). Boston: College-Hill.

Catts, H. W. (1989b). Speech production deficits in developmental dyslexia. *Journal of Speech and Hearing Disorders, 54,* 422–428.

Catts, H. W. (1991a). Early identification of reading disabilities. *Topics in Language Disorders, 12* (1), 1–16.

Catts, H. W. (1991b). Facilitating phonological awareness: Role of speech-language pathologists. *Language, Speech, and Hearing Services in Schools, 22,* 196–203.

Catts, H. W. (1993). The relationship between speech-language impairments and reading disabilities. *Journal of Speech and Hearing Research, 36,* 948–958.

Catts, H. W. (1996). Defining dyslexia as a developmental language disorder: An expanded view. *Topics in Language Disorders, 16* (2), 14–29.

Catts, H. W., Hu, C-F, Larrivee, L., & Swank, L. (1994). Early identification of reading disabilities in children with speech-language impairments. In R. V. Watkins & M. L. Rice (Eds.), *Specific language impairments in children* (pp. 145–160). Baltimore: Paul H. Brookes.

Chaney, C. (1992). Language development, metalinguistic skills, and print awareness in 3-year-old children. *Applied Psycholinguistics, 13,* 485–514.

Chapman, R. S. (1991). Models of language disorders. In J. Miller (Ed.), *Research on child language disorders: A decade of progress* (pp. 287–297). Austin, TX: Pro-Ed.

Clark-Klein, S., & Hodson, B. W. (1995). A phonologically based analysis of misspellings by third graders with disordered-phonology histories. *Journal of Speech and Hearing Research, 38,* 839–849.

Cochran, P. S., & Masterson, J. J. (1995). NOT using a computer in language/assessment intervention: In defense of the reluctant clinician. *Language, Speech, and Hearing Services in Schools, 26,* 213–222.

Cole, K. (1995). What is the evidence from research with young children with language disorders? Paper presented on Discrepancy Models and the Discrepancy between Policy and Evidence at the Annual Convention of the American Speech-Language-Hearing Association, Orlando, Florida, December 1995.

Crago, M. B., & Gopnik, M (1994). From families to phentotypes: Theoretical and clinical implications of research into the genetic basis of specific language impairment. In R. V. Watkins & M. L. Rice (Eds.), *Specific language impairment in children* (pp. 35–51). Baltimore: Paul H. Brookes.

Crais, E. R. (1992). Fast mapping: A new look at word learning. In R. S. Chapman (Ed.), *Processes in language acquisition and disorders* (pp. 159–185). St. Louis, MO: Mosby.

Crais, E. R., & Chapman, R. S. (1987). Story recall and inferencing skills in language/learning-disabled and non-disabled children. *Journal of Speech and Hearing Disorders, 52,* 50–55.

Damico, J. S. (1991). Descriptive assessment of communicative ability in limited English proficient students. In E. V. Hamayan & J. S. Damico (Eds.), *Limiting bias in the assessment of bilingual students* (pp. 157–217). Austin, TX: Pro-Ed.

Damico, J. S. (1993). Language assessment in adolescents: Addressing critical issues. *Language, Speech, and Hearing Services in Schools, 24,* 29–35.

Donahue, M. L. (1994). Differences in classroom discourse styles of students with learning disabilities. In D. N. Ripich & N. A. Creaghead (Eds.), *School discourse problems (second edition)* (pp. 229–261). San Diego: Singular.

Duchan, J. F. (1995). *Supporting language learning in everyday life.* San Diego: Singular.

Dunn, L. M., & Dunn, L. M. (1981). *Peabody picture vocabluary test-revised.* Circle Pines, MN: American Guidance Service.

Ehren, B. (1994). New directions for meeting the academic needs of adolescents with learning disabilities. In G. P. Wallach & K. G. Butler (Eds.), *Language learning disabilities in school-age children and adolescents: Some principles and applications* (pp. 393–417). Boston: Allyn & Bacon.

Ehri, L. C. (1989a). Movement into word reading and spelling: How spelling contributes to reading. In J. M. Mason (Ed.), *Reading and writing connections* (pp. 65–81). Boston: Allyn & Bacon.

Ehri, L. C. (1989b). The development of spelling knowledge and its role in reading acquisition and reading disability. *Journal of Learning Disabilities, 22,* 356–365.

Ehri, L. C. (1991). Learning to read and spell words. In L. Rieben & C. A. Perfetti (Eds.), *Learning to read: Basic research and its implications* (pp. 57–73). Hillsdale, NJ: Lawrence Erlbaum.

Englert, C. S., Tarrant, K. L., Mariage, T. V., & Oxer, T. (1994). Lesson talk as the work of reading groups: The effectiveness of two interventions. *Journal of Learning Disabilities, 27,* 165–185.

Feagans, L., & Short, E. J. (1984). Developmental differences in comprehension and production of narratives by reading-disabled and normally achieving children. *Child Development, 55,* 1727–1736.

Fey, M. E., Catts, H. W., & Larrivee, L. S. (1995). Preparing preschoolers for the academic and social challenges of school. In M. E. Fey, J. Windsor, & S. F. Warren (Eds.), *Language intervention: Preschool through the elementary years* (pp. 3–37). Baltimore: Paul H. Brookes.

Fujuki, M., & Brinton, (1994). Social competence and language impairment. In R. V. Watkins & M. L. Rice (Eds.), *Specific language impairment in children* (pp. 123–143). Baltimore: Paul H. Brookes.

Garnett, K. (1986). Telling tales: Narratives and learning-disabled children. *Topics in Language Disorders, 6* (2) 44–56.

Gathercole, S. E. (1993). Word learning in language impaired children. *Child Language Teaching and Therapy, 9,* 187–199.

German, D. J. (1986). *Test of word finding (TWF).* Chicago: Riverside.

German, D. J. (1987). Spontaneous language profiles of children with word-finding problems. *Language, Speech, and Hearing Services in Schools, 18,* 217–230.

German, D. J. (1990). *Test of adolescent/adult word finding skills (TAWF).* Chicago: Riverside.

German, D. J. (1994). Wordfinding difficulty in children and adolescents. In G. P. Wallach & K. G. Butler (Eds.), *Language learning disabilities in school-age children and adolescents: Some principles and applications* (pp. 323–351). Boston: Allyn & Bacon.

Gilger, J. W. (1995). Behavioral genetics: Concepts for research and practice in language development and disorders. *Journal of Speech and Hearing Research, 38,* 1126–1142.

Gillam, R., & Johnston, J. R. (1992). Spoken and written language relationships in language/learning-impaired and normally achieving school-age children. *Journal of Speech and Hearing Research, 35,* 1303–1315.

Gillam, R., McFadden, T. U., & van Kleeck, A. (1995). Improving narrative abilities: Whole language and language skills approaches. In M. E. Fey, J. Windsor, & S. F. Warren (Eds.), *Language intervention: Preschool through the elementary years* (pp. 145–182). Baltimore: Paul H. Brookes.

Goodman, Y. M., Watson, D. J., & Burke, C. L. (1987). *Reading miscue inventory: Alternative procedures.* Katonah, NY: Richard C. Owen.

Graham, S., Harris, K. R., MacArthur, C. A., & Schwartz, S. (1991, Spring). Writing and writing instruction for students with learning disabilities: Review of a research program. *Learning Disability Quarterly, 14,* 89–114.

Graybeal, C. M. (1981). Memory for stories in language-impaired children. *Applied Psycholinguistics, 2,* 269–283.

Griffith, P. L., Ripich, D. N., & Dastoli, S. L. (1986). Story structure, cohesion, and propositions in story recalls by learning-disabled and nondisabled children. *Journal of Psycholinguistic Research, 15,* 539–555.

Gutierrez-Clellen, V., & Quinn, R. (1993). Assessing narratives if children from diverse cultural/linguistic groups. *Language, Speech, and Hearing Services in Schools, 24,* 2–9.

Halliday, M. A. K. (1987). Spoken and written modes of meaning. In R. Horowitz & S. J. Samuels (Eds.), *Comprehending oral and written language* (pp. 55–82). San Diego: Academic Press.

Hammill, D. D., Brown, L., & Bryant, B. R. (1992). *A consumer's guide to tests in print.* (2nd ed.). Austin, TX: Pro-Ed.

Hammill, D. D., Brown, V. L., Larsen, S. C., & Wiederholt, J. L. (1994). *Test of adolescent and adult language: Assessing linguistic aspects of listening, speaking, reading, and writing* (3rd ed.). Austin, TX: Pro-Ed.

Hart, B., & Risley, T. R. (1995). *Meaningful differences in the everyday experiences of young American children.* Baltimore: Paul H. Brookes.

Haynes, W. O., Pindzola, R. H., & Emerick, L. L. (1992). *Diagnosis and evaluation in speech pathology* (4th ed.). Englewood Cliffs, NJ: Prentice-Hall.

Heath, S. B. (1982). What no bedtime story means: Narrative skills at home and school. *Language in Society, 11,* 49–76.

Heath, S. B. (1983). *Ways with words: Language, life, and work in communities and classrooms.* New York: Cambridge University Press.

Heath, S. B. (1986). Taking a cross-cultural look at narratives. *Topics in Language Disorders, 7* (1), 84–94.

Hedberg, N. L., & Stoel-Gammon, C. (1986). Narrative analysis: Clinical procedures. *Topics in Language Disorders, 7* (1), 58–69.

Hedberg, N., & Westby, C. E. (1993). *Analyzing story telling skills: Theory to practice:* Tucson, AZ: Communication Skill Builders.

Hewitt, L. E., & Duchan, J. F. (1995). Subjectivity in children's fictional narrative. *Topics in Language Disorders, 15* (4), 1–15.

Hicks, D. (1991). Kinds of narratives: Genre skills among first graders from two communities. In A. McCabe & C. Peterson (Eds.), *Developing narrative structure* (pp. 55–87). Hillsdale, NJ: Erlbaum.

Hodson, B. W. (1994). Helping individuals become intelligible, literate, and articulate: The role of phonology. *Topics in Language Disorders, 14* (2), 1–16.

Hoffman, P. R. (1990). Spelling, phonology, and the speech-language pathologist: A whole language perspective. *Language, Speech, and Hearing Services in Schools, 21,* 238–243.

Hogan, K. C., & Strong, C. J. (1994). The magic of "once upton a time": Narrative teaching strategies. *Language, Speech, and Hearing Services in Schools, 25,* 76–89.

Hummel, L. J., & Prizant, B. M. (1993). A socioemotional perspective for understanding difficulties of school-age children with language disorders. *Language, Speech, and Hearing Services in Schools, 24,* 216–224.

Hunt, K. W. (1965). *Grammatical structures written at three grade levels.* Urbana, IL: National Council of Teachers of English.

Jenkins, R., & Bowen, L. (1994). Facilitating development of preliterate children's phonological abilities. *Topics in Language Disorders, 14* (2), 26–39.

Johnson, C. J. (1995). Expanding norms for narration. *Language, Speech, and Hearing Services in Schools, 26,* 326–340.

Johnston, J. R. (1994). Cognitive abilities of children with language impairment. In R. V. Watkins &

M. L. Rice (Eds.), *Specific language impairments in children* (pp. 107–121). Baltimore: Paul H. Brookes.

Kamhi, A. G. (1989). Causes and consequences of reading disabilities. In A. G. Kamhi & H. W. Catts (Eds.), *Reading disabilities: A developmental language perspective* (pp. 67–99). Boston: College-Hill.

Kamhi, A. G. (1992). Response to historical perspective: A developmental language perspective. *Journal of Learning Disabilities, 25,* 48–52.

Kamhi, A. G. (1996). Linguistic and cognitive aspects of specific language impairment. In M. D. Smith & J. S. Damico (Eds.), *Childhood language disorders* (pp. 97–116). New York: Thieme.

Kamhi, A. G., & Catts, H. W. (1989). Language and reading: Convergences, divergences, and development. In A. G. Kamhi & H. W. Catts (Eds.), *Reading disabilities: A developmental language perspective* (pp. 1–34). Boston: College-Hill.

Kushinoff, B. E., & Creaghead, N. E. (1994). Literacy in elementary school: Getting started. In D. N. Ripich & N. A. Creaghead (Eds.), *School discourse problems* (2nd ed.) (pp. 29–62). San Diego: Singular.

Lahey, M. (1988). *Language development and language disorders.* New York: Macmillan.

Lahey, M. (1990). Who shall be called language disordered? Some reflections and one perspective. *Journal of Speech and Hearing Disorders, 55,* 612–620.

Lahey, M. (1995). Who shall be called language disordered? Paper presented on discrepancy models and the discrepancy between policy and evidence at the Annual Convention of the American Speech-Language-Hearing Association, Orlando, Florida, December 1995.

Lahey, M., & Bloom, L. (1994). Variability and language learning disabilities. In G. P. Wallach & K. G. Butler (Eds.), *Language learning disabilities in school-age children and adolescents: Some principles and applications* (pp. 354–372). Boston: Allyn & Bacon.

Lahey, M., & Edwards, J. (1995). Specific language impairment: Preliminary investigation of factors associated with family history and with patterns of language performance. *Journal of Speech and Hearing Research, 38,* 643–657.

Larson, L. L., McKinley, N. L., & Boley, D. (1993). Service delivery models for adolescents with language disorders. *Language, Speech, and Hearing Services in Schools, 24,* 36–42.

Lawrence, C. W. (1992). Assesing the use of age-equivalent scores in clinical management. *Language, Speech, and Hearing Services in Schools, 23,* 6–8.

Leonard, L. B. (1994). Some problems facing accounts of morphological deficits in children with specific language impairments. In R. V. Watkins & M. L. Rice (Eds.), *Specific language impairments in children* (pp. 91–105). Baltimore: Paul H. Brookes.

Lewis, D. J., & Windsor, J. (1996). Children's analysis of derivational suffix meanings. *Journal of Speech and Hearing Research, 39,* 209–216.

Liberman, I. Y., & Shankweiler, D. (1991). Phonology and beginning reading: A tutorial. In L. Rieben & C. A. Perfetti (Eds.), *Learning to read: Basic research and its implications* (pp. 3–17). Hillsdale, NJ: Lawrence Erlbaum.

Liles, B. Z. (1987). Episode organization and cohesive conjunction in narratives of children with and without language disorder. *Journal of Speech and Hearing Research, 30,* 185–196.

Liles, B. Z. (1993). Narrative discourse in children with language disorders and children with normal language: A critical review of the literature, *Journal of Speech and Hearing Research, 36,* 868–882.

Liles, B. Z., Duffy, R. J., Merritt, D. D., & Purcell, S. L. (1995). Measurement of narrative discourse ability in children with language disorders. *Journal of Speech and Hearing Research, 38,* 415–425.

Liles, B. Z., & Purcell, S. (1987). Departures in the spoken narratives of normal and language-disordered children. *Applied Psycholinguistics, 8,* 185–202.

Locke, J. L. (1994). Gradual emergence of development language disorder. *Journal of Speech and Hearing Research, 37,* 608–616.

Long, S. H., & Masterson, J. J. (1993). Computer technology: Use in language analysis. *Asha, 35* (8), 40–44, 51.

Lund, N. J., & Duchan, J. F. (1993). *Assessing children's language in naturalistic contexts* (3rd ed.). Englewood Cliffs, NJ: Prentice-Hall.

MacLachlan, B. G., & Chapman, R. S. (1988). Communication breakdowns in normal and language learning-disabled children's conversation and narration. *Journal of Speech and Hearing Disorders,* 53, 2–7.

Mann, V. A. (1993). Phonemic awareness and future reading ability. *Journal of Learning Disabilities,* 26, 259–269.

Mann, V. (1994). Phonological skills and the prediction of early reading problems. In N. C. Jordon & J. Goldsmith-Phillips (Eds.), *Learning disabilities: New directions for assessment and intervention* (pp. 67–84). Boston: Allyn & Bacon.

McCabe, A., & Rollins, P. R. (1994). Assessment of preschool narrative skills. *American Journal of Speech-Language Pathology,* 3, 45–55.

McCauley, R. J., & Swisher, L. (1984a). Psychometric review of language and articulation tests for preschool children. *Journal of Speech and Hearing Disorders,* 49, 34–42.

McCauley, R. J., & Swisher, L. (1984b). Use and misuse of norm-referenced tests in clinical assessment: A hypothetical case. *Journal of Speech and Hearing Disorders,* 49, 338–348.

McFadden, T. U. (1996). Creating language impairments in typically achieving children: The pitfalls of "normal" normative sampling. *Language, Speech, and Hearing Services in Schools,* 27, 3–9.

McGregor, K. L., & Leonard, L. B. (1995). Intervention for word finding deficits in children. In M. E. Fey, J. Windsor, & S. F. Warren (Eds.), *Language intervention: Preschool through the elementary years* (pp. 85–105). Baltimore: Paul H. Brookes.

McTear, M. F., & Conti-Ramsden, G. (1992). *Pragmatic disability in children.* San Diego: Singular.

Mehan, H., Hertweck, A., & Meihls, J. L. (1986). *Handicapping the handicapped: Decision making in students' educational careers.* Stanford, CA: Stanford University Press.

Meitus, I. J., & Weinberg, B. (Eds.) (1983). *Diagnosis of speech and language disorders.* Baltimore: University Park Press.

Mentis, M. (1994). Topic management in discourse: Assessment and intervention. *Topics in Language Disorders,* 14 (3), 29–54.

Mentis, M., Briggs-Whittaker, J., & Gramigna, G. D. (1995). Discourse topic management in senile dementia of the Alzheimer's type. *Journal of Speech and Hearing Research,* 38, 1054–1066.

Merritt, D. D., & Liles, B. Z. (1987). Story grammar ability in children with and without language dis-

order: Story generation, story retelling, and story comprehension. *Journal of Speech and Hearing Research,* 30, 539–552.

Merritt, D. D., & Liles, B. Z. (1989). Narrative analysis: Clinical applications of story generation and story retelling. *Journal of Speech and Hearing Disorders,* 54, 438–447.

Miller, J. (1981). *Assessing language production in children: Experimental procedures.* Austin, TX: Pro-Ed.

Miller, J. F., & Paul, R. (1995). *The clinical assessment of language comprehension.* Baltimore: Paul H. Brookes.

Milosky, L. M. (1987). Narratives in the classroom. *Seminars in Speech and Language,* 8, 329–343.

Milosky, L. M. (1994). Nonliteral language abilities: Seeing the forest for the trees. In G. P. Wallach & K. G. Butler (Eds.), *Language learning disabilities in school-age children and adolescents: Some principles and applications* (pp. 275–303). Boston: Allyn & Bacon.

Miranda, E., McCabe, A., & Bliss, L. S. (1994). Jumping around and leaving things out: Assessing impaired narration. Miniseminar presented at the Annual Convention of the American Speech-Language-Hearing Association, New Orleans, LA.

Montague, M., Maddux, C. D., & Dereshiwsky, M. I. (1990). Story grammar and comprehension and production of narrative prose by students with learning disabilities. *Journal of Learning Disabilities,* 23, 190–197.

Morine-Dershimer, G. (1985). *Talking, listening, and learning in elementary classrooms.* New York: Longman.

Morrow, L. M. (1993). *Literacy development in the early years: Helping children read and write* (2nd ed.). Boston: Allyn & Bacon.

Morrow, L. M., & J. K. Smith (1990). Introduction. In L. M. Morrow & J. K. Smith (Eds.), *Assessment for instruction in early literacy* (pp. 1–6). Englewood Cliffs, NJ: Prentice-Hall.

Naremore, R. C., Desnmore, A. E., & Harman, D. R. (1995). *Language intervention with school-aged children: Conversation, narrative, and text.* San Diego: Singular.

Nation, J. E., & Aram, D. M. (1991). *Diagnosis of speech and language disorders (second edition).* San Diego: Singular.

Nelson, N. W. (1993). *Childhood language disorders in context: Infancy through adolescence.* New York: Merrill-Macmillan.

Nelson, N. W. (1994). Curriculum-based language assessment and intervention across the grades. In G. P. Wallach & K. G. Butler (Eds.), *Language learning disabilities in school-age children and adolescents: Some principles and applications* (pp. 104–131). Boston: Allyn & Bacon.

Nippold, M. A. (1988a). The literate lexicon. In M. Nippold (Ed.), *Later language development: Ages nine through nineteen* (pp. 29–47). Boston: College-Hill.

Nippold, M. A. (1988b). Linguistic ambiguity. In M. Nippold (Ed.), *Later language development: Ages nine through nineteen* (pp. 211–223). Boston: College-Hill.

Nippold, M. A. (1992). The nature of normal and disordered word finding in children and adolescents. *Topics in Language Disorders, 13* (1), 1–14.

Nippold, M. A. (1993). Developmental markers in adolescent language: Syntax, semantics, and pragmatics. *Language, Speech, and Hearing Services in Schools, 24,* 21–28.

Nippold, M. A. (1995). School-age children and adolescents: Norms for word definitions. *Language, Speech, and Hearing Services in Schools, 26,* 320–325.

Nippold, M. A., & Fey, S. H. (1983). Metaphoric understanding in preadolescents having a history of language acquisition difficulties. *Language, Speech, and Hearing Services in Schools, 14,* 171–180.

Nippold, M. A., & Taylor, C. L. (1995). Idiom understanding in youth: Further examination of familarity and transparency. *Journal of Speech and Hearing Research, 38,* 426–433.

Owens, R. E., Jr. (1996). *Language development: An introduction* (fourth edition). Boston: Allyn & Bacon.

Palincsar, A. S., Brown, A. L., & Campione, J. C. (1993). First grade dialogue for knowledge acquisition and use. In E. A. Forman, N. Minick, & C. A. Stone (Eds.), *Contexts for learning: Sociocultural dynamics in children's development* (pp. 43–57). New York: Oxford.

Palincsar, A. S., Parecki, A. D., & McPhail, J. C. (1995). Friendship and literacy through literature. *Journal of Learning Disabilities, 28,* 503–510, 522.

Parnell, M. M. (1995). Characteristics of language disordered children. In H. Winitz (Ed.), *Human communication and its disorders: A review* (Vol. 4, pp. 171–275). Timonium, MD: York Press.

Paul, R. (1995). *Language disorders from infancy through adolescence.* St. Louis: Mosby.

Paul, R., & Smith, R. L. (1993). Narrative skills in 4-year-olds with normal, impaired, and late-developing language. *Journal of Speech and Hearing Research, 36,* 592–598.

Peterson, H. A., & Marquardt, T. P. (1994). *Appraisal and diagnosis of speech and language disorders* (3rd ed.). Englewood Cliffs, NJ: Prentice-Hall.

Plante, E., & Vance, R. (1995). Diagnostic accuracy of two tests of preschool language. *American Journal of Speech-Language Pathology, 4,* 70–76.

Pressley, M., Brown, R., El-Dinary, P. B., & Afflerbach, P. (1995). The comprehensive instruction that students need: Instruction fostering constructively responsive reading. *Learning Disabilities Research and Practice, 10,* 215–224.

Pressley, M., & McCormick, C. B. (1995). *Cognition, teaching, and assessment.* New York: HarperCollins.

Rees, N. S., & Gerber, S. (1992). Ethnography and communication: Social role relations. *Topics in Language Disorders, 12* (3), 15–27.

Reid, D. K., & Button, L. J. (1995). Anna's story: Narratives of personal experience about being labeled as learning disabled. *Journal of Learning Disabilities, 28,* 602–614.

Ricciardelli, L. A. (1993). Two components of metalinguistic awareness: Control of linguistic processing and analysis of linguistic knowledge. *Applied Psycholinguistics, 14,* 349–367.

Rice, M. L. (1994). Grammatical categories of children with specific language impairments. In R. V. Watkins & M. L. Rice (Eds.), *Specific language impairments in children* (pp. 69–89). Baltimore: Paul H. Brookes.

Rogoff, B. (1995). Observing sociocultural activity on three planes: participatory appropriation, guided participation, and apprenticeship. In J. V. Wertsch, P. Del Rio, & A. Alvarez (Eds.), *Sociocultural studies of mind* (pp. 139–164). New York: Cambridge University Press.

Romaine, S. (1984). *The language of children and adolescents.* New York: Basil Blackwell.

Roth, F. P. (1986). Oral narrative abilities of learning-disabled students. *Topics in Language Disorders, 7* (1), 21–30.

Roth, F. P., & Spekman, N.J. (1986). Narrative discourse: Spontaneously generated stories of learning disabled and normally achieving students. *Journal of Speech and Hearing Disorders, 51,* 8–23.

Salvia, J., & Yesseldyke, J. E. (1991). *Assessment* (5th ed.). Boston: Houghton Mifflin.

Sawyer, D. (1987). *Test of awareness of language segments.* Austin, TX: Pro-Ed.

Scott, C. M. (1988a). Producing complex sentences. *Topics in Language Disorders,* 8 (2), 42–62.

Scott, C. M. (1988b). Spoken and written syntax. In M. Nippold (Ed.), *Later language development: Ages nine through nineteen* (pp. 49–95). Boston: College-Hill.

Scott, C. M. (1988c). A perspective on the evaluation of school children's narratives. *Language, Speech, and Hearing Services in Schools,* 19, 67–82.

Scott, C. M. (1989). Problem writers: Nature, assessment, and intervention. In A. G. Kamhi & H. W. Catts (Eds.), *Reading disabilities: A developmental language perspective* (pp. 303–344). Boston: College-Hill.

Scott, C. M. (1994). A discourse continuum for school-age students: Impact of modality and genre. In G. P. Wallach & K. G. Butler (Eds.), *Language learning disabilities in school-age children and adolescents: Some principles and applications* (pp. 219–252). Boston: Allyn & Bacon.

Scott, C. M. (1995). Syntax for school-age children: A discourse perspective. In M. E. Fey, J. Windsor, & S. F. Warren (Eds.), *Language intervention: Preschool through the elementary years* (pp. 107–143). Baltimore: Paul H. Brookes.

Scott, C. M., & Stokes, S. L. (1995). Measures of syntax in school-age children and adolescents. *Language, Speech, and Hearing Services in Schools,* 26, 309–319.

Semel, E., Wiig, E. H., & Secord, W. A. (1995). *Clinical evaluation of language fundamentals* (3rd ed.). San Antonio, TX: The Psychological Corporation.

Shulman, B. B., Katz, K. B., & Sherman, T. (1995). Language and assessment: Current issues and anticipated trends. *Diagnostique,* 20 (1–4), 53–69.

Seidenberg, P., & Bernstein, D. (1986). The comprehension of similes and metaphors by learning-disabled and non-learning disabled children. *Language, Speech, and Hearing Services in Schools,* 17, 219–229.

Siegel, G., & Broen, P. (1976). Language assessment. In L. Lloyd (Ed.), *Communication, assessment and intervention strategies* (pp. 74–122). Baltimore: University Park Press.

Silliman, E. R. (1989). Narratives: A window on the oral substrate of written language disabilities. *Annals of Dyslexia,* 39, 125–139.

Silliman, E. R., & Wallach, G. P. (1991, November). *The communication process model for language learning disability children: Making it work.* Short course presented at the American Speech-Language-Hearing Association Convention, Atlanta, GA.

Silliman, E. R., & Wilkinson, L. C. (1991). *Communicating for learning: Classroom observation and collaboration.* Gaitherburg, MD: Aspen.

Silliman, E. R., & Wilkinson, L. C. (1994a). Discourse scaffolds for classroom intervention. In G. P. Wallach & K. G. Butler (Eds.), *Language learning disabilities in school-age children and adolescents: Some principles and applications* (pp. 27–52). Boston: Allyn & Bacon.

Silliman, E. R., & Wilkinson, L. C. (1994b). Observation is more than looking. In G. P. Wallach & K. G. Butler (Eds.), *Language learning disabilities in school-age children and adolescents: Some principles and applications* (pp. 145–173). Boston: Allyn & Bacon.

Silliman, E. R., Wilkinson, L. C., & Hoffman, L. C. (1994). Progress in language and literacy learning: Ongoing assessment in the classroom. In K. G. Butler (Ed.), *Best practices I: The classroom as an assessment arena* (pp. 101–124). Gaithersburg, MD: Aspen.

Silliman, E. R., Wilkinson, L. C., & Hoffman, L. P. (in press). *Children's journeys through school: Assessing and building competence in language and literacy learning.* San Diego: Singular.

Sleight, C. C., & Prinz, P. M. (1985). Use of abstracts, orientations, and codas in narration by language-disordered and non-disordered children. *Journal of Speech and Hearing Disorders,* 50, 361–371.

Snow, C. E. (1994). What is so hard about learning to read?: A pragmatic analysis. In J. F. Duchan, L. E. Hewitt, & R. M. Sonnenmeir (Eds.), *Pragmatics: From theory to practice* (pp. 164–184). Englewood Cliffs, NJ: Prentice-Hall.

Snyder, L., & Downey, D. M. (1991). The language reading relationship in normal and reading disabled children. *Journal of Speech and Hearing Research,* 34, 129–140.

Snyder, L. S., & Godley, D. (1992). Assessment of word finding in children and adolescents. *Topics in Language Disorders,* 13, (1), 15–32.

Society for Visual Education (1989). *Max in motion: Developing language skills* and *Adventuresome Max: Discovering the world* [videotapes]. Chicago: SVE Videoplus.

Spear-Swerling, L., & Sternberg, R. J. (1994). The road not taken: An integrative theoretical model of reading disability. *Journal of Learning Disabilities,* 27, 91–103, 122.

Stallman, A. C., & Pearson, P. D. (1990). Formal measures of early literacy. In L. M. Morrow & J. K. Smith (Eds.), *Assessment for instruction in early literacy* (pp. 7–44). Englewood Cliffs, NJ: Prentice-Hall.

Stein, N. L. (1983). On the goals, functions, and knowledge of reading and writing. *Contemporary Educational Psychology,* 8, 261–292.

Stein, N. L., & Glenn, C. G. (1979). An analysis of story comprehension in elementary school children. In R. O. Freedle (Ed.), *New directions in discourse processing* (pp. 53–120). Norwood, NJ: Ablex.

Sternberg, R. J. (1987). A unified theory of intellectual exceptionality. In J. D. Day & J. G. Borkowski (Eds.), *Intelligence and exceptionality: New directins for theory, assessment, and instructional practices* (pp. 135–172). Norwood, NJ: Ablex.

Strong, C. J., & North, K. H. (1996). *The magic of stories: Literature-based language intervention.* Eau Claire, WI: Thinking Publications.

Strong, C. J., & Shaver, J. P. (1991). Stability of cohesion in the spoken narratives of language impaired and normally developing school-aged children. *Journal of Speech and Hearing Research,* 34, 95–111.

Swank, L. K., & Catts, H. W. (1994). Phonological awareness and written word decoding. *Language, Speech, & Hearing Services in Schools,* 25, 9–14.

Terrell, B. Y. (1994). Emergent literacy: In the beginning there was reading and writing. In D. N. Ripich & N. A. Creaghead (Eds.), *School discourse problems* (2nd ed.) (pp. 9–28). San Diego: Singular.

Terrell, S. L., & Terrell, F. (1993). African-American cultures. In D. E. Battle (Ed.), *Communication dis-*orders in multicultural populations (pp. 3–37). Boston: Andover Medical Publishers.

Tomblin, J. B. (1989). Familial concentration of developmental language impairment. *Journal of Speech and Hearing Disorders,* 54, 287–295.

Treiman, R. (1993). *Beginning to spell.* New York: Oxford University Press.

Tyack, D. L., & Gottsleben, R. H. (1986). Acquisition of complex sentences. *Language, Speech, and Hearing Services in Schools,* 17, 160–174.

van Dijk, T. A. (1987). Episodic models in discourse processing. In R. Horowitz & S. J. Samuels (Eds.), *Comprehending oral and written language* (pp. 161–196). San Diego: Academic Press.

van Kleeck, A. (1990). Emergent literacy: Learning about print before learning to read. *Topics in Language Disorders,* 10 (2), 25–45.

van Kleeck, A. (1994). Metalinguistic development. In G. P. Wallach & K. G. Butler (Eds.), *Language learning disabilities in school-age children and adolescents: Some principles and applications* (pp. 53–98). Boston: Allyn & Bacon.

van Kleeck, A. (1995). Emphasizing form and meaning separately in prereading and early reading instruction. *Topics in Language Disorders,* 16 (1), 27–49.

van Kleeck, A., & Schuele, C. M. (1987). Precursors to literacy: Normal development. *Topics in Language Disorders,* 7 (2), 13–31.

Vellutino, F. R., Scanlon, D. M., & Tanzman, M. S. (1994). Components of reading ability: Issues and problems in operationalizing word identification, phonological coding, and orthographic coding. In G. R. Lyon (Ed.), *Frames of reference for the assessment of learning disabilities* (pp. 279–332). Baltimore: Paul H. Brookes.

Vigil, A., & van Kleeck, A. (1996). Clinical language teaching: Theories and principles to guide our responses when children miss our language targets. In M. D. Smith & J. S. Damico (Eds.), *Childhood language disorders* (pp. 64–96). New York: Thieme.

Wallach, G. (1990). Magic buries Celtics: Looking for broader interpretations of language learning and literacy. *Topics in Language* Disorders, 10 (2), 63–80.

Wallach, G. P., & Butler, K. G. (1994). Creating communication, literacy, and academic success. In G. P. Wallach & K. G. Butler (Eds.), *Language learning disabilities in school-age children and adolescents: Some principles and applications* (pp. 2–26). Boston: Allyn & Bacon.

Wallis, V. (1993). *Two old women: An Alaskan legend of betrayal, courage, and survival.* New York: HarperCollins.

Watkins, R. V., Kelly, D. J., Harbers, H. M., & Hollis, W. (1995). Measuring children's lexical diversity: Differentiating typical and impaired language learners. *Journal of Speech and Hearing Research,* 38, 1349–1355.

Weaver, C. (in press). Understanding and helping Jaime with reading and with language: A psycholinguistic and constructivist perspective. In E. R. Silliman, L. C. Wilkinson, & L. P. Hoffman (Eds.), *Children's journeys through school: Assessing and building competence in language and literacy learning.* San Diego: Singular.

Wells, G. (1985). *Language development in the preschool years.* New York: Cambridge University Press.

Westby, C. E. (1984). Development of narrative language abilities. In G. P. Wallach & K. G. Butler (Eds.), *Language learning disabilities in school-age children* (pp. 103–127). Baltimore: Williams & Wilkins.

Westby, C. E. (1985). Learning to talk—talking to learn: Oral-literate language differences. In C. S. Simon (Ed.), *Communication skills and classroom success: Therapy methodologies for language-learning disabled students* (pp. 181–213). San Diego: College-Hill Press.

Westby, C. E. (1989). Assessing and remediating text comprehension problems. In A. G. Kamhi & H. W. Catts (Eds.), *Reading disabilities: A developmental language perspective* (pp. 199–259). Boston: College-Hill.

Westby, C. (1990). Ethnographic interviewing: Asking the right questions to the right people in the right ways. *Journal of Childhood Communication Disorders,* 13, 101–111.

Westby, C. E. (1994). The effects of culture on genre, structure, and style of oral and written texts. In G. P. Wallach & K. G. Butler (Eds.), *Language learning disabilities in school-age children and adolescents: Some principles and applications* (pp. 180–218). Boston: Allyn & Bacon.

Westby, C. (1995). Culture and literacy: Frameworks for understanding. *Topics in Language Disorders,* 16 (1), 50–66.

Westby, C. (in press). Working in the zone of proximal development. In E. R. Silliman, L. C. Wilkinson, & L. P. Hoffman (Eds.), *Children's journeys through school: Assessing and builing competence in language and literacy learning.* San Diego: Singular.

Westby, C. E., & Rouse, G. R. (1993). Facilitating text comprehension in college students: The professor's role. In L. Clark (Ed.), *Faculty and student challenges in facing cultural-linguistic diversity.* Springfield, IL: Thomas.

Westby, C. E., Van Dongen, R., & Maggert, Z. (1989). Assessing narative competence. *Seminars in Speech and Language,* 10, 63–76.

Wiig, E. H., Jones, S. S., & Wiig, E. D. (1996). Computer-based assessment of word knowledge in teens with learning disabilities. *Language, Speech, & Hearing Services in Schools,* 27, 21–28.

Wiig, E. H., & Secord, W. A. (1989). *Test of Language Competence—Expanded.* San Antonio, TX: Psychological Corporation.

Wiig, E. H., & Secord, W. (1990). *Test of word knowledge.* San Antonio, TX: Psychological Corporation.

Wiig, E. H., & Secord, W. A. (1991). *Measurement and assessment: Making sense of test results.* Lockport, NY: Educom.

Wilkinson, L. C., & Silliman, E. R. (1994). Assessing students' progress in language and literacy learning: A classroom approach. In L. M. Morrow, J. K. Smith, & L. C. Wilkinson (Eds.), *Integrated language arts: Controversy to consensus* (pp. 241–269). Needham Heights, MA: Allyn & Bacon.

Wilkinson, L. C., Silliman, E. R., Nitzberg, L. A., & Aurilio, M. (1993). Narrative analysis: Filtering individual differences in competence. *Linguistics and Education,* 5, 195–210.

Windsor, J. (1994). Children's comprehension and production of derivational suffixes. *Journal of Speech and Hearing Research,* 37, 408–417.

Wolf, M., & Segal, D. (1992). Word finding and reading in the developmental dyslexias. *Topics in Language Disorders,* 13 (1), 51–65.

Yopp, H. K., & Yopp, R. H. (1996). *Literature-based reading activities (second edition).* Boston: Allyn & Bacon.

Chapter 8

Planning Language Intervention for Young Children

AMY L. WEISS
University of Iowa

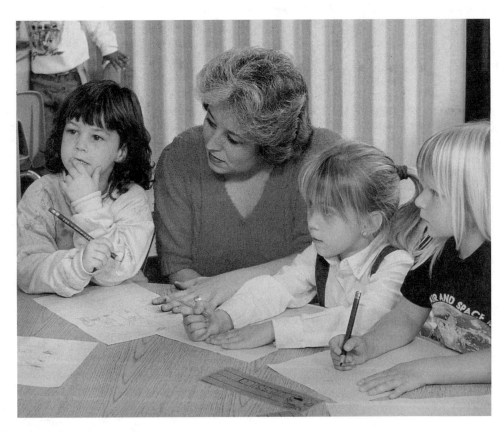

In this chapter, readers will be challenged to think about language intervention planning and implementation as dynamic processes that are driven by a young client's changing abilities and needs, the clinical skills and experience of the speech-language clinician and those of additional support personnel, as well as the less easily measured environmental factors that impinge on language development and use, such as caregiver input and the child's opportunities for social interaction with peers. In addition, the alternatives for intervention context will be explored, including suggestions for choosing among those alternatives. A case will also be made for the importance of thorough generalization planning when we first design our treatment protocols; the reader will be introduced to several methods useful for increasing the likelihood that generalization will occur as a result of the language intervention provided. The following questions will be addressed in this chapter:

1. How do speech-language clinicians develop language intervention programs for young children?
2. How have changes in legislation mandating provision of services for young children with disabilities affected the role and responsibilities of the speech-language clinician?
3. How can speech-language clinicians facilitate generalization of language goals from therapeutic contexts to nontreatment settings?

What Is Language Intervention?

The Demographics of Early Language Disorder

According to research findings compiled by the American Speech-Language-Hearing Association (1995), language disorders are found in approximately 2 to 3 percent of the preschool population and 1 percent of the school-age population. Estimates of the occurrence of Specific Language Impairment (SLI), where other systems (e.g., cognitive, socioemotional, and physical), appear to be intact and functioning within normal limits, average around 5 percent of the preschool population. These percentages translated to approximately 490,000 students in the 0-to-5-year range who were diagnosed with disabilities and who received special education services for the 1991–92 school year. Additional studies that have examined the development of speech and language in late talkers have reported that the majority of these children, identified prior to their second birthdays and who remained delayed in language development when 4 years of age, carried with them a very high risk for a learning disability. This latter finding is particularly important to consider because it supports the need for aggressive and comprehensive programs for early identification and intervention.

In addition to facing the challenges posed by the numbers of service recipients as intimated above, speech-language pathologists have been made increasingly aware over the last decade of the changing make-up of the national caseload in terms of cultural diversity (Cole, 1989). Specifically, Cole (1989) noted that as professionals we need to be aware that a set of multicultural issues or challenges face the profession, among them: (1) the fact that in the coming years there will be more individuals representing minorities on caseloads; (2) more minority children are born at-risk for communication disorders; (3) that the non–European American presents with different etiologies and prevalences for disorders; (4) there is less normative data available for nonmajority populations; (5) there will be different perspectives on the concepts of health and disorder to be addressed; (6) there is greater opportunity for conflicts in the intervention context based on cultural differences; (7) there are differences in service delivery preference from the mainstream; and (8) there is a greater incidence of linguistic differences within nonmajority populations. These facts represent challenges because as of 1993 the vast majority (94 percent) of the speech-language clinicians who were members of the American Speech-Language-Hearing Association described themselves as members of the majority culture (Screen & Anderson, 1994) and monolingual. As will be discussed later in this chapter, the issue of cultural differences is a critical one in developing appropriate intervention programming.

The difficulties of providing appropriate service delivery are truly national in scope. Roseberry-McKibben & Eicholtz (1994) reported findings from their national survey investigating how children who were Limited English Proficient (LEP) are served in the schools. They found that although treatment focusing on language was what was most often provided by the more than 1100 speech-language clinicians who replied to the survey, more than 90 percent of them did not speak the language (most often Spanish) spoken by their clients well enough to provide treatment in that language. In addition, the authors noted that more than three quarters of their respondents indicated that they had not completed any course work designed to prepare them for working with children who were LEP. Clearly, our profession needs to continue to emphasize ways of infusing multicultural information into the curricula of our graduate programs and continuing education opportunities.

Why Language Intervention Is Needed

We know that the vast majority of speech-language pathologists—89.3 percent of them according to the 1988 Omnibus Survey conducted by the American Speech-Language-Hearing Association (Shewan, 1988)—serve children with language disorders on their caseloads. This percentage is formidable but should not be too surprising given research findings that suggest that disorders of language first identified in childhood often continue to be a part of the social and communicative life of the individual and are not easily outgrown (Aram, Ekelman, & Nation, 1984; Hall & Tomblin, 1978; King, Jones, & Lasky, 1982). So language disorders in children not only exist, but they have the potential to be a problem of long standing for the children themselves, their families, school personnel, clinicians charged with the responsibility of teaching them, and perhaps society as a whole.

Moreover, because the needs for competent language use are pervasive in our daily lives, if a person's language abilities are just functional, that person will likely lead a life that is compromised in some respect. Consider the role played by language in establishing and maintaining relationships between friends, colleagues, and loved ones, or in functioning as a productive member of a society through one's career, civic, and social activities. It is because language is such an integral part of our lives that the development of techniques to augment the language learning abilities of young children who exhibit language disorders is a very important charge to the language interventionist.

A Definition of Language Intervention and Interventionists

What is language intervention and who provides these services? The field of speech-language pathology has periodically engaged in debate over the appropriateness of its name and the name of those who provide its services. Are we speech-language pathologists, or clinicians, or therapists, or teachers, or correctionists? At one time or another in our history one of these terms has been in vogue (Miller, 1989).

There have been at least two recent changes in how we perceive our roles and enact them. With the advent of collaborative consultation models, the responsibility for language facilitation is often shared with classroom teachers. We will discuss that in more depth later in this chapter. Further, transdisciplinary teaming models, where multiple professionals are involved in the planning and provision of treatment programs, the concept of "role release" allows for team members to transcend their disciplinary training where necessary to provide clients with comprehensive service delivery. For example, the speech-language pathologist working to facilitate accurate articulatory productions in a child with cerebral palsy may work to reduce the child's hypertonicity prior to speech activities, a goal usually reserved for the physical therapist. In both situations the roles and responsibilities of the speech-language pathologist have shifted to meet the demands posed by changes in service delivery models.

The term **intervention,** as applied to the field of speech-language pathology, has also met with less than universal acceptance as a descriptor of one of the services we provide to our clients. As noted by Schiefelbusch (1983), the term intervention has been used to describe what it is we do to bring about changes in the behavior of our clients. He says that language intervention "denotes an act of assistance" (p. 15). When language intervention for young children is considered, that assistance takes the form of helping "the child to develop the social/communicative competence for achieving both immediate and long-term purposes" (p. 15).

For the purposes of this chapter, language intervention is defined as the use of instructional contexts designed to facilitate language learning. Depending on the needs and abilities of the client and his or her family, programs of language intervention will differ in terms of who is involved in the intervention, where the intervention takes place, and the degree of structure imposed on the client within the instructional context.

It is important for beginning clinicians to recognize that the goal of language intervention, or any type of intervention, is to make itself obsolete. That is, the objective of any language intervention program is to eliminate its rationale for existence by demonstrating that the client is ready for dismissal. This can be done in at least two ways. One is to help the client become his or her own clinician through the development of accurate self-monitoring skills. The client must therefore learn strategies to facilitate new learning. Once the client demonstrates correct discrimination between acceptable and unacceptable language productions (or effective and ineffective communication), one of the essential competencies necessary for achieving generalization to new, untrained contexts has been acquired. Once self-monitoring is established, the client can extend learning without the clinician's input.

Another approach to planned obsolescence involves demonstrating that the client has the language competencies typically observed in normally developing individuals similar to the client in age, education, and culture. Here, techniques for future learning do not appear to be as important as being able to show that the client is presently a successful communicator in all settings in which language is used. Unfortunately, we still know far too little about what constitutes appropriate dismissal criteria in speech-language intervention (Fey, 1988; Olswang & Bain, 1985). Appropriate dismissal criteria are those that indicate that treatment services can be removed without an appreciable loss of the gains made by the client through therapy and that additional intervention services are not likely to be needed in the future.

This chapter serves as an introduction to some of what we *do* know about language intervention with young children and the thinking that takes place when a speech-language clinician formulates a plan for a young child with a language disorder.

The Role of Speech-Language Clinicians in Early Language Intervention

The Efficacy of Early Language Intervention

It is generally agreed that where identification of communication and language disorders is concerned, earlier is better, whether the etiology of the problem is genetic or due to environmental agents (Warren & Kaiser, 1988). Bricker (1986) noted that it is generally accepted that what the child learns early on is needed to support the more sophisticated learning that will follow and that early intervention allows the opportunity for clinicians to set up "proper support systems for families and children to inhibit the development of secondary or associated disabilities" (p. 30). Because speech-language disorders have been shown to have both a pervasive a cumulative effect on children's growth and development, waiting to begin intervention may mean that the problem will be significantly greater by the time a program is instituted. Although delays in getting started are sometimes unavoidable, the child stands to lose valuable time in the language-learning process.

Support for the efficacy of early intervention also comes from research studies demonstrating that development during the prelinguistic period is crucial to the acquisition of linguistic competence (Leonard, 1991). In addition, advanced research technologies have allowed investigators to determine that infants know much more about the world around them by the end of the first year of life than had been previously suspected (Mandler, 1990). Thus, delays in beginning intervention have the potential effect of putting the young child with a language disorder even further behind than had been previously thought.

Legislative Mandates for Service Delivery

Additional support for early intervention is reflected in the passage and implementation of legislation mandating educational services for young children with disabilities. One such important legislative action, the Education of the Handicapped Act Amendments of 1986 (Public Law 99-457), focuses on making special services available to children from birth through 5 years of age. It serves as an addendum to PL 94-142, passed in 1975 and generally known as the Education for All Handicapped Children Act. More recently, PL 101-576 (1990) or Individuals with Disabilities Education Act (IDEA) was passed and its function was to reauthorize PL 94-142 and update it by including two additional categories for service delivery: traumatic brain injury and autism.

One innovative feature of PL 99-457 was its focus on the role that the family plays in the service delivery system for very young children. The law calls for an Individualized Family Service Plan (IFSP) to be developed by the speech-language clinician with input from the child's parents. Parents are also called on to help prioritize the child's goals (Lowenthal, 1987). Some language intervention programs for this young population are centered around teaching parents how to interact communicatively with their at-risk or disordered infants and toddlers so that they can capitalize on the infants' capabilities (Klein & Briggs, 1987; MacDonald & Carroll, 1992a; Sparks, 1989). Although to carry out this type of program the speech-language clinician must carefully evaluate the infant or toddler, the focus of direct training will often primarily be on the parents, who will be trained to become the therapeutic agents. In classroom programs for preschool-aged children with disabilities, it is also not unusual to find support groups or ancillary programs designed to teach families how best to work with their children to carry over classroom learning into the home environment.

A Continuum of Language Difficulties

Another reason for the burgeoning interest in early language intervention probably came from the recognition that individuals identified in the preschool years as having language disorders are often the same students diagnosed as language learning disabled later on in their academic careers (Aram et al., 1984; King et al., 1982). The problem may persist despite the fact that language intervention is provided to many of these children. The findings from follow-up studies of young children who were identified as speech-language disordered consistently demonstrated that the majority of these children were still showing signs of language disorders or additional problems with learning many years after their initial diagnoses. As noted by Maxwell and Wallach (1984), "one myth, that the majority of children 'outgrow' their early language disabilities, is dispelled by this research" (p. 20). Recent studies of very young children identified as language delayed (Rescorla & Schwartz, 1990; Scarborough & Dobrich, 1990) have indicated that catching up to their peers may take longer than once expected.

If language-learning difficulties are resistant to change in the long term, how are the lives of our clients affected? Records, Tomblin, and Freese (1992) studied the quality of life experienced by young adults with life-long language-learning disorders. Interestingly, these investigators found that when asked about their perceptions of their own life quality, including issues of personal happiness, satisfaction with their lives, and perceived status with regard to education, their occupations and their families, the subjects' responses were not significantly different from those of a matched control group of young adults with no history of language-learning disorders. However, when these two groups of subjects were compared objectively according to income levels and educational achievement, they were clearly different, with the language disordered group having achieved to a significantly lesser degree. The authors noted that this result led them to conclude that "language impairment seems to be associated with the objective aspects of life, but not with the subjective aspects" (p. 49).

One of the reasons for the long-term effects of language-learning difficulties undoubtedly is related to the connection between a child's oral language competencies and acquisition of literacy skills. The connections between the two systems are complicated and are not the same all the way through the developmental process (Wallach & Butler, 1994) so that at times spoken language exerts an influence on literacy learning and at other points in the process, the development of literacy competencies influences production of spoken text. An example of this would be the situation where a young child, having become familiarized with literate storytelling style through book reading at school, begins to generalize it to accounts of school activities when she is at home. Even when assembling language intervention programs for young children, which are usually focused on expressive oral language production, we should probably keep in mind that we should be setting the stage for literacy learning. Snyder (1980) put some of the blame for the longevity of language disorders on the type of intervention services provided. She suggested that the language intervention provided to school-age children diagnosed as language disordered had little effect on making the children sufficiently "mobilized for reading" (p. 40). Specifically, she noted that the ability to make syntactic predictions and inferences were two skills necessary to reading success and that these were not usually addressed in language intervention programs for young children. The author acknowledged that some of the more specific competencies needed to learn reading and writing have been neglected by speech-language clinicians who work with preschoolers. More recently, Fey, Catts, and Larrivee (1995) discussed the academic and social demands placed on children in school and suggested ways to prepare preschool-aged children with language impairments for meeting those demands.

Determining the "Wheres" and "Hows" of Language Intervention

As already noted, attitudes and "fashion" with regard to what speech-language clinicians call themselves and the clinical services they perform have changed over time (Miller, 1989). Similarly, the settings where speech-language clinicians most commonly perform language intervention have changed. In fact, the change in typical settings for clinical service has been dramatic over the past several years. This should not be surprising given that the changes are in keeping with a more general shift in the perception of the role of the speech-language clinician as well as increases in the demand for services. Table 8-1 presents the benefits and drawbacks inherent in three different language intervention settings: (a) the pull-out model, (b) the classroom model, and (c) the collaborative-consultation model. Professionals in the field of speech-language pathology have attempted to address weaknesses in each of the models by developing new models or revising present models, as shown in Figure 8-1.

The Pull-Out Model.   Traditionally, speech-language clinicians engaged in the "pull-out" model of service delivery for children attending school programs. With classroom programs for preschoolers with disabilities becoming more commonplace, it is likely that this approach has also been used with very young children. In the pull-out model, students are removed from their classrooms to work with a clinician either individually or in groups, usually consisting of other children who exhibit similar problems. Pull-out therapy was typ-

TABLE 8-1   Benefits and Drawbacks of Service Delivery Models

Model	Benefits	Drawbacks
Pull-Out	Child less distracted by classroom activities Child given opportunities to learn/practice in a less threatening, less competitive atmosphere	Setting for language learning is decontextualized May be stigmatizing to child to be withdrawn from class Child misses important class time
Classroom	Clinician experiences child's language difficulties as they happen "Where the action is"	May be distracting to other students or the teacher May be stigmatizing to the child to be observed receiving special assistance
Consultation (general)	Intervention strategies taught to the teacher by the clinician Teacher is primary intervention agent	Teacher may perceive clinician as language expert to deliver intervention services Teacher may perceive self as too busy
Collaborative Consultation	Teacher and clinician share mutual respect and mutual responsibility for the child's program	[same as above]

ically performed in small rooms or areas away from the child's classmates. The rationale for this model probably stemmed from the belief that separating the child from the rest of the class would provide a quiet location where the specific goals of therapy could be addressed. There should be less opportunity for the child to become distracted, and the therapy would not disrupt the classroom program of classmates who did not have language disorders.

One potential "down" side to this approach is that it singles out a child for having a problem and possibly stigmatizes him as being different from the classmates who stay behind (Brush, 1987). Furthermore, the child is removed from the very setting in which he is likely to use the language features being taught. Through the pull-out model, language is taught without context or at least taught in a rather contrived, unrealistic context. One very important facet for ensuring generalization—context validity—is eliminated. It should also be noted that for the child receiving therapy in a community clinic or private practice, language intervention can also resemble the decontextualized setting of the pull-out model. Unless steps are taken by the clinician to help the young child recognize that the clinical

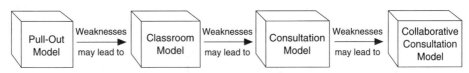

FIGURE 8-1   **Relationships among models of language intervention service delivery.**

setting and other frequently experienced settings (e.g., home, school) have some communicative similarities, there is no reason to expect the child to apply the structures and strategies learned in therapy outside of the clinic.

The move away from the pull-out model has been accelerated by legislation mandating that children with disabilities receive appropriate services in the least restrictive environment possible. Sequestering a child from his or her classmates for language intervention represents a very restrictive environment, only justified if shown to be essential for the success of an individual child's treatment.

Intervention in the Classroom.   An appreciation for the social foundations of language development and the need for context support in learning has led to attempts to remedy the problems posed by the pull-out model. One solution has been to provide speech-language intervention in the classroom itself. Whether a preschool, a kindergarten, or a grade school classroom, it is the classroom context where language problems, if they exist, are likely to manifest themselves. The classroom is also likely to offer more naturally occurring opportunities for conversational exchanges between teachers and students, and between students and their peers. The speech-language clinician who provides treatment in the classroom will have a better chance to observe problem situations as they unfold for the child and to provide on-line assistance or suggestions for remedying communication breakdowns.

One of the difficulties with a classroom-based approach is that the classroom routine could be affected by the presence of another adult who may be working at cross purposes with the classroom teacher. That is, the classroom teacher presents information for all of the children, whereas the speech-language clinician is usually presenting information that is relevant for just one or maybe a few students. The speech-language clinician's interaction with the child draws attention to itself and away from the classroom teacher when attention paid to the classroom teacher would be beneficial for completing class projects. Further, the child with a language disorder is still the recipient of extra assistance in the classroom, and the child or the child's classmates may see this difference in a negative light (Jenkins & Heinen, 1989). So, although working in the classroom eliminates some of the problems presented by the pull-out approach, it may create others for the clients being served.

Collaborative Consultation.   A third option is the collaborative consultation model for service delivery (Frasinelli, Superior, & Meyers, 1983). Actually, when we use the term *consultation,* we are referring to a family of possible models for interaction between the speech-language clinician and school personnel (Marvin, 1987). By serving as a consultant to a classroom, a speech-language clinician can eliminate some of the drawbacks to the pull-out and in-class models. In addition, both professionals end up learning more about the other's area of expertise; the classroom teacher should end up learning more about how communication can be facilitated, and the speech-language clinician learns more about the classroom curriculum and its demands (Prelock, Miller, & Reed, 1995). Assuming the role of language expert, the speech-language clinician provides the classroom teacher with techniques for addressing the language difficulties of the children in the class diagnosed with language disorders. Although the speech-language clinician may interact directly with a child, direct intervention may be limited to the evaluation phase of service delivery, and the classroom teacher serves as the language disordered child's "primary interventionist"

(Marvin, 1987, p. 5). Speech-language clinicians may spend more of their time observing the child in the classroom, studying the classroom curriculum, and giving suggestions for using the classroom as a language learning environment.

There is probably an endless variety of ways in which the collaborative consultation model can be implemented. Prelock et al. (1995) describe a Language in the Classroom (LIC) program involving collaborative partnerships between speech-language clinicians and classroom teachers. In this particular program collaborative efforts include assessment, "goal setting, planning, and implementation of intervention for students with communication disorders as well as for those students who are at risk for language and learning problems" (p. 286). In another approach to service delivery, Farber, Denenberg, Klyman, and Lachman (1992) describe what they call the Language Resource Room Level of Service, incorporating aspects of "the classroom, a team teaching model, itinerant support, and consultative services" (p. 293). Farber et al. (1992) suggest that with the speech-language clinician potentially assuming roles of co-teacher, consultant, or direct service provider depending on programming needs, a greater number of treatment options is possible (p. 293).

The collaborative consultation model is often promoted as an efficient way to use the speech-language clinician's time (Marvin, 1987). By using a classroom teacher as the intervention agent, the speech-language clinician typically spends less time in the classroom working directly with children. The classroom teacher can apply the language intervention techniques learned to more than just the targeted child, so that the clinician's suggestions may be useful for more than one child in the same classroom at the same time. This model may be more effective because the child's intervention is delivered within the classroom setting when the need for it arises and in the context where it makes the most sense.

Speech-language clinicians have reported that some classroom teachers are at least initially resistive to implementation of the collaborative consultation model. They may view the speech-language clinician as the language expert who is abdicating responsibility in favor of turning the work over to the classroom teacher, who is less comfortable with focusing on language facilitation. Classroom teachers may also believe that they are too busy with the needs of their other students to spend the time needed to accommodate classroom routines for several children who require specialized assistance with language learning. Further, they may not view themselves as competent service providers for children with special needs or not recognize the importance of language intervention delivered in the classroom context.

All of these potential concerns on the part of the classroom teacher are logical ones and should they be expressed, they need to be addressed carefully by the speech-language clinician who wants to work as a collaborative consultant. Collaborative consultation may be more easily implemented if the following perspectives are maintained. First, intervention planning should be carried out in an atmosphere of mutual respect and where the participants have a similar level of involvement in terms of the plan's implementation and success, although their responsibilities may differ considerably. It should be understood by the classroom teacher and speech-language clinician that their individual roles may shift during the course of a child's language intervention program. In other words, at some point the teacher may spend more time serving as the speech-language clinician's consultant—explaining classroom teaching techniques and routines—than the other way around. School-based speech-language clinicians sometimes report slow progress in implementing collaborative consultation models. So, if the classroom teacher can be shown to benefit by switching to this model, either because the child makes more progress or that implementation of classroom techniques is not too time consuming or too difficult, speech-language clinicians may meet with less resistance from other teachers in the school.

The Full Inclusion Model.   No discussion of collaborative consultation or provision of speech and language services in the classroom would be complete without an acknowledgment of the "bigger picture" of the regular education initiative (REI), more commonly referred to as *inclusion* or *full inclusion* (Wolery & Wilbers, 1994). Following federal legislation mandating the provision of appropriate education to all children in the "least restrictive environment" (PL 94-142, 1975; PL 99-457, 1986; PL 101-576, 1990), many state departments of education and individual school districts have interpreted these laws in ways that more or less conform to the notion of the REI, whereby special education and regular education are melded into one (Stainback & Stainback, 1990). By definition, supporters of full inclusion believe that the "least restrictive environment" is a mainstreamed classroom for all children regardless of level of ability. That is, promoters of the full inclusion standpoint, Stainback, Stainback, and Forest (1989) view the concept of "inclusion" as the logical outcome of the practice of providing children with the least restrictive educational environment; there should be no differentiated, segregated, special education classrooms. However, these authors believe that inclusion is more than just mainstreaming. They note that "an inclusive school is a place where everyone belongs, is accepted, supports, and is supported by his or her peers and other members of the school community in the course of having his or her educational needs met" (p. 3). Within an inclusive classroom model "the focus is on how to operate supportive classrooms and schools that include and meet the needs of everyone" (p. 4). This model is not to be construed as dismissing the important role of the special educator, however, and Stainback and Stainback (1990) maintain that "students cannot be successfully integrated without integrating personnel and resources" (p. 5). In order for the inclusion model to work, therefore, it is imperative that special educators and regular classroom teachers provide classroom instruction cooperatively and collaboratively, guided by the needs of the individual children in their classroom. This focus on service delivery obviously necessitates the development of exemplary teaming skills on the part of each of the participants in the teaming process. Further, there is a strong emphasis on the involvement of the family in all decision making and prioritizing of goals as is also mandated by law.

It is easy to understand the motivation for the full inclusion approach. Children with disabilities are believed to benefit because they are not labeled as different and placed in separate educational settings, with the accompanying stigma of not being like their normal peers. In addition, these children are provided with the opportunity to learn social, communicative, and academic skills from competent peers as well as to develop friendship ties with these more competent classmates. Their normally developing classmates are also believed to benefit from inclusion because they, in turn, are provided with opportunities to learn about individuals who are different from themselves and to do so in a positive venue. Overall, both groups of children are given the chance to operate in a context that inclusion supporters view as a more ecologically valid community than the one afforded through segregated classroom settings. Similarly, the families of children with disabilities should benefit from participation in the inclusion model because doing so promotes inclusion into the rest of the community, educational and otherwise. This provides all families, whether or not they have a child with a disability, with greater opportunities to make positive and supportive contacts with each other. Certainly not to be discounted is the further belief that there are both short-term and long-term economic advantages to the community from the practice of inclusion. There are benefits in the short-term because when children are taught within the inclusion model, the need for specialized classroom programs is eliminated and resources can be more prudently used. The perceived long-term benefits come from starting children with disabilities off in inclusion programs at the preschool level, which should increase the likelihood that they will be appropriately educated in mainstream classrooms for the rest of their educational lives. This movement should make the need for more expensive special schooling negligible. In fact, some people who question the wisdom of the full-inclusion approach argue that much of its attraction stems from the fact that school administrators view it as an "economically feasible way to see to their requirements to serve children with disabilities" (Newhoff, 1995, p. 4).

Although in theory there is little to argue with, there have been a number of practical problems with the enactment of the full inclusion model, most of which stem from its **exclusion** of any alternative education placements. The potential "down" sides to the inclusion model need to be understood by any practitioner who may be faced with participation. To begin with, the practice of full inclusion eliminates the variety of educational contexts that had been formerly available to children with special needs, which for some individual children may represent an education team's best guess regarding the setting in which a particular child can best learn. In essence, full inclusion provides one choice only: the mainstreamed classroom. For some children with significant communication, sociobehavioral, physical, and intellectual challenges, the full inclusion context in reality could be identified as "very restrictive" as the child who needs maximal individual assistance and structure attempts but fails to succeed in a regular classroom although receiving support from special educators and other resources. Opponents of full inclusion are quick to point out that there are many children with disabilities who can be appropriately educated in a regular classroom with special support services and for those children the notion of inclusion is highly appropriate and long overdue for some. Unfortunately, there are others who cannot achieve success, despite all of the dedication and motivation of the special and regular educators assigned to a regular classroom. There is also the issue in extreme cases of the disruption of the learning environment for the other classmates (Newhoff, 1995).

Because of the strength of the inclusion movement, it has become extremely difficult to staff a child who has experienced consistent failure in a mainstreamed classroom into what appears to be a more restrictive learning environment, if that option even exists (Idelstein, 1995). In many communities the continuum of special services that was once available for staffing options no longer exists. Thus some educators have been put in the position of being unable to provide what they believe to be the most appropriate educational setting for a particular child, something they say more essentially violates the spirit of the Individuals with Disabilities Education Act (PL 101-576) than does the existence of segregated classrooms. Those who oppose inclusion appear to do so primarily because they claim that no one solution, in this case the regular classroom, can be the best solution for all children given the diversity of disabilities. As Zigler and Hall (1995) note, "Ironically, the very law that was designed to safeguard the options of handicapped children and their parents may, in the end, act to constrict their choices and result in disservice to the very children the legislators sought to help, by forcing schools to place them in programs that are not equipped to meet their needs" (p. 295). It is primarily for this reason that the American Federation of Teachers; the Association for Persons with Severe Handicaps; the Consumer Action Network of, by, and for Deaf and Hard of Hearing Americans; the Council of Administrators of Special Education, Inc.; the Council for Learning Disabilities; and the Council for Exceptional Children, among others, have published position statements supporting the provision of a continuum of special services, and stating their concerns regarding the inappropriate uses of the full-inclusion model (Kauffman & Hallahan, 1995).

There are additional difficulties with the implementation of full inclusion that stem from the lack of specialized training on the part of regular and special educators to make the collaborations necessary in the classroom a reality. Although we can hypothesize that changes in university curricula for teacher training and enhanced opportunities for continuing education will eventually alleviate this problem, one problem that is not likely to be alleviated is the already identified shortages of special education personnel nationwide and the dwindling financial support in many school districts to hire the special educators needed.

The Speech-Language Clinician's Responsibilities for Language Intervention

A Systems Approach to Evaluating Treatment Outcome.   If you take a comprehensive point of view, the responsibility for language facilitation and remediation falls to some extent on everyone who has contact with the child diagnosed with a language disorder. This section presents a synopsis of what parents, classroom teachers, and the speech-language clinician are most typically expected to bring to language intervention. Obviously, speech-language clinicians are trained to provide intervention services. Therefore, it is important for them to have a strong background in language development as well as in the assessment of language disordered individuals (Weiss, Tomblin, & Robin, 1994). An appreciation for the fact that language development represents only one aspect of the growing child's development is also important as is an understanding of normal cognitive, social-emotional, and physical development patterns. An understanding of learning theory is also essential along with more specific knowledge of language treatment programs, techniques, and their rationales. Because the study of treatment efficacy is a burgeoning area of research, speech-language clinicians should be prepared to update their internalized data continuously bases with regard to which strategies for language facilitation have been shown to be both effective and efficient for which types of clients.

Success in the area of language intervention takes more than a wealth of background knowledge, however. In discussing the meaning of clinicianship, Nelson and Blakeley (1989) delineated several personal characteristics that they believe are essential in clinicians. In their experience, successful clinicians were energetic, creative, flexible, dramatic, and realistic (p. 104). These are qualities that develop over time and with varied experiences, according to these authors. Goldberg (1993) suggests that taken together, lists of desirable clinical characteristics typically describe an individual who is "a nondefensive, confident, and accepting individual" (p. 40).

In addition, because our nation is demographically changing in substantive ways, along with these changes have gone changes to the distribution of our clients in terms of their cultural backgrounds. Recognizing this pattern, Hanson (1992) suggested that "an appreciation and respect for cultural variations, as well as group and individual differences, is crucial for the interventionist" (p. 5). Lynch (1992) added that interventionists working with families from cultures other than their own will enhance their communicative effectiveness if they focus on the other culture as a potential learning experience and remain open to the different perspectives that will be shared by virtue of working together to develop a workable treatment program.

Along with having basic knowledge about language development and disorders, the speech-language clinician should know how to use that information to decide which children are developing language normally and which ones are not. Once the decision that a problem exists has been made, it must be decided whether language intervention is warranted. Olswang and Bain (1991) describe three methods: profiling, the static determination of what a client knows at a particular time; dynamic assessment, an analysis of the extent to which a client can benefit from cues and support in the environment; and monitoring (or tracking), a systematic evaluation of progress over time that allows for a prediction of future development, which can be incorporated into the decision-making process to facilitate appropriate recommendations for treatment (p. 255). According to the authors, the two critical determiners for treatment readiness are the exhibition of a significant difference between competencies of different language components, or between linguistic and cognitive competencies; and evidence that the client is ready to make changes in language performance. Specifically, profiling and dynamic assessment are most useful in providing clues as to when to begin intervention, and tracking or monitoring can be used retrospectively to evaluate whether the decision to intervene had been a good one.

If the speech-language clinician believes that intervention is warranted, then decisions must be made about a specific plan of action. Many variables are called in for consideration to develop a plan of action for a child. Of course, how much language the child already has and how much of it is typically used will need to be considered. The clinician must also consider how the child best learns, as well as the degree to which the parents and others who have significant contact with the child will cooperate with the program and can be called on to carry over the intervention program in the home environment. A listing of additional questions that should glean useful information for decision-making purposes is presented in Table 8-2.

Clinical Judgment.   Information derived from answers to the questions listed in Table 8-2 will not be sufficient to develop an appropriate intervention program. Skilled speech-language clinicians recognize that good decision-making and intervention planning result from a blend of objective information and good clinical "feel" for the therapeutic situation. There is an art to clinical practice that is difficult to specify but that is most likely a product of clinical experience tempered by the facts of clinical science (Records & Weiss, 1990). Given this subjective portion of clinical judgment, clinicians must guard against falling victim to unsubstantiated biases as they make decisions. Because there is still too little efficacy

TABLE 8-2   **Selected Information Needed to Develop a Language Intervention Plan**

1. Is the child cooperative and able to comply with structured tasks?
2. Is the child willing to separate from the parent or caregiver to work with the clinician?
3. Are pictures meaningful to the child, or should three-dimensional objects be used?
4. Does the child exhibit both receptive and expressive language disorders?
5. Do any members of the child's immediate family also have a language disorder?
6. Have the parents expressed interest in participating in their child's language intervention program?
   a. If so, how much time could they reasonably devote to specific activities?
   b. If so, how knowledgeable are the parents regarding language development milestones?
   c. If so, is their typical interaction style with their child directive? egalitarian?
7. Does the child show any awareness of the language disorder?
8. Has the child been reported to become frustrated in his/her attempts to communicate?
9. Will intervention activities hold the child's attention for 5 minutes? 10 minutes? 15 minutes?
10. Is the child involved in a classroom program?
    a. If so, what is the focus of the classroom (e.g., academic, pre-academic, daycare)?
    b. If so, does the child's language disorder compromise the child's interactions with classmates?
    c. If so, does the child appear to enjoy the classroom experience?
    d. If so, are there other children in the child's class with language difficulties? other developmental problems?
    e. If so, has the child's teacher(s) expressed concern about the child's language abilities? willingness to participate in language intervention?

research pointing to which intervention programs are best suited to which children, there is a danger in assuming that one intervention plan that appears to have worked well with one child will necessarily work well with all children.

One way to help overcome a tendency toward bias in selecting intervention approaches is to focus on our rationales for choosing certain clinical methods and to maintain a healthy skepticism until supporting data become available (Newhoff, 1995). Continuing to collect objective data to substantiate client progress or lack of progress helps prevent clinicians from becoming too complacent with one or another therapeutic technique.

A Sample Decision Tree.   Figure 8-2 delineates an example of one type of decision-making process, a decision tree. S. Ellis Weismer (1988) developed this particular decision tree for the speech-language clinician who must undertake the planning of an intervention program for a child with "specific language learning problems" (p. 43). Notice that the clinician is called on to incorporate all of the information gleaned from the case history and a "comprehensive communication profile" (p. 42) to determine what needs to be taught and the relative priority for each need (Step A). Ellis Weismer (1988) suggested that "as a general guideline, early stages of training should focus on the functions language serves and its content, with emphasis on the form of the message coming later" (p. 42).

The next step in the decision tree is to determine ways to help the child adequately make use of language input provided during intervention (Step B). If the child is demonstrating a language problem and has been unable to learn the rule structures of language, then maybe the language input presented has not been sufficiently structured for that pur-

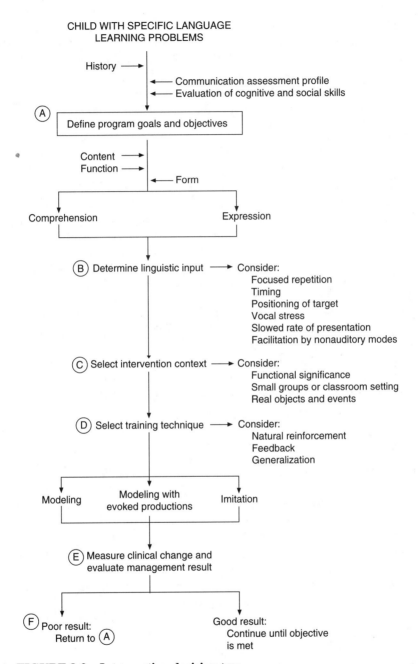

FIGURE 8-2 Intervention decision tree.

(From: D. Yoder, E. David, & Raymond D. Kent, *Decision making in speech-language pathology,* Philadelphia, B. C. Decker, 1988, Reproduced by permission of Mosby-Year Book, Inc., St. Louis.)

pose. Notice that Ellis Weismer (1988) made specific suggestions about how linguistic input might be altered to achieve greater success. Any of these alterations of the input signal (e.g., timing, slowed rate of presentation) could make the difference between the child's understanding or misunderstanding of language both in and out of intervention.

It is also important for the clinician to determine the best setting for intervention (Step C). Ellis Weismer (1988) suggested that an appropriate setting for intervention is one where "a legitimate reason for communication underlies therapy activities" (p. 42). Certainly the settings selected will differ according to each child's special circumstances and the availability of intervention services. The clinician may have many alternatives to choose from or may be relegated to only one option.

Once the methods for language input and the intervention context have been determined, the clinician must then choose the specific training technique to be used (Step D). Although there is evidence supporting the usefulness of many different language intervention techniques, Ellis Weismer (1988) cautioned that clinicians must carefully select the technique depending on the area of language targeted for intervention. Decisions concerning use of reinforcers, how feedback will be provided, and how generalization will be promoted also should be considered at this early point in planning (p. 42).

The speech-language clinician's role as a decision maker does not end with the actual implementation of the intervention program. To determine whether or not the early decisions made have been appropriate ones, it is critical for the clinician to collect data systematically to support or refute the contention that progress has been made (Step E). If the data show that progress has been made, the intervention program appears to have been effective and should be continued. If no measurable progress has been demonstrated, then the clinician will need to return to Step A and troubleshoot the program for errors in decisions already made.

Others Who Share in the Provision of Language Intervention

It has already been mentioned that, to some extent, anyone in contact with a child in need of language intervention can share in the responsibility for intervention. Most individuals who come in contact with the child provide language modeling (input) or opportunities for interaction where language can be used and learned. All interactions can potentially provide language learning experiences. In fact, one of the challenges to beginning student clinicians is to start viewing every interaction with a client in terms of its language facilitation potential. Given the pervasiveness of language-learning contexts, children's parents, other caregivers, classroom teachers, siblings, and peers can share in the intervention process to a greater or lesser extent depending on the specifics of the client's needs, abilities, and circumstances. There are two aspects of the intervention process with which these "others" are most closely associated. The first is in promoting generalization, either stimulus or response generalization to untrained contexts (Hughes, 1985). The second is in the facilitation of language learning itself, where these more knowledgeable language users consider what the child already knows in creating low-risk language learning experiences (van Kleeck & Richardson, 1988). This is sometimes called **scaffolding** (Bruner, 1985) and is closely related to the concept of **dynamic assessment,** already referred to as a technique to determine readiness for intervention (Olswang & Bain, 1991).

The Role of Parents

As mandated by 99-457, parents are integral members for both the planning and executing of the IFSPs drawn up with substantive assistance from professionals representing many different disciplines. The implication of this legislation is that parents have been deemed highly responsible parties in intervention planning, although of the team's members, they probably do not possess the most information about language intervention. The need to bring parents into the circle of service providers in a manner that builds mutual respect and consensus for the duration of service delivery has led to a substantial literature on the best ways to accomplish this (Crais, 1991). Crais (1991) noted that the involvement of parents in service delivery has shifted, which is apparent in the changing terminology, where terms referring to the family-focused or family-centered nature of treatment are commonplace. She further suggested that all of these approaches share a set of common underlying assumptions, among them "that families are equal partners in assessment and intervention, that families will be encouraged and allowed to choose their own level of involvement in decision making and implementation of both assessment and intervention practices, and that supporting the family in the ways they consider useful is a primary goal of intervention services (Crais, 1991, p. 2)."

Speech-language clinicians should note that the notion of incorporating parents into the decision making process, while implemented as a means to empower family members and acknowledge their important role in service delivery, operates as a culturally sensitive phenomenon. That is, when working with families from some nonmajority cultures (e.g., Asian, Hispanic), the practitioner may be viewed as the expert to whom the child has been brought for the express purpose of deciding on a course of action. If the parents are then asked to take part in the decision-making process by giving advice and setting priorities, this may signal that the so-called experts are less than competent and the professionals' credibility is diminished. In a general sense, when the speech-language clinician is a member of a different culture from that of the family, it is important to be cognizant of potential misunderstandings brought on by differences in belief systems surrounding healthcare, child-care routines, wellness management, and so on. Hanson (1992) refers to these misunderstandings as potentials for "cultural clashes" (pp. 4–5).

Lynch (1992) noted that cultures differ along the preferred mode of information transfer, with some cultures exhibiting a preference for explicit transfer through oral language and others preferring to transmit information implicitly by means of the contextual cues inherent in a situation, the relationship that holds between the participants, and nonlinguistic cues (p. 44). This difference in style translates into two culture types, according to the author. There is a "high-context" culture type that is observed to be more formal than the "low-context" culture type, which is more informal and which demonstrates a tendency toward more egalitarian interaction (Lynch, 1992, p. 45). The use of a cultural style by a clinician that does not match that of the family may result in unintended communications of insensitivity, which are likely to impede the working relationships of the participants. Therefore, it would be worthwhile for the speech-language clinician to attempt to determine as early in their interactions as possible, the level of context-based communication that will be comfortable for the family in question.

The amount of time that parents spend with their children will vary from family to family, but it is very likely that they spend more time with the child than does the speech-language clinician. That means that in addition to their legal role as decision makers for their child, they also are likely to have a great deal of influence over their child's language intervention by virtue of the importance of language input and their frequent presence as language interactants. The speech-language clinician should find some way to use the parents' proximity and interest in helping their child who has a language disorder. The parental role in intervention will also vary from parent to parent depending on the parent's facility or willingness or availability to learn intervention techniques, reporting skills for monitoring the child's language use at home, and ability to follow through at home with the therapeutic contingencies used in the clinic. Techniques for making the home environment more like the intervention setting and the intervention setting more like home have been suggested by Hughes to promote generalization outside the treatment setting. Parents are the perfect consultants for putting these suggestions into practice.

It is also important for speech-language clinicians to remember that as important as the development of speech-language competence is, it may be considered a lower priority than some of the other concerns parents may have. In families where having sufficient food and shelter are daily worries, or catastrophic health issues are present, following through on a language intervention program may take a back seat. Just as it is important not to set children up to fail by instituting impossible goals, it is also important when incorporating parents into an intervention plan not to ask them to do more than can be reasonably expected. Asking a parent to spend a half hour per night engaged in a specific language task is often too much to ask. Most parents want to be as helpful as possible, but for many such a request would seriously compromise other familial duties.

One approach that might solve this problem is to work with parents on ways to facilitate their child's participation in naturally occurring language "happenings," perhaps during quiet times when the child and parent are the only participants, or when the entire family can participate in some group activity. Promoting conversations at mealtimes is one suggestion that parents frequently say works well. Here the parent can serve to reinforce the child's attempts to communicate. Better still, the parent does not necessarily have to be put in a position of doling out performance-based rewards or punishments.

In a recent study, Fey, Cleave, Long, and Hughes (1993) compared two techniques for facilitating grammatical productions in children with language impairments, one of which utilized the child's parents for service delivery. The authors noted that although both the parent-administered technique and a more traditional clinician-administered technique appeared to yield positive results, it was the clinician-administered approach that provided more consistently positive treatment effects. This led the authors to caution their readers that parent-administered programs may require clinicians to more closely monitor client change over time and institute changes to the program if the child's progress falls below what would be expected. This conclusion by Fey and colleagues (1993) may provide support for the notion that although parents are generally highly useful resources for implementing some language programs, they do not take the place of trained speech-language clinicians. In a similar vein, results reported by Girolametto, Tannock, and Siegel (1993) revealed that parents' subjective judgments of the post-therapeutic improvements of their children bore little relationship to the objective data chronicling pre- to post-therapy changes in the same children's performances. This again suggests that parents are very interested in their children's successes but are likely, because of the bias of wanting to see progress as well as their lack of specialized training in speech-language pathology, will not take the place of the speech-language clinician's eyes, ears, and expertise.

Other investigators suggest that parents can be given rather specific goals in terms of providing their children with language-learning experiences. Pierce and McWilliams (1993) noted that the parents of children with severe speech and physical impairments who indicate willingness to participate can be given specific suggestions for increasing the literacy and preliteracy experiences of their young children.

The Role of Classroom Teachers

Classroom teachers play an important role in language intervention. By understanding their young student's language deficiencies, and usually with some assistance from the speech-language clinician, the teacher can provide frequent language learning experiences in the classroom and make these experiences more relevant to the child's ongoing classroom curriculum (Fujiki & Brinton, 1984).

As the expert on the classroom curriculum, the classroom teacher is a valuable resource for the clinician who is working in the classroom itself or serving as a classroom consultant. Classroom teachers can help to pinpoint the situational demands on language that occur during the classroom routine and they are in a good position to monitor the child's successes and failures in generalizing the language features targeted in intervention. Teachers also have the knowledge and expertise to facilitate success in the classroom. For example, by periodically changing the child's seating arrangement to promote interactions with a variety of classmates (some of whom may be more willing to interact with a child who has a language disorder than others), the child may have more opportunities to practice and perfect new communication skills. The classroom teacher has expert understanding of the classroom members' social dynamics, and this information can be used to advantage by those planning language intervention.

The Role of Classmates

Young, normally developing children seem to learn quickly which of their classmates have difficulties with communicating. This can be demonstrated by their ability and willingness to accommodate their own language to the less sophisticated abilities of their classmates (Guralnick & Paul-Brown, 1977). It is also clear that normally developing children are preferred when a peer wants to initiate contact or when children in a classroom are asked to indicate with whom in the classroom they would prefer to play (Craig & Washington, 1993; Rice, 1993; Rice, Sell, & Hadley, 1991). Further, when children with language difficulties do communicate, they tend to do so with adults perhaps because they historically have found more acceptance in such interactions.

Rice, Hadley, and Alexander (1993) suggested that data describing the interactions of preschool-age children with different abilities within classroom settings point to a pattern of social consequence for children with language impairment or limitations in language use. That is, if a child demonstrates limited language abilities, he or she will be less likely to be involved in experiences that will facilitate peer initiation abilities or to practice the language competencies that are needed to develop friendships. Furthermore, when a child discovers that he or she is not a likely candidate for friendships with classmates, there is probably less motivation for the child to work to develop those needed language skills. After a short period of time in classrooms where young children with disabilities are mainstreamed, it is not unusual for the normally developing children to ignore their classmates with language impairments in favor of interacting with their normally developing peers (Snyder, Apolloni, & Cooke, 1977). With very young children, some of this behavior results from immature socialization skills, but with older children it seems that the children are being ignored because of their poor language skills. As Craig (1993) noted with reference to children with Specific Language Impairment, "it appears that the amount of their peer interaction is limited and that, when it does occur, it probably is reduced in quality compared to that of children with normal language development" (p. 214). Children from nonmajority cultures may present both language and socialization challenges to the speech-language clinician (Damico & Damico, 1993), Given that so much important language learning is closely tied with the development of children's social skills, it will be important for the speech-language clinician (as well as the classroom teacher) to learn how to assist the culturally different children in their classrooms "in becoming more empowered in their social and educational contexts" (p. 241).

These findings lead us to believe that clinicians and classroom teachers must not assume that beneficial language learning interactions take place between all children in classrooms and instead, need to figure out ways to facilitate the opportunities for interaction both inside and outside of the classroom. Rice (1993) additionally suggested that teachers and others specifically not only redirect the requests and statements made to adults by children with language difficulties to classmates but also teach the children specific strategies to do so. This technique makes it less likely that the child with limited language abilities will use the adults in the classroom as the "default" interactant.

Even in classroom situations where language "models" are employed, it cannot be taken for granted that these children, by virtue of their language normal status and presence in the classroom, are providing adequate language modeling for their classmates with limited language. Weiss and Nakamura (1992) investigated the extent to which normally developing children serving as "model" children in a class of language disordered children interacted with their classmates. They found that two of the three model children spent very little, if any time, with their peers who had language disorders. Unfortunately, the purpose of this classroom's reverse mainstreaming plan was to promote interactions between the models and their classmates so that those with language disorders would benefit from competent language input provided by the models. The failure on the part of the models in this study to interact with their language disordered classmates was not an isolated finding (Odom & McEvoy, 1988). The authors recommended that teachers should take the lead in putting groups of child conversants together and give them less opportunity to form their own interactant groups based on language competencies. Taking this thought one step further, Venn, Wolery, Fleming, DeCesare, Morris, and Cuffs (1993) reported on the use of a mand-model procedure to teach normal classroom peers to interact with their classmates who had language disorders. Not only did the normal classmates easily learn to incorporate the mand-model appropriately, but the children with disabilities with whom they were paired increased both the frequency of their responses to their peers and in the production of their own unprompted requests!

Facilitating Language Change

The Connection of Theories to Treatment

Speech-language clinicians need methods for critically assessing and choosing among the many approaches to language intervention. Johnston (1983) proposed that to develop intervention procedures that work, each clinician must determine his or her own theory of language development/disorders and design treatment approaches, or select from among those already available, that are consistent with those beliefs. Therapy plans cannot be successful if they reflect a confused sense of either theory or the factors that affect language development and language change, according to Johnston (1983). The development of intervention strategies for children demonstrating disorders in language have paralleled the changes in the theories proposed to explain child language acquisition. Although changes in therapeutic approaches have somewhat lagged behind major shifts in perspectives on language acquisition theory, a review of the history of language intervention reveals strong connections between the two (McLean, 1983).

A good theory accounts for the course of language development by empirical research and careful observation. To date, no theory of language acquisition has been proposed that satisfactorily explains all observations. A discussion of language theories has been presented elsewhere inn this text and will not be discussed here. However, it is important to recognize that adherence to one or another theory has implications for how the clinician views her role in intervention. Different language theories also influence clinical decision making in different ways.

For example, the clinician who follows the nativist perspective, or innateness hypothesis (see Psycholinguistic/Syntactic Approach, Chapter 1, p. 13), probably views herself in the role of facilitator but not trainer. That is, the job of the clinician is to assist the child in recognizing the systematicity and the rule-governed nature of language structures. The clinician presents a child with sets of sentences organized in such a way that the ungrammatical examples are highlighted as different from those that follow a targeted rule. Therefore, the rule becomes the target to be inferred from the examples provided; the examples themselves are not the targets.

One influence of the cognitivists' point of view (see Semantic/Cognitive Approach, Chapter 1, pp. 14–15) may be observed in formulas devised by school systems or clinics to determine who is an appropriate candidate for language intervention. Some professionals believe that children who demonstrate equitable levels of cognitive and linguistic attainments should not be eligible to receive language intervention, even if the degree of language competence achieved is less than expected for the child's chronological age (Lyngaas, Nyberg, Hoekenga, & Gruenewald, 1983). The rationale for this decision stems from the belief that expectations for language abilities cannot exceed what has been demonstrated cognitively. Not all clinicians agree with this approach to eligibility (Fey, 1986). Leonard (1983) suggested that "language ability can be facilitated through intervention to a point at which it surpasses the level of the child's other abilities" (p. 111).

In a third example, the social-interactionist viewpoint (see Pragmatic Approach, Chapter 1, pp. 15–16) has placed emphasis on early intervention services by suggesting that children begin to learn language long before they produce their first words. Sometimes medical or social problems upset the possibility for natural caregiver-child interactions, as may be the case with prolonged hospitalizations following premature birth or other birth complications. Speech-language clinicians may be asked to analyze infant behaviors and abilities to develop a program demonstrating to family members how to capitalize on their infant's limited capabilities for early communication (Ensher, 1989; Sparks, 1989). Similarly, the importance of early childhood special education programs for children developing more slowly than their peers has received support due to the popularity of the social-interaction approach. The passage of PL 99-457, which mandates services to children ages 3 to 5 who have disabilities, was probably an outcome of the interest in the language learning that goes on during the preschool years.

The transition to the collaborative consultation model from the more traditional pull-out model of therapy could also be traced to the social-interaction approach. The language milieu in the classroom has been shown to be quite different from that in the home environment. To be successful conversationalists in school, children need to learn the rule systems of both; where they are similar and where they are different. Instead of learning discourse conventions of the classroom in a third setting, the therapy room, treatment in the classroom itself provides immediate occasions for using the new structures and strategies targeted in therapy.

Getting Started

The speech-language clinician's role in facilitating language change proceeds from a series of decisions. The first major decision involves a "best guess" about where to begin in therapy; this will come from the results of standardized and nonstandardized tests and measures completed in the child's diagnostic evaluation. Added to this will be the observations of parents and other caregivers who will be able to contribute information relevant to how well the child can use the language he or she does have to best advantage and who will also be able to provide input with regard to the language demands in the child's life. Along with determining whether a problem exists, the clinician should determine the scope of the problem and how the child can best learn language. Often these last two features of the case are not determined until after a period of diagnostic therapy (Goldberg, 1993; Weiss, Tomblin, & Robin, 1994).

During diagnostic therapy, a variety of materials can be employed, and different combinations of input stimuli are emphasized while the child's performance is carefully monitored for changes. Questions concerning the breadth of the problem and most useful methods for remediation are important and need to be answered by the clinician because their answers will furnish useful insights for designing treatment plans that have a greater chance of success. Answers to these questions supply the "hows" of the therapy plan's implementation. Here are four examples:

1. *What presentation methods-facilitate the child's ability to demonstrate new language targets?* That is, should the clinician embed the targets in a story retelling task or use sentence contexts? If the child is supplied with opportunities to produce targeted structures in natural conversation exchanges, will the child tend to take advantage of these with little prompting?
2. *How much stimulus support does the child need to be successful?* For example, are auditory cues alone sufficient to result in production of the targeted language structures or are combinations of auditory and visual cues necessary? Does the child benefit from orthographic cues (letter symbols), or are these confusing? For some young children, orthographic cues may not be meaningful and present more of a hindrance than a help.
3. *Is the child willing to risk being wrong?* Does the child refuse to incorporate newly targeted structures and forms unless provided with imitative prompts so that he is left with little guesswork when formulating language? Or is this young child willing to quickly try to incorporate new language targets in his own spontaneous language? If the latter is true, under what circumstances is spontaneous usage more likely to occur?
4. *What motivates the child to improve language performance?* Does the child demonstrate any awareness of her own difficulties in being understood or in understanding others? When placed in a situation where a communication breakdown is likely to occur, and then occurs, does the child exhibit any understanding of what happened? What strategies does the child use, if any, to remedy a breakdown in communication?

Obviously, along with the "hows," the "whats" of the therapy plan also need to be determined. Goals that emerged from formal testing and therefore appear to be appropriate should be targeted in baseline testing before their final selection. That is, several trials containing a number of examples of the potential structure or forms to be targeted for therapy should be administered so that the clinician can determine whether test results were artifacts of the testing process, of the test itself, or truly represent the child's specific deficits. Sometimes baseline trials are administered within one session; sometimes they are administered over the course of several days. The point is that a stable baseline of the child's performance should be established so the clinician knows the child's level of competence before therapy begins. Failure to have this information leaves open the possibility that time will be wasted either by targeting "goals" already established and leaving other appropriate goals untargeted, or incorrectly crediting the child's miraculous progress to the therapy program. See Hegde (1985) for a detailed discussion of implementing baseline testing.

Selecting Goal Attack Strategies

If the goals are bona fide, the clinician is ready to designate a goal attack strategy (Fey, 1986), which will provide a framework for the intervention program. A **goal attack strategy** is a pattern of goal sequencing and emphasis used in a treatment program where more than one goal will be targeted. Fey (1986) noted that selecting a goal attack strategy is an important decision worthy of careful consideration. To make this selection, clinicians need to answer several pertinent questions in light of the goal attack strategies available:

1. What characteristics of the language learner may render one or another of the strategies more or less successful?

2. Will the specific goals selected for the child have a particular impact on attack strategy chosen?
3. What is the theory of the clinician with regard to language learning?

Fey (1986) described three different goal attack strategies: vertical, horizontal, and cyclical. In the **vertical goal attack strategy,** one goal is worked on until a predetermined criterion level of performance is reached. This criterion may have been set at 80 percent correct or 90 percent or 100 percent by the clinician. Criterion level percentages are arbitrary but typically are set at a level the clinician believes will ensure adequate learning by the child for either generalization of that goal or success at the next higher level of difficulty. When the criterion performance level is met, the next goal becomes the focus of treatment. Entire sessions are often devoted to the teaching of one goal, and it is likely that this goal will remain the focus of intervention for a considerable period of time. Because of the intensive nature of the vertical strategy, some children are less likely to become distracted or confused when it does come time to change goals. This approach is believed to be less cognitively demanding and ensures concentrated practice on one goal that the child learns well before moving on to the next one. A potential negative feature of the vertical strategy is that the child may become bored with a session due to its narrow focus. Another is that the child may have more difficulty seeing generalities across different speech/language behaviors. The child doesn't recognize the shared features of Goal 1 and Goal 2 because work on these goals is separated in time. Because generalization may be impeded, some clinicians suggest that the vertical approach is the least time efficient of the three for some children in certain clinical situations.

The **horizontal goal attack strategy** prescribes work on more than one goal within the same session. These goals may be closely related to each other (e.g., all conversation act types) or quite dissimilar (e.g., plural morpheme -*s,* tag questions, and responses to clarification requests). The underlying principle is that this strategy better reflects normal language learning because many different language forms and structures are experienced and learned at the same time. The horizontal strategy may be more time efficient: General insights and skills in language learning gained from working on Goal 1, such as learning to correctly monitor self-performance, may benefit progress on Goal 3. Children known to be distractible may not be considered good candidates for this strategy because they might not recognize when a different goal, with different expectations for acceptability, is being targeted. It is also less likely that individual goals will be overlearned or become routine, because less time is devoted to each. For children who have particular problems with language learning, overlearning may be necessary for success, and for them the vertical goal attack strategy may be a wiser selection.

In the **cyclical goal attack strategy,** a number of different goals are worked on within a particular time unit of treatment (e.g., month, semester, or school year), but unlike the horizontal goal attack approach, each goal is presented individually within a session. After each of the goals has been worked on sequentially over the time frame of interest, the targets within the cycle are reevaluated and the cycle is revised (goals may be added or subtracted) or repeated if need be. Cyclical approaches suggest that much of the child's learning takes place when the clinician is not present. The child takes what is learned in the therapy setting, considers it, and practices it when outside of therapy. Therefore, intensive ongoing client-clinician contact often duplicates effort or wastes time because its benefits may be as easily derived by the child alone, provided that the clinician has successfully taught the necessary tools for teaming language. According to proponents of the cyclical goal attack strategy, true changes in language competencies occur only after the child has figured out how to incorporate new language goals into his repertoire over time.

Figure 8-3 lists some of the variables a clinician must consider when selecting a goal attack strategy.

Selecting Intervention Settings

Beginning clinicians often fail to recognize that many of the decisions dealing with the disposition of a treatment plan need to be tentatively decided at the beginning stages of treatment. That is, the clinician needs to know where the young child with a language disorder uses language and plan treatment so that the child's new language competencies will be incorporated in an ever-widening set of daily circumstances. In short, the clinician should start therapy having already made some decisions concerning where therapy should take place, with whom, and the amount of structure to be imposed. In addition, there should be some general plan for increasing the "degree of difficulty" for the child as progress is made. One conceptualization for making these sorts of decisions was described by Fey (1986) as a "naturalness continuum" (Figure 8-4).

Common sense dictates that for language intervention to be considered successful, the goals targeted for intervention must be apparent in the child's spontaneous language repertoire. So, at some point in the intervention process, the clinician will need to be sure that the therapeutic environment closely resembles the child's natural environment, or vice versa (Hughes, 1985). If this is not done, generalization of newly learned language competencies to the child's activities of daily living may not be easy. Some clinicians wait until the closing stages of intervention before introducing activities specifically aimed at promoting generalization. Others develop intervention programs that account for the generalization of

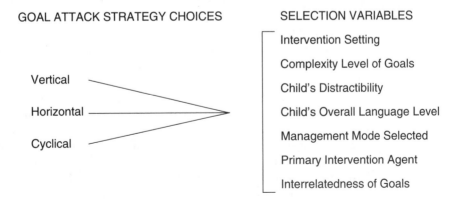

FIGURE 8-3   Variables involved in goal attack strategy selection.

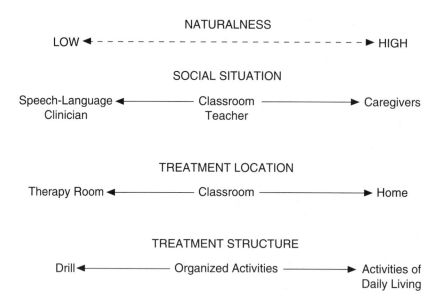

FIGURE 8-4   Components of naturalness along a naturalness continuum.

(Adapted from Fey, 1986)

language goals from the very start of treatment. Growing sentiment in the field of speech-language pathology supports the latter approach.

As shown in Figure 8-4, Fey (1986) delineated three features of naturalness on his naturalness continuum: the activity devised by the clinician, the physical context used for intervention, and the social context in which the intervention transpires. For each of these parameters, he suggested that a continuum exists, ranging from more to less naturalness. Taken together, the relative naturalness of the therapy plan can be estimated. The treatment program that incorporates daily activities in the child's home with parents would be perceived as possessing a very high degree of naturalness. That means that the therapeutic setting closely resembles a *non*therapeutic setting. When the child achieves success in this type of a treatment milieu, the clinician can be more comfortable that the transition to generalization will be accomplished with less directed effort. If the child already views the two settings as similar, he or she should view their language opportunities and requirements as similar as well.

Just because a highly natural treatment setting appears to have a major advantage for generalization purposes does not mean that all intervention programs should be designed in the same way As with selecting the most appropriate goal attack strategy for a particular child, there are client characteristics that may steer the clinician to one or another location along the naturalness continuum. Imposing more structure and very little naturalness in the therapy setting on some children early on may better ensure that they learn new structures. However, generalization will eventually need to be addressed in the therapy program for these children as well. To some degree, an increase in naturalness will have to be incorporated.

Selecting Management Modes: One Example

One way for speech-language clinicians to arrive at a general framework for intervention plan is by carefully looking at the essential component parts of therapy and assembling them logically and creatively according to the child's needs and the clinician's own philosophy of management. Most clinicians can tell that "drill" is more structured than "play" but the specifics of how the two treatment methods differ and in what ways they are similar are less widely understood. By understanding these specifics, we have a better chance of matching a child to an appropriate treatment approach and knowing which components may need to be altered when and if a change in our initial therapy plan becomes necessary.

In their germinal article discussing therapy modes useful in the management of phonological disorders, Shriberg and Kwiatkowski (1982) described four categories of treatment components:

1. Target responses: including what the clinician intends the target response to be, and the client's actual response.
2. Training stimuli: the stimuli that will be used to elicit responses from clients, which may be presented individually or in sets; and the termination criterion for moving on to higher degrees of difficulty in the treatment plan.
3. Instructional events: the clinical teaching we do is referred to as an antecedent instructional event while the **feedback** we provide to our clients following their responses is referred to as a subsequent instructional event.
4. Motivational events: are employed to "accelerate learning by heightening a child's receptivity to all instructional events" (Shriberg & Kwiatkowski, 1982, p. 245) and can be incorporated as antecedent motivational events prior to the client's attempts at a response, or as subsequent motivational events, also referred to as **reinforcement.**

The authors arranged these component parts into four management modes which they called: **drill, drill play, structured play,** and **play.** The modes exist along a continuum from "most structured" (drill) to "least structured" (play). It should also be noted that as one moves from the more structured end of the management mode continuum to the less structured end, the treatment focus moves from being clinician centered to client centered (which in this case is also child centered). That is, on the less structured end of the continuum, the child exerts more influence on the pace and focal point of therapy.

By incorporating the components described by Shriberg and Kwiatkowski (1982) as the entire set of options for the four modes, you can observe the ways in which the four management modes are related to one another. Figure 8-5 illustrates these differences.

Note that structured play and play are quite similar, as are drill play and drill. For example, drill and drill play are identical with one exception. In drill play there is an antecedent motivational event that is missing in drill. That is, something is added to the drill play approach to increase the likelihood that the child will comply with the task. The antecedent motivational event, then, represents a small shift away from the most structured end of the continuum. In both of these modes, drill and drill play, there is a subsequent motivational event (a reinforcer), but this will be presented only in cases where the child's actual response is equivalent to the response definition delineated. Said another way, the child is not

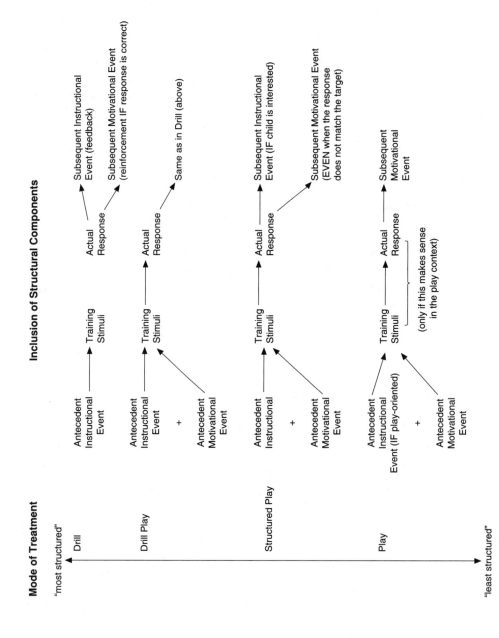

FIGURE 8-5   Differences between four management modes.

Adapted from Shriberg, L. & Kwiatkowski, J. (1982). Phonological disorders II. A conceptual framework for management. *Journal of Speech and Hearing Disorders, 47,* 242–256.

being reinforced for willingness to participate; the reinforcer is directly tied to the adequacy of the response.

As the structure of the management mode decreases, there is less emphasis on the antecedent instructional event. This means that formalized teaching of the target becomes a less important part of the treatment. For example, in the play management mode, the definition of an acceptable response and the criterion needed for terminating therapy are not even brought to the child's attention in therapy. This is quite a contrast to the way proponents of drill view therapy, but this management mode is considered equally viable and is more appropriate than drill for certain children in certain therapeutic situations. In structured play, which is closer to the clinician-centered end of the continuum than play, the child is presented with information about response definition if he is interested in that information. What is more important in structured play is that the clinician will spend time emphasizing the enjoyability of the therapy activity.

Shriberg and Kwiatkowski (1982) also reported the results of studies that incorporated their taxonomy in the treatment of children with phonological disorders. Their findings from 22 children who received these different treatment approaches indicated that the drill and drill play modes were more effective and efficient than were the structured play and play modes. Clinicians who had participated in the studies reported that they (a) believed drill play was the most effective and efficient mode, (b) also preferred to use the drill play approach, and (c) believed that their clients preferred drill play, structured play, or play over drill. One study focused on determining what specific client characteristics would indicate a better match with one or another management mode but yielded inconclusive results. Obviously, this information is critical for us to be accountable to the children we serve. Clinical researchers should be encouraged to seek out answers to this important question.

Using Information about Caregiver-Child Interactions in Therapy

Once the goals for therapy have been selected and arranged according to the chosen goal attack strategy, and the management mode has been developed, the clinician must decide how interactions with the child will teach or facilitate the learning of these goals. Research based on how caregivers and young children interact serves as a basis for some language therapy techniques; these techniques are sometimes called **experiential language intervention techniques.** Researchers have noted recurring patterns of language use, usually in mother-child dyads, and have hypothesized that these play an important role in facilitating infants' developing linguistic competence. It has been suggested that these patterns should have a similar effect on the child who is not learning language normally. Therefore, patterns such as expansion, expatiation, modeling, and scaffolding have been discussed in the literature of language development as well as that of language intervention (Connell, 1982; Leonard, 1981; Ratner & Bruner, 1978; Snow, 1986; Weiss, 1981). In terms of management mode, most of the natural caregiver-child techniques fit better with the less structured modes—structured play and play—because they are usually embedded within conversations.

This is probably an appropriate point to insert a cautionary note having to do with the cultural biases inherent in the caregiver-child research used as a basis for much of this branch of language intervention. The vast majority of research done on caregiver-child interactions has been done with families from the mainstream culture. As a result, it is very likely (and in fact we know this to be true) that there are significant enough cultural differences from one culture to another in terms of child rearing practices, view of children's talking with adults, and so on. that the techniques to be described may not be typical for many of the clients we see professionally. Van Kleeck (1994) reported on a number of the cultural differences that could lead to misunderstandings when we as clinicians attempt to teach caregivers how to interact "appropriately" with their children for therapeutic purposes. For example, in some cultures where young children are not encouraged to initiate conversations with their elders, teaching parents strategies for responding to their child's initiations probably would not be a particularly fruitful approach.

Adopting caregiver-child interaction techniques in therapy has been challenged by some clinicians. Their view is that because most caregivers engage their young children in similar types of language interaction, the language disordered child has probably already been exposed to these techniques. If the usual caregiver-child patterns had been sufficient to effect language development for the child, they would have done so. Opponents to using natural caregiver-child interaction techniques suggest instead that natural and more directive bombardment with examples of acceptable structures is needed. They believe that, by definition, the child diagnosed as having a language disorder probably possesses some sort of deficit that makes it more difficult to benefit from natural interaction patterns. Thus, reliance on these natural intervention techniques alone has little reasonable chance for success. Despite this controversy, experiential language intervention techniques have been widely used and deserve consideration.

Remember that experiential language intervention techniques have their roots in natural caregiver-child interactions and that their use in therapy should not seriously compromise the naturalness of the treatment. Although the manner in which they are presented by the clinician is prescribed, in practice they are supposed to sound less like a contrived script and more like the normal course of conversational events. The following techniques are commonly used in programs that emphasize conversation development in children who are severely limited in their ability to express themselves (MacDonald & Gillette, 1984; Weiss, 1981).

Imitation.   The clinician's use of imitation appears to accomplish several things. First, it has been hypothesized that it validates for the child the acceptability of his own production. It also gives the child an opportunity to reimitate for emphasis by copying what the clinician said. That is, the child may believe that if the clinician repeated what he said first, it must be acceptable. When the child is expected to imitate the clinician, it represents a less risky attempt at contributing to a conversation. Although imitation has been used widely in operant programs as the main means for eliciting responses from clients, the discussion here refers to a less structured use. Imitation occurs frequently in language samples collected from normally developing children and their caregivers (Cross, 1978).

Definitions of what constitutes an imitation differ. Imitations may refer to a verbatim reiteration of what was said or only part of it (a partial imitation). An imitation called for by the clinician may require an immediate imitation or a delayed imitation, where either a pause or some intervening dialogue is imposed. Imitation by the clinician also serves as a topic maintainer, letting the child know that the clinician acknowledges the topic established by the child.

Expansion.   Expansion refers to the clinician's embellishment of a young child's immature production so that it reflects the adult version of what the child was attempting to produce. The clinician is not supposed to extend the boundaries of the child's original production, so that if the child produced "kitty go," an appropriate expansion would be "The kitty goes." To extend beyond the verb (e.g., "The kitty goes in the car") would constitute the use of expatiation, a slightly different experiential language intervention technique.

The clinical assumption is that expansion, like imitation, provides some useful feedback to the child. Here the message is not necessarily that the child's contribution was acceptable but that its value as a contribution to the conversation structure has been acknowledged. That is, the clinician has accepted the child's contribution as a turn that served to initiate, maintain, or bring to a close an already established topic. Furthermore, the clinician has modeled a *more* acceptable version of the child's production, possessing the same communicative intention but with a different surface structure.

The latter rationale hints at one danger with expansion use. Unless the clinician carefully uses the linguistic and nonlinguistic information available from the context of the ongoing conversation—what was happening at the time of the child's utterance, what constituted the clinician's linguistic turn just before the child spoke, and so on—the clinician may misinterpret what the child was attempting to convey.

Expatiation.   This technique is closely related to expansion in that the clinician produces an adult-appropriate version of what the child was attempting to produce. However, in expatiation, the clinician's version of the child's utterance extends beyond the apparent limits of the child's original utterance. Again, the clinician must carefully consider the context of the child's utterance to produce something that reflects the child's intent. If the main goal of expressive language development is to enable the child to encode the relationships among the people, places, things, and events in the world, then what is said must match closely with the child's own perceptions. This is not always easy to do, especially when clinicians operate in situations where contextual information can be compromised, as in a therapy room.

Modeling.   Definitions of the modeling technique abound. For our purposes, a very broad definition has been adopted. Modeling can be thought of as an utterance that attempts to demonstrate one viable linguistic option that could be used in that situation. Unlike imitation, expansion, and expatiation, the basis for the modeled utterance does not have to be something said by the child.

Sometimes the clinical expectation in modeling is that the child will imitate the clinician's production. In other clinical applications, modeling provides the child with examples of the acceptable target structure, either in a structured setting or within quasinatural conversation, and no response from the child is expected. What is expected is that the child will listen carefully and observe how the clinician's utterances "work" in the situation. In still others, reinforcers are given to the speaker-model for acceptably modeled utterances. Sometimes the speaker is a third participant (Leonard, 1975), and the client is asked to consider all of the examples provided and then determine what made some of the modeled utterances acceptable and others unacceptable. In this way, the child is led along a path of rule induction.

In some language intervention programs, self-talk and parallel talk are described as separate techniques, but under the broad definition used here, they are both more specific types of modeling. **Self-talk** refers to the clinician's monologue about what she is doing. **Parallel talk** refers to the clinician's running commentary describing what the child is doing. Neither situation necessitates that the child says anything in response. Instead, it is hypothesized that the client is being provided with opportunities to match up ongoing activity with appropriate linguistic encoding in a nonthreatening manner.

Scaffolding.   Bruner (1985) and others have used the term *scaffolding* to describe a pattern of interaction noted in mother-child dyads. It is a description of what Vygotsky may have been referring to when he suggested that children learn through the assistance of competent confederates (Bruner, 1985). Caregivers become well versed in their children's abilities, whether language or motor skills, so that when they request action or information from their children they can predict whether or not their child will be able to successfully comply. It has been generally observed that parents want to see their children succeed. Knowing their child's capabilities is useful not only because caregivers like to have their children "show off" but also because they want to be able to *reasonably* increase the degree of difficulty in the tasks they request of their children. In this way, they can maintain the challenge of the interaction (and thus their child's attention) and promote success at the same time. These two characteristics of a language task will help to ensure their child's continued participation and learning (Kirchner, 1991).

This sort of scaffolding interaction has been demonstrated in repetitions of storybook readings observed between young children and their caregivers. Often children request readings of the same book night after night. When examples of these separate readings were analyzed in a controlled study, Snow and Goldfield (1983) found that the dialogue between caregiver and child changed as the child became more familiar with the book. Specifically, the mother in the study was asking new and more challenging questions of her child when she was reasonably sure the child would answer correctly.

Scaffolding also serves as a useful metaphor for speech-language intervention. That is, treatment goals should always represent achievements still beyond the child's easy grasp. If they are too easily achieved or cannot be achieved, the goals are inappropriate. Reaching an easily achieved goal does not represent true growth, and improbable goals only frustrate the child. Prerequisite skills for achieving selected goals should be in place, making the eventual reaching of the goal reasonable with sufficient teaching and practice. A good clinician constantly monitors a client's performance for evidence that tasks and goals have been appropriately chosen.

S.O.U.L.   S.O.U.L. (*S*ilence, *O*bservation, *U*nderstanding, and *L*istening) is a technique developed in conjunction with the INREAL (Inclass Reactive Language Therapy) program (Weiss, 1981) to establish an empathetic relationship with the child. The four portions of S.O.U.L. are part of the general reactive approach espoused by INREAL clinicians who are taught to "follow the child's lead" rather than impose structure on the client. Remaining silent at least initially in your dealings with a young child, observing what the child is able to do and is interested in, attempting to make sense of the observations you have made, and listening to what the child says whether or not you are involved in the conversation should permit you and the young child to get to know each other. According to the INREAL approach, that is the way an adult earns the right to enter into a therapeutic relationship with a child (Weiss, 1981).

See Table 8-3 for examples of these six techniques carried out in context.

Current Intervention Approaches

This section is divided into three parts, each of which reflects an aspect of the current intervention literature. In one, Fey's (1986) assertiveness-responsiveness scheme will be explained in some detail because underlying it presents a focus on intervention that is functionalist; in other words, it is pragmatic in its orientation and thus very current in its approach. Second, a model useful in treatment focusing on caregiver-child interactions will be discussed (MacDonald & Carroll, 1992a, b). Because the area of treatment efficacy research has burgeoned of late in the area of language intervention for young children, the third section will deal with some of the most recent findings in this very necessary area of research endeavor.

Fey's Assertiveness-Responsiveness Scheme

In his text, *Language Intervention with Young Children,* Fey (1986) described four different types of language impaired children, a method used to delineate these types, and a prescription for planning appropriate intervention based on the characteristics of each. A traditional approach would have been to take the child's production of language form as the basis of

---

TABLE 8-3   Dialogue Excerpts Illustrating Language Intervention Techniques

---

Setting: A preschool classroom at snacktime. A speech-language clinician and a child with a language disorder are seated next to each other. They talk while consuming grape juice and celery sticks spread with peanut buffer.

S.O.U.L.: Before joining the child at the snack table and engaging the child in conversation, the clinician spent several minutes silently observing the child. Listening carefully, the clinician realized that the child had some concerns about the snack. He had never eaten celery before and was told by his teacher that he had to at least try some. The child appeared to be quite apprehensive as the clinician approached.

Imitation
CHILD: Don't want more juice.
CLINICIAN: Don't want more juice?

Expansion
CHILD: That crunchy one.
 (*referring to celery*)
CLINICIAN: You're right. That's a crunchy one.

Expatiation
CHILD: Gimme more uh that.
CLINICIAN: Give me some more of that celery
 because it's *good.*

Modeling (parallel talk)
CLINICIAN: You've licked all the peanut butter out of that
 celery stalk. Now you're chewing that
 celery very carefully. Oh, you're done with it.

Scaffolding
CLINICIAN: That peanut butter is crunchy. That
 celery is crunchy. That snack is crunchy. That
 peanut butter is _____ .
CHILD: Crunchy.
CLINICIAN: Yeah. It sure is. Tell me about that celery.
CHILD: Celery is crunchy.

the classification system by prioritizing analysis of syntax and morphological performance. instead, Fey suggested that the child's ability to *use* the language he has in his productive repertoire is the key for delineating impairment type. This is clearly a functional approach to clinical intervention as evidenced by the fact that the author strongly encourages that data used for diagnostic decision making be collected in a number of natural speaking situations where the child interacts with different co-conversationalists. The child's home and classroom environments should both be carefully scrutinized so that conversational competencies exhibited by the language impaired child in the clinic do not bias the diagnosis of impairment type.

Fey (1986) used two distinctive features of conversational participation as his primary diagnostic variables: conversational assertiveness, which refers to the child's propensity or ability to take a turn in a conversation even when one has not been specifically solicited by the child's co-conversationalist, and conversational responsiveness, the child's propensity or ability to provide appropriate responses to the requests made by the child's conversation partner. If the child exhibits the feature, it is assigned a positive value; if the child does not exhibit the feature, it is assigned a negative value. Four combinations of the two features and their respective values are possible, each describing a different type of language impairment:

Conversational Characteristics	*Description of Child*
+ Assertiveness, + Responsiveness	Active conversationalist
– Assertiveness, + Responsiveness	Passive conversationalist
+ Assertiveness, – Responsiveness	Verbal noncommunicator
– Assertiveness, – Responsiveness	Inactive communicator

Methods for analyzing assertiveness and responsiveness within a child's language sample and cautions for making diagnoses of each of these four language impairment types are presented by the author.

Once the child has been described as exhibiting one or another of these impairment types, intervention programming goals based on the child's conversational characteristics can be implemented (Fey, 1986, p. 99). The basic premise for devising intervention plans for each of these four separate groups is that the general goals for each impairment type are closely related to how the child does and does not use language in conversations. For example, consider a child who has been diagnosed as an active conversationalist by demonstrating that he is assertive and responsive in conversations. This means that the child places himself in situations where conversations are occurring and participates in them even though the language form or content used may not be as sophisticated as would be expected, given the child's age. Nevertheless, this child has demonstrated an appreciation for the assertiveness and responsiveness expected of a conversational partner. It is also likely that the child will recognize the conversational utility of learning new forms. In fact, this is a child for whom spontaneous generalization to using newly trained forms in conversation may occur because the underlying knowledge of conversational speech acts is present and put into practice.

Table 8-4 contains a delineation of basic intervention goals for the four classifications of language impaired children described by Fey (1986). As shown in the table, active con-

TABLE 8-4   Goals Suggested for Children Exhibiting Fey's Patterns of Language Use

Impairment Type	Goals
Active conversationalist (+ assertive, + responsive)	1. New content-form interactions are trained for use with conversation acts already acquired. 2. Child will use old forms to express different conversation acts.
Passive conversationalist (– assertive, + responsive)	1. Child will make more frequent use of acquired assertive conversation acts in social contexts. 2. Child will increase the variety of requestive conversation acts used. 3. New linguistic forms will be learned to express assertive conversation acts.
Verbal noncommunicators (+ assertive, – responsive)	1. The child's responses will demonstrate more relatedness to assertives produced by the co-conversationalist. 2. Topically related utterances will be produced more often. 3. Referents will be indicated more clearly.
Inactive communicators (– assertive, – responsive)	1. Both verbal and nonverbal social bids will occur more frequently in many different social contexts. 2. Add goals for the passive conversationalist.

Adapted from Fey (1986).

versationalists have demonstrated use of a number of different conversation acts (e.g., requests for information, comments, response for clarification, etc.) but need new structures to fulfill them in conversation. According to Fey (p. 99), these children will also need opportunities to recognize that forms already in their repertoire may satisfy a number of different conversational acts (Goal 2). In contrast to active conversationalists, inactive communicators demonstrate a lack of both assertiveness and responsiveness in conversation. These children need to learn their roles in conversation first before specific forms are targeted. Unlike with active conversationalists, it cannot be assumed that these children have an underlying appreciation for conversational act usage.

It is helpful to view the basic goals outlined by Fey as a general umbrella under which more client-specific goals can be listed. Once the classification of the child has been established, treatment may begin because the clinician then has a better understanding of the conversational role(s) typically played by the child and what the child's conversational needs are. Note that conversational competence is the goal for all clients served by this approach.

Use of a Conversational Framework for Treatment

As noted earlier in this chapter, the incorporation of parents into treatment programs is not necessarily a new focus for language interventionists working with young children. Caregivers presumably spend a significant amount of time with their children, involved in daily routine activities that can be used as background for a foreground of language-learning opportunities. MacDonald and Carroll (1992a, b) have delineated a systematic approach for teaching parents, as well as whoever else typically interacts with children, how to facilitate conversational exchanges with young partners who are very limited in how they can make conversational contributions. Their overriding rationale for this program is that when a child with a language disorder can communicate successfully with adults, all developmental areas will benefit, not just the development of the child's communication skills (p. 47).

MacDonald and Carroll (1992a) refer to their approach as the ECO model, signifying that when involving young children with language deficits in conversations it is important also to involve "their social ecology, including the relationships and play contexts and provide natural support for communication and language learning" (p. 39). This approach is highly reminiscent of the framework supplied by the scaffolding technique, discussed above, where a more knowledgeable interactant provides assistance to the degree needed to ensure the less competent participant's success. In this case, all potential language-competent conversation partners can serve as the supportive, enabling participants for the child with language disorders. Notice how the heart of the intervention is in the most social of venues: conversation.

The authors suggest that it is important to teach children to be initiators in their conversational interactions as well as to be adequate responders. Remember from the discussion of work reported by Rice and colleagues (1993) that children with language deficits rarely initiate and only infrequently are they selected to receive the social/conversational bids of their peers. It was this finding that led Rice and colleagues to suggest that classroom teachers intervene directly to redirect the children's adult-directed conversation turns to their classmates. MacDonald and Carroll's (1992a, b) program may represent a prerequisite step in this process in as much as it focuses more directly on the adult-child communications. It provides guidance for adults who want to figure out how to increase the likelihood that children with limited language will be successful communicators in these interactions. Part of the battle may first involve increasing the likelihood that the child will be willing to communicate with the adult.

The following five interactive styles of communication are suggested by MacDonald and Carroll (1992a) as successful for facilitating communication with young children. Adults are told that **balance,** as it relates to the egalitarian nature of sharing the responsibility for conversation, should be a goal. That is, neither partner should be expected to carry the burden of the conversation; similarly, no one participant should dominate the conversation. Adults are also told to promote **responsiveness,** meaning that as rudimentary as a child's early attempts at conversation turn taking are, efforts should be made by the adult to fit these turns within a meaningful conversation framework. It is also important for the adults to **match** the child's current linguistic repertoire with the expectations for conversation participation. This should ensure a maximum of participation on the part of the child because he or she will be less likely to feel overwhelmed with the conversation task and more likely to risk participation. Another interactive style is that of **nondirectiveness,** meaning that the child's lead is followed by the adult where the former clearly has a topic or focus. In addition, nondirectiveness has to do with the adult's demonstrated willingness to allow the child to direct the interaction (i.e., changing or shading topics). Finally, **emotional attachment** refers to the stage of participation in the dyad when the adult begins to converse with the child because the activity is rewarding in and of itself, rather than because the particular conversation serves as a means to an end.

Recent Findings in Intervention Research

There appear to be at least two main focuses for the research involving language intervention with young children. In one branch of the research literature, investigators are attempting to determine whether one service delivery mode is more efficacious than another (Wilcox, Kouri, & Caswell, 1991). In the other branch of intervention research, investigators are comparing two or more treatment methods to determine which work, which may work better, and if there is a differential effect of the treatments, and which children seem to benefit more from which treatment (Weismer, Murray-Branch, & Miller, 1994). Related to this second focus are studies that have attempted to study the relationships that may exist between treatments provided for phonological or grammatical deficits (Tyler & Sandoval, 1994).

A Comparison of Classroom vs. Individual Intervention.   Wilcox, Kouri, & Caswell (1991) reported the results from a study of 20 children roughly between a year and a half and four years of age who were learning their first vocabularies. All of the children had been diagnosed with language delays; half received treatment within a classroom setting and half received individual treatment. Treatment measures of vocabulary growth indicated that neither service delivery situation had yielded superior results until the investigators looked at the children's abilities as measured by generalization to their home environments. Specifically, the children taught the new targeted vocabulary items in the classroom were significantly more likely to generalize these vocabulary words to the home environment than were the children who had received individual instruction (pull-out). Therefore, the researchers concluded that for the purpose of early vocabulary training, the classroom environment is not only a viable location for service delivery but it is also a superior one.

In another study that looked at differences between service delivered within the classroom and outside of the classroom setting, Roberts, Prizant, and McWilliam (1995) focused on the communication dynamics of the clinician-client dyads in both venues. Although they looked carefully at a number of potential differences in conversation behaviors, only two reached significance. Their findings revealed that during the within-class interactions, children were less responsive to the clinicians, showing a significantly greater degree of compliance during the out-of-class sessions. On the other hand, their speech-language clinicians tended to contribute more turns to conversations conducted during out-of-class sessions than those held within the classroom. Given that only these two differences were discovered, the authors suggested that decisions concerning selection of in-class versus out-of-class service delivery should be made on the basis of more than just these differences in communication dynamics.

Treatment Efficacy: Selecting between Treatment Options.   Weismer, Murray-Branch, and Miller (1994) attempted to determine the effects of two procedures—modeling only, and modeling with an evoked production—on teaching new vocabulary items to three young children identified as late talkers. Two of the three subjects demonstrated learning that could be attributed to the treatment procedures but interestingly one of the two children appeared to benefit from one of the techniques and the other benefited from the remaining technique. Unfortunately, attempts to utilize dynamic assessment methods to determine if it would have been possible to predict ahead of time which subject would have done better with which treatment technique failed to yield helpful results. The third subject did not appear to make gains from implementation of either treatment method.

In a study by Camarata, Nelson, and Camarata (1994) two methods, one employing imitation and one employing conversational recasting, were employed to teach a number of different grammatical structures to young children diagnosed with Specific Language Impairment. Although both of the techniques appeared to be effective for facilitating the subjects' productions of the majority of the targeted structures, it was the conversational recasting procedure that was more facilitative when both spontaneous productions of the trained targets and generalized, spontaneous productions of untrained structures were considered. These findings suggest that a method that is less structured and more naturalistic could be better able to foster generalization, specifically to conversational settings.

In a study utilizing the techniques of verbal routines and expansions, Yoder, Spruytenburg, Edwards, and Davies (1995) found that their four subjects, who ranged in age from two years to four and a half years, made gains as measured by mean length of utterance (MLU) over the duration of the treatment. However, looking retrospectively at the results, which included assessing generalization across trainers, interaction styles, and modalities, the authors noted that it was the children in the earlier stages of language development who appeared to make the greater gains than those subjects who were in the later stages, which may have had to do with the measure of progress chosen (MLU), which is less sensitive to gains in language development after the MLU reaches 3.0.

Differential Effects of Phonological and Language Treatment.   Fey, Cleave, Ravida, Long, Dejmal, and Easton (1994) were interested in examining the effects of two grammar-focused treatment programs on the phonological abilities of their group of subjects, all of whom were diagnosed with deficits in both grammatical and phonological development. Given that phonology is a bona fide component of language, exploring the potential connectedness for treatment purposes between syntax and phonology makes sense but represents an area where there is little information to clinicians. Despite the fact that both treatment procedures were shown to have had a positive effect on facilitation of the subjects' grammar performance, there were no obvious effects on the children's phonological skills. The authors concluded that their results do not support a shared effect between language treatment focused on grammar and phonological gains and that difficulties with the speech sound system should be addressed directly with preschool-aged children.

In a study similar in focus, Tyler and Sandoval (1994) reported the findings of their treatment study from preschool-aged subjects who were diagnosed with both language and phonological deficits. There were three possible treatment methods received by the subjects and they yielded significantly different results. Specifically, subjects who were recipients of direct intervention on their phonology targets ended up demonstrating moderate gains for both their phonology and language goals; those who were recipients of language treatment only showed some small language gains but little improvement in their phonology targets. Those subjects who were the recipients of a combined program focusing on both language and phonology demonstrated appreciable positive gains in both areas. The authors suggested that in most cases, if you can only focus on one of the two treatment areas, treating phonology is more likely to provide you with carryover effects to language than the other way around. However, when children are observed to have deficits in both areas the most efficacious route would probably be to treat both phonology and language at the same time. Tyler and Sandoval (1994) noted that it was their least severely involved subjects who benefited the most from the combined speech and language treatments.

Intervention with Children from Multicultural Populations

Providing language intervention services to children from nonmajority populations can represent a challenge to the speech-language clinician who may not share the same cultural background and/or first language with the client. However, Seymour (1991) noted that when speech-language clinicians are forced to think carefully about the potential points of bias in the construction of intervention programs or selection of appropriate assessment tools, they are really not doing anything new and different from the processes they go through to ensure quality service delivery for all of their clients—even those with whom they share cultural background and language. For example, as Terrell and Hale (1992) noted, cultural differences may be manifested as differences in individual learning styles. It will be important for the speech-language clinician to determine what that learning style difference is and how it can be best utilized for language learning purposes. Certainly it is the case that paying attention to how our clients learn best should always be of paramount concern to speech-language clinicians.

When interacting with children from cultures other than one's own, it is critical that the clinician convey both "respect for and appreciation of the child's L1 and culture" (Roseberry-McKibben, 1994, p. 84). Given the system's nature of treatment management for young children, it is very likely that the parents and/or the child's extended family will be involved with the treatment program. Therefore, it will be necessary to determine the family's attitude toward intervention provided by someone from outside their cultural milieu and more generally how they approach the notion of a disorder of communication and treatment for same. Knowing something of the family's cultural beliefs and attitudes will facilitate appropriate communication exchange between the clinician and the family.

We will assume that the readers of this chapter are well aware of the language difference versus language disorder issue, that we should not be providing speech-language therapy for children demonstrating normal development in their first language although they may not yet be competent English language speakers. For those readers who may want some good reference materials to more fully understand this important conceptual point as well as references that specifically address intervention with nonmajority populations, there are several useful references provided in the Suggested Readings section at the end of this chapter.

For children with bona fide language disorders in their first language, treatment should be provided in that first language. Unfortunately, most speech-language clinicians are not bilingually competent, which means that provision of services may need to rely on the teaming of the speech-language clinician with someone who does possess linguistic competence in the child's first language. This person may already be a member of the child's treatment team (e.g., a resource room specialist), or may be a paraprofessional person hired because of bilingual competence. When the speech-language clinician works "through" another person, the type of working relationship that develops may range from one similar to the collaborative consultation model already discussed to one that is very directive, as in the case of the paraprofessional.

Facilitating Generalization

Generalization is such an important topic in the consideration of language intervention that it deserves its own section for discussion. Generalization is the hallmark of a successful intervention program and serves as one of the best ways, if not the best way, for speech-language clinicians to demonstrate the benefits of the programs they execute. As already mentioned, the seasoned clinician will develop a language intervention program with generalization in mind and not "train and hope" (Hughes, 1985, p. 1) that it will occur. If generalization did not occur, language intervention programs would be interminably long because clinicians would have to teach every possible occurrence of every goal.

Generalization is usually described as the use of trained responses in untrained situations. It is evidence that the child actually learned something in intervention, although as will be discussed, that "something" may not always be what was intended by the clinician! Note the use of the term *response* here. Much of the work done concerning generalization has come out of the learning theory tradition with its historical roots in behaviorism (Baer, 1981, cited in Hughes, 1985). Therefore, the child's participation in language exchanges is most often viewed as a response to the stimuli presented by the world, whether by the parent, teacher, peer, sibling, or speech-language clinician.

Generalization Types

There are two basic types of generalization: stimulus generalization and response generalization, and the possibilities for both occurring should be considered. **Stimulus generalization** refers to the use of trained responses in: (a) new settings (e.g., at school when the intervention took place at home or in the playground at school when intervention occurred in the classroom), (b) with new people (e.g., with the classroom teacher when the speech-language clinician provided intervention, with a classmate when the classroom teacher provided intervention, or with a new clinician during the spring semester when the child had been taught the goal by last fall's clinician), and (c) with new materials (e.g., the child responds to the clinician's use of pictures when only object stimuli had previously been used in intervention or the child who was taught narrative skills in intervention using sequencing cards now displays those skills when shown a video tape). In each case, the child exhibits command over language goals that had been taught in a different situation.

Response generalization refers to learning that has transcended a language complexity level or that has extended to untrained examples at the same level of complexity. For example, if a language goal was targeted at the sentence level and the child demonstrates production (or comprehension) of that goal in text (e.g., a narrative or an expository paragraph), response generalization has been achieved. Similarly, if in spontaneous interactions with the clinician the child uses request forms that were never specifically targeted in therapy, response generalization has occurred, provided that *different* request types had been targeted in therapy. If the new request forms in this last example were produced in conversation with the child's classroom teacher, both response and stimulus generalization could be said to have occurred. That is, there were new response types produced (response generalization), and they were produced with a new person (stimulus generalization). Table 8-5 lists some of the differences between stimulus and response generalization.

Why Attempts to Teach Generalization Fail

When generalization does not occur, there are several probable explanations. Just because the clinician has an agenda to enhance generalization through teaching does not mean that the agenda has been conveyed to the child. What may seem perfectly well connected and logical to a competent adult language user may not be quite as logical when perceived by a young child with a language disorder.

In the case of response generalization, what we are really hoping to convey to our young clients is that we are teaching them general rules that can be applied in multiple examples. We do this by teaching a subset of examples that are drawn from all possibilities and that we hope are good, representative examples. Sometimes we use only a few examples of the targeted rule; this has been referred to as "training deep" (Elbert & Gierut, 1985). For some children, the commonality that exists between these few examples cannot be understood. So, in some cases where generalization does not occur, training too deeply may be the problem.

At other times we may make use of too many examples, and the rule may be lost on the young child. Using a large number of exemplars has been referred to by Elbert and Gierut (1985) as "training broad." Training broad may be the problem standing in the way of generalizations for some children in some language learning situations, Speech-language clinicians sometimes must struggle to find that "just right" mixture where we do not burden the child with too many examples or undercut his or her ability to find the general rule by providing too few examples. Sometimes, too, the examples are poor or nonrepresentative, and that may be another reason why generalization fails to occur.

TABLE 8-5   Example Showing Differences between Stimulus and Response Generalization

Scenario: Child, age 5, receives language intervention at school twice weekly in individual sessions. The clinician uses picture cards with action illustrations to prompt child to form past tense of verbs. Child enters the house and announces: "Mom, I walk*ed* home with Joe."

Stimulus Generalization	*Response Generalization*

Use with:
   a new person (with mother),
      or
   in a new setting (at home)
      or
   new materials
   (spontaneous production)
	Use at a different language complexity level (in a sentence, not a single word)
	      or
	Use of an untrained example at the same language complexity level (*walked* was never targeted)

Some empirical data have been forthcoming to assist clinicians in making these kinds of choices. Elbert, Powell, and Swartzlander (1991) noted that the number of exemplars needed for generalization to occur varied significantly among their 19 phonologically impaired subjects. The majority of these children needed three exemplars (59 percent), but 14 percent required 10 exemplars to reach the generalization criterion specified by these investigators.

Response Sets

Another possibility for explaining generalization failure has to do with not knowing the appropriate response set for the examples taught. A **response set** is the extension of a language rule that can be reasonably expected.

For example, few clinicians would expect that by targeting -*ing,* the present progressive morpheme, one could logically expect the client to then generalize to learning to correctly use nominative and objective case pronouns. Because these two goals seem to be entirely unrelated, generalization between them appears to be unlikely. What about teaching the initial /s/ sound and testing for generalization to the final /s/? That seems to be logical and could be expected, although there are a number of possible mitigating variables. If it turned out that probe testing revealed generalization to final /s/, it could be said that for that child initial /s/ and final /s/ belonged to the same response set.

This discussion of response set is important because it is possible to become overzealous in the quest for generalization and to expect generalization where generalization is not likely to occur. Clinicians must remember to try to take the child's perspective and to keep the expectation for generalization from exceeding what is reasonable. Children who have language disorders have already experienced too much failure. Often, their failure to generalize can be traced back to the clinician's own faulty planning. More specifically, the child's failure to generalize could be the result of expecting generalization where none should be expected; using exemplars in intervention that are poor representatives of the rule, principle, or construct being taught; using too few or too many examples; or not having spent enough time in intervention to rightfully expect generalization learning to have occurred in the first place.

Planning for Generalization

As stated throughout this chapter, clinicians must plan strategies for generalization from the very start of intervention planning. Remember that to some extent concerns about generalization and context-appropriate treatment led to the movement toward classroom-based language intervention. Providing intervention in a context (the classroom) where newly taught gains in language competencies could be frequently utilized should make it more likely that generalization to the classroom *without* the presence of the clinician will occur. Opportunities for using the new language abilities should occur whether or not the clinician is present. The speech-language clinician who wants to encourage generalization would be wise to spend substantial time pointing out to the child what the identifying characteristics of these opportunities are.

Hughes's (1985) text, *Language Treatment and Generalization,* contains many thoughtful and thought-provoking suggestions for generalization planning. The author presents two

TABLE 8-6 Ways to Make Therapy Situations More Like Natural Environments

1. Alter the physical attributes of the setting; e.g., move tables and chairs, add carpeting and posters, to simulate natural environments where the target language behaviors are expected to occur. Conduct therapy in a variety of nontherapy settings, e.g., hallways, classrooms, playground.

2. Alter the visual stimulus materials used: e.g., use photographs taken of the client in various places. Use popular magazines, toys, entertainment items (radio, stereo, watch, video game), board games, clothing, jewelry, grooming items.

3. Alter the language used by the clinician: e.g., reduce the frequency of direct instructions. Try role-playing various scenes that simulate experiences within a variety of natural environments.

4. Move from one-to-one interaction between clinician and client to small-group interaction. Use turn-taking in dialogues on a given topic, with feedback given to individuals after the dialogue is done or after a certain time period.

5. Use less direct and less artificial consequences for correct and incorrect production of the language target behaviors. Instead of verbal consequences such as "No, say 'She is baking a cake'" try a more subtle cue to prompt a self-correction of grammatical structure, such as "What did you say?" with a puzzled facial expression.

From D. Hughes, *Language Treatment and Generalization: A Clinician's Handbook* (p. 157), San Diego: College-Hill Press, 1985. Reprinted by permission.

sets of these suggestions, one for making therapy more like natural environments (p. 157) and one for making the natural environment more like therapy (p. 158). These appear in Tables 8-6 and 8-7. In each case, the clinician attempts to give the client a broader perspective of where it is appropriate to use his new language skills. It is not uncommon to hear a young, noncompliant child tell a parent who is trying to do carryover work in the home: "I don't do that with you. I do that with [name of child's speech-language clinician]." In these cases, the child appears to categorize language functioning according to setting. Certain language is used in one setting and not in another. If the child "knows" this, then we may have fostered it, and we will have to spend time presenting counterevidence to *un*teach it.

Clinicians should also recognize that some goals will be more easily generalized than others due to the inherent, functional nature of the goal. These more easily generalized goals should be considered priorities in intervention because they may assist the young child in understanding the gist of generalization. Consider, for example, the goal of demonstrating consistent production of request forms (e.g., "Can I have that?") versus the goal of spontaneously producing superlative adjective forms (e.g., *fluffiest*). Being able to produce a variety of request forms (e.g., "What did you say?" "Tell me another story" "Do you know where Marc is?") will permit a child to specifically request the information or action desired. Request forms are produced frequently in conversations and allow speakers to exert some control over an ongoing conversation and the immediate world. On the other hand, having a firm grasp on how to form superlative adjective forms is less functional—this ability represents one more piece of the language puzzle. Superlative adjective forms are neither as common nor as critical to communication as the request form.

Last, as the child begins to grasp the specified language goal within a task or intervention structure, generalization can be facilitated if the speech-language clinician will begin to systematically alter the teaching situation. Hughes (1985) referred to this as "teaching loosely" (p. 160). Within the teaching phase of intervention, the clinician adds some change to the proceedings. Perhaps this will mean that another person, maybe a parent, begins to sit in on the treatment sessions. It could mean that feedback is given on every other attempt at the teaching task made by the child, so that the intervention more closely resembles life outside the therapy room. Outside the therapy room, it is rare indeed to receive a pat on the back for a well-constructed sentence! Regardless of how the clinician attempts to loosen up the intervention process, the end result should be the same: intervention that more closely resembles something other than intervention.

A Final Word on Generalization

These basic suggestions for promoting generalization apply whether intervention takes place in or outside a classroom and whether a teacher collaborates with the speech-language clinician or the speech-language clinician provides direct service delivery. The variables involved in enhancing generalization (e.g., settings, providers, targets for generalization) will differ from case to case depending on how intervention was originally de-

TABLE 8-7   Ways to Make Natural Environments More Like Therapy Situations

1. Alter the verbal and nonverbal behaviors of parents, siblings, and other family members. For example, teach parents to ask the kinds of questions that will provide opportunities for display of the language target behavior. Teach parents and siblings to recognize and give positive responses to the language target and to ignore or give negative responses to errors in language target production.
2. Alter the verbal and nonverbal behaviors of peers, friends, teachers, and other people found frequently in nontreatment environments. For example, teach peers and teachers to provide prompts for production of language targets and to respond appropriately to correct and incorrect productions of language targets.
3. Alter the physical environment within the living space of the client. For example, the dining arrangements in group homes or the recreational spaces within institutional settings might be altered to provide more opportunities for display of the language target behaviors. Arrange the physical setting to promote social interaction among groups of clients or among clients and staff.
4. Alter the visual stimuli available to talk about. For example, plan to change toys or games available for recreation or plan and take trips to interesting places to provide topics for discussion and social interaction. Remember, we often talk about *new* information and events or *changes* in routines.
5. Teach the client self-monitoring and self-reinforcement behaviors that can be used within natural environments. This may include self-reminders to produce the language target—e.g., wearing a Band-Aid or marking a spot that will be noticed frequently—in order to remind the client to produce and monitor the behavior.

From D. Hughes, *Language Treatment and Generalization: A Clinician's Handbook* (p. 158), San Diego: College-Hill Press, 1985. Reprinted by permission.

vised. However, no matter what the format of the language intervention may be, there is no excuse for not promoting generalization from the very first intervention session.

Some Thought-Provoking Questions for the Future

When we consider language intervention for young children, it seems that we continue to have at least two critical questions left to finish answering. The first has to do with our ability as professionals to predict language-learning outcomes and the second can be best described as an issue of treatment efficacy. That is, we need to be better able to predict on the basis of their earliest behaviors which children, who present themselves as at-risk for language-learning problems, will actually experience difficulties and what will be the magnitude of those problems. The logical concomitant question has to do with how do we then go about selecting the most efficient and most effective treatment plan for each individual client on our caseload.

Note that the twin questions of enhancing our powers of predictability and the efficacy of the treatment we provide both carry with them sets of underlying assumptions. The predictability question, for example, presupposes the availability of valid and reliable measures for evaluating a child's early language, social, and motor behaviors and the existence of adequate information concerning how these behaviors relate to normal developmental expectations. Questions of efficacy also have several underlying assumptions. In order to select a most efficacious treatment plan, preliminary studies will first have to establish that each option is efficient and effective in its own right. Additional research will then have to determine which intervention plans are best suited to individual children based on carefully constructed profiles of each child's language-learning strengths and weaknesses.

Answering questions that will allow us to serve as reliable predictors of future speech and language performance as well as provide the most efficient and effective intervention for our clients represents a challenge to clinicians and researchers alike. In fact, it is likely that it will take many years to be able to approach a comprehensive answer to either one. However, the answers to these questions are not luxuries. Rather, they are necessary if we are to continue to provide our clients and patients with the best possible clinical services.

Summary

This chapter described the speech-language clinician's role in the development of language intervention programs for young children. It is important to understand the challenging nature of the many decisions the clinician must make along the way, the different options available for selection, and the rationales behind those selections. Given the changing demographics of the young clients we serve as speech-language clinicians, it is additionally important that we acknowledge the ways in which cultural differences should affect the treatment choices we make.

Further, an understanding of the different theories of language acquisition allows the speech-language clinician to appreciate the evolution of the speech-language clinician's role in the therapeutic process itself. Specifically, many clinicians have moved from viewing themselves as language "trainers" to language "facilitators." This change can be directly credited to belief in the child as an active participant in the language development process and the view that learning language involves the learning of a generative rule system.

Language intervention may be accomplished in many different settings. The speech-language clinician should acknowledge the benefits and drawbacks to each service delivery model in terms of client progress. In addition, the roles of the classroom teacher and the child's parents in the successful completion of the language intervention program should be considered. It is rarely the case that language intervention for a child can afford to be viewed as the responsibility of the speech-language clinician alone.

Finally, the concept of generalization is one of the most essential to the development of appropriate language intervention procedures. Because language is generalizable, we are able to assume that a small and carefully chosen subset of all of the possible examples of a goal form or structure will be sufficient to teach a more general rule. For language intervention programs to work, clinicians must pay close attention to how they expect the child to generalize their learning from the first intervention contact. Troubleshooting the expected course of generalization from the very first planning stages will allow the speech-language clinician a greater chance for succeeding in increasing the language competence of the young child with a language disorder.

Study Questions

1. How do parents and classroom teachers serve indispensable functions in the success of language intervention programs developed for young children?
2. Assume that a speech-language clinician has the luxury of determining which service delivery model will be used in each of her cases. Delineate the pros and cons of choosing a pull-out, classroom-based, or collaborative consultation service delivery model.
3. If generalization is essential to the success of any language intervention program, clinicians should account for it as early as possible in their planning. List five general strategies for enhancing the generalization observed in a young language-disordered child. Indicate the child's age, a particular goal for consideration, and the service delivery model through which the child receives language intervention.
4. You are planning a language intervention program for a young child from a culture other than your own. What information would you want to have prior to developing the plan that would assist you in designing an appropriate program? What information would you be able to collect during a diagnostic therapy phase that would help you to fine-tune your treatment approach?
5. Which information, collected during the evaluation/assessment phase of service delivery to a particular client, would help you to develop an appropriate treatment plan?

Suggested Readings

Fortunately for those of us who practice in the area of speech-language pathology, the literature pertinent to the planning of language intervention with young children is a burgeoning one, with excellent new sources of information available almost continually. What follows is a listing of what I believe to be some of the best sources of information currently available.

Fey, M. (1986). *Language intervention with young children.* Needham Heights, MA: Allyn & Bacon.

Fey, M., Windsor, J., & Warren, S. (1995). (Eds.), *Language intervention: Preschool through the elementary years.* Baltimore: Paul H. Brookes.

Lynch, E., & Hanson, M. (1992). (Eds.), *Developing cross-cultural competence: A guide for working with young children and their families.* Baltimore: Paul H. Brookes.

MacDonald, J., & Carroll, J. (1992). Communicating with young children: An ecological model for clinicians, parents, and collaborative professionals. *American Journal of Speech-Language Pathology,* 1(4), 39–48.

van Kleeck, A. (1994). Potential cultural bias in training parents as conversational partners with their children who have delays in language development. *American Journal of Speech-Language Pathology,* 3, 67–78.

References

American Speech-Language-Hearing Association (1995). *Prevalence of communication disorders in the United States.* Rockville, MD: ASHA Science and Research Department.

Aram, D., Ekelman, B., & Nation, J. (1984). Preschoolers with language disorders: 10 years later. *Journal of Speech and Hearing Research,* 27, 232–244.

Bricker, D. (1986). An analysis of early intervention programs: Attendant issues and future directions (pp. 28–65). In R. Morris and B. Blatt (Eds.), *Special education: Research and trends.* New York: Pergamon Press.

Bruner, J. (1985). Vygotsky: A historical and conceptual perspective. In J. Wertsch (Ed.), *Culture, communication, and cognition: Vygotskian perspectives.* Cambridge: Cambridge University Press.

Brush, E. (1987, November). Public school language, speech and hearing services in the 1990's. Paper presented to the annual convention of the American Speech-Language-Hearing Association, New Orleans.

Camarata, S., Nelson, K., & Camarata, M. (1994). Comparison of conversational-recasting and imitative procedures for training grammatical structures in children with Specific Language Impairment. *Journal of Speech and Hearing Research,* 37, 1414–1423.

Cole, L. (1989). E pluribus pluribus: Multicultural imperatives and the 1990s and beyond. *ASHA,* 31, 65–70.

Connell, P. (1982). On training language rules. *Language, Speech and Hearing Services in Schools,* 13, 231–248.

Craig, H. (1993). Clinical forum: Language and social skills in the school-age population, social skills of children with specific language impairment: Peer relationships. *Language, Speech, and Hearing Services in Schools,* 24, 206–215.

Craig, H., & Washington, J. (1993). Access behaviors of children with specific language impairment. *Journal of Speech and Hearing Research,* 36, 311–321.

Crais, E. (1991). *A practical guide to embedding family-centered content into existing speech-language pathology coursework.* Chapel Hill, NC: Carolina Institute for Research in Infant Personnel Preparation.

Cross, T. (1978). Mothers' speech adjustments: The contribution of selected child listener variables. In C. Snow & C. Ferguson (Eds.), *Talking to children: Language input and acquisition.* Cambridge: Cambridge University Press.

Damico, J., & Damico, S. (1993). Language and social skills from a diversity perspective: Considerations for the speech-language pathologist. *Language, Speech, and Hearing Services in Schools,* 24, 236–243.

Elbert, M., & Gierut, J. (1985). *Handbook of clinical phonology.* San Diego: College-Hill Press.

Elbert, M., Powell, T., & Swartzlander, P. (1991). Toward a technology of generalization. How many exemplars are sufficient? *Journal of Speech and Hearing Research,* 34 (1), 81–87.

Ellis Weismer, S. (1988). Specific language learning problems. In D. Yoder & R. Kent (Eds.). *Decision making in speech-language pathology.* Toronto: B. C. Decker.

Ensher, G. (1989). The first three years: Special education perspectives on assessment and intervention. *Topics in Language Disorders,* 10 (1), 80–90.

Farber, J., Denenberg, M., Klyman, S., & Lachman, P. (1992). Language Resource Room Level of Service: An urban school district approach to integrative treatment. *Language, Speech, & Hearing Services in Schools,* 23, 293–299.

Fey, M. (1986). *Language intervention with young children.* Needham Heights, MA: Allyn & Bacon.

Fey, M. (1988). Dismissal criteria for the language-impaired child. In D. Yoder & R. Kent (Eds.), *Decision making in speech-language pathology.* Toronto: B. C. Decker.

Fey, M., Catts, H., & Larrivee, L. (1995). Preparing preschoolers for the academic and social challenges of school (pp. 3–34). In M. Fey, J. Windsor & S. Warren (Eds.), *Language intervention: Preschool through the elementary years.* Baltimore: Paul H. Brookes.

Fey, M., Cleave, P., Long, S., & Hughes, D. (1993). Two approaches to one facilitation of grammar in children with language impairment: An experimental evaluation. *Journal of Speech and Hearing Research,* 36, 141–157.

Fey, M., Cleave, P., Ravida, A., Long, S., Dejmal, A., & Easton, D. (1994). Effects of grammar facilitation on the phonological performance of children with speech and language impairments. *Journal of Speech and Hearing Research,* 57, 594–607.

Frasinelli, L., Superior, K., & Meyers, J. (1983). A consultation model for speech and language intervention. *ASHA,* 25 (11), 25–30.

Fujiki, M., & Brinton, B. (1984). Supplementing language therapy: Working with the classroom teacher. *Language, Speech and Hearing Services in Schools,* 15, 98–109.

Girolametto, L. Tannock, R., & Siegel, L. (1993). Consumer-merited evaluation of interactive language intervention. *American Journal of Speech-Language Pathology,* 2, 41–51.

Goldberg, S. (1993). *Clinical intervention: A philosophy and methodology for clinical practice.* New York: Macmillan.

Guralnick, M. & Paul-Brown, D. (1977). The nature of verbal interactions among handicapped and non-handicapped preschool children. *Child Development,* 48, 254–260.

Hall, P., & Tomblin, J. (1978). A follow-up study of children with articulation and language disorders. *Journal of Speech and Hearing Disorders,* 43, 227–241.

Hanson, M. (1992). Ethnic, cultural, and language diversity in intervention settings (pp. 1–18). In E. Lynch & M. Hanson (Eds.), *Developing cross-cultural competence: A guide for working with young children and their families.* Baltimore: Paul H. Brookes.

Hegde, M. (1985). *Treatment procedures in communicative disorders.* San Diego: College-Hill Press.

Hughes, D. (1985). *Language treatment and generalization: A clinician's handbook.* San Diego: College-Hill Press.

Idelstein, P. (1995). Swimming against the mainstream. In J. Kauffman & P. Hallahan (Eds.), *The illusion of full inclusion: A comprehensive critique of a current special education bandwagon.* Austin, TX: Pro-Ed.

Jenkins, J., & Heinen, A. (1989). Students' preferences for service delivery: Pull-out, in-class, or integrated models. *Exceptional Children,* 55 (6), 516–523.

Johnston, J. (1983). What is language intervention? The role of theory. In J. Miller, D. Yoder, & R. Schiefelbusch (Eds.), *Contemporary issues in language intervention (ASHA Reports No. 12).* Rockville, MD: American Speech-Language-Hearing Association.

Kauffman, J., & Hallahan, D. (1995). Toward a comprehensive delivery system for special education. In J. Kauffman & D. Hallahan (Eds.), *The illusion of full inclusion: A comprehensive critique of a current special education bandwagon.* Austin, TX: Pro-Ed.

King, R., Jones, C., & Lasky, E. (1982). In retrospect: A fifteen-year follow-up report of speech-language disorders in children. *Language, Speech and Hearing Services in School,* 13, 24–32.

Kirchner, D. (1991). Using verbal scaffolding to facilitate conversational participation and language acquisition in children with developmental disorders. *Journal of Childhood Communicative Disorders,* 14, 81–98.

Klein, M., & Briggs, M. (1987). Facilitating mother-infant communicative interaction in mothers of high-risk infants. *Journal of Childhood Communicative Disorders,* 14, 81–98.

Leonard, L. (1975). Modeling as a clinical procedure in language training. *Language, Speech and Hearing Services in Schools,* 6, 72, 85.

Leonard, L. (1981). Facilitating linguistic skills in children with specific language impairment: A review. *Applied Psycholinguistics,* 2, 89–118.

Leonard, L. (1983). Discussion: Part II: Defining the boundaries of language disorders in children. In J. Miller, D. Yoder, & R. Schiefelbusch (Eds.), *Contemporary issues in language intervention (ASHA Reports No. 12).* Rockville, MD: American Speech-Language-Hearing Association.

Leonard, L. (1991). New trends in the study of early language acquisition. *American Speech-Language-Hearing Association,* 33 (4), 43–44.

Lynch, E. (1992). Developing cross-cultural competence. In E. Lynch & M. Hanson (Eds.), *Developing cross-cultural competence.* Baltimore: Paul H. Brookes.

Lowenthal, B. (1987). Public Law 99-457: An ounce of prevention. (ERIC Document 293 300).

Lynch, E. (1992). Developing cross-cultural competence. In E. Lynch & M. Hanson (Eds.). *Developing cross-cultural competence.* Baltimore: Paul H. Brookes.

Lyngaas, K., Nyberg, B., Hoekenga, R., & Gruenewald, L. (1983). Language intervention in the multiple contexts of the public school setting. In J. Miller, D. Yoder, & R. Schiefelbusch (Eds.), *Contemporary issues in language intervention (ASHA Reports No. 12).* Rockville, MD: American Speech-Language-Hearing Association.

MacDonald, J., & Carroll, J. (1992a). Communicating with young children: An ecological model for clinicians, parents and collaborative professionals. *American Journal of Speech-Language Pathology,* 1 (4), 39–48.

MacDonald, J., & Carroll, J. (1992b). A social partnership model for assessing early communication development: An intervention model for preconversational children. *Language, Speech, & Hearing Services in Schools,* 23, 113–124.

MacDonald, J., & Gillette, Y. (1984). Conversation engineering: A pragmatic approach to early social competence. *Seminars in Speech and Language,* 5, 171–183.

Mandler, J. (1990). A new perspective on cognitive development in infancy. *American Scientist,* 78 (3), 236–243.

Marvin, C. (1987). Consultation services: Changing roles for SLPs. *Journal of Childhood Communication Disorders,* 11, 1–15.

Maxwell, S., & Wallach, G. (1984). The language learning disabilities connection: Symptoms of early language disability change over time. In G. Wallach & K. Butler (Eds.), *Language learning disabilities in school-age children.* Baltimore: Williams & Wilkins.

McLean, J. (1983). Historical perspectives on the content of child language programs. In J. Miller, D. Yoder, & R. Schiefelbusch (Eds.), *Contemporary issues in language intervention (ASHA Reports No. 12).* Rockville MD: American Speech-Language-Hearing Association.

Miller, L. (1989). Classroom-based language intervention. *Language, Speech and Hearing Services in Schools,* 20, 153–169.

Nelson, C., & Blakeley, R. (1989). Clinicianship: What is it? *Seminars in Speech and Language,* 10 (2), 102–112.

Newhoff, M. (1995). So many fads, so little data. *Clinical Connection,* 8 (3), 1–5.

Odom, S., & McEvoy, M. (1988). Integration of young children with handicaps and normally developing children. In S. Odom & M. Karnes (Eds.), *Early intervention for infants and children with handicaps.* Baltimore: Paul H. Brookes.

Olswang, L., & Bain, B. (1985). Monitoring phoneme acquisition for making treatment withdrawal decisions. *Applied Psycholinguistics,* 6, 17–37.

Olswang, L., & Bain, B. (1991). Clinical Forum: Treatment efficacy: When to recommend intervention. *Language, Speech, and Hearing Services in Schools,* 22, 255–263.

Pierce, P., & McWilliams, P. (1993). Emerging literacy and children with severe speech and physical impairments (SSPI): Issues and possible intervention strategies. *Topics in Language Disorders,* 1 (2), 47–57.

Prelock, P., Miller, B., & Reed, N. (1995). Collaborative partnerships in a language in the classroom program. *Language, Speech, and Hearing Services in Schools, 26,* 286–292.

Ratner, N., & Bruner, J. (1978). Games, social exchange and the acquisition of language. *Journal of Child Language, 5,* 392–401.

Records, N., Tomblin, J., & Freese, P. (1992). The quality of life among young adults with histories of Specific Language Impairment. *American Journal of Speech-Language Pathology, 1* (2), 44–53.

Records, N., & Weiss, A. (1990). Clinical judgment: An overview. *Journal of Childhood Communication Disorders, 13* (2), 153–165.

Rescorla, L., & Schwartz, E. (1990). Outcome of toddlers with specific expressive language delay. *Applied Psycholinguistics, 11,* 393–407.

Rice, M. (1993). Social consequences of specific language impairment. In H. Grimm & H. Skowranek (Eds.), *Language acquisition problems and reading disorders: Aspects of diagnosis and intervention* (pp. 111–128). New York: de Gruyter.

Rice, M., Hadley, P., & Alexander, A. (1993). Social biases toward children with speech and language impairments: A correlative causal model of language limitation. *Applied Psycholinguistics, 14,* 445–471.

Rice, M., Sell, M., & Hadley, P. (1991). Social interactions of speech and language impaired children. *Journal of Speech and Hearing Research, 34,* 1299–1307.

Roberts, J., Prizant, B., & McWilliam, R. (1995). Out-of-class versus in-class service delivery in language intervention: Effects on communication interaction with young children. *American Journal of Speech-Language Pathology, 4* (2), 87–94.

Roseberry-McKibben, C. (1994). Assessment and intervention for children with Limited English Proficiency and language disorders. *American Journal of Speech-Language Pathology, 3* (3), 77–88.

Roseberry-McKibben, C., & Eicholtz, G. (1994). Serving children with Limited English Proficiency in the schools: A national survey. *Language, Speech, & Hearing Services in the Schools, 25,* 156–164.

Scarborough, H., & Dorbrich, W. (1990). Development of children with early language delay. *Journal of Speech and hearing Research, 33,* 70–83.

Schiefelbusch, R. (1983). Language intervention in children: What is it? In J. Miller, D. Yoder, & R. Schiefelbusch (Eds.), *Contemporary issues in language intervention (ASHA Reports No. 12).* Rock-

ville, MD: American Speech-Language-Hearing Association.

Screen, R., & Anderson, N. (1994). *Multicultural perspectives in communication disorders.* San Diego: Singular.

Seymour, H. (January, 1991). Language acquisition and disorders. A presentation to the Multicultural Literacy in Communication Disorders Conference, Sea Island, GA.

Shewan, C. (1988). Omnibus Survey: Adaptation and progress in times of change. *ASHA, 30* (8), 27–30.

Shriberg, L., & Kwiatkowski, J. (1982). Phonological disorders II: A conceptual framework for management. *Journal of Speech and Hearing Disorders, 47,* 242–256.

Snow, C. (1986). Conversations with children. In P. Fletcher & M. Garman (Eds.), *Language acquisition* (2nd ed.). New York: Cambridge University Press.

Snow, C., & Goldfield, B. (1983). Turn the page please: Situation-specific language acquisition. *Journal of Child Language, 10,* 551–569.

Snyder, L. (1980). Have we prepared the language disordered child for school? *Topics in Language Disorders, 1* (1), 29–45.

Snyder, L., Apolloni, T., & Cooke, T. (1977). Integrated settings at the early childhood level: The role of non-retarded peers. *Exceptional Children, 43,* 262–266.

Sparks, S. (1989). Assessment and intervention with at-risk infants and toddlers: Guidelines for the speech-language pathologist. *Topics in Language Disorders, 10* (1), 43–56.

Stainback, S., Stainback, W., & Forest, M. (Eds.). (1989). *Educating all students in the mainstream of regular education.* Baltimore: Paul H. Brookes.

Stainback, W., & Stainback, S. (1990). Support networks for inclusive schooling: Independent integrated education. Baltimore: Paul H. Brookes.

Terrell, B., & Hale, J. (1992). Serving a multicultural population: Different learning styles. *American Journal of Speech-Language Pathology, 1* (2), 5–8.

Tyler, A., & Sandoval, K. (1994). Preschoolers with phonological and language disorders: Treating different linguistic domains. *Language, Speech, and Hearing Services in Schools, 25,* 215–234.

van Kleeck, A. (1994). Potential cultural bias in training parents as conversational partners with their children who have delays in language development. *American Journal of Speech-Language Pathology,* 3, 67–78.

van Kleeck, A., & Richardson, A. (1988). Language delay in the child. In N. Lass, L. McReynolds, J. Northern, & D. Yoder (Eds.), *Handbook of speech-language pathology and audiology.* Toronto: B. C. Decker.

Venn, M., Wolery, M., Fleming, L., DeCesare, L., Morris, A., & Cuffs, M. (1993). Effects of teaching preschool peers to use the mand-model procedure duing snack activities. *American Journal of Speech-Language Pathology,* 2 (1), 38–46.

Wallach, G., & Butler, K. (1994). Creating communication, literacy, and academic success (pp. 2–26). In G. Wallach and K. Butler (Eds.), *Language learning disabilities in school age children and adolescents: Some principles and application.* New York: Macmillan.

Warren, S., & Kaiser, A. (1988). Research in early language intervention. In S. Odom & M. Karnes (Eds.), *Early intervention for infants and children with handicaps.* Baltimore: Paul H. Brookes.

Weismer, S., Murray-Branch, J., & Miller, J. (1994). A prospective longitudinal study of language development in late talkers. *Journal of Speech and Hearing Research,* 37, 852–867.

Weiss, A., & Nakamura, M. (1992). Language-normal children in preschool classrooms for children with language impairments. *Language, Speech and Hearing Services in Schools,* 23, 64–70.

Weiss, A., Tomblin, J., & Robin, D. (1994). Language Disorders. In J. Tomblin, H. Morris, & D. Spriesterbach (Eds.). *Diagnosis in Speech-Language Pathology.* San Diego: Singular.

Weiss, R. (1981). INREAL intervention for language handicapped and bilingual children. *Journal of the Division of Early Childhood,* 4, 40–51.

Wilcox, M., Kouri, T., & Caswell, S. (1991). Early language intervention: A comparison of classroom and individual treatment. *American Journal of Speech-Language Pathology,* 1 (1), 49–62.

Wolery, M., & Wilbers, J. (Eds.). (1994). Including children with special needs in early childhood programs. *Research Monograph of the National Assocation for the Education of Young Children,* 6, NAEYC, Washington, D.C.

Yoder, P., Spruytenburg, H., Edwards, A., & Davies, B. (1995). Effect of verbal routine contexts and expansions on gains in the Mean Length of Utterance in children with developmental delays. *Language, Speech, and Hearing Services in Schools,* 26, 21–32.

Zigler, E., & Hall, N. (1995). Mainstreaming and the philosophy of normalization. In J. Kauffman and D. Hallahan (Eds.), *The illusion of full inclusion.* Austin, TX: Pro-Ed.

Chapter 9

Language Intervention in School Settings

NICKOLA WOLF NELSON
Western Michigan University

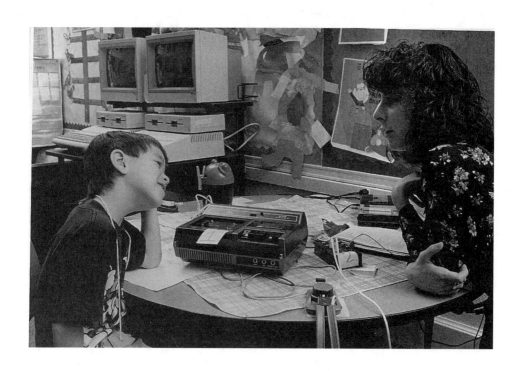

Serving children with communication disorders in school settings is both demanding and rewarding. School is where children spend most of their days. Experiences in school influence how students define themselves, what they know, how they think, how they communicate orally and in writing, and how they live their lives. Students who can handle the specialized language demands of formal education have an important tool for success and failure both in school and beyond. Providing services in school settings allows professionals to collaborate across territorial boundaries and to design programs that are relevant to students' functional communicative needs as they continue to learn language and to use language to learn.

Children with language disorders make up the largest proportion of school speech-language pathology caseloads. Data gathered by the American Speech-Language-Hearing Association (S. Dublinske, personal communication, March 18, 1987) showed that 53 percent of children on caseloads in the schools had language disorders, compared with only 28 percent with articulation disorders. Infants, toddlers, and preschoolers who have language disorders, or who are at risk for developmental delays of various types, may also receive services from professionals employed by school systems. However, because the policies and procedures for providing services to infants and young children are discussed elsewhere, this chapter is confined to a discussion of the language assessment and intervention needs of school-age children.

Working with children in school settings requires a tremendous breadth of knowledge on the part of speech-language pathologists and other language specialists (e.g., teachers or consultants for students with learning disabilities). Professionals in school settings must be knowledgeable about normal development and learning, varied types of communicative and learning disorders (both developmental and acquired), curriculum development and teaching methodology, and participating as members of collaborative teams. They cannot afford to specialize in any one area of development to the exclusion of others. The problems are too complex.

Children with language disorders may have concomitant voice problems or fluency disorders; they may have physical disabilities that make it difficult to produce intelligible speech or to write with a pencil; they may have developmental delays in multiple areas; or they may have social interaction problems with teachers and peers—as well as countless other possibilities. As discussed throughout this book, individuals with language and communicative disorders may have related impairments involving learning disabilities; mental retardation; hearing impairment; autism; social-emotional, attentional, or behavior problems—again, among numerous other possibilities.

In this chapter, two sets of multiple factors are considered that influence school programming for children and adolescents with language disorders: one set derives from influences of "best practice," and the other derives from influences of "public policy." Of course, the ideal situation is when best practice and public policy are perfectly compatible, but this is not always the case. When the implementation of best practice is impeded by misguided public policy, professionals need to recognize the problem and to know how to advocate for change.

This chapter is divided into three sections, followed by a case example. The first offers a brief overview of some recent changes in educational practices. The second is a summary of five principles of best practice to guide service delivery for school-age children and adolescents with language and communicative disorders. The third is a review of public policies that influence the provision of services to school-age children in schools in the United States, presented as a series of eight procedural steps. At the conclusion of these three sections a case example is presented to illustrate best practice and public policy and some of the challenges to be overcome in implementing them.

Recent Shifts in Educational Practices

The Context of Educational Reform

The provision of speech-language and audiology services to children with communication disorders in school settings can only be understood within the broader context of educational systems. Public education is never out of a nation's public focus. As "school reform" has become a watchword in the United States, local school districts and national policy makers have implemented change processes with implications for all school children. Local school districts do so through such strategies as "site-based management" (David, 1995–1996), and the nation does so through federal legislation, such as the Educate America Act (Public Law 103-227, 1994). That law established Goals 2000, which included goals of literacy and successful completion of high school for all students. These goals are not equally accessible to all students, however, especially students whose language and learning disabilities stand in the way of their school success. Professionals who understand the specialized language learning needs of such students must work side by side with educators with general education responsibilities if the nation is to come closer to meeting the broader goals of universal school success.

A look at past success rates can be discouraging—or it can be taken as a challenge by the next generation of school professionals. At the present, a whopping 24.4 percent of youth in the general population fail to complete high school, and even higher dropout figures have been reported for students with learning disabilities (36.1 percent), speech impairments (including language impairments; 32.5 percent), and serious emotional disturbance (54.8 percent; Council for Exceptional Children, 1994).

How to turn these dismal success rates around is, of course, the ultimate question. Although there are no simple answers, a primary purpose of the current chapter is to show how to help students with language problems fit better in the general educational system and to support them in their quests for success. Serving this purpose requires looking at students with special needs first as people with abilities, rather than simply as people with impairments. Recent changes in educational and special educational practices have been designed to foster this shift in perspective.

Legislation Passed as IDEA

As a major component of this shift, the Education for All Handicapped Children Act (originally passed by the U.S. Congress in 1975 as PL 94-142) was renamed the Individuals with Disabilities Education Act when it was reauthorized in 1990 as Public Law 101-476. This change reflected a shift in attitude from considering the needs of *handicapped children* to considering the needs of *children with disabilities*. Now, throughout the law, children with special needs are referred to as *having disabilities* rather than as *being handicapped*. The new terminology emphasizes that children with disabilities are individuals first; their disabilities do not constitute their identities.

The change also reflects the increased recognition of disabilities as contextually based. The World Health Organization defines *disability* as a reduced ability to *meet daily living needs* (Wood, 1980). That is, as daily living needs change under different contexts and in varied stages of life, degree of disability may vary as well (Frey, 1984; Wood, 1980). This means that children may be relatively more disabled in some contexts because the mismatches between their abilities and the communicative demands of the context are relatively greater. In other contexts, children may be relatively less disabled, either because the communicative demands of the situation are closer to their reach or because an adult facilitator is aware of the mismatch and consciously builds a bridge or "scaffold" to help children attain communicative access they would not otherwise have.

Focus on Inclusion

Traditional approaches to special education have not ignored this relationship. In fact, most special education classrooms and center programs (i.e., school buildings specially adapted for individuals with severe disabilities) have been designed to provide special contexts with different standards and curricula for children who could not meet the demands of regular school settings. The problem is that when children are removed from general education settings, they are also removed from opportunities to participate with peers in other ways and to learn the skills they need to compete in society (Calculator & Jorgenson, 1994). The implications are more far reaching than anyone originally expected. Now, parents and professionals are rethinking special education strategies that remove children from learning contexts with their peers. Greater emphasis is placed on providing opportunity for youngsters to be included in regular classrooms, even when they have severe disabilities (Calculator & Jorgensen, 1991; Lipsky & Gartner, 1989), necessitating that professionals' roles be redefined as part of the process (Hoskins, 1990).

This shift in philosophy about the role of special education means that special educators and regular educators must work together more closely in the common cause of educating all children. Rather than "mainstreaming" children only for limited activities (and often with limited success), new ways are being sought to "modify the mainstream" so that more students have true access to it. This position was advocated by Stainback, Stainback, Courtnage, and Jaben (1985):

> *In order to foster change in regular education, special educators need to reduce the current emphasis on classifying, labeling, and offering "special" programs for students who do not fit within the present regular education structure. Instead, they should put more emphasis on joining with regular educators to work for a reorganization of regular education itself so that the needs of a wider range of students can be met within the mainstream of regular education. (p. 148)*

The practice of including students with disabilities of varying severity in their home schools and in general education classrooms continues to grow. The National Center for Educational Restructuring and Inclusion (1995) reported a three-fold increase in school districts reporting inclusive education programs from 1994, in which 267 districts reported such programs, to 1995, in which 891 districts reported them. Although the reasons for this explosion, and its wisdom, are still debated, there is little question that:

> *Inclusion is on the rise. Spurred by changing public attitudes, court cases, and the work of advocates, inclusion of children with disabilities in regular classrooms is becoming increasingly common in schools across North America. Yet experts differ on whether inclusion is proceeding in ways that best meet children's varied needs. (Willis, 1995, p. 1)*

How inclusion appears in practice varies depending on the motivations and philosophies of those implementing it, as well as the individualized needs and abilities of the students being served in this manner. The American Speech-Language-Hearing Association (1995) has passed a position statement that recognizes the value of "inclusionary practices," emphasizing that they may take a variety of forms in actual implementation. Decisions to address students' needs in the contexts of their general education classrooms should be made because that is the best place to meet those needs, not to save money (Roberts & Mather, 1995).

An Expectation That All Children Can Learn

Services to children with milder impairments who may not have qualified for special education services are also being reexamined. Allington (1991) reviewed the history of educational efforts for children who were less adept than their peers at learning to read:

> *It was near the end of this period (1910–1930) that the concept of "slow learners" emerged; slow learning was viewed as limited aptitude as defined by performance on the new tests of "intelligence." Research into diagnostic procedures was by now well established and the differentiation of "remedial readers" (children who would benefit from intervention), from slow learners (children who would not), became a matter for substantial study. The primary strategy of slowing the pace, delineating specific skills deficits, and teaching components of the reading process separately and in isolation became standard practice in remedial instruction, as had the practice of employing teaching methods different from those used in the classrooms. (p. 20)*

Allington's (1991) main point was that unexamined, long-held beliefs like these can limit progress and drive current policies and programs in state and federal education agencies. As an alternative, he recommended developing new frameworks that recognize the learning potential of all children and the power of instruction that is aimed at higher levels of learning, even for children with limitations. For example, rather than slowing down instruction and presenting oral and written language instruction in small, meaningless pieces, professionals might seek new ways to help students with oral and written language problems gain access to interesting, meaningful language, used for real communicative purposes.

New Roles for Special Educators and Speech-Language Pathologists

In this chapter, it is suggested that speech-language-hearing professionals need to be prepared to provide language intervention services to individuals with a wide variety of language-related learning deficits and within a continuum of service delivery models. Professionals must function as members of teams that make decisions for youngsters based on their individualized needs but also recognize the ultimate goal of helping them become full-fledged members of society. Perhaps the most critical characteristics a speech-language pathologist or other language specialist can bring to a position in a school setting are solid knowledge of language systems and communicative behaviors, sensitivity and flexibility in working with people, and ability to establish and work cooperatively toward goals. As school systems work toward "school improvement" objectives, communication specialists need to participate in plans to improve schools for all children.

As noted in these discussions, the latest shift in philosophy of service provision represents only one of many changes that have occurred since professionals first began to serve children with communicative impairments in schools (Miller, 1989). Some changes seem to result from theoretical shifts, grounded in thoughtful analysis and research; others spring forth dramatically, taking on characteristics of fads; still others (sometimes resulting from either theoretical shifts or faddish appeals) receive public support and become mandated as policy. All changes take place within larger sociopolitical contexts that influence how needs are defined and addressed by a society.

For example, as part of the inclusion movement, a current trend is to limit the amount of time that children receive pull-out services, in which they are removed from their regular classrooms for special education services, such as speech and language intervention. Many good reasons may be found for keeping children in their regular classrooms and in the regular curriculum as much as possible. Sometimes, however, it may be in the best interests of children to remove them intermittently from the classroom for specialized work. Some students even express a preference for being pulled out (Guterman, 1995). The point intended in this chapter is that professionals should avoid making simplistic "always" or "never" judgments about practices of this kind. Rather, they should attempt to achieve a balanced perspective in which many variables are considered and collaborative processes are used to arrive at decisions that best serve individual children. This is part of developing procedures that can be considered "best practice."

Using Technology to Support School Services

Another change that affects service provision in school settings is the increased availability of technology and the extended functions it serves. Consider the many uses of computer-based technologies (Cochran & Masterson, 1995). Report writing and other paperwork chores can be greatly facilitated by using word processing programs and other software.

Many school districts have set up automized data management systems to assist with the legal requirements associated with service provision, such as meeting timelines and writing individualized education plans (Masterson, 1995a). Data banks of program planning objectives also support this process (eg., Nelson & Snyder, 1990). E-mail and the internet access new connections to outside professional and collegial resources, supporting consultation with colleagues and access to new ideas (Masterson, 1995b).

Microcomputer applications for direct clinical work continue to expand as well. Cochran and Masterson (1995) categorized them into six types: (a) a *context for treatment* may be established as an adult interacts with one or more students to "create a picture from existing graphics libraries, write or narrate a story, make a sign or greeting card, or solve a puzzle" (p. 217); (b) a microcomputer and software can provide a *tool for learning*, as when an adult works with a student on the student's written language at a computer, perhaps using a program that provides spelling- or grammar-checking assistance; (c) software can support *language (including phonological) sample analysis*; (d) computers can assist in performing *data collection and storage* functions to measure change in therapy; (e) a computer can act as a *treatment materials generator*, either supporting the development of customized materials or access to a data base of pre-established materials (e.g., *Picture Gallery* [Psychological Corporation, 1994] allows one to select from over 1,000 full color pictures stored on CD-ROM to correspond with students's phonological targets); and (f) a microcomputer, software, and peripheral system can serve as a *biofeedback device*, reflecting evidence of physiologic variation and providing motivating feedback.

Another primary function of technology in today's schools is to augment the oral and written communication abilities of students with severe motor speech impairments, language and learning disabilities, and other multiple impairments (Beukelman & Mirenda, 1992). Provision of low- and high-technology supports for students with severe speech and language impairments is complex and demanding, but no longer the province of only a few specially trained experts. With the inclusion of more students with severe disabilities in their home schools, increasing numbers of "local experts" are developing skill and confidence in establishing a variety of augmentative and alternative communication supports for students who need them. Possibilities include adaptations that permit alternative access to standard microcomputers and software programs, as well as dedicated electronic devices and alternative symbol systems that support users with particular needs. For example, a child with cerebral palsy whose speech is largely unintelligible might need a device with a single switch activation and scanning to create unique messages with synthetic speech or built-in printer output to participate in class discussions and do homework. This same student's supports might also include low technology picture boards and a range of more rapid communication strategies (e.g., natural gesture, vocalizing, and yes/no strategies) for use in other contexts, such as socializing with friends on the playground or in the gymnasium.

Children with hearing impairments often benefit from specialized technological supports as well. The technology of personal hearing aids continually improves and now can provide access to auditory information for children who previously would have had little or none (Northern & Downs 1991). FM units, in which a primary speaker wears a microphone that transmits an FM signal directly to a receiver worn by the student, offer enhanced signal-to-noise ratios, and can assist students with severe to profound losses in "learning sports activities, driver's education, and large group theatre or auditorium activities" as well as participating in academic lessons (Northern & Downs 1991, p. 315). Tactile sensory aids are used by some students whose profound deafness prevents then from receiving acoustic information from auditory channels (Northern & Downs, 1991), and increasing numbers of children are benefiting from cochlear implants, whose technology is constantly improving as well (Nevins & Chute, 1996). Even children with minimal or no hearing losses benefit from having sound field amplification systems in their classrooms. Such systems employ a microphone worn by the teacher (or a peer doing show-and-tell or reading aloud) and multiple speakers around the room enhance the signal-to-noise ration slightly to make it easier for all students to hear, whether or not they are in the front or back of the room, or happen to have middle ear fluid blocking the important sounds of learning on a particular day (Carlson & Nelson, 1994; Crandell, Smaldino, & Flexer, 1995).

Five General Principles of Best Practice

In this section, five principles of best practice are suggested for guiding the design of language intervention programs for children regardless of service delivery setting. They are:

1. Language is an integrated system.
2. Developmental validity is not a simple concept.
3. Contextual relevance leads to functional outcomes.
4. Individualization requires frequent updates and cultural sensitivity
5. Collaboration is a problem-solving mode, not a service delivery model.

Language Is an Integrated System

Language is not something that can be fractured into small pieces and retain its essence. It is largely through language that people learn to know themselves, each other, and something about the world. They use language to accomplish purposes that are functional for them. It is perhaps because children *need* language that they learn it at all. When children fail to learn language normally on their own in naturalistic surroundings, language intervention needs to be designed in such a way as to foster the integrated acquisition of its various aspects.

An integrated model of language that has been widely accepted by clinicians is the content, form, and use model (Bloom & Lahey, 1978; Lahey, 1988), discussed in Chapter 1. According to this model, language rules (sometimes listed as rules of phonology, morphology, syntax, semantics, and pragmatics) are learned as intersecting subsystems (see Figure 1–1). It is during the school-age years that many of the fine touches of language learning are added to each of these systems and especially to the ways they work together.

Language *content* rules include the set of conventions for talking about shared meanings (semantics) in ways that can be understood by other members of the same linguistic community. Proficiency with language content in the school-age years, for example, means that individuals have an adequate lexicon (internalized vocabulary), including later learned words, many of which are abstract. School-age language learners also master inflectional variations in word forms even when the relationships are irregular (e.g., *mouse* and *mice*;

buy and *bought*), along with derivational morphemes (e.g., *-tion, -ly, un-,* and *per-*) to modify word meanings (e.g., *tie* to *untie*; *hundreds* to *hundredths*) and to change their parts of speech (e.g., *official* to *officiate*). Such knowledge about words allows language users to function creatively when producing and understanding unfamiliar words. Language content knowledge also allows users to combine words to create and comprehend abstract and relational meanings that go beyond the meanings of their individual components. In addition, competent language users are sensitive to multiple layers of meaning, going beyond literal meaning to manipulate and interpret discourse conveying emotional tone and metaphoric, idiomatic, or other figurative meanings. They are able to integrate their knowledge of the world with their knowledge of texts to infer meaning from oral or written discourse even when they are not sure of the meanings of all of the individual words. In the process, they "fast-map" meanings onto new words and elaborate those meanings in subsequent encounters with the same words. When formulating language for speech or writing, they can use their semantic knowledge to recall and produce just the right words to fulfill their communicative purposes.

Language *form* rules allow a person to combine syntactic rules with modality-specific rules for producing intelligible words, phrases, and sentences that are either spoken (with morpho-phonologic rules) or written (with morpho-phonologic-graphemic rules). Competent language users can produce and recognize different syntactic forms (paraphrases) for conveying the same meaning. They can recognize basic sentence elements and can comprehend or produce sentences they have never encountered before. They can do this even when elements are moved around, added, or deleted as they are in complex sentences, negatives, questions, or passives. School-age language learners gain increasing ability to manipulate multiple sentence like meanings (propositions) into a single complex unit by embedding and combining parts to convey a variety of logical relationships (e.g., similarity or contiguity with *and*; contrast or disjunction with *but, or, although,* and *except*; temporal order with *after, before, then,* and *when*; conditionality with *if . . . then*). They can use rules for auxiliary verb formation and syntactic construction for varied purposes, such as to convey complex temporal meanings (e.g., from "He has been working there for 2 weeks" to "He had been working there for 2 weeks when he got fired"), subjunctive mood (e.g., "I wouldn't do that if I were you"), and to soften their requests (e.g., from "Give me that book" to "I sure would like to see that book when you're done with it"). They also have some sense of the structure of larger units of text, such as stories (narratives) and informational (expository) texts. Within those texts, they know semantic-grammatic rules that can be used to build cohesion, make reference, and construct smooth transitions from one sentence or paragraph to the next (e.g., pronoun reference and word replacement strategies in sentences like "The pilgrims arrived on the shore at daybreak. They knelt and prayed before they fixed their first meal in the new land"). Furthermore, school-age language users can apply their knowledge of the form of language to help them understand or produce connected discourse to learn about things and experiences they have never encountered before except through language.

Language *use* rules allow a person to communicate within social networks, both immediate and far reaching. They include the pragmatic rules for accomplishing varied communicative purposes and for modifying language form and content to meet particular contextual demands for social appropriateness (e.g., speaking more formally with persons in authority and using the latest slang with peers). Language use rules allow school-age language learners to interpret or convey meanings in which the speaker's underlying intentions are masked somewhat by the language structures actually produced (e.g., "That's just wonderful!" spoken sarcastically). To fit language into a particular context, a language user must be sensitive to the language capabilities and shared informational backgrounds of communicative partners (even preschool-age children adjust their language for toddlers, for instance). As they develop full competence during the school-age years, language users become increasingly sensitive to the informational needs of their communicative partners. As they learn to write for audiences that are absent or even largely unknown, they learn how to encode enough of the context linguistically to make sense. As they learn how to act appropriately in varied social settings, they learn to modify the ways they speak or write for accomplishing varied purposes (e.g., writing social notes to friends and writing a polished draft of a formal term paper).

When school-age language learners have difficulty with one or more of the language subsystems—content, form, and use—it is helpful to analyze where breakdowns are occurring. An individual may have relatively more difficulty with one subsystem than another. This first principle of best practice, however, is meant to warn against artificially fragmenting language in the assessment and intervention process. After all, the hallmark of language acquisition in the school-age years is not the acquisition of new rules so much as it is increased ability to do several things at once and to do them increasingly well. It is during the school-age years that children learn to apply multiple grammatical rules in the same piece of discourse and to control them with more flexibility to achieve desired communicative purposes (Hunt, 1965; Loban, 1963; Scott, 1988, 1994), to think consciously about how they are using language (Nippold, 1988), and to use multiple memory, inferential, and audience awareness strategies while constructing or comprehending written texts (Calkins, 1983; Muth, 1989; Van Kleeck, 1994).

One of the problems traditionally faced by speech-language pathologists has been planning activities that encourage their clients to *use* their newly acquired content and form rules in natural communication events. This first general principle of language assessment and intervention suggests that programs should be planned to encourage integration among these various aspects from the beginning. That is, activities for encouraging functional use of new language content and form rules should be built into all phases of intervention, not just the final ones.

Damico (1988) provided a case example of what can happen when the guiding principle of viewing language as an integrated system is not put into practice. Debbie was initially on Damico's school caseload as a first grader. Damico's analysis showed her language difficulty to involve primarily grammatical rules for pronouns, plurals, and auxiliary verbs. Debbie responded well to an intervention program targeting these features and was dismissed from therapy at the end of her first-grade year. However, at the beginning of her seventh-grade year, Damico encountered Debbie again in another school. This time, instead of a bright and interested communicative partner, Debbie was "less friendly and somewhat introverted" (p. 54). She was reading four grades below grade level and had few friends. She was experiencing severe difficulties using the semantic and pragmatic rules of language to do such things as judge the amount of information to provide to a listener, give appropriate answers to questions, maintain conversational topics, and produce language without excessive revision errors and nonfluencies. By overlooking the initial indicators of these problems when they appeared in Debbie's earlier communicative behaviors and by focusing instead on syntactic rules as an isolated system of language, Damico was influenced by what he later called the "fragmentation fallacy." Although other factors were also involved, Damico believed that the fragmentation involved in discrete-point language assessment, which "breaks the elements of language apart and tries to test them separately with little or no attention to the way those elements interact in a larger context of communication" (p. 56), played a major role in the failure of Debbie's intervention program.

Developmental Validity Is Not a Simple Concept

The second general principle for guiding best practice in any setting is that, although normal developmental sequences almost always provide the best blueprint for designing language intervention programs, developmental validity is not a simple concept. According to this principle, earlier developing aspects of language content, form, and use generally can be acquired more easily by children having difficulty learning language, just as they are by younger children learning language normally. However, selecting goals and objectives to meet the test of developmental validity requires more than just targeting behaviors in the order in which they occur in a standard developmental sequence. Two reasons suggest the need for caution. The first has to do with patterns of developmental scatter often observed among children with language disorders. The second has to do with addressing needs related to chronological age as well as developmental sequence.

The issue of developmental scatter has been addressed by researchers seeking to differentiate language disability from language delay. This research has revealed that development in children with language disabilities is sometimes uneven across domains (Leonard, 1972). That is, some children with language disabilities seem to have difficulty with earlier developing forms at a point when they have partial control of skills usually mastered later in normal development. When the linguistic characteristics of children with language disabilities are considered singly, they may not differ appreciably from those of younger children developing normally, but when the relationships across areas of language development are considered, differences are more likely to appear (Leonard, 1987). Such children are not simply late in reaching linguistic milestones "but have limitations in their language abilities that are long standing, at least in the absence of intervention" (Leonard, 1987, p. 31).

Observations of developmental scatter have several implications for language assessment and intervention practices. First, relatively intact later developing skills in one language area may be used to support development in other areas in which a child may be experiencing difficulty. For example, children with reading decoding difficulties who have higher level vocabulary knowledge may use that vocabulary to help predict word meanings as they read a paragraph. Using word prediction strategies for reading would only be unwise if children failed to use other methods and produced numerous substitution errors that led them away from the intended meaning (Roth & Perfetti, 1980). Then, the best intervention plan might involve two types of activities. In one activity, children would be given instruction and practice in making deliberate sound-symbol associations without concern for larger meanings and without the help of contextual associations. Later in the same day or session children would be expected to use their newly acquired decoding skills in meaningful contexts to check their word predictions. This plan would ensure the integration of word recognition and accurate meanings.

Developmental scatter may also make it appropriate to violate normal developmental sequences in some instances. For example, in oral and written language development, a strictly developmental sequence might suggest that acquiring relatively mature listening and speaking skills should always precede learning to read and write. However, for some children, written language skills may actually help them acquire aspects of spoken language processing that are typically acquired earlier but with which they have had difficulty (Nelson, 1981). For example, when children demonstrate multiple articulation and speech-sound discrimination problems, the relative permanence of written representations of sound sequences may help them begin to sort out some of those relationships in speech.

The second reason for exercising caution when making decisions about developmental validity relates to the complex interaction between life stage needs based on chronological age and those based on developmental levels. Developmental milestones, when used to establish "readiness standards," may inadvertently limit the access of some children to opportunities to participate with their normally developing peers in real-life contexts. For example, when children have severe physical disabilities and cannot speak, a strictly developmental approach might lead to a plan that emphasizes self-help and dressing skills because such skills are generally acquired in the preschool years, before learning to read and write. In another example, adolescents with preschool-level language skills might experience social communication needs that are more commensurate with their chronological ages than their language stages. Such individuals might benefit more from learning how to make small talk with co-workers and how to ask clarification questions of job coaches and supervisors than from learning to produce perfectly well formed sentences. The willingness to communicate and the ability to make sense (even with imperfectly formed syntactic structures) have greater validity for the developmental life stages of such individuals than a narrowly ordered linguistic sequence would.

Contextual Relevance Leads to Functional Outcomes

The purpose of language intervention is to improve real-life functioning, but this fact may be obscured by language assessment and intervention practices that are not contextually relevant. When formal tests are used as the sole means to identify intervention needs, a danger arises that only isolated and trivial behaviors will be targeted. For example, if formal testing shows deficits in such processing abilities as memory span for related or unrelated syllables, discrimination of individual phonemes, or other auditory perceptual skills, clinicians may be tempted to focus on such "splinter skills" in remediation on the assumption that their improvement may be prerequisite to further language acquisition. However, the evidence for the success of approaches aimed at improving "prerequisite" processing skills has been disappointing (Bloom & Lahey, 1978; Hammill & Larsen, 1974).

The first step in achieving contextual relevance is to collaborate with those who know the child well (usually teachers, parents and caregivers, and the children themselves) to identify several key contexts where communicative problems are evident. For a kindergartner who has trouble approaching peers socially and participating with them in play interactions, the context might be free play time. For a third grader, one problematic context might involve understanding the teacher's directions for each new activity during the day. Another might be making an oral presentation during show-and-tell. For a ninth grader, the most problematic context might involve reading the American history textbook and answering written discussion questions provided by the teacher. This student may also have difficulty recalling information from the science textbook when taking tests.

The second step of this process is to observe the student within the chosen contexts. During observation, the language specialist seeks three kinds of information.

1. A description of the language and communicative demands of the context. What language and communication skills and strategies does a child need in this situation to participate successfully in it?
2. A description of what the child actually does when attempting the task without support. What kinds of language skills and communicative strategies does the child currently use in this context when participating independently?
3. A description of forms of support that will help the student function at a level more like that of her peers. What kinds of scaffolding support are required for the child to appear more competent in this context, and how readily does the child respond to them? (Scaffolding is discussed further later in this chapter.)

Contextually based communication assessment activities can be conducted with individuals of any age and stage of life. When used with school-age children in contexts relevant to functioning in school, they may be identified as curriculum-based language assessment (Nelson, 1989, in 1992, 1994) because they address the child's functioning in various areas of the academic and nonacademic curriculum.

Contextually based communication assessment and intervention activities are consistent with the first two principles of best practice because they encourage an integrated view of language functioning. They also involve selection of intervention targets based on developmental relevance for functioning at the level of peers as well as reaching the next rung on some narrowly defined developmental ladder of isolated skills.

For example, observation of the kindergarten child during free play might reveal the child's need to use questions socially to enter the group (e.g., "Can I play too guys?" "Wanna play house?"), to find appropriate props to fit into other children's play schemes (e.g., being a patient in the doctor's office), and to negotiate disputes with communicative strategies other than screaming and hitting. This child may also be having trouble because her speech is unintelligible to the other children. Intervention therefore might include some direct attention to improving articulation skill. Articulatory targets might be based on analysis of developmental phonological processes (Hodson & Paden, 1991). Rather than using a strictly developmental sequence to select stimuli, however, stimulus words could be selected for functional relevance in favorite play routines (Hillard & Goepfert, 1979). This therapy could be provided in the kindergarten room or in a pull-out room, individually or in small groups, but the words should be prompted during the actual play time as well as in isolated practice sessions. By scheduling part of the child's intervention program during free-play time in the classroom, the language specialist might also act as a participant-observer on the edge of the children's play group. The specialist would not direct play but would provide scaffolding through strategically placed prompts, questions, suggestions, and articulatory cuing to make appropriate participation in the group easier for the target child. The term *scaffolding* was introduced by Bruner (1978) to describe how adults systematically modify language learning contexts and help children focus their attention to make it possible for them to function at higher levels. Scaffolding would be gradually withdrawn as the target child acquired new skills. In this way, independent functioning can be encouraged from the start, and desired functional outcomes can be achieved most efficiently.

Similar strategies might be used to serve the third grader and ninth grader mentioned previously, but with modifications appropriate to their developmental levels. For the third grader, for example, the classroom teacher and speech-language pathologist might collaborate to provide some whole-class instruction about show-and-tell. It is common to assume that children can abstract the rules for acting appropriately in such classroom routines without direct instruction, but not all children do (Creaghead, 1990). To make some of the key characteristics of a successful show-and-tell experience explicit, the language specialist might lead a whole-class brainstorming session about them, using the class discussion to organize the key characteristics into a chart that could be posted in the classroom and later included in the target child's speech and language notebook for review. The list might include: (a) talk loudly enough so everyone can hear you; (b) tell the name of the thing you brought; (c) tell several interesting things about it; (d) look at the audience some of the time; and (e) ask if anyone has any questions or comments. Because the whole-class experience might not provide enough opportunity for practice by the child with the language disorder, she might be given extra chances to rehearse in individual or small-group pull-out sessions before taking a turn in front of the class.

To address the problems related to direction following, the speech-language pathologist and the classroom teacher might observe the student to identify several variables that influence successful performance. In the process, the teacher could move the child's seat to the side-front of the room, where the child could observe other students but still hear clearly and where the teacher could check for signs of step-by-step comprehension (e.g., by noting whether the child selects the appropriate textbook and page when so directed). The teacher might try to make the orienting cues for beginning a directional sequence stronger, to stress key pieces of information deliberately, to reduce the numbers of directions given in one sequence, and to ask the student to repeat important steps privately before beginning to work (perhaps until some predetermined criterion is reached for encouraging independence). Meanwhile, in separate sessions, the speech-language pathologist could be helping the child acquire some of the previously misunderstood directional terminology that is important in the classroom. The child could also be taught to be a better observer of other aspects of classroom routine so that the processing load is lightened (Creaghead, 1990).

As students advance in grade level, they become more sensitive about having services provided in their classrooms (Jenkins & Heinen, 1989). For the ninth grader having difficulty with her history and science textbooks, therefore, all services might be provided in pull-out sessions with other students with similar needs in a regularly scheduled study hall time-slot or in a "communication strategies" class for which students get course credit and letter grades (if the particular state and school system allow such an arrangement; see Anderson & Nelson, 1988, for an example). Observation might reveal several sources of difficulty that arise when the student is paraphrasing key sections of the textbook or answering questions about the text. For example, even a student who can read aloud with few decoding errors might have difficulty understanding the pronoun references or complex syntax of her text. Intervention for this student and her peers might be aimed at teaching them strategies for finding appropriate sections in their textbooks, identifying subsections and paragraphs relevant to the study questions, using advanced strategies for understanding complex syntax and pronoun reference, and paraphrasing appropriate passages when answering questions. Several sessions might be spent helping them tune-in to the meaning of key words in discussion questions, such as *describe*, *compare*, *contrast*, *list*, and *discuss*. Examples of how textbooks are structured may be drawn from several classes. For example, semantic hierarchies are often used as primary organizing strategies in science textbooks. To improve comprehension and recall, students might be taught to construct graphic organizer charts to illustrate the hierarchical relationships. A variety of sources illustrate how such charts may be constructed (Calfee & Chambliss, 1988; Pehrsson & Denner, 1988; Richgels, McGee, Lomax, & Sheard, 1987; Westby, 1994). One rather simple strategy is illustrated in Figure 9-1. The students might use the charts to ask each other questions about the topics they are studying "backward and forward." That is, first they might give each other the name of a hierarchical category and ask for examples to fit that category; then they might give the names of examples, asking which category they fit and why.

These examples stress the principle of contextual relevance. That is, in each case, language intervention provides an opportunity for the student to use language in forms and contexts that are as intact as possible for real communicative and educational purposes. The analytical breakdowns that occur are mostly in the mind of the adult who guides the intervention process, not in the activities used for intervention. By alternating focus on various aspects of communicative events in holistic contexts, the adult can help the child acquire more mature language knowledge and skills in targeted areas without fragmenting them.

Individualization Requires Frequent Updates and Cultural Sensitivity

The fourth general principle of best practice is that language intervention should be individualized. Part of this principle is that individualization requires frequent updates and sensitivity to the child's world beyond the school setting.

The group of children with language disorders is a heterogeneous one, and it is heterogeneous in a number of ways. As noted previously, some children have relatively greater difficulty with the content of language, others with its form or use. Children also have varied talents and abilities in areas that may have little to do with language processing (Miller, 1990) but much to do with their ability to develop positive self-images. Variation may also occur within children as they develop across the age span from infancy through adolescence, and planning needs to be continuously updated to take such changes into account.

Children and families of children with language disorders may vary in other ways as well. Cultural and linguistic variation related to ethnic heritage and socioeconomic characteristics of families are particularly critical to consider when individualizing services for children. Public policy mandates that language assessment be free from bias related to linguistic or cultural difference (see discussion later in this chapter, and also Chapter 10), but it

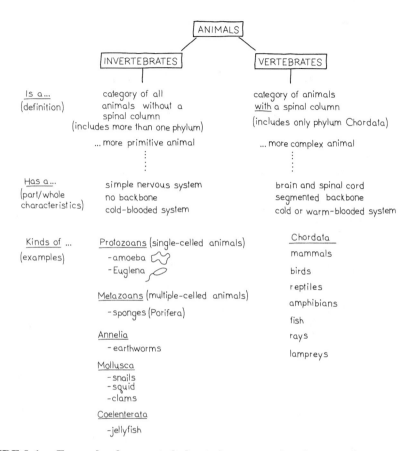

FIGURE 9-1   **Example of a way to help students organize the macrostructure of a science lesson.**

is easier to state the mandate than to meet it. This is partially because of the lack of standardized measures for conducting valid nonbiased assessment of culturally and linguistically different children (Taylor & Payne, 1983; Vaughn-Cooke, 1983) and partially because of traditional reliance on standardized assessments as the most valid measures of language development. No matter how well they are standardized with one population, tests are not valid when used with another, different population. The lack of appropriate assessment devices may lead to problems of overidentification—identifying children as language disordered when they are not—or underidentification—not identifying children who actually have valid needs for language intervention services (Damico & Hamayan, 1991; Kretschmer, 1991; Ortiz & Maldonado-Colon, 1986; Terrell & Terrell, 1983).

Part of the solution is for the language specialist to be sensitive to test bias and to multiple measures, including informal ones to determine the need for service. In addition, the first three principles of best practice—treating language as an integrated system, basing determination of developmental validity on comparison with local peer groups, and using contextually based observations of functional competency for assessment and intervention

—each contribute something to the process of individualization and nonbiased service provision for all children.

Collaboration Is a Problem-Solving Mode, Not a Service Delivery Model

This fifth and final principle of best practice is that collaboration is an essential part of effective language assessment and intervention. Language is not learned in isolation but in meaningful contexts in communication with others. As has been noted in the preceding discussions, family members and regular and special education teachers are important participants in all stages of the process. Other professionals, such as school psychologists, school social workers, and occupational therapists, may be members of intervention teams in school-based programs as well. No team functions efficiently without strong support from administrators. Building principals are particularly important when designing comprehensive service delivery plans for children with language disorders.

An important corollary of the collaboration principle is that collaboration is not a kind of service delivery to be selected in some cases and not others, as consultation might be. Rather, collaboration is a problem-solving mode that is appropriate regardless of the service delivery model selected for an individual. The term *collaborative consultation* is often used to characterize this approach. It is frequently defined as:

> *. . . an interactive process that enables teams of people with diverse expertise to generate creative solutions to mutually defined problems. The outcome is enhanced, altered, and produces solutions that are different from those that the individual team members would produce independently (Idol, Paolucci-Whitcomb, & Nevin, 1986, p. 1)*

Such an approach differs from consultation as a service delivery model, in which a relationship is set up so that someone other than the consultant acts as the primary intervention agent. For example, "when discussing consultation services for speech-language problems in the public schools, the SLP can be viewed as the consultant and the classroom teacher designated as primary interventionist" (Marvin, 1987, p. 5).

An important feature of the collaborative process is the mutual definition of problems and goals. If other participants are included in the process of identifying real-life contexts where problems are occurring, they are more likely to participate in designing plans that will lead to comprehensive solutions. A teacher who feels some ownership of the process of language intervention will be more likely to assist in making environmental modifications to support the target student's learning and growth, as did the third-grade teacher in the example described previously.

When disagreements arise about how best to serve children, interfering with the spirit of collaboration, it often helps to take a step back to a prior level of goal setting. For example, if parents and school personnel disagree about a child's classroom placement, rather than focusing immediately on where the student should be placed, the intervention team might collaborate first to create lists of expectations for the student ten years in the future, 5 years in the future, and then, in the coming year. Asking participants to talk separately about what they consider "idealistic goals," as well as "realistic goals," might also help them to achieve perspective as a collaborative group. Then, it may be easier to come to mutually agreeable decisions about meeting the child's needs in the coming year.

Planning to include students with severe disabilities in general education classrooms brings a special set of complexities that require a collaborative approach. Several problem-solving systems have been designed specifically to support such planning (Calculator & Jorgensen, 1994). These systems can offer a different way to look at assessment as a group problem-solving activity, rather than as a way of testing the individual to isolate areas of difficulty. Two decision-making systems currently in widespread use are M.A.P.S. and C.O.A.C.H. (Calculator & Jorgensen, 1994). The M.A.P.S. approach (McGill Action Planning System; Vandercook, York, & Forest, 1989) is conducted within one or more collaborative sessions in which the student, family members, and friends collaboratively answer seven questions about: (a) who the person is (avoiding special education jargon); (b) the individual's history; (c) the nature of his or her dream; (d) the person's nightmare if the dream does not come true; (e) the person's gifts; (f) what the person needs right now (this year) to have a good life; and (g) what everyone (student, parents, teachers, peers, other support staff) will do to meet those needs. The C.O.A.C.H. process (Choosing Options and Accommodations for Children with Handicaps; Giangreco, Cloninger, & Iverson, 1993) is also family-centered decision-making approach. It yields for components of an individualized plan: (a) a set of annual goals, which are based on the individual's needs rather than the disciplines of the professionals who will provide service; (b) measurable short-term objectives that lead toward the goals; (c) a list of supports the individual will need within an inclusive regular classroom to reach the goals; and (d) preliminary plans for facilitating the individual's participation within the regular curriculum in the regular classroom.

Collaborative problem-solving modes should also extend to relationships between language specialists and children or adolescents who need language learning assistance. Rather than a doctor-patient relationship, or even a teacher-pupil relationship, the relationship between professionals and persons needing assistance should be collaborative. From the first contact with the child or adolescent, the professional should attempt to convey the attitude of coconspirator *with* the child in figuring out what needs to be done to make life better. The child should be an active participant in the process, not a passive recipient. The professional, rather than acting primarily as examiner, or as a person who sets up small tests for the child to pass or fail, acts as a colearner, whose main job is to help the child figure out how to make sense out of the world and how to make sense in it. Even when giving formal tests, the language specialist should make it clear that the purpose is to figure out what makes it easier or harder for the person to do well, not to assign a label. Consistent with this principle, results of tests should be explained in ways that examinees can understand, with honesty, but with a sensitivity toward protecting the individual's sense of underlying competence. Most children and adolescents should also play a major role in selecting the contexts for intervention. If they do so, they are more likely to assume some ownership of the process of change.

Summary of Best Practice Principles

Because of the need for individualization, it may seem presumptuous to claim that the five principles presented here constitute best practice principles for serving all children with language and communicative disorders regardless of setting. It is because the principles are based on a recommendation for contextual relevance that this claim can be made.

To review, language assessment and intervention should be based on principles that recognize: (a) language as an integrated system, (b) complex ways of establishing developmental validity when setting goals, (c) definition of communicative contexts for intervention that are relevant to desired functional outcomes, (d) frequent updates of individualization and sensitivity to cultural and linguistic difference, and (e) collaboration as a problem-solving mode, regardless of service delivery model.

The key to using these five principles in school settings as a specialized context is that the decisions made must relate to needs that arise in educational settings. For example, recognizing language as an integrated system in schools means that both written and oral language are considered appropriate assessment and intervention targets. Also in schools, language for formal educational purposes as well as for social interaction purposes must be considered. In school settings, grade level expectations and formal definitions of curricula may be used to assist in establishing developmentally valid performance criteria for students with disabilities. By using such standards, programs may be designed to help students with special needs stay as close to their normally developing peers as possible. Teachers, as well as parents and students, become key participants when defining contextually relevant goals in school settings. Schools also provide special opportunities for addressing intervention targets in the settings where they will be needed. Study after study has shown that school presents special challenges for children from socioeconomically limited families regardless of their ethnic status (e.g., see Loban, 1963, 1976; Wells, 1986), and such differences must be considered without discriminating against children on the basis of those differences. Children who come from homes where cultural and linguistic expectations are distinct from those that underly most formal schooling and language tests must have their individualized needs and experiences considered in determining their competence as communicators. Finally, the collaborative process needs to be fit into the institutions of schooling. To some extent, the activities required by public policy may be used to meet these purposes. Principals who are committed to building collaborative teams that work well can help teams find time and space to meet in their schools. Practitioners who make collaborative strategies work for them, however, often note that they do most of their collaborating in classroom doorways and school parking lots, looking for opportunity wherever they can find it.

Public Policy Influences

In the United States, Congress has determined not only that speech and language intervention in schools is desirable for children with communicative disorders but also that it is part of their right to "free appropriate public education." This right has been guaranteed since 1979, when the **Education for All Handicapped Children Act of 1975** (PL 94-142) was first implemented. In the **Education of Handicapped Act Amendments of 1986** (PL 99-457), the federal government added a commitment to serve the needs of infants and toddlers, birth through age 2, with identified disabilities as well as those who are at risk for developing disabilities. The amendments also gave added support for states to provide preschool programs to serve 3- to 5-year-olds with disabilities. Programs for 3- to 5-year-olds had been optional under PL 94-142.

PL 99-457 also changed the definition of qualified personnel. The amendments specified that the highest qualification standard in the state must be used to determine eligibility to provide services in public education settings. This means that if the state requires individuals in health care settings or private practice to hold master's degrees, those providing services in school settings must also hold master's degrees. As state education agencies revise and resubmit their state's plans for implementing the federal legislation, they are required to indicate the steps they are taking to retrain or hire professionals who meet the highest standards of the state.

The **Education of the Handicapped Amendments of 1990** (PL 101-476) reauthorized PL 94-142 and renamed the law the Individuals with Disabilities Education Act (IDEA), along with a number of other changes. As noted previously, this is the act that replaced the word *handicapped* with *disabilities*. Other aspects of the IDEA amendments address materials and training for parents, programs for children exposed prenatally to maternal substance abuse, programs for ethnically and culturally diverse children with disabilities, and the elimination of illiteracy among individuals with disabilities. The reauthorization also expanded the general definition of children with disabilities to include separate categories for children with autism and traumatic brain injury. When the revised law was being drafted, considerable controversy was raised over whether attention deficit disorder (ADD) (also called attention-deficit hyperactivity disorder, ADHD; American Psychiatric Association, 1987) should also be added as a separate category or subcategory of disability. After much debate, it was decided not to include ADD as a new category, but to consider children with ADHD as "otherwise health impaired". Children with ADHD also qualify for special services in schools under Section 504 of the Rehabilitation Act if they need those services to benefit from education. Section 504 is a civil rights statute that was passed in 1973 and amended with the Rehabilitation, Comprehensive Services and Developmental Disabilities Amendments of 1978. It guarantees freedom from discrimination on the basis of handicap in programs that receive federal funds. In Section 504, *handicap* is defined as a physical or mental impairment that substantially limits one or more major life activities, including learning.

The regulatory influences discussed here are based on federal laws, which, like all policies, are subject to change. The provision of services in school settings is also influenced by regulatory controls at several other levels. First, at the most immediate level, local districts, referred to in the laws as local education agencies (LEAs), have direct responsibility for providing appropriate educational programs for all children, whether they have disabilities or not. Second, some states have intermediate educational agencies at a level between local and state agencies. These districts, which often span one or two counties, consolidate services and coordinate communication between state and local agencies. Third, state departments of education, regulated by state boards of education and/or legislatures, determine the policies of states regarding provision of regular and special education services. State education agencies (SEAS) write state plans (with public input), which describe policies and procedures they will use to meet federal requirements. State plans are submitted to the United States Department of Education, Office of Special Education and Rehabilitation Services (OSERS), for approval. This is the federal agency charged with seeing that the IDEA is implemented to provide "free appropriate public education" (FAPE) for all children with disabilities.

The information in this chapter about legal requirements for provision of special education programs is drawn from publications regarding PL 94-142, PL 99-457, and PL 101-476 in the *Federal Register.* Most of the procedures have been implemented for a number of years, and they are generally appropriate in any area of the United States but are often interpreted differently across regions. For a detailed understanding of procedures in any particular district, the professional is referred to the special education office in that district, where copies of state, intermediate (if any), and local policy statements should be available. Awareness of the distinction between regulations arising from different administrative levels is also important. When state and local requirements consume professionals' time yet have little positive effect on children, it is the responsibility of professionals to participate in the processes needed to change the requirements. Most of the basic federal requirements are no more extensive than those required for any good clinical practice.

The next reauthorization of IDEA is likely to include a number of modifications relating to planning and monitoring progress of students with special needs (A. Amiot, personal communication, December 21, 1995). For example, the group of individuals who are designing a student's Individualized Education Plan (IEP) may need to be more specific about justifying why a student cannot participate in certain areas of the regular curriculum. Such a policy would be consistent with the best practice principle discussed previously for relating a student's language intervention needs to the student's difficulties in handling the language demands of the regular curriculum. Another change might be a requirement for reporting periods to coincide with the reporting periods of general education, rather than occurring only once per year. Again, if a student's IEP goals are tied directly to the student's ability to function in the regular curriculum, collaborative monitoring by the general education teacher and the speech-language pathologist or other special educator will make sense. Changes noted on a student's report card might include such functional, classroom-based outcomes as "now speaks loudly enough so other children can hear him during show-and-tell," or "scored 8 of 10 correct on last test in which social studies vocabulary was pre-taught."

Procedures

Procedures for service provision in the schools are presented here in the order in which they are usually implemented as steps of a process. They include (a) identifying students with language disorders, (b) notifying parents, (c) conducting a multidisciplinary evaluation, (d) holding an individualized education planning meeting, (e) selecting a service delivery model, (f) writing and implementing an Individualized Education Plan (IEP), (g) documenting progress, and (h) reevaluating the student's needs comprehensively at least every three years. A flowchart outlining these general procedures is presented in Figure 9-2.

Identifying Students with Language Disorders

Both PL 94-142 (Part B) and PL 99-457 (Part H) require that states implement comprehensive "Child Find" systems to identify children in need of services. However, a distinction

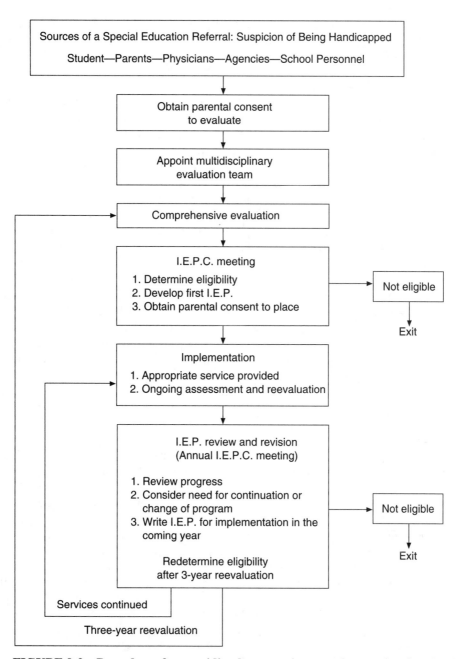

FIGURE 9-2 **Procedures for providing language intervention services in school settings consistent with federal policies.**

(From *Program Suggestions for Speech and Language Services* [p. 2] by the Michigan Department of Education, 1982, Lansing, MI: Special Education Services. Reprinted by permission.)

occurs in the types of children to be identified in the two instances. Under Part H, which relates to infants and toddlers, children eligible for services include not only those who are clearly disabled but also those who are at risk of experiencing developmental delays, depending on decisions made within each state. The definition of developmental delay is to be determined by each state.

Part B of PL 94-142 relates to school-age children. According to its requirements, educators have a responsibility to identify all and only the children in the district who have disabilities and need special education. Before passage of PL 99-457, states differed as to the age levels of disabled children to be served as part of public education. Now, because of PL 99-457, all states have agreed to provide coordinated services from birth. This requires increased interagency cooperation.

Children who experience developmental delays may be referred to Child Find teams by physicians, parents, community health agencies, family courts, early detection centers, or school personnel. Speech-language pathologists and audiologists should be members of such teams. The original impetus for referring children in their preschool years is often delay or abnormality in learning to talk, but other disabilities may be apparent in early childhood as well. As children advance in school, early appearing language disorders usually do not disappear. However, because federal guidelines specify "unduplicated counts" of children with different disabilities (i.e., an individual child can be counted in only one category), the prevalence of "speech impairments" (the official federal label for all kinds of speech, language, and communicative disorders) appears to diminish, as shown in Figure 9-3. Based on data from the "Tenth Annual Report to Congress on the Implementation of The Education of the Handicapped Act (EHA)" (USDE, 1988), this figure (Gerber & Levine-Donnerstein, 1989) shows proportions of students with learning disabilities, speech impairments, mental retardation, and emotional disturbance within four age groups: preschool (3–5 years), primary (6–11 years), secondary (12–17 years), and postsecondary (17–21 years).

The appearance that the proportion of children with communicative disorders reduces dramatically over the ages from 3 to 21 years is deceiving. Longitudinal studies show that language disorders generally do not disappear over time, but that many children who start out with language disorders become a major part of the group identified as having learning disabilities (Maxwell & Wallach, 1984). Scarborough and Dobrich (1990) summarized the results of longitudinal studies that showed that from 28 percent to 75 percent of children with language impairments in their preschool years continue to exhibit residual speech and language problems in later childhood, and that 52 percent to 95 percent of them show impairments in reading achievement (Aram, Ekelman, & Nation, 1984; Aram & Nation, 1980; Levi, Capozzi, Fabrizi, & Sechi, 1982; Padgett, 1988; Stark et al., 1984).

Identifying children who should receive speech and language services is one of the major challenges facing speech-language pathologists in schools, and this is one area where service provision may differ markedly from service in other settings. For example, in community clinics and hospitals, clients and their families often seek services themselves, approaching professionals directly. In schools, teachers make most referrals, and professionals sometimes have to inform families that a communicative disorder may exist and that evaluation is recommended. Parents may also refer their children for diagnostic services in schools, and this happens, particularly at the preschool level, when community Child Find

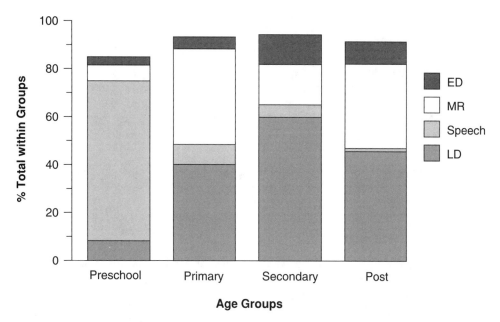

FIGURE 9-3   **Proportions of students identified with learning disabilities (LD), speech impairments, mental retardation (MR), and emotional disturbance (ED) within four age groups.**

(From "Educating All Children: Ten Years Later" by M. M. Gerber & D. Levine-Donnerstein, *Exceptional Children,* 56, 1989, 17–27. Copyright 1989 by the Council for Exceptional Children. Reprinted with permission.)

programs make it clear that children have a right to receive such services in their local schools if needed. At the secondary-school level, students might also be encouraged to refer themselves for assessment (Larson & McKinley, 1987).

Identifying Elementary School Students.   Before federal mandates were set in place, elementary-age children with communicative disorders traditionally were identified by screening whole grades of students and placing those who failed the screening on a caseload. This activity usually took place at the beginning of each schoolyear, with new placement decisions made each fall. Such a practice is no longer routinely followed for several reasons, the primary one being that children now must be considered as individuals. The IDEA requires that children be provided services outlined in IEPS, which are based on comprehensive multidisciplinary evaluations. IEPs are reviewed and revised at least annually until it is determined at an IEP meeting that the student no longer needs the program. While an IEP is in place, the services defined in it must be provided.

Unilateral decision making is also inappropriate because the law requires that decisions about children with disabilities must be made by more than one person. Classroom teachers generally have the best opportunity to observe students using language in a variety of ways. Classroom teachers are also best suited to determine effects of children's speech and language impairments on educational performance, a further requirement of the law. They are, therefore, important members of multidisciplinary identification and evaluation teams.

Although teachers are often the best sources of referrals, they may need guidance about making them. Teachers will generally pick up a student's surface errors in grammatical usage and articulatory production, but interactions of language impairment and educational problems are not always apparent (Damico & Oller, 1980). When children do not make obvious errors, perhaps because earlier problems of spoken language have been remediated or expressive deficits do not characterize the child's language difficulty, signs of language disorder may be overlooked. When children speak spontaneously, they make choices about how to express their ideas. They may choose to use relatively simple forms and may speak about concrete content without making obvious errors. When children do not attempt to use more complex forms, it may not be apparent that they *cannot* use such forms or that they cannot understand abstract content. However, when the same children are expected to process the more complex language forms and content used by teachers and in textbooks, they may experience increasing difficulties as the contextual demands of school language increase (Maxwell & Wallach, 1984; Nelson, 1984).

To help teachers identify children with language disorders, both in-service educational activities and consultation regarding specific children may be appropriate. The process may be facilitated by providing teachers with checklists to help them identify students who should be referred for evaluation. The introduction of the checklists may create a context for more general in-service on the types of educational problems that can involve communicative disorders. Such checklists help teachers look beyond the usual error-based criteria for identifying children in need of special services.

For students in grades 1 through 5, Damico and Oller (1980) suggested the following signs for teachers to use in determining that a child might need to be referred:

1. *Linguistic nonfluency*—in which children's speech production is disrupted by a disproportionately high number of repetitions, unusual pauses, and excessive use of hesitation forms

2. *Revisions*—in which speech production includes numerous false starts or self-interruptions and revisions as if children keep coming to dead ends in a maze

3. *Delays before responding*—in which communication attempts initiated by others are followed by pauses of inordinate length

4. *Nonspecific vocabulary*—in which children use expressions such as "this" or "that," "then," "he," "over there," without making references clear or use all-purpose words such as "thing:" "stuff," "these," and "those" when more specific referring expressions would be better

5. *Inappropriate responses*—in which children appear to be operating on an independent discourse agenda—not attending to the prompts or probes of adults or others

6. *Poor topic maintenance*—in which children make rapid and inappropriate changes in the topic without providing transitional clues to their listeners

7. *Need for repetition*—in which children request multiple repetitions but do not show improvement in comprehension

Damico and Oller (1980) evaluated the success of criteria like these against more traditional morpho-syntactic criteria for language referrals. The results showed that teachers who were taught to use the pragmatic criteria listed here identified significantly more children and were more often correct in their identification than teachers taught to use syntactic criteria. Both groups identified significantly fewer children as grade level increased.

Identifying Secondary School Students

Larson and McKinley (1987) suggested a similar set of criteria for identifying secondary-level students who may need language intervention services. Their referral form, which appears as Figure 9-4, includes criteria divided into five categories: thinking, listening, speaking, nonverbal communication, and survival language. Like Damico and Oller's (1980) referral criteria for elementary children, these criteria may help teachers focus on interactions of language processing with educational expectations.

Pre-Kindergarten Screening

Although referral by teachers currently is considered to be a more valid means of identifying school-age children with speech-language impairments than whole-grade screening, large-group screening still is used in some districts, particularly for children entering kindergarten. If screening procedures are comprehensive, they may help to identify children who need early intervention to prevent or reduce later problems of educational performance related to language weakness. No child may be placed in special education, however, including speech-language intervention, on the basis of screening results alone.

Identifying Disability When Culture Varies

A nonbiased comprehensive multidisciplinary evaluation must be provided to ensure that only children who have true speech-language impairments are placed in special programs. Children who score below norms, not because they are speech and language impaired, but because they have language experiences that do not match those measured by most evaluation tools, must not be labeled as disabled. On the other hand, children from diverse cultural communities who have true language disorders must be identifiable (Hamayan & Damico, 1991; Taylor & Payne, 1983; Terrell & Terrell, 1983). Speech-language pathologists may be required to use specialized techniques, to become bilingual themselves, or to use interpreters in evaluating children who come from different cultural and linguistic backgrounds who are suspected of being speech and language impaired (Anderson, 1992). Parental reports about communicative problems children have in their home community are critical in making decisions about the potential need for intervention services.

Identifying Language Disorder When Other Disabilities Are Present

As noted previously, children who need speech-language intervention may have other disabilities as well. Communicative disorders are often integrally related to such other conditions as learning disabilities, mental retardation, autism, and hearing impairment (Nelson, 1993c). When children do have some other primary disability, they may qualify for speech-language intervention as a related service, which is listed on their IEP. Deciding which children need such service, however, is not easy. For example, all children with mental retardation probably have language skills that are inappropriate for their chronological

SECONDARY-LEVEL REFERRAL FORM:
COMMUNICATION DISORDERS

Course or Specialty: _____   Educator: _____

Date Completed: _____   Total of All Ratings: _____

Using the following scale, mark the following statements regarding the
communication behavior of _____ in your classroom.

(student)

> 5 - Almost Always
>
> 4 - Frequently
>
> 3 - Sometimes ("50 - 50")
>
> 2 - Infrequently
>
> 1 - Almost Never
>
> NA - Not Applicable/No Chance to Observe

Thinking

____ **1.** The student organizes and categorizes information.

____ **2.** The student sequences data in a logical order.

____ **3.** The student identifies and solves problems independently.

____ **4.** The student finds, selects, and utilizes information for assignments.

____ **5.** The student thinks about ideas and events that are not just in the "here and now."

____ TOTAL

Listening

____ **1.** The student understands complex sentences and multiple meaning words.

____ **2.** The student indicates comprehension of main ideas presented.

____ **3.** The student follows a sequence of directions even if asked only once.

____ **4.** The student identifies relevant supporting details and records then in a
notebook and/or systematically retrieves them on request.

____ **5.** The student uses critical listening skills such as detecting fact form opinion,
evaluating a speaker's argument, and recognizing propaganda.

____ **6.** The student effectively listens by asking questions and making comments
during conversations.

____ TOTAL

Speaking

____ **1.** The student plans what to say, sequences it in a logical way, and produces the
resultant sentence(s) with few verbal mazes.

____ **2.** The student uses grammatically intact sentences; sentence fragments are
appropriate to the context (e.g., the student answers with a single word in
response to a question such as, "Where is he going?").

____ **3.** The student easily finds words to communicate as precisely and accurately as
possible and avoids use of low informational words (e.g., "stuff," "things,"
"whatchamacallit").

____ **4.** The student gives directions, makes reports, tells or retells stories, and
explains processes in detail with clarity and accuracy.

____ **5.** The student provides relevant and complete answers to questions.

____ **6.** The student interacts orally with educators and other students, being considerate of their feelings, taking turns speaking and listening, and initiating and maintaining conversations.

____ **7.** The student displays normal voice characteristics with regard to pitch, volume, and quality (e.g., lack of chronic hoarseness, breathiness).

____ **8.** The student displays normal fluency characteristics (i.e., lack of word or syllable repetitions, prolongations of sounds, silent gaps within words).

____ TOTAL

Nonverbal Communication

____ **1.** The student interprets and uses correct body movements and facial expressions.

____ **2.** The student follows rules for social distance when talking.

____ TOTAL

Survival Language

____ **1.** The student demonstrates comprehension of basic spatial and temporal concepts.

____ **2.** The student demonstrates the ability to obtain and to keep a job with his/her present level of communication skills (i.e., Would you hire this student given the way the individual talks and listens?).

____ **3.** The student demonstrates sufficient language to cope with daily living situations such as job applications, shopping, using the telephone, and interpreting signs and labels.

____ **4.** The student understands and uses figurative language acceptable to the peer group.

____ TOTAL

Thinking Total: _____

Listening Total: _____

Speaking Total: _____

Nonverbal Communication Total: _____

Survival Language Total: _____

TOTAL OF ALL RATINGS (A): _____

TOTAL NUMBER OF POINTS POSSIBLE (B): _____

PERCENTAGE ([A÷B] × 100):

I feel confident in this student's ability to function independently once his/her school experience is over. ____

If you rate this item "1" or "2," please comment on how the student's oral communication is contributing to the problem: _____

FIGURE 9-4   Referral form for secondary students suspected of having communication disorders.

(From: *Communication Assessment and Intervention Strategies for Adolescents* by V. L. Larson & N. L. McKinley, 1987, Eau Claire, WI: Thinking Publications. Copyright 1987 by Thinking Publications. Reprinted by permission.)

ages by virtue of their retardation. The question is whether they need specialized intervention from a speech-language pathologist or whether their language development needs can be met within a classroom curriculum (regular or special education). One criterion for recommending specialized services is that there should be a discrepancy between the child's language age and the child's mental age. Discrepancy criteria are also frequently recommended for identifying the presence of specific language impairment (Tallal, 1988). A number of problems exist in the use of discrepancy criteria, however (Aram, Morris, & Hall, 1992; ASHA, 1989; Casby, 1992; Lahey, 1988; Nelson, 1993). They imply that the results of two different tests, standardized on two different samples at two different times, are directly comparable. They also imply that results of tests that yield mental age scores are not confounded with those that yield language age scores. The similarity of items on the two types of tests, however, leads one to question this assumption. The decision to provide specialized speech-language intervention services to an individual with multiple impairments is best based on a combination of formal test results along with informal observations and interviews designed to determine whether the student *needs* the services (Nelson, 1993).

Another way of addressing the problem of whether a child with severe or multiple disabilities should receive speech and language services is to broaden the concept of those services. Rather than viewing services as occurring within a single model, in which children are removed from their classrooms and taken down the hall to receive a half-hour of individualized therapy on objectives related only marginally to classroom activities, the service guaranteed on the student's IEP might be to receive consultation within the classroom setting (e.g., see Hoskins, 1990; Marvin, 1987; Simon, 1987). Such a plan could make it easier to meet the needs of the child who does not have the skills to function effectively within the classroom (Calculator & Jorgensen, 1991, 1994).

Rather than involving work on an isolated set of separate speech and language skills, the plan might involve collaboration between the speech-language pathologist and classroom teacher to identify communicative demands of regular classroom activities that are problematic for the student and to devise ways to make those activities more accessible to the student. In some instances, speech-language pathologists might demonstrate a way to prompt a desired behavior or to notice occasions for particular communicative behaviors to occur, which the teacher could encourage throughout the day. In others, children might need some direct instruction about a skill such as articulatory placement. In still others, teachers and speech-language pathologists might plan to coteach special lessons to elicit language content and forms needed by all children in a classroom. Ultimately, however, the program is the joint responsibility of an intervention team, not several individuals working separately. When children have multiple disabilities, evaluation of speech and language should be conducted as part of comprehensive multidisciplinary assessment activities. It is much easier to include speech-language services in the initial IEP than to hold a meeting later to add them, and services can only be provided in areas that have been evaluated.

Parent Notification and Consent

The IDEA requires signed, informed parental consent to be obtained at two points in the service delivery process: (a) before conducting a preplacement evaluation and (b) before initial placement of a child in a program of special services. Procedures involve informing parents of their legal rights to due process as well as informing them about specific planned activities. For requesting permission before an initial evaluation, most school districts use preprinted forms with descriptions of language, speech, and hearing evaluations and blank spaces for individualization. Parents sign and return one copy of the form and keep the other for their records.

If evaluation shows a need for special services, an IEP meeting is scheduled to explain the results of the evaluation and to determine what kinds of services the student should receive. Parental signature is required before the student's first placement in a special education program. Thereafter, the educational agency must notify the parents about evaluation activities that might change the child's identification as speech and language impaired or modify the IEP Parents must also be given opportunity to participate in decision making (and this must be documented), but their signatures are not required during the notification process.

Several regulations apply to formal notification. Information must be presented in a form understandable by parents, using translators when parents do not speak English or cannot read. Parents must understand that their consent is voluntary and may be retracted later. They also should be informed of their rights to request a review of their child's IEP more frequently than mandatory 1-year intervals if they are concerned about its appropriateness. Finally, parents are informed of their rights under the Family Rights and Privacy Act to have access to their children's school records and to grant permission before information in those records is shared with anyone outside the school district.

Comprehensive Evaluation

Once parental permission has been obtained, the comprehensive evaluation process can begin. Evaluation of children suspected of having language disorders has two major purposes: (a) determining eligibility for placement in a speech-language intervention program and (b) identifying specific intervention needs, when service is required. These two goals are considered separately in the following sections, but they overlap in actual practice.

Determining Eligibility
Eligibility for special services is determined by practices and criteria guided by state rules and regulations. These are generally more specific than requirements in the federal IDEA. Most states establish eligibility criteria and service delivery guidelines for each of the categories of disability. Although efforts are currently under way in some areas to reduce the labeling that accompanies a categorical approach to special education, teacher certification and program reimbursement often depend on the use of such categories, so the categorical approach is unlikely to be abandoned soon.

Definitions for determining language disorders vary, but most specify that to qualify for service, children must show language deficits in one or more of the systems of language—phonology, morphology, syntax, semantics, or pragmatics. Sometimes deficits are defined in psychometric terms (e.g., more than 1 or 1.5 standard deviations from the mean on at least 2 tests or 2 subtests designed to measure language learning). In addition, activities to be included in the evaluation process may be specified, such as requiring a spontaneous language sample in addition to formal test results. As a minimum, the federal regulations for the IDEA specify that a full and individual evaluation must be conducted with more than one procedure, each of which has been validated for the purpose for which it is used. Procedures must also be selected and administered so as not to be racially or culturally discriminatory. A child must be evaluated in all areas related to the suspected disability, and the evaluation must be conducted by a multidisciplinary team.

For children with multiple disabilities, the requirement for comprehensive preplacement evaluations means that when communicative problems are involved, the need for speech-language assessment should not be overlooked. For children in regular education classrooms, the multidisciplinary team requirement means that someone other than the speech-language pathologist must participate. In such instances, classroom teachers typically play a role in the evaluation, not administering formal tests but providing information about the child's speech and language behaviors (both oral and written) in classroom contexts. Other team members may include special education teachers, particularly learning disability specialists, psychologists, occupational therapists, and others knowledgeable about the child or the suspected impairment.

Often the quantitative requirements of comprehensive language evaluation are met by starting with a broad language assessment instrument with a number of subtests. Using a single score to represent a child's language functioning is generally not enough, however. Broad comprehensive testing often must be followed by specific evaluation in areas suspected to be relatively more intact or impaired, perhaps using samples of oral and written communication behaviors as well as formal tests. Many children with language disorders show uneven profiles of relative strengths and weaknesses. Identifying areas of strength, as well as weakness, is an important function of the evaluation process. It also contributes to meeting the second, more qualitative goal of assessment, determining individualized intervention needs.

Determining Intervention Needs

The second goal of individualized assessment is to describe the communicative processes and needs of children with language disorders in enough detail to allow determination of appropriate intervention contexts and content. As discussed, to be relevant to children's needs, this process should be conducted in collaboration with important participants (e.g., teachers, parents, and children themselves), who can identify significant contexts for use in assessment and intervention processes (Nelson, 1990). IEPs may then be written with appropriate descriptions about present levels of performance in those contexts so that goals, short-term objectives, and program details may be relevant to functional outcomes.

Collaborative evaluation activities involve participant interviews and classroom observations as well as traditional standardized tests. When school-age children experience communicative problems, teachers, parents, and the students themselves should be interviewed. For example, they might be asked, "If you could change one thing about the way this child [your child/you] communicates, what would it be?" and "If you could pick one kind of situation where changes need to occur, what would that be?" Abilities and contexts that teachers, parents, and students name in response to such questions may not be the only ones to consider in the assessment and intervention process, but they definitely should be some of them. These "zones of significance" (Nelson, 1992, 1993) are critical to this particular student because changes in these contexts will determine whether the student attains functional outcomes through intervention. Many of the targeted areas involve problems of functioning that determine whether or not the student will be able to keep up with peers in the regular curriculum.

"Curriculum-based language assessment" (Nelson, 1989, 1990, 1994) has some things in common with techniques of more general "curriculum-based assessment" used by educators to measure children's progress within the local curriculum (Rosenfield & Rubinson, 1985; Tucker, 1985), but it differs in its specific focus on the language demands of the curriculum and children's abilities to meet those demands. Contextually based assessments help IEP committees design interventions to help students acquire specific language knowledge, skills, and strategies leading to desired functional outcomes. Artifacts of students' work (e.g., worksheets, math assignments, journal writing, and written assignments from textbooks) in significant curricular contexts may be used when conducting assessments like these. Both previously completed samples and new, interactive ones might be gathered to develop a comprehensive picture of the multiple rule systems, modalities, linguistic levels, and contexts that are relevant to the evaluations. Some of the key elements of this process are listed in Table 9-1 (Nelson, 1986).

Both onlooker observation and participant observation may be used to develop ecologically valid descriptions of the problem elements, once the student's particular zones of significance have been identified. Onlooker observation involves observing from a distance without direct participation. Alternatively, the participant observation approach of ethnographic researchers (e.g., see Green & Wallat, 1981) might be used to investigate a student's use of language in a particular targeted academic activity by participating with the student in the activity. For example, when direction following has been reported as problematic, onlooker observation strategies might be used to observe the student's attentional and communicative behaviors during regular classroom activities. Later, the professional might use a tape recording of the teacher's directions to probe with the student whether breakdowns are occurring in misunderstanding of key vocabulary, syntactic decoding, length overload, or a combination of factors. The professional participant might also probe for metacogni-

TABLE 9-1   Key Elements of Comprehensive Speech-Language Assessments

Rule Systems	Modalities	Linguistic Levels	Contexts
Phonological	Listening	Sound	Formal tests
Morphological	Speaking	Syllable	Spontaneous samples
Syntactic	Reading	Word	Academic materials
Semantic	Writing	Sentence	• Workbook pages
Pragmatic	Thinking*	Complex sentence	• Reading text
		Text	• Grade level
			• Reading level
			• Science text
			• Problem solving

Adapted from Nelson (1986).

*"Thinking language" is observed as verbal mediation ability. The ability to consciously "talk through" an academic task, or classroom routine, represents metacognitive, metapragmatic, and metalinguistic skill (depending on the task), and is an important part of the individualized assessment of a student having difficulty in classroom contexts.

tive strategies the student could use to compensate for memory deficits. For example, the student might not know that most students do not remember directions verbatim but chunk the material into relevant pieces. For example, they attend only to topic, workbook, and page numbers, knowing that the teacher usually writes assigned problem numbers on the chalkboard.

Participation observation of this nature extends beyond the cultural descriptions of anthropological ethnographers. Part of the advantage of participation is that the professional may begin to explore ways to facilitate the student's communicative performance, perhaps asking strategically placed questions or focusing the student's attention on key aspects of the activity. Such strategies have been called "dynamic assessment" (e.g., see Feuerstein, 1979; Feuerstein, Rand, & Rynders, 1988) because they avoid static description of what "is" and consider "what might be." That is, they consider not only what a person can do without assistance but also what the individual might be able to do if scaffolding is provided. Vygotsky (1934/1962) first introduced the idea that children can sometimes perform tasks with support from an adult at a developmental level that is impossible without the support. He called the difference between what children could do by themselves and what they could do with assistance the "zone of proximal development." By identifying the developing edge of competence for individual children in several key contexts, professionals can then identify scaffolding techniques (Applebee & Langer, 1983; Bruner, 1978; Cazden, 1988; Silliman & Wilkinson, 1994; Nelson, 1995) appropriate in those contexts. These are techniques of best practice (described previously) that serve the functional needs of children.

Placement Decisions and Planning

Comprehensive assessment results, including information from parents and teachers, guide decisions about placing children in special education programs and selecting models of service delivery. No one type of service delivery is right for all children, even when they have similar disabilities (Robert & Mather, 1995). Furthermore, federal requirements dictate that placement decisions be made collaboratively by an IEP team that includes the child's parents and that they be based on the needs of children, not on the availability of programs. The trouble is that all participants do not always agree on what kinds of service would best serve the child.

As noted previously, one of the primary tensions in current service delivery decisions is whether "full inclusion" options are best for children with severe disabilities. Should special classroom contexts be provided for these children or should regular classrooms be adapted to include such children no matter how severe their disabilities? Some parents and professionals believe that education in the "least restrictive environment" (LRE), guaranteed by the IDEA, means that their children should be educated in their local schools with same-age peers (Flynn, 1990; Markus, 1988), noting that integrated programs have benefits for children with and without disabilities (Knoll & Meyer, 1987). For example, a high school student with Down syndrome (who previously had ridden a bus many miles to attend a special school) became manager of the football team when his placement was changed to the local high school. A nondisabled student who got to know the newcomer was quoted by Ruben (1988) as saying, "You used to see those kids in the mall or something, and you'd shy away. . . . Now you just go up and talk to 'em without worrying about it" (p. 121). Social benefits like these may be critical to the ultimate inclusion of many people with disabilities in society.

Other parents and professionals identify different factors that determine which environments are "least restrictive" for their children. This second viewpoint was exemplified by a mother from Michigan (Lord, 1991), who wrote about her 15-year-old daughter who was born profoundly deaf. Throughout her early education, this girl attended a total communication program in a regular school in her local community. Although she learned Signed English well, she had virtually no audible speech and could communicate with few of her classmates and with few adults, except her mother, who had become an expert in sign language. As a result, this teenager had become increasingly isolated socially. Recent school testing showed her to be educable mentally impaired (i.e., to have mild mental retardation), and the girl's mother reported that "her frequent temper tantrums and out-of-control behavior would certainly qualify her as emotionally impaired" (p. 4). Questions of LRE for this adolescent were extremely complex. Previously, her mother had known vaguely about the Michigan School for the Deaf in Flint, but, along with local school personnel, had viewed it as unnecessarily restrictive. That opinion changed when mother and daughter visited the school. The mother described the experience:

> *We were taken on a tour of the facility by the school's principal. Although he himself is profoundly hearing impaired, he is very skilled in communicating in spoken English and in sign. Wherever we went, students, teachers, and support staff spoke easily with him in spoken language and simultaneously in sign. The warm, relaxed, and friendly atmosphere and the natural ease of communication was one of the delights of our visit.*
>
> *My often sullen and angry daughter was in her glory. From the principal's first greeting, she fell into step with him, joking, teasing, and conversing comfortably as we walked down corridors full of the evidence of students of all ages doing the kinds of things that nonhandicapped students do. We visited classrooms where small groups of students, intent on their work, interrupted themselves for brief greetings and introductions. Much to my surprise, my daughter was outgoing and friendly, exchanging questions and information of the usual teenage sort. She was wearing her Camp Chris [a special camp for children with hearing impairments] sweatshirt, and that generated a lot of discussion. In the computer room, a girl got up and greeted my daughter with a warm and enthusiastic hug. A friend from Camp Chris! I was surprised and taken aback. At home my daughter has never had friends her own age with whom she could truly communicate. . . . In this setting she didn't look either dull or disturbed. In fact, I have never seen her so happy, so lively, or so interested and involved. (p. 4)*

Actual decisions regarding placement are finalized at initial IEP meetings. At those meetings, parental permission is obtained for the initial placement in a special education program. When conflicts arise about what placement might be "least restrictive" for a given child, the courts sometimes become involved (Osborn & Dimattia, 1994). A less combative problem-solving approach is for the collaborative team to move back a step from the placement decision and attempt to clarify their goals and values. One set of values concerns parental desires about the appropriateness of including their children in classrooms where they might not be academically competitive, no matter how much support they are given. Beukelman and Mirenda (1992) discussed a system for value clarification in which decisions could be made based on academic and social functioning on three levels:

1. *Competitive*—children with disabilities compete as equals with peers (perhaps using compensatory techniques and devices), attempting the same activities and influencing the choices made by the group
2. *Active*—children with disabilities participate actively in classroom academic and social activities, learning some things and having their ideas be considered in making decisions, but not being fully competitive members of the group
3. *Involved*—children interact successfully in classrooms and with peers largely through the efforts of adult facilitators and peers who have adopted the value system of inclusion

By building a chart of academic and social areas and identifying the level on which the planning team members view the child functioning in each area, it may be possible to clarify the decisions to be made for this student and to select an appropriate service delivery model.

Service Delivery Options

Possible service delivery model options are listed in Table 9-2, as summarized by the ASHA Committee on Language, Speech, and Hearing Services in the Schools (1984). In this summary, service delivery models are divided into four basic types: (a) consultant, (b) intermittent or itinerant, (c) resource room, and (d) self-contained classroom. Actually, many more options exist, including several forms of "integrated service delivery" approaches (Elksnin & Capilouto, 1994). Models may also be used in combination with one another to create new options. The key to service provision is individualization.

Consultant Services.   A certain amount of collaborative consultation is necessary in the intervention programs for all children to keep activities relevant to individuals' functional needs. As noted in the previous discussion of principles of best practice, collaboration is a decision-making mode with broader implications than defining a single service delivery model. The consultation model uses collaborative strategies heavily, but it is also a service delivery model with a number of special characteristics of its own.

As noted in Table 9-2, the consultant model of service delivery may be appropriate for children with all degrees of impairment, from those with mild to severe disabilities. When consultation is used as an alternative to direct service by speech-language pathologists, consultant services may take many forms. All of them involve collaboration to enhance the language learning opportunities of natural environments with individuals who spend time with the target student. The defining feature of consultant speech-language services is that others (primarily teachers and parents) implement objectives established collaboratively with, and monitored by, speech-language pathologists. Those other individuals, who are in more frequent direct contact with the child, thus become the primary agents of communicative change (Frassinelli, Superior, & Meyers, 1983; Marvin, 1987; Simon, 1987).

TABLE 9-2   Recommended Caseload Sizes for Four Kinds of Service Delivery in Schools

	Consultation Program (Indirect Service)	Itinerant Program (Intermittent Direct Service)	Resource Room Program (Intensive Direct Service)	Self-Contained Program (Academically Integrated Direct Service)
Cases Served	All communicative disorders All severities (mild to severe)	All communicative disorders All severities (mild to severe)	All communicative disorders, particularly language and articulation All severities	Primary handicap: communication Severe/multiple disorders particularly language and articulation
Services Provided	Program development, management, coordination Indirect services	Program development, management, coordination, evaluation Direct services Coordination w/educators	Program development, management, coordination, evaluation Direct service/self-study/aide Coordination w/teachers(s) Teacher has academic responsibilities	Program development, management, coordination, evaluation Direct services plus academic instruction
Group Size	Individual or group (indirect service)	Individual or small group (up to 3 students/session)	Individual or small group (up to 5 students/ session)	Up to 10 students/speech-language pathologist Up to 15/speech-language pathologist w/supportive personnel
Time per Day	Variable: Possible range ½ hour (mild) to 3–4 hours/day	½ to 1 hour/day	1 to 3 hours/day	Full school day
Times per Week	1 to 5 times/week	2 to 5 times/week	4 to 5 times/week	Full-time placement
Rationale for Caseload Size	Time necessary by organization Variable needs	Complex cases demand lower caseloads Approximates national average	Cases require intensive services Consistent w/regulations	Consistent w/regulations Provides for intensive services
Caseload Maximums*	Up to 15–40 students	Up to 25–40 students	Up to 15–25 students	Up to 15 students w/aide Up to 10 students w/out aide

From "Guidelines for Caseload Size for Speech-Language Services in the Schools" by the ASHA Committee on Language, Speech, and Hearing Services in Schools, 1984, *ASHA, 26,* pp. 53–58. Copyright 1984 by the American Speech-Language-Hearing Association. Adapted by permission.

*Maximums are not additive across programs and do not account for travel time.

Such an approach may be identified as "indirect service," but this does not mean that the service is haphazard, or even less time-consuming than direct service. When consultative services are written on a child's IEP, it is expected that the professional will have regularly scheduled contact with the primary intervention agent, including observation of the student in targeted activities.

Consultant services may be an appropriate intervention model for children with milder impairments whose needs are best met in the context of regular classroom activities. Even when disabilities are more severe, in particular when children are extremely low functioning and demonstrate prelinguistic stages of development, consultant services provided by a speech-language pathologist to classroom teachers and aides may be most appropriate. In such instances, consultants may focus on assisting those who spend the most time with the child "tune in" to primitive communication attempts and to encourage the cognitive underpinnings of language. Home programs might also provide appropriate means of delivering language intervention services to infants and preschoolers with severe disabilities or developmental risks who are too young for classroom placement and would be served best by their own parents or other caregivers at home.

Intermittent Services.   "Itinerant" or intermittent services are considered the traditional service delivery model for children with speech-language impairments. This model has been called itinerant because it usually is delivered by speech-language pathologists traveling from school to school, serving children in several different buildings. This model is still prevalent in most communities, but it may be replaced gradually as more speech-language pathologists become based in single buildings, serving children with moderate to severe impairments in special classrooms, resource rooms, or regular classrooms housed together. When that happens, a school staff may be more likely to develop a collaborative synergy that will benefit the communicative development needs of all students and that involves a variety of types of interactions among students and professionals.

The traditional approach also has been called a "pull-out" approach because youngsters have been pulled out of their regular classrooms to be taken to a quiet room down the hall for half-hour sessions of individual or small-group therapy two or three times per week. For some children with language disorders, pull-out contexts are helpful because the children have more opportunity to talk than in their regular classrooms and they can practice difficult speech and language skills without interruption. However, special contexts may not be best for learning other aspects of contextually based communication. Many children with subtle but significant language disorders, for example, can handle regular educational experiences if language intervention is provided early enough and with enough intensity to allow them to acquire the psycholinguistic foundations for much of later learning. Intermittent direct services for such youngsters do not necessarily have to be provided in pull-out classrooms. Some sessions may be scheduled with speech-language pathologists providing direct service in the classroom. This approach might be recommended not only for children who receive no other special education services but also for children who spend time in a resource room with a special education teacher.

Regardless of the service delivery setting, language specialists must make plans with parents and teachers to encourage children to generalize newly learned skills and strategies to a variety of contexts. For example, kindergarten children might be engaged in snack preparation or art activities designed to encourage the use of newly acquired language content and forms for real communicative purposes (e.g., requesting materials or describing actions). Older students might benefit from activities in cooperative learning groups (e.g., see Johnson, Johnson, & Holubec, 1988; Slavin, 1983) used for such purposes as group discussion of curricular topics, role-playing social situations, and completing classroom assignments. Although studies of cooperative learning groups involving students with disabilities have produced equivocal results regarding academic achievement benefits (Tateyama-Sniezek, 1990), their benefits have yet to be explored systematically. Other values may justify such services as well. In any case, less structured, in-class activities give speech-language pathologists a chance to probe newly acquired behaviors in situations that are more like those of real life. This allows them to judge whether targeted behaviors are sufficiently automatic to be maintained outside the relatively protective environment of the pull-out room.

Team Teaching and Other Forms of "Integrated Service Delivery." Children with language disorders accompanying other disabilities may also benefit from close interaction between speech-language pathologists (SLPs) and classroom teachers (CTs). For example, as discussed in Chapter 13, communicative disorders are an integral part of the syndrome of autism. Children with autism need a program in which more than 30 minutes two times per week are devoted to meeting their needs for communication intervention. Team teaching is one way of meeting these needs. Using classroom contexts, teachers and speech-language pathologists can work together to provide comprehensive programs. Manual communication systems or microcomputer-based learning experiences may provide initial access to language for some autistic children. Meaningful, but structured communication experiences can be devised and repeated in classroom contexts many more times than in a pull-out room.

Team teaching may be called for when serving children with learning disabilities or mental impairments or isolated speech-language impairments. It may also be provided in collaboration with regular classroom teachers as whole-class sessions on special topics like direction-following, story retelling, or semantic mapping. Integrated service delivery models in which a speech-language pathologist (SLP) and classroom teacher (CT) work in a single classroom at the same time can take several forms. Options include: (a) *one teach, one observe*, gathering onlooker observation data that may be useful in future planning (b) *one teach, one "drift,"* assisting individual students who need help; (c) *station teaching,* with movement of students among stations to work with both the SLP and CT at different times; (d) *parallel teaching*, with the SLP and CT each teaching the same content to half the class; (e) *remedial teaching*, in which one adult works with the students who have not mastered a concept to remediate its meaning for them; (f) *supplemental teaching*, in which one adult provides extra support to students who have not mastered key material, and (g) team teaching, in which adults share responsibility equally for lecturing and experiential learning (Elksnin & Capilouto, 1994).

Resource Rooms or Alternative Classrooms. Some children with language impairments need services that are more intensive than those provided on an intermittent, twice-a-week basis. A resource room model, similar to that used with many learning disabled children, may best meet their needs. Enrollment in a resource room for part of the day may provide access to the language arts curriculum for children with moderate to severe language learning disabilities, particularly at middle-school to secondary-school levels. Alternate language classes for adolescents, for example, might meet 5 days per week in a regularly scheduled time slot and allow students to earn course credit as they do for any other class. Activities would mirror and augment those of the regular curriculum, and students would be systematically taught strategies to help them cope with the language expectations of their other classes, with the goal to return to those classes full time (Anderson & Nelson, 1988; McKinley & Lord-Larson, 1985).

Self-Contained Classroom Programs.   In some educational systems, speech-language pathologists serve as primary teachers for children with severe speech-language impairments. The advantage of self-contained classrooms is that all academic and social interaction activities can be exploited to their fullest extent for encouraging language in its most relevant and communicative forms. Language intervention generally proceeds best in meaningful contexts, and children with severe disabilities need clear examples and repetitive opportunities to practice new skills and strategies.

Speech-language pathologists serving as classroom teachers (and sometimes in itinerant roles) generally are required to hold teaching credentials in addition to their clinical certificates. When they do assume the role of classroom teachers, speech-language pathologists accept responsibility for meeting students' total developmental and educational needs. For example, preschoolers need activities aimed at developing gross and fine motor skills and cognitive abilities as well as language and communication. School-age youngsters need to learn all aspects of the academic curriculum in addition to receiving specialized instruction in spoken and written language (e.g., see Nelson, 1981).

IEP Meetings

Decisions regarding a particular type of program for an individual student are not made unilaterally. They are made on the basis of a multidisciplinary evaluation by an IEP committee. Regulations exist for specifying the kinds of individuals who must be present at the IEP meeting. These include:

1. *A representative of the public agency, other than the child's teacher, who is qualified to provide or supervise the provision of special education.* This person may be the special education coordinator for the district, the building principal, or another speech-language pathologist or special education teacher.

2. *The child's teacher.* This person may be the speech-language pathologist; in some states, however, if a school-age child is in a regular education classroom, the child's regular education teacher must attend the IEP meeting. For secondary students, only one teacher need attend, but collaborative planning may proceed best if several teachers provide information about the student's functioning in their classrooms.

3. *One or both of the child's parents or guardians.* The regulations for implementing the IDEA are specific about ensuring that parents be afforded opportunity to participate in their child's IEP meeting. Steps include notifying parents of the meeting early enough, scheduling the meeting at a mutually agreed on time and place, taking care that parents know the purpose of the meeting and who will be there, and providing special assistance to help them understand the proceedings if necessary. Meetings may be held without parents if school districts can show that, although repeated attempts were made, they were unable to convince the child's parents to attend the meeting. Fulfilling requirements for parental participation in the planning process can be one of the most time-consuming aspects of providing language intervention services in school settings. However, the expectations are no greater than those that would generally be a part of service provision in any other environment. Quite apart from meeting legal requirements, they are also important to best practice.

4. *The child, where appropriate.* Modifying communicative behaviors entails the shaping of skills that are largely automatic, although never trivial nor simple. The active and self-motivated involvement of the individual being served greatly increases the likelihood of success. When children can be appropriately included in goal-setting phases of program planning, goal-directed learning may be enhanced. Children who are old enough to recognize that they have problems deserve to have explanations for those problems. If left to draw their own conclusions, they too often conclude that they are too dumb, or otherwise inferior, to be good in school. Providing children with some simple explanations of their problems and the special services they receive is an important function of the school speech-language pathologist.

5. *Other individuals.* Either the child's parents or educational agency may invite other individuals to the IEP meeting. If the agency invites additional individuals, the parents must be informed of who will be there. At the first IEP meeting, the law requires that someone be present to explain any of the evaluation procedures and results. If the IEP meeting is scheduled for a child who has some other primary impairment accompanied by a language disorder, the speech-language pathologist who performed the evaluation should make every effort to be at the meeting. In this way, not only can the language evaluation process and results be explained, but also the collaborative context may make it easier to sort out confounding influences of language, cognition, and cultural environmental factors as the IEP committee decides whether a child or adolescent needs language intervention services.

IEP Content and Review under PL 94-142

The format for writing IEPs varies widely from district to district across the United States. Most districts have designed their own forms, and the same form is used regardless of type of disability. Some forms feed easily into computerized information processing systems. Others are processed with a number of manual steps to meet accountability needs. Regardless, each IEP must include information in six areas:

1. *A statement of the child's present levels of education performance.* This statement generally records the highlights of the comprehensive multidisciplinary evaluation. This information may be entered on the form before the IEP meeting, or it may be recorded while the child's current functioning is being discussed at the meeting. For a child with a language disorder who is functioning generally at grade level, language assessment data plus anecdotal evidence that the child can handle the regular curriculum except for the noted areas of difficulty are sufficient. Formal test scores of academic achievement are not necessary. For a child with learning disabilities or mental retardation, psychological and educational assessments are frequently conducted as part of preplacement evaluations but again, curriculum-based assessment information may be the most useful. For a child with emotional impairment, a social work evaluation may be involved. For a child with physical impairments, physical therapy and occupational therapy evaluations may be conducted. A summary of the results of the multidisciplinary assessment is included for describing present levels of education performance in all relevant areas.

The degree of detail in this statement depends on the philosophy of the district. If greater detail is included to provide baseline or criterion-referenced data, the information may be used as a point of comparison for the evaluation plan, a required component of the IEP. The primary purpose of this part of the IEP is to provide an accurate sketch of the total child at a particular point in development. With this in mind, a microscopic look at some of the critical aspects related to the disability is appropriate, but not at the expense of a macroscopic view of the child as a whole person.

2. *A statement of annual goals, including short-term instructional objectives.* This component provides a time frame for the process. The challenge facing individuals who gather at IEP meetings is to establish goals that are broad enough to be significant (avoiding triviality), yet specific enough to be manageable (avoiding lack of clarity). The goals and short-term objectives must be revised within at least 1 year.

The leveling between goals and short-term objectives in the regulations for the IDEA contributes to the decision-making process. Using both formal and informal evaluation results, individuals at IEP meetings set goals. Within goal areas, individual behaviors might be targeted because they are: (a) next in developmental sequence and ripe for change, (b) particularly impaired, (c) potential catalysts for other delayed processes, or (d) functionally significant.

Frequently, the team members establish separate goals for implementation by each of the specialists who will be working with the child. Teams who work collaboratively are also likely to establish collaborative goals. At the very least, teams should coordinate their efforts so that students will not receive fragmented programs using multiple curricula and approaches. The speech-language pathologist will usually need two or three goals to define a meaningful program. For example, a single goal, such as "to improve communication skill," may focus the group on the need to be concerned about communication in general, but including language intervention as a specific service to be provided to the child probably accomplishes as much. The specialist can more efficiently use IEP space by indicating several annual goals, such as: (a) use new conceptual vocabulary to understand science, social studies, and language arts texts; (b) produce sentences of greater length and complexity than current oral and written language samples show; and (c) take active turns in cooperative group discussions with peers. More than three goal areas may be targeted, depending on the time available to implement the plan and keeping in mind the principles of best practice, but three areas is usually a manageable, appropriate size.

Short-term objectives are more precise than goals and add detail to them. Objectives are sufficiently detailed to guide intervention efforts, and they include measurement criteria for determining whether a program is bringing a child closer to appropriate targets. The targets may be chronologically "normal" skills for some children, or functional, independent living skills for others. Whereas goals are based on macroscopic views of what is important for the individual, short-term objectives offer a relatively more microscopic view of how to meet those goals.

More than one short-term objective must be provided under each of the established goals. Objectives may be written for relatively more structured or naturalistic activities by operationally defining the desired skill as an observable, quantifiable behavior. Writing objectives behaviorally does not mean that behavior modification techniques must be used to implement them. For example, Figure 9-5 is a portion of a sequence of objectives for encouraging "later listening, speaking, reading, writing, and thinking skills" (Nelson, 1988). It is based on Bloom's (1956) taxonomy for encouraging higher level language processing skills, including: (a) knowledge of specifics about who, what, when, and where; (b) comprehension by using the known to predict the unknown using translation, interpretation, and extrapolation; (c) application to new contexts; (d) analysis that extends beyond the immediate material; (e) creative synthesis of new ideas; and (f) evaluation of those ideas. (see also Wiig & Wilson, 1994).

The short-term objectives in these examples are written to include three kinds of information: (a) what the student will do, (b) the conditions of performance, and (c) how well the student must perform. Each of these objective components provides important information about the design of a student's individualized language intervention program.

The *"do" statement* in these objectives is the behavioral one. It refers to the student's behavior, not the speech-language pathologist's. The focus is on establishing behaviors that demonstrate progress in targeted areas. If written in terms of what the speech-language pathologist or teacher will do, the student-oriented focus is diminished. It is also important that the behavior in the "do" statement is observable and measurable. In the examples in Figure 9-5, behaviors such as question answering (see Statement 3) provide observable means of measuring comprehension. An objective stating only that the child must "understand" or "discriminate" gives no behavior that can be documented. When the speech-language pathologist determines that skills such as understanding and discrimination are important, operational definitions of such abilities must be written.

The *conditions* portion of short-term objectives indicates the type of approach and environmental contexts that will be used in documenting that the child has acquired the new behavior. Conditions statements can specify content for a number of different variables. Among these, kinds and complexity of stimuli may be described, along with the degree of structure or spontaneity to be provided or expected in the communicative exchanges. Also important are environmental contexts and people with whom the new behavior is to be demonstrated. In the examples in Figure 9-5, several different communicative contexts are specified ("Listening and Discussing in Practice Activities:" etc.) The objectives may be initiated in all or only some of these contexts.

Short-term objectives written into IEPs are intended to provide measurement points and not to outline an entire intervention program. In fact, it may be desirable to leave them slightly more open-ended to allow flexibility as the program is implemented. Some states do require more specific, step-by-step programs of performance objectives to be written to supplement the IEP If so, additional time after the initial IEP meeting is usually allowed before this requirement must be met. Computerized lists of objective sequences may facilitate this process as well (Nelson & Snyder, 1990).

The third component of well-written short-term objectives is a specification of *how well* the student must perform. These are criteria for determining when an objective has been met. Criteria are integrally tied to descriptions of conditions. Being able to demonstrate a new behavior spontaneously in a classroom without any modeling by the speech-language pathologist is quite different from demonstrating it in a highly supportive pull-out environment. Criteria may also specify how complete, how frequent, or how rapid correct responses must be. For example, the speech-language pathologist must decide how many occurrences of a new behavior must be observed on how many occasions in order to be confident that the current objective has been met and the child is ready to move on to a higher level. For example, in Figure 9-5, the student must complete the task in Statement 3 in "4 of 5 units of discourse"

Percentages (e.g., 80 to 90 percent correct) are often used for this purpose. However, percentages have little meaning unless a time frame or number of trials is specified as a ba-

INFORMATION PROCESSING: LATER LISTENING,
SPEAKING, READING, WRITING, AND THINKING SKILLS

Date: _____
Child: _____

SHORT-TERM OBJECTIVES: THE CHILD WILL:	LISTENING AND DISCUSSING IN PRACTICE ACTIVITIES		LISTENING AND DISCUSSING IN REAL CLASSROOM AND OTHER NATURALISTIC ACTIVITIES		READING AND WRITING IN PRACTICE ACTIVITIES		READING AND WRITING IN REAL CLASSROOM AND OTHER NATURALISTIC ACTIVITIES		DESCRIPTION OF STIMULI AND RESPONSES	COMMENTS/ TECH- NIQUES/ EVALUATION
	Date In.	Date Ac-com.	Date In.	Date Accom.	Date In.	Date Accom.	Date In.	Date Accom.		
3. demonstrate *comprehension* of passages by answering the following kinds of questions for each type of task (appropriate responses should be given in each category for a mixture of questions regarding 4 of 5 units of discourse of varying types):										
a. *translation* (How else can it be said/written? Can you summarize what was said/written? Can you show how to follow oral/written directions for such things as cooking, fixing a car, setting up a VCR unit? [observe strategies for doing so])										
b. *interpretation* (What does it mean? How does it relate? What is the main idea? Can you relate one idea to another? What is the speaker's/writer's purpose? Is there more than one purpose?)										
c. *extrapolation* (What came before? What is next? Given part of the story, can you infer what happened before? Can you suggest a plausible ending?)										
4. demonstrate *application* of verbal material to extended contexts of the following types (appropriate responses given for 4 of 5 units of discourse):										
a. *common applications* (How do you use it? How do you use it in still another way?)										

FIGURE 9-5 Portion of a sequence of short-term objectives for building information processing skills.

(From *Planning Individualized Speech and Language Intervention Programs*—Revised and Expanded, by Nickola Wolf Nelson, copyright 1988 by Communication Skill Builders, Inc., PO Box 42050, Tucson, AZ 85733. Reprinted with permission.)

sis for computing them. Otherwise, 80 percent may mean 4 out of 5 possible occurrences, or it may mean 40 out of 50 possible occurrences. The speech-language pathologist must decide whether the total number of trials is significant in a particular instance and, if so, what number is most appropriate for determining the acquisition of a particular skill.

By considering what the student will do, under what conditions, and how well, IEP team members can write meaningful short-term objectives that will move children closer to their longer-term goals. By writing at least two short-term objectives under each goal, movement toward the goal can be measured at more than one point during the year that each IEP is in effect.

3. *A statement of the specific special education and related services to be provided to the child and the extent to which the child will be able to participate in regular education programs.* These components describe the placement of the child in a particular program and the amount of time the child will spend in the program and in the regular classroom. Federal regulations require that the type of delivery model recommended for a particular child be recorded on the IEP (e.g., consultation, intermittent therapy, resource room placement, or placement in a specially designed self-contained classroom program). The time to be spent in the program must also be specified. Possible examples are "1 hour per week," "1 hour per day," or "full time except for art, music, and gym with regular education classes." Parents are often particularly concerned with this part of the IEP, because it is the component that ensures that their children will receive the services they need.

4. *The projected dates for initiation of services and the anticipated duration of services.* Federal regulations specify that an IEP meeting must be held within 30 calendar days of the determination that a child needs special education and related services. States have differing rules for meeting the placement decision and first IEP requirements. Some districts combine these two functions in the same meeting. Other requirements may be established by states for timelines between the initial IEP meeting and the start of services. It is a federal requirement, however, that an IEP must be in effect before special education and related services are provided to a child. If the evaluation has included a qualitative analysis as well as a quantitative one, it will have been possible to write meaningful objectives to be included in this first IEP. Although details of programming method and style may be added later, when zones of significance for the student are identified in the preplacement evaluation, relevant goals and short-term objectives may be written in the initial IEP. Most districts require that children begin to receive the services outlined in their IEPs within a few days after the initial IEP meeting.

Within 1 year, another IEP meeting must be convened to revise the IEP and to consider whether the child still needs the special education and related services outlined in the plan. This 1-year interval is usually used to define the "anticipated duration of services," as is required in this component of the IEP. Some states interpret the law as requiring that the IEP team establish prognosis for the child's need for special education over a number of years. The more common interpretation is that the team must enter a date on the IEP form indicating that the IEP will be reviewed and revised before a year has passed. When the IDEA is reauthorized, more frequent reporting may be required.

Districts use different management schemes for spreading IEP annual review meetings throughout the year. An IEP must be implemented all the time it is in effect. That is, children must begin receiving speech and language intervention services when school begins in the fall if an IEP is in effect for them from the previous school year, and they must continue to receive that service until another IEP meeting is held to terminate it.

5. *Appropriate objective criteria and evaluation procedures and schedules for determining whether the short-term instructional objectives are being achieved.* If short-term instructional objectives have been written to be measurable, this requirement will have been partially met. Criterion statements form an integral part of short-term objectives—and evaluation plans. In addition, pretest and posttest formats may have been adopted for determining progress. Formal tests may be selected and may be identified by name or generically (e.g., "a standardized vocabulary test") as part of the evaluation plan on the IEP form, or criterion-referenced procedures, including curriculum-based language measurements, based on samples of oral and written work, may be used to document progress. Teacher and parental reports are usually important components of an evaluation plan.

6. *A statement of the needed transition services for students beginning no later than age 16 and annually thereafter (and when determined appropriate for the individual, beginning at age 14 or younger), including, when appropriate, a statement of the interagency responsibilities or linkages.* This final requirement was added by the amendments to the IDEA in the federal law (PL 101-476). That law defines *transition services* as a coordinated set of activities designed to be outcome oriented. Transition services should promote movement from school to postschool activities, including postsecondary education, vocational training, integrated employment (including supported employment), continuing and adult education, adult services, independent living, or community participation.

This new requirement is for the IEP team to plan a coordinated set of activities based on the individual student's needs, taking into account the student's preferences and interests, including such things as instruction, community experiences, and the development of employment and other postschool adult living objectives. When appropriate, as when individuals have severe disabilities, the transition plan should address acquisition of daily living skills and functional vocational evaluations. If some agency other than an educational agency fails to provide agreed upon services, the educational agency is responsible for reconvening the IEP team to identify alternative strategies to meet the transition objectives.

Speech-language pathologists and other language learning specialists might fill important roles in implementing transition plans. Language and communication skills contribute to the success of such plans whether they are aimed primarily toward higher education or employment. Language assessment activities, for example, might include contextually based observation of functional communication demands of targeted employment contexts. Then intervention goals and activities could be coordinated with other activities to prepare students to meet such functional communication requirements as they begin their work-study or supported-employment activities.

Reevaluation

Reevaluation is the final requirement of the IDEA to be considered in this discussion of language intervention in school settings. To be certain that students continue to receive the most appropriate education possible, it is necessary to step back occasionally and take a comprehensive look at their abilities, needs, and functional outcomes.

An implicit goal for many students with language disorders is to function as much like normally developing same-age peers as possible, remaining "competitive" in academic activities as well as in social interactions. As noted previously, goals for students may be written with the intention for them to be "active" with classmates even though they may not be truly competitive, or to be "involved," even though they may not hope to compete on the same level with their peers (Beukelman & Mirenda, 1992). It is easy to lose sight of such broad goals in the day-to-day details of meeting behavioral objectives. Re-evaluation at specified intervals allows a team to determine whether broader goals are still appropriate.

When the goal is for a student with a relatively mild disability to remain competitive with peers, professionals must keep an eye on what peers without language problems are doing, to prevent the student from falling further and further behind. Although true competitiveness may never be possible, if the language professional never looks at the relationship, it is impossible to see where it is going.

To ensure that professionals maintain a broad perspective as well as a detailed one, the IDEA requires comprehensive reevaluation at least every 3 years. This comprehensive reevaluation must meet all of the requirements of the original preplacement evaluation. Parental permission is not required before testing, but the district must notify parents in writing that their child is undergoing a reevaluation that will determine whether the child is still identified as having a disability. Following the comprehensive reevaluation, another meeting is scheduled, possibly coinciding with the regularly scheduled annual review, to explain the results of the evaluation and to make further plans (see Figure 9-2).

The suggestion here is that, in addition to administering formal tests, this also might be a time to assess where students stand relative to peers in meeting the curricular demands of regular education. It is possible for a student to score within normal limits on formal tests and still be unprepared to meet regular classroom language demands. Conversely, it is possible for a student to score low on some formal language measures but to function well in regular classroom settings. These kinds of information about language functioning in classroom contexts should be considered along with formal test data about the need to provide continued intervention services.

Summary of Public Policy Procedures

Both best practices and public policies influence language intervention in school settings. Public policies influence procedures for identifying students suspected of having disabilities; notifying parents and obtaining their permission for preplacement evaluations and initial special education placement; conducting a comprehensive, nonbiased multidisciplinary evaluation; holding an IEP meeting; selecting a service delivery model; writing and implementing an IEP; documenting progress; and performing a comprehensive reevaluation at least once every 3 years. The requirements for these procedures may seem extensive, but they can be implemented in such a way to be consistent with best practices for children if those goals are kept in mind.

Case Study

This case study is based on data for a real child who has been given a fictitious name. It is presented, not as a model of all that is perfect about providing services in school settings, but to illustrate some of the challenges that need to be overcome before best practices become commonplace. Janet Sturm's contributions to this case study are gratefully acknowledged.

Background Information

Barbie was an 11½-year-old fourth grader who met the requirements of her school district as "physically and otherwise health impaired" (POHI). As a secondary impairment, she received speech-language services from her school speech-language pathologist. Barbie's pediatrician diagnosed her as having attention-deficit disorder, temporal sequential disability, and language deficit secondary to temporal lobe seizure disorder. The temporal lobe seizures occurred since Barbie was 3 years old, with unknown etiology. Currently, Barbie's mother noted that the seizures were controlled by medication and she could go months without having one. When they occurred, the seizures resulted in tremors in Barbie's face and mouth with occasional drooling and tingling, but with no loss of consciousness.

At school, Barbie was placed in a regular fourth-grade classroom for science and social studies and special curricular activities, such as music and physical education. She was also placed in a special education resource room 2½ hours per day, where she received instruction in reading, math, language, and spelling. Barbie's IEP also included speech-language intervention services twice a week.

Language Assessment

Assessment of Barbie's language indicated both receptive and expressive deficits on the Clinical Evaluation of Language Fundamentals—Revised (Semel, Wiig, & Secord, 1987). On the Story Construction Subtest of the Detroit Tests of Learning Aptitude—2 (Hammill, 1985), Barbie earned a raw score of 7, placing her at the 16th percentile. Barbie's "stories" consisted mostly of picture description. For example, when telling a story about a picture of a bear cub walking near a tourist bus, Barbie said:

> *A baby cub is chewing on a cart and his mama or his papa is getting him off that cart because he doesn't want him to get hurt. The people are looking happy and that was a bus and they're in traffic.*

A sample of spontaneous self-formulated language gathered throughout the evaluation session showed a mean length of utterance of 5.8 morphemes. Barbie demonstrated few problems in the area of expressive syntax, using utterances up to 15 morphemes in length: "When she hits the door, she just wants to get that tail off." The content of many of her utterances, however, lacked clarity. For example, in describing play with her cat, Barbie used many pronouns without cohesive ties. She was attempting to convey that her pet cat enjoyed playing with a stuffed cat's tail, but it was difficult for a listener to discern which cat was being discussed.

Barbie also had difficulty conveying temporal concepts. For example, when discussing the cat, the clinician asked, "Is it a baby or is it grown up?" Barbie replied, "I really don't know. We got it pretty much in the summer." Clinician: "Last year?" Barbie: "I really don't know. Her name is Pepper. It's a black one with green eyes."

To explore Barbie's understanding of spatial, temporal, and quantitative conceptual vocabulary, the Boehm Test of Basic Concepts (Boehm, 1971) was given. Even though Barbie was above the second-grade ceiling level of the test, the test was administered because Barbie was having difficulty understanding conceptual vocabulary in classroom contexts. On the test, she scored at the 35th percentile for second graders, misunderstanding such terms as *beside*, *skip*, and *fewest*.

During informal conversations of later sessions, the clinician noted a number of discourse-related problems. Specifically, Barbie had trouble with word retrieval, topic management, responding to *wh-* questions, and using specific vocabulary in response to questions. Pragmatic assessment of Barbie's communication acts using Fey's (1986) communication acts profiling revealed that the majority of Barbie's utterances were statements. Barbie demonstrated strong ability to extend topics she initiated, but between topics, utterances were related tangentially, contributing to communication breakdowns. During these, Barbie appeared to be insensitive to her listener's needs and did not repeat or rephrase utterances following requests for clarification. Of six requests in one conversation with the clinician, she responded to none. When asked to read aloud, Barbie exhibited frustration, saying, "I can't" and "My mouth hurts."

Although no consistent articulatory problems were noted, Barbie did demonstrate some difficulty with phonological sequencing in spontaneous oral communication. For example, instead of "pie filling," Barbie said "pilling fie."

Current Functioning in Classroom Settings

Observation in Barbie's regular classroom showed her able to sit at her desk for 10 minutes listening to her teacher read a story. After reading the story, the teacher said that English would be next. Writing compound sentences was the topic for the day. Students were asked to refer to their "key word cards" and locate compound predicates. During a task that involved each student writing a sentence with a compound predicate, the teacher cued the task with "power words." These included indent, punctuation, capitals, and "power one words" used in forming compound sentences like "Stations look like barns and look like cellars."

While her classmates were completing this assignment, Barbie wrote numbers in a grid from 1 to 132 and completed a worksheet that involved following directions like "Give the bird a yellow beak." Barbie also worked on a written assignment entitled, "My Favorite Rocks." It was a topic she had chosen herself to correspond with her "rock collection," a set of rocks she had glued into a box lid. When asked about the meaning of this topic choice, Barbie's teacher suggested that Barbie was emulating an assignment the rest of the class had completed earlier in the semester. The "story" she had written to go with the rock collection had many incomplete sentences, which Barbie's teacher had corrected. Her current task was to recopy the corrected story. During the independent work session, Barbie's teacher checked her work on two occasions and provided verbal feedback. Barbie worked independently and did not experience difficulty during any one task.

The clinician held a collaborative session with Barbie's special education teacher when Barbie was not present. This teacher commented on academic difficulties experienced by Barbie on tasks requiring discrimination of word patterns such as *fits* and *fists*. She also had difficulty with morphological word endings, such as -*s*, -*ed*, and -*ing*. Addition was her most difficult area in math. When the special education teacher was asked to indicate her primary concern regarding speech and language, she said she hoped Barbie could learn to "repeat exactly," because this ability played a major role in the design of her special curriculum for learning to read.

IEP Objectives

These goals and objectives were established for Barbie:

1. To demonstrate increased self-monitoring and self-confidence by
   a. Participating in selection of intervention topics and activities, the order of activities in a session, and books or topics to be used in the activities
   b. Using a verbal or gestural sign to indicate recognition of her own success during I or more points in each activity
   c. Evaluating and revising her own work when given the opportunity
2. To demonstrate increased skill in reading by
   a. Predicting the main idea of a story from only its title, for 4 of 5 stories, and explaining discrepancy accurately when it occurs
   b. Responding to miscue feedback appropriately when the clinician says things like, "I heard you reading 'that' and I'm seeing 't' 'h' 'i' 's' [spelling aloud]:" self-correcting 80 to 90 percent of reading miscues (Goodman, 1969, 1973; Goodman, Watson, & Burke, 1987)
   c. Answering 8 of 10 questions correctly after reading a story aloud or hearing a story read aloud
3. To demonstrate increased skill in oral and written expression by
   a. Recounting an event or describing an object or experience using at least 10 complete sentences with appropriately specific vocabulary by either initiating a topic or responding to a request for information by the clinician
   b. Composing at least 10 event narrations over the duration of the IEP, with at least 5 logically sequenced, grammatically complete sentences, and specific references

Intervention Program and Progress in the First Semester

To increase self-confidence and willingness to attempt new tasks, Barbie was given a voice in deciding the topics and order of intervention activities. Potential written language topics were generated in collaboration with the resource room teacher, and Barbie could select from these or generate her own. Topics chosen ranged from "How to Make Orange Juice" to "What I Did over Spring Break."

At the beginning of the year, Barbie did not greet the clinician upon arrival for therapy sessions, put her head on the table, closed her eyes, and did not respond to the clinician's request for information. Following a 2–5 minute period, Barbie consistently became an active participant for all therapy tasks by attending, initiating, and responding. Being told that the story generated would be put on the computer (if time allowed) was especially motivating to her.

The computer program used was *Cue-Write: Word Processing With Spelling Assistance and Practice* (Beukelman, Tice, Garrett, & Lange, 1988). It allowed Barbie to see words on the bottom half of the screen as she entered them on the top half of the screen, helping her develop confidence and independence, but with support in an area of significant disability.

By the end of the semester, Barbie had become an active and enthusiastic participant, demonstrating confidence in each activity by smiling, acting eager to begin, and initiating many ideas during each task. She asked many appropriate questions during each task, demonstrating reduced fear of "not knowing" and recognition that it is OK to ask questions. She also developed a healthy intrapersonal sense of humor about her difficulties, saying, "Sometimes things don't go through my brain quite right" and "I was just checking to see if you were paying attention" (when a spelling error was noted by the clinician).

Early in the year, Barbie struggled with the writing task, having difficulty organizing her ideas, generating complete sentences, and being motivated by the task. By the end of the semester, she appeared eager to start a new story each week, generating ideas before arriving for the intervention session and formulating grammatically complete sentences. She composed 12 stories, each with 10–15 grammatically complete sentences, ordered logically. Barbie enjoyed taking the role of leader during the activity, using the clinician as a "secretary" to jot down notes during the idea formulation stage. She also cued the clinician to use appropriate writing skills and strategies (reinforcing her own skills). For example, while Barbie was typing in a story, she asked the clinician to "Repeat my sentence for me and say the whole thing please."

Because of time constraints and Barbie's aversion to reading, her own stories provided the context for work on reading decoding. The objectives on story prediction and written language comprehension were modified. Barbie became increasingly confident about reading her stories once she had experienced some success. Whereas early in the semester she refused to read her first story aloud, saying "I can't," by the end of the semester she read each story aloud without hesitating.

Barbie was able to describe objects or pictures using 10 or more adjectives when asked by the clinician to "tell me about it" at random points during sessions when appropriate topics arose. Barrier tasks were also used to encourage Barbie to be sensitive to her listener's need for sufficient information. In these activities, Barbie described an object or picture to the clinician, whose view of the object was blocked by a barrier and who gave nonverbal cues to indicate noncomprehension. Throughout the semester, Barbie's descriptions became longer and more relevant. Although she continues to use nonspecific vocabulary and to have difficulty connecting ideas across utterances, she has become increasingly aware of communication breakdowns and now repeats or rephrases when breakdowns occur. She has met the objective of recounting events and experiences using at least 10 complete sentences, when encouraged to provide additional information by the clinician.

Evaluation and Recommendations
for Additional Intervention

Functional changes in Barbie's language and communication skills have been noted by both her special education and regular education teachers in classroom contexts. Neither classroom was especially conducive to meeting Barbie's needs at the outset. A good example was the lack of connectedness Barbie felt in her regular classroom. Barbie's teacher kept her from participating with her classmates in the regular curriculum, and she was consigned to working on boring and meaningless worksheets provided by the special education teacher. Barbie was sensitive to this and complained about not being allowed to remove from the room the unused textbooks that lay in her desk. She tried to resolve the problem of curricular relevance on her own, by attempting the rock collection project after her classmates had finished theirs. In the resource room, Barbie had reacted to the highly structured remedial reading approach that required her to repeat meaningless, phonetically regular sentences by not wanting to read at all.

Although some collaboration is evident in this program, it could be stronger. Barbie's clinician is new to the building and is not in a position to suggest major changes in the special education reading curriculum or in Barbie's participation in the classroom. She has begun to work with these two teachers to identify more meaningful learning contexts, however. Now, the regular education teacher allows Barbie to join the rest of the class for special projects, to follow along when they read aloud from their textbooks, and to participate in group discussions. The special education teacher has instituted more spontaneous writing assignments, in which the students write their own ideas and read their work to each other for feedback. She has also begun to encourage real communication in the children's journals (rather than just having the students copy sentences like "I had lunch" from the chalkboard). For example, when children write such sentences in their journals, the teacher might respond, "Who do you like to sit beside at lunch?"

Future goals are to use meaningful literature selections that Barbie chooses to address reading decoding and comprehension objectives. She will be encouraged to discard a book if she starts reading it and does not like it. Barbie's clinician plans to use "communicative reading strategies" (Norris, 1988; 1989) in collaboration with her teachers to encourage reading confidence and the ability to draw inferences from text. Barbie's program in the three learning contexts should become increasingly integrated, as the clinician has arranged to demonstrate the communicative reading strategies technique in the special education classroom. Although Barbie's program is still not perfect, its efficacy can be demonstrated by real changes in the way she functions in multiple settings. She has come a long way from avoiding interactions by putting her head on the table or saying her mouth hurts. Further improvement can be expected.

Summary

This chapter provides a comprehensive, although abbreviated, view of the provision of language intervention in the schools. It encourages a primary emphasis on best practices for meeting the needs of individual children and a secondary emphasis on the use of federal and state regulations to do so. Best practices relate to viewing language as an integrated system, appreciating the complexity of developmental validity, using contextual relevance to achieve functional outcomes, individualizing programs through frequent updates and cultural sensitivity, and using collaboration as a problem-solving mode.

Procedures for implementing such practices are guided by public policies at federal, state, intermediate, and local levels. When compliance with regulations is emphasized to the point that service to children becomes incidental, individualized needs may not be met.

To be effective, speech-language pathologists in schools are encouraged to become involved with program planning at all levels. This involves becoming more knowledgeable about local, state, and federal regulations and the political process for changing them when they are counterproductive to providing appropriate services. Membership in state and national professional associations provides a mechanism for staying informed and for increasing awareness of the needs of speech and language impaired children.

A number of problems associated with identifying best practices for the provision of services in school settings remain to be solved. Among these are needs to increase the precision of determining which students qualify for language intervention programs; to expand the continuum of service delivery models in all areas of the country, both rural and urban; to clarify the role of speech-language pathologists in evaluating and serving individuals with severe and multiple disabilities in varied settings, including integrated regular classrooms; to foster awareness of the professional skills of speech-language pathologists by others and to build collaborative relationships; and to ensure that regulations, including those related to maximum caseload size, allow best practices to be implemented. Addressing these concerns will be the challenge of the coming years.

Study Questions

1. In what ways is language intervention in school settings unique, and in what ways should it be similar to the provision of services in other settings?
2. List the sequential steps for placing a child in a special education program and for planning, implementing, and reviewing an IEP.
3. What are some best practice principles for planning language intervention regardless of setting, and how might the school setting be used to plan intervention activities using these principles?
4. What are the levels of regulatory influence on the provision of programs in school settings, and what should the role of the speech-language pathologist be in attempting to ensure that the regulatory influences are facilitative?
5. Formulate at least two well-written, short-term objectives, and suggest intervention contexts (use your imagination) for each goal area identified for the following two children:

a. A 7-year-old boy with Down syndrome and mild mental retardation who interacts well with peers in his first-grade classroom and resource room most of the time, but who demonstrates language problems involving

   (1) Plural and possessive morphological endings

   (2) Comprehension and production of constructions with three or more components (e.g., agent + action + object, and agent + action + location)

   (3) Understanding stories his teacher reads aloud

b. A sixth-grade girl with language learning disabilities who is having academic difficulty in most subjects and needs to develop

   (1) Comprehension and production of complex sentence forms (e.g., with conjunctions *since, while, if...then, because,* and *except*)

   (2) Ability to organize ideas and present them orally or in writing

   (3) Ability to recognize and use abstract and multiple word meanings associated with other academic areas

6. What new regulations did later laws (PL 99-457 and PL 101-476) add to those already existing under PL 94-142?

References

Allington, R. L. (1991). The legacy of "Slow it down and make it more concrete." In G. Zutell & S. McCormick (Eds.), *Learner factors/teacher factors: Issues in literacy research and instruction* (pp. 19–30). Chicago: National Reading Conference.

American Psychiatric Association. (1987). *Diagnostic and statistical manual of mental disorders, third edition, revised* (DSM III-R). Washington, DC: American Psychiatric Association.

American Speech-Language-Hearing Association. (1995). Position statement on "inclusionary practices." Policy established at the Annual Convention of the American Speech-Language-Hearing Association, Dec. 8–10, Orlando, FL.

Anderson, G. M., & Nelson, N. W. (1988). Integrating language intervention and education in an Alternate Adolescent Language Classroom. *Seminars in Speech and Language, 9*(4), 341–353.

Anderson, N. B. (1992). Understanding cultural diversity. *American Journal of Speech-Language Pathology, 1*(2), 11–12.

Applebee, A. N., & Langer, J. A. (1983). Instructional scaffolding: Reading and writing as natural language activities. *Language Arts, 60,* 168–175.

Aram, D. M., Ekelman, B. L., & Nation, J. E. (1984). Preschoolers with language disorders: 10 years later. *Journal of Speech and Hearing Research, 27,* 232–244.

Aram, D. M., Morris, R., & Hall, N. E. (1992). *Validity of discrepancy criteria for identifying children with developmental language disorders.* Manuscript submitted for publication.

Aram, D. M., & Nation, J. E. (1980). Preschool language disorders and subsequent language and academic difficulties. *Journal of Communication Disorders, 13,* 159–170.

ASHA Committee on Language Learning Disorders (F. M. Cirrin, Chair). (1989). Issues in determining eligibility for language intervention. *Asha,* 31(3), 113–118.

ASHA Committee on Language, Speech, and Hearing Services in the Schools. (1984). Guidelines for caseload size for speech-language services in the schools. *ASHA,* 26, 53–58.

Beukelman, D. R., & Mirenda, P (1992). *Augmentative communication: Management of children and adults with severe communication disorders.* Baltimore: Paul H. Brookes.

Beukelman, D. R., Tice, R., Garrett, K., & Lange, U. (1988). *Cue-write: Word processing with spelling assistance and practice* [Computer program]. Tucson, AZ: Communication Skill Builders.

Bloom, B. S. (Ed.). (1956). *Taxonomy of educational objectives. Handbook I: Cognitive domain.* New York: David McKay.

Bloom, L., & Lahey, M. (1978). *Language development and language disorders.* New York: Wiley.

Boehm, A. (1971). *Boehm Test of Basic Concepts.* San Antonio: Psychological Corp.

Bruner, J. (1978). The role of dialogue in language acquisition. In A. Sinclair, R. J. Jarvella, & W. J. M. Levelt (Eds.), *The child's conception of language: Springer series in language and communication* (pp. 242–256). New York: Springer-Verlag.

Calculator, S. N., & Jorgensen, C. M. (1991). Integrating AAC instruction into regular education settings: Expounding on best practices. *Augmentative and Alternative Communication,* 7, 204–213.

Calculator, S. N., & Jorgensen, C. M. (1994). *Including students with severe disabilities in schools.* San Diego: Singular.

Calfee, R., & Chambliss, M. (1988). Beyond decoding: Pictures of expository prose. *Annals of Dyslexia,* 38, 243–257.

Calkins, L. M. (1983). *Lessons from a child: On the teaching and learning of writing.* Portsmouth, NH: Heinemann.

Carlson, C. C., & Nelson, N. W. (1994). Classroom amplification, middle ear pathology, and academic success. Paper presented at the annual convention of the American Speech-Language-Hearing Association, November 19, 1994, New Orleans.

Casby, M. W. (1992). The cognitive hypothesis and its influence on speech-language services in schools.

Language, Speech, and Hearing Services in Schools, 23, 198–202.

Catts, H. W., & Kamhi, A.G. (1986). The linguistic basis of reading disorders: Implications for the speech-language pathologist. *Language, Speech and Hearing Services in Schools,* 17, 329–341.

Cazden, C. B. (1988). *Classroom discourse: The language of teaching and learning.* Portsmouth, NH: Heinemann.

Cochran, P. S., & Masterson, J. J. (1995). NOT using a computer in language assessment/ intervention: In defense of the reluctant clinician. *Language, Speech, and Hearing Services in Schools,* 26, 213–222.

Council for Exceptional Children. (1994, January). Supplement to *Teaching Exceptional Children,* 26(3), 1–4.

Crandell, C. C., Smaldino, J. J., & Flexer, C. (Eds.). (1995). *Sound-field FM amplification.* San Diego: Singular.

Creaghead, N. A. (1990). Mutual empowerment through collaboration: A new script for an old problem. *Best Practices in School Speech-Language Pathology,* 1, 29–36.

Damico, J. S. (1988). The lack of efficacy in language therapy: A case study. *Language, Speech and Hearing Services in Schools,* 19, 51–66.

Damico, J. S., & Hamayan, E. V. (1991). Implementing assessment in the real world. In E. V. Hamayan & J. S. Damico (Eds.), *Limiting bias in the assessment of bilingual students* (pp. 303–316). Austin, TX: Pro-Ed.

Damico, J., & Oller, J. W., Jr. (1980). Pragmatic versus morphological/syntactic criteria for language referrals. *Language, Speech and Hearing Services in Schools,* 11, 85–94.

David, J. L. (1995–1996). The who, what, and why of site-based management. *Educational Leadership,* 53(4):4–9.

Elksnin, L. K., & Capilouto, G. J. (1994). Speech-language pathologists' perceptions of integrated service delivery in school settings. *Language, Speech, and Hearing Services in Schools,* 25, 258–267.

Feuerstein, R. (1979). *The dynamic assessment of retarded performers.* Austin, TX: Pro-Ed.

Feuerstein, R., Rand, Y., & Rynders, J. E. (1988). *Don't accept me as I am: Helping "retarded" people to excel.* New York: Plenum Press.

Fey, M. E. (1986). *Language intervention with young children.* Austin, TX: Pro-Ed.

Flynn, G. J. (1990, February/March). Quality education: Community or custody. *Newsletter of the Michigan Society for Autistic Citizens,* pp. 1, 5–6.

Frassinelli, L., Superior, K., & Meyers, J. (1983). A consultation model for speech and language intervention. *ASHA,* 25(11), 25–30.

Frey, W. (1984). Functional assessment in the '80s. In A. Halpern & M. Fuhrer (Eds.), *Functional assessment in rehabilitation* (pp. 11–43). Baltimore: Paul H. Brookes.

Gerber, M. M., & Levine-Donnerstein, D. (1989). Educating all children: Ten years later. *Exceptional Children,* 56, 17–27.

Giangreco, M., Cloninger, C., & Iverson, V. (1993). *Choosing, options and accommodations for children (C.O.A.C.H.): A guide to planning inclusive education.* Baltimore: Paul H. Brookes.

Goodman, K. S. (1969). Analysis of oral reading miscues: Applied psycholinguistics. *Reading Research Quarterly,* 5(1), 9–30.

Goodman, K. S. (1973). Analysis of oral reading miscues: Applied psycholinguistics. In F. Smith (Ed.), *Psycholinguistics and reading* (pp. 158–176). New York: Holt, Rinehart & Winston.

Goodman, Y. M., Watson, D. J., & Burke, C. L. (1987). *Reading miscue inventory: Alternative procedures.* New York: Richard C. Owen.

Green, J. L., & Wallat, C. (1981). *Ethnography and language in educational settings.* Norwood, NJ: Ablex.

Guterman, B. R. (1995). The validity of categorical learning disabilities services: The consumer's view. *Exceptional Children,* 62, 111–124.

Hamayan, E. V, & Damico, J. S. (Eds.). (1991). *Limiting bias in the assessment of bilingual students.* Austin, TX: Pro-Ed.

Hammill, D. (1985). *Detroit Tests of Learning Aptitude—2.* Austin, TX: Pro-Ed.

Hammill, D., & Larsen, S. (1974). The effectiveness of psycholinguistic training. *Exceptional Children,* 40, 5–13.

Hillard, S. W., & Goepfert, L. P (1979). Articulation training: A new perspective. *Language, Speech and Hearing Services in Schools,* 10, 145–151.

Hodson, B. W., & Paden, E. P (1991). *Targeting intelligible speech: A phonological approach to remediation* (2nd ed.). Austin, TX: Pro-Ed.

Hoskins, B. (1990). Collaborative consultation: Designing the role of the speech-language pathologist in a new educational context. *Best Practices in School Speech-Language Pathology* (Vol. 1). San Antonio: Psychological Corp.

Hunt, K. W. (1965). *Grammatical structures written at three grade levels.* Urbana, IL: National Council of Teachers of English.

Idol, L., Paolucci-Whitcomb, P., & Nevin, A. (1986). *Collaborative consultation.* Rockville, MD: Aspen.

Jenkins, J. R., & Heinen, A. (1989). Students' preferences for service delivery: Pull-out, in-class, or integrated models. *Exceptional Children,* 55, 516–523.

Johnson, D. W., Johnson, R. T., & Holubec, E. (1988). *Cooperation in the classroom* (rev. ed.). Edina, MN: Interaction Book Co.

Knoll, J. A., & Meyer, L. (1987). Integrated schooling and educational quality: Principles and effective practices. In M. S. Berres & P. Knoblock (Eds.), *Program models for mainstreaming: Integrating students with moderate to severe disabilities* (pp. 41–59). Rockville, MD: Aspen.

Kretschmer, R. E. (1991). Exceptionality and the limited English proficient student: Historical and practical contexts. In E. V. Hamayan & J. S. Damico (Eds.), *Limiting bias in the assessment of bilingual students* (pp. 1–38). Austin, TX: Pro-Ed.

Lahey, M. (1988). *Language disorders and language development.* New York: Macmillan.

Larson, V. L., & McKinley, N. L. (1987). *Communication assessment and intervention strategies for adolescents.* Eau Claire, WI: Thinking Publications.

Leonard, L. (1972). What is deviant language? *Journal of Speech and Hearing Disorders,* 37, 427–447.

Leonard, L. B. (1987). Is specific language impairment a useful construct? In S. Rosenberg (Ed.), *Advances in applied psycholinguistics: Vol. 1. Disorders of first language acquisition* (pp. 1–39). New York: Cambridge University Press.

Levi, G., Capozzi, E, Fabrizi, A., & Sechi, E. (1982). Language disorders and prognosis for reading disabilities in developmental age. *Perceptual and Motor Skills,* 54, 1119–1122.

Lipsky, D. K., & Gartner, A. (Eds.). (1989). *Beyond separate education: Quality education for all.* Baltimore: Paul H. Brookes.

Loban, W. (1963). *The language of elementary school children* (Research Report No. 1). Champaign, IL: National Council of Teachers of English.

Loban, W. (1976). *Language development: Kindergarten through grade twelve* (Research Report No. 18). Champaign, IL: National Council of Teachers of English.

Lord, W. (1991, November). Parent point of view: What is the least restrictive environment for a deaf child? *Statewide Newsletter,* p. 4. (Published by the Statewide Communication and Dissemination System [SCADS], Michigan Department of Education, Special Education Services, Lansing, MI.)

Markus, D. (1988, November). Out of the shadows. *Parenting,* pp. 113–114.

Marvin, C. A. (1987). Consultation services: Changing roles for SLPS. *Journal of Childhood Communication Disorders,* 11, 1–15.

Masterson, J. J. (1995a). Computer applications in the schools: What we *can* do—What we *should* do. *Language, Speech, and Hearing Services in Schools,* 26, 211–212.

Masterson, J. J. (1995b). Future directions in computer use. *Language, Speech, and Hearing Services in Schools,* 26, 260–262.

Maxwell, S. E., & Wallach, G. P. (1984). The language-learning disabilities connection: Symptoms of early language disability change over time. In G. P. Wallach & K. G. Butler (Eds.), *Language learning disabilities in school-age children* (pp. 15–34). Baltimore: Williams & Wilkins.

McKinley, N. L., & Lord-Larson, V. (1985). Neglected language-disordered adolescent: A delivery model. *Language, Speech and Hearing Services in Schools,* 16, 2–15.

Miller, L. (1989). Classroom-based language intervention. *Language, Speech and Hearing Services in Schools,* 20, 153–169.

Miller, L. (1990). *The smart profile: A qualitative approach for describing learners and designing instruction.* Austin, TX: Smart Alternatives.

Muth, K. D. (1989). *Children's comprehension of text.* Newark, DE: International Reading Association.

National Center for Educational Restructuring and Inclusion. (1995). Study of Inclusive Education. Unpublished report available from the Graduate School and University Center, City University of New York.

Nelson, N. W. (1981). An eclectic model of language intervention for disorders of listening, speaking, reading and writing. *Topics in Language Disorders,* 1, 1–24.

Nelson, N. W. (1984). Beyond information processing: The language of teachers and textbooks. In G. Wallach & K. Butler (Eds.), *Language learning disabilities in children* (pp. 154–178). Baltimore: Williams & Wilkins.

Nelson, N. W. (1986). Individual processing in classroom settings. *Topics in Language Disorders,* 6(2), 13–27.

Nelson, N. W. (1988). *Planning individualized speech and language intervention programs* (2nd ed.). Tucson, AZ: Communication Skill Builders.

Nelson, N. W. (1989). Curriculum-based language assessment and intervention. *Language, Speech and Hearing Services in Schools,* 20, 170–184.

Nelson, N. W. (1990). Only relevant practices can be best. *Best Practices in School Speech-Language Pathology,* 1, 15–27. (Published by The Psychological Corporation, Inc., San Antonio.)

Nelson, N. W. (1992). *Collaborative consultation and curriculum-based assessment and intervention.* Kalamazoo, MI: Author.

Nelson, N. W. (1992). Targets of curriculum-based language assessment. *Best Practices in School Speech-Language Pathology* (Vol. 2, pp. 73–85). San Antonio: Psychological Corp. (pp. 104–131).

Nelson, N. W. (1993). *Childhood language disorders in context: Infancy through adolescence.* Boston: Allyn & Bacon.

Nelson, N. W. (1994). Curriculum-based language assessment and intervention across the grades. In G. P. Wallach & K. G. Butler (Eds.), *Language learning, disabilities in school-age children and adolescents* (pp. 104–131). Boston: Allyn & Bacon.

Nelson, N. W, & Snyder, T. [programmer]. (1990). *Planning individualized speech and language intervention programs: Software version* (rev. ed.) [Computer program]. Tucson, AZ: Communication Skill Builders.

Nevins, M. E., & Chute, P. M. (1996). *Children with cochlear implants in educational settings.* San Diego: Singular.

Nippold, M. A. (Ed.). (1988). *Later language development: Ages nine through nineteen.* Boston: College-Hill Press.

Norris, J. A. (1988). Using communication strategies to enhance reading acquisition. *The Reading Teacher,* 47, 668–673.

Norris, J. A. (1989). Providing language remediation in the classroom: An integrated language-to-reading intervention method. *Language, Speech and Hearing Services in Schools,* 20, 205–218.

Northern, J. L., & Downs, M. P. (1991). *Hearing in children* (4th ed.). Baltimore: Williams & Wilkins.

Ortiz, A. A., & Maldonado-Colon, E. (1986). Reducing inappropriate referrals of language minority students to special education. In A. C. Willig & H. F. Greenberg (Eds.), *Bilingualism and learning disabilities* (pp. 37–52). New York: American Library Publishing Co.

Osborne, A. G., & Dimattia, P. (1994). The IDEA's least restrictive environment mandate: Legal implications. *Exceptional Children,* 61, 6–14.

Padgett, S. Y (1988). Speech- and language-impaired three and four year olds: A five year follow-up study. In R. L. Masland & M. W. Masland (Eds.), *Preschool prevention of reading failure* (pp. 52–77). Parkton, MD: York Press.

Pehrsson, R. S., & Denner, P. R. (1988). Semantic organizers: Implications for reading and writing. *Topics in Language Disorders,* 8(3), 24–37.

Psychological Corporation. (1994). Picture gallery: articulation and phonology [Computer software]. San Antonio, TX: author.

Public Law 94-142. (1977, August 23). Implementation of Part B of the Education of the Handicapped Act. *Federal Register.*

Public Law 99-457. (1986, October 8). Education of Handicapped Amendments of 1986. *Federal Register.*

Public Law 101-476. (1991, August 19). Proposed regulations for implementation of Part B of the individuals with Disabilities Education Act. *Federal Register.*

Public Law 103-227. (1994, March). Goals 2000: Educate America Act: *Federal Register* (108 Stat. 125). Washington, DC: Superintendent of Documents, U.S. Government Printing Office.

Richgels, D., McGee, L. M., Lomax, R., & Sheard, C. (1987). Awareness of four text structures: Effects on recall of expository text. *Reading Research Quarterly,* 22, 177–196.

Roberts, R., & Mather, N. (1995). The return of students with learning disabilities to regular classrooms: A sellout? *Learning Disabilities Research and Practice,* 10, 46–58.

Rosenfield, S., & Rubinson, F. (1985). Introducing curriculum-based assessment through consultation. *Exceptional Children,* 52, 282–287.

Roth, S. R., & Perfetti, C. A. (1980). A framework for reading, language comprehension, and language disability. *Topics in Language Disorders,* 1(1), 15–27.

Ruben, D. (1988, November). Triumph of the heartland: How two mothers and their disabled sons made their Iowa town a beacon for the nation. *Parenting,* 120–126.

Scarborough, H. S., & Dobrich, W. (1990). Development of children with early language delay. *Journal of Speech and Hearing Disorders,* 33, 70–83.

Scott, C. M. (1988). Spoken and written syntax. In M. A. Nippold (Ed.), *Later language development: Ages 9–19* (pp. 49–95). Austin, TX: Pro-Ed.

Scott, C. M. (1994). A discourse continuum for school-age students: Impact of modality and genre. In G. P. Wallach & K. G. Butler (Eds.), *Language learning, disabilities in school-age children and adolescents* (pp. 219–252). Boston: Allyn & Bacon.

Semel, E., Wiig, E. H., & Secord, W. (1987). *Clinical Evaluation of Language Fundamentals—Revised.* San Antonio: Psychological Corp.

Silliman, E. R., & Wilkinson, L. C. (1994). Discourse scaffolds for classroom intervention. In G. P. Wallach & K. G. Butler (Eds.), *Language learning disabilities in school-age children and adolescents* (pp. 27–52). Boston: Allyn & Bacon.

Simon, C. S. (1987). Out of the broom closet and into the classroom: The emerging SLP. *Journal of Childhood Communication Disorders,* 11, 41–66.

Slavin, R. E. (1983). *Cooperative learning.* New York: Longman.

Stainback, W, Stainback, S., Courtnage, L., & Jaben, T. (1985). Facilitating mainstreaming by modifying the mainstream. *Exceptional Children,* 52, 144–152.

Stark, R. E., Bernstein, L. E., Condino, R., Bender, M., Tallal, P, & Catts, H. (1984). Four-year follow-up study of language impaired children. *Annals of Dyslexia,* 34, 49–68.

Tallal, P. (1988). Developmental language disorders. J. F. Kavanagh & T. J. Truss, Jr. (Eds.), *Learning disabilities: Proceedings of the National Conference* (pp. 181–272). Parkton, MD: York Press.

Tateyama-Sniezek, K. M. (1990). Cooperative learning: Does it improve the academic achievement of students with handicaps? *Exceptional Children,* 56, 426–437.

Taylor, O. L., & Payne, K. I. (1983). Culturally valid testing: A proactive approach. *Topics in Language Disorders,* 3(3), 8–20.

Terrell, S. L., & Terrell, F. (1983). Distinguishing linguistic differences from disorders: The past, present, and future of nonbiased assessment. *Topics in Language Disorders,* 3(3), 1–7.

Tucker, J. A. (1985). Curriculum-based assessment: An introduction. *Exceptional Children,* 52, 199–204.

U.S. Department of Education (USDE), Office of Special Education and Rehabilitation Services. (1988). *Annual report to Congress on the implementation of the Education for All Handicapped Children Act.* Washington, DC: Author.

van Kleeck, A. (1994). Metalinguistic development. In G. P. Wallach & K. G. Butler (Eds.), *Language learning disabilities in school-age children and adolescents* (pp. 53–98). Boston: Allyn & Bacon.

Vandercook, T., York, J., & Forest, M. (1989). The McGill action planning system (M.A.P.S.): A strategy for building the vision. *Journal of the Association for Persons with Severe Handicaps,* 14, 205–215.

Vaughn-Cooke, R. B. (1983). Improving language assessment in minority children. *ASHA,* 25(9), 29–34.

Vygotsky, L. S. (1962). *Thought and language* (E. Hanfmann & G. Vakar, Eds. and Trans.). Cambridge: MIT Press. (Original work published 1934)

Wells, G. (1986). *The meaning makers: Children learning language and using language to learn.* Portsmouth, NH: Heinemann.

Westby, C. E. (1994). The effects of culture on genre, structure, and style of oral and written texts. In G. P. Wallach & K. G. Butler (Eds.), *Language learning, disabilities in school-age children and adolescents* (pp. 180–218). Boston: Allyn & Bacon.

Wiig, E. H., & Wilson, C. C. (1994). Is a question a question? Passage understanding by preadolescents with learning disabilities. *Language, Speech, and Hearing Services in Schools,* 25, 241–250.

Willis, S. (1995). Inclusion gains ground. *Education Update* (Newsletter of the Association for Supervision and Curriculum Development), 37(9), 1, 6, 8.

Wood, P. (1980). Appreciating the consequences of disease: The classification of impairments, disabilities, and handicaps. *The World Health Organization Chronicle,* 34, 376–380.

Language and Communication Disorders in Culturally and Linguistically Diverse Children

DOLORES E. BATTLE
Buffalo State College

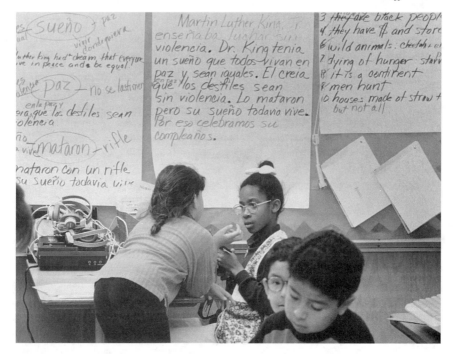

The United States has been from its beginning a nation of immigrants who came primarily from European countries that shared a common cultural and linguistic background. Since the 1980s, however, the nation has had a major increase in cultural and linguistic diversity resulting from the immigration of people from Central and South America, the Caribbean, and the Asian and Pacific Island countries, as well as from the Middle Eastern countries and the African diaspora. The new immigrants have changed the demographic picture of this country.

According to the 1990 census (U.S. Bureau of the Census, 1990), one in four people in the United States defines himself or herself as a nonwhite. Of the 248 million people in the country, nearly 25 percent, or 61.5 million, identify themselves as nonwhite. African Americans make up the largest group (12.1 percent) followed by Hispanic Americans (9.0 percent), Asian Americans (2.9 percent) and Native Americans (.8 percent). If current birth rates and immigration patterns continue, by the end of the 20th century, not only will there be continued increases in the number of culturally and linguistically diverse people, there will be an increase in the diversity represented within the groups themselves.

With the increase in immigration, there has been an increase in the number of children in the schools who speak a language other than English at home. According to the 1990 census, there are 32 million people (13 percent) in the United States who speak a language other than English at home. Many children entering the public schools speak little or no English and are considered Limited English Proficient (LEP). This presents a tremendous challenge for those charged with identification and treatment of children with communication and language disorders.

The American Speech-Language-Hearing Association (ASHA, 1991) and the National Deafness and Other Communication Disorders Advisory Board (1991) estimate that 10–15 percent of the U.S. population has a speech-language hearing disorder. The prevalence of communication disorders among the culturally and linguistically diverse is difficult to determine; however, based on census data, it is estimated that more than 6 million racial/ethnic minorities have a communication disorder. These may be a conservative estimates because of the greater risk for disability and communication disorders among those from below the poverty level, which includes a disproportionate number of racial/ethnic minorities. Socially and economically disadvantaged populations are more likely than other groups to be predisposed to the communication disorders related to environmental factors; traumatic factors; and teratogenic factors such as low birthweight related to poor prenatal nutrition and health care, high lead levels, and drug and alcohol abuse; as well as to other types of communication disorders such as stroke due to increased prevalence of high blood pressure and the effects of sickle-cell anemia in African Americans (Marge, 1993).

An estimated 6 million children under the age of 18 have a speech or language disorder (Office of Scientific and Health Reports, 1988). In the 1992–1993 school year 4.6 million children with disabilities received services in the public schools under IDEA Part B (U.S. Department of Education, 1994). Of these, 1,000,154 (21.6 percent) children received services for speech and language disorders and 60,896 (1.3 percent) received services for hearing disorders. Language disorders are prevalent in the 3 million children with mental retardation, learning disabilities, and other disabilities. If estimates concerning the prevalence of communication disorders among culturally and linguistically different persons are correct, over 500,000 culturally and linguistically diverse school-aged children received services for speech-language or hearing disorders in the public schools in the 1992–1993 school year.

To have a thorough understanding of the factors affecting communication disorders in culturally and linguistically diverse populations is necessary to understand (1) the relationship between culture and language, (2) the relationship between language, dialects, and disorders, (3) the nature of language development versus disorders of the specific language or dialect, (4) specific issues related to assessment, and (5) intervention.

Language and Culture

Culture is composed of the values, norms, beliefs, attitudes, folkways, behavioral styles, and traditions linked to form an integrated whole that functions to preserve a society (Terrell & Terrell, 1993). It encompasses a set of behaviors, institution, beliefs, technologies, values, and worldview passed on and maintained by an identifiable group in order to sustain what they believe to be a high quality of life and to negotiate their environment. Cultural variables influencing speech-language behavior include ethnic origin, race, place of birth and subsequent relocations, age, gender, socioeconomic status, educational level, language and/or dialects spoken, religious beliefs, health beliefs and practices, and family network.

Language, the primary mode of communication utilized by members of a culture to express their fundamental thoughts, principles, and attitudes, is enveloped within the culture. It is defined by the rules governing its form, content, and use and is the boundary for establishing the boundaries of a culture and the unification of its members (Taylor & Clarke, 1994). Any discussion of language disorders must emanate from an understanding of the set of presumptions or beliefs pertaining to normal communication and language behavior within a culture.

Culture, Family, and Language

A major force in the culture of a people is the family, including the structure of the family unit and the roles and expectations of individual members within the family. Children acquire language within the context of the family. The language systems acquired by children reflect the language behaviors, norms, and expectations of the family.

The role of the family in child rearing and the development of language differ across cultures (Anderson & Battle, 1993; Haynes & Shulman, 1994). According to Farran (1982) and Heath (1983b), the differences in interfamily communication affect the emergent communication and literacy behavior of young language learners. Each culture has its own communication rules and accepted ways of communicating to others in the group, its own beliefs about the existence and nature of language and communication, and its own expectations about the role of the family in the development of language.

The structure of the family and the roles of individual members within the family vary across cultures. These cultural differences affect feeding and sleeping patterns, and toileting, as well as the development of communication. For example, European-American families are usually structured as nuclear families, defined as the parents and their children. The mother is the prime caretaker and prime communicant with the child. She has primary responsibility for child rearing and for transmitting cultural norms and linguistic behavior to the child. The children are often in dyadic language environments where the parents participate in primarily dyadic verbal exchanges and actively encourage their children to develop communication and language skills at an early age. (Heath, 1983a, 1986)

Hispanic families are often both nuclear and extended family environments. Extended families, which include the parents, children, and other relatives living in the home or nearby, often provide multiparty communication environments where children are indirect participants in communication. Hispanic mothers, assisted by the maternal grandmother, are the prime communicant with the child. They do less teaching and give more nonverbal instructions to their children than European mothers and do not see themselves as teachers (Owens, 1992; Kayser, 1993). In Native American families, the extended family, defined as the entire tribe, is responsible for transmitting cultural rules or linguistic behaviors to the child (Harris, 1993). Middle Eastern children learn cultural rules by watching interactions among the extended family members. Verbal stimulation comes from adults other than the parents. There is much storytelling, rhyming, poems, and encouragement of communication from early ages (Lynch & Hanson, 1993). Cultural differences in child rearing result in differences in communication style.

Languages, Dialects, and Language Disorders

Dialects and Languages

A dialect is a variety of a language that is shared by a particular speech community for purposes of interaction (Taylor, 1986). A language difference or dialect is a rule-governed variation in a language used by racial, ethnic, geographical, or socioeconomic groups and reflects the phonological, semantic, syntactic, and pragmatic rules used by a particular speech community. Dialects reflect basic behavioral differences between groups of individuals within a society and are as natural as any other cultural manifestation of group differences. Although dialects of the same language may differ in form, pronunciation, vocabulary, and/or grammar, they are enough alike to be understood by other speakers of different dialects of the same language.

The 32 million Americans who speak a primary language other than English use more than 300 different languages and dialects (U.S. Bureau of the Census, 1990). The dialects of English commonly identified as Standard American English (SAE), African-American English (AAE), Appalachian English, Southern White Standard English, and numerous other regional dialects are mutually intelligible. When a person speaks a dialect of a primary language, it is referred to by the primary identification feature of the users of the dialect (e.g., African-American English). People who are able to speak two dialects of a single language (e.g., Standard American English and African-American English) are called bidialectal. A person who has native or near native fluency in two languages is called bilingual.

In addition to the dialects of American English there are many totally different languages spoken in the United States. By far the most common language other than English spoken by children at home is Spanish (17,339,172) followed by French, German, Italian,

Chinese, and 8.6 million persons who speak a language identified as "other" (U.S. Bureau of the Census, 1993). Each language has several dialects. Spanish, the principal minority language in the United States, is spoken by immigrants from as many as 20 different countries and has as many different mutually intelligible dialects. Each language in Asia and the Pacific Islands has several dialects. Of the Chinese population in the United States, 94 percent speak Han or one of its seven dialects, which include Cantonese and Mandarin. There are 87 mutually unintelligible Philippine languages and dialects. Although there are hundreds of dialects in India, the majority of Asian Indians living in the United States speak a dialect of Hindi or Kannada (Cheng, 1995). Arabic, the sixth most common first language spoken in the world and the chief language in 18 countries in the Middle East and North Africa, has a number of dialects that are so different as to preclude communication unless standard Arabic is used. The 500 Native American tribal entities in the United States speak as many as 200 distinct languages and dialects, some of which are mutually intelligible but most of which are mutually unintelligible to other Native American speakers (Harris, 1993).

When a person applies the rules of one language or dialect to a second language or dialect, the rules become mixed. For example, Indian-English refers to dialects of English spoken within Native American communities. Because of the similarity of some syntactic characteristics of the two languages, speakers may mix syntactic rules of the two languages. In Navajo, for instance, possession is expressed by personal pronouns prefixed to the noun or possessor noun plus possessive prefix plus possessed object (e.g., boy his hat). In English possession is expressed by possessive pronouns (e.g., my book) or by suffixes 's or -s' added to the noun. Navajo children who express possession according to the Navajo rule may be identified as having difficulty with syntax when they apply Navajo rules to Standard American English.

Language Disorders versus Language Differences and Dialects

As defined by the American Speech-Language-Hearing Association (1993), a language disorder is "impaired comprehension and/or use of spoken, written and/or other symbol systems. The disorder may involve (1) the form of language (phonology, morphology, syntax), (2) the content of language (semantics), and/or (3) the function of language in communication (pragmatics) in any combination."

Since language is embedded in culture, a definition of language disorder must be defined by the parameters established by the community of which the child is a member. As culturally defined, a language disorder is the impaired comprehension and/or use of spoken, written, and/or other symbol systems used by the child's indigenous culture or language group. The disorder may involve (1) the form of language (phonology, morphology, syntax), (2) the content of language (semantics), and/or (3) the function of language in communication (pragmatics) in any combination such that it interferes with communication within the indigenous culture of language group.

According to ASHA (1983):

> *No dialectal variety of English (or any other language) is a disorder or pathological form of speech or language. Each social dialect is adequate as a functional*

and effective variety of English. Each serves a communication function as well as a social solidarity function. It maintains the communication network and the social construct of the community of speakers who use it. (pp. 23–24)

Second Language Acquisition: Bilingualism

When a child is developing the use of English in a bilingual or bidialectal environment, he or she must learn two linguistic systems. The development of the two linguistic systems interact with each other and affect the acquisition of each system. Although most discussions of bilingualism focus on second-language learning among Spanish-speaking children, the principles of second-language acquisition apply to other languages as well. According to Saville-Troike (1986), nearly one-fourth of the Navajo children living on reservations in the Southwest learn the Navajo language as their first language and English as a second language. Although there is considerable information about the linguistic features of African-American English, there is very little information about the development of bidialectalism in African-American children. Discussion of second-language acquisition will for these reasons focus on the development of English as a second language among Spanish speakers (bilingualism) and later the development of features in African-American English (bidialectalism).

The acquisition of two languages can be either simultaneous or successive. Simultaneous bilingualism occurs when a child develops two languages from the onset of language, usually before the age of 3 years. Children learning two languages simultaneously acquire both languages at a normal rate (Dulay, Hernàndez-Chàvez, & Burt, 1978; Doyle, Champagne, & Segalowitz, 1978). While there may be interference with syntactic organization, lexical forms, or phonology, the children become genuinely bilingual by age 7 (Ambert, 1986). They are able to codeswitch—alternately switch between the two languages at the word, phrase, or sentence level—or use each language with equal facility depending on the language of their communication partners or the situational context. Codeswitching between two languages may occur when the child attempts to use a form that has not been learned in the second language or a concept that is more appropriately expressed in one language or the other.

Successive or sequential bilingualism occurs when a child acquires a second language (L2) after the basic linguistic acquisition of the primary language (L1) has been acquired. In successive bilingualism, children generally learn simple structures first, followed by more complex structures. Errors in the first language are similar to errors found in first-language learning. Common differences include omission and overextension of morphological inflections, double marking, misordering of sentence constituents, and the use of archiforms (using one member of a word class for all members, such as "that" for all demonstratives) or free alternation (using all members of a word class without concern for the different meanings) (Owens, 1996).

Successive bilingualism often results in language loss, which occurs when the child either losses ability in the original language (L1) or does not progress in the development of L1 while becoming more proficient in the second language being learned (L2), primarily because of lack of use (Wong-Fillmore, 1991b).

A child who learns two languages becomes most capable with the language that is used the most. If a child is exposed to L2 after the development of L1 and exposure to the first language is concurrently reduced, the rate of learning the first language is slowed or stopped. Proficiency in both L1 and L2 will show significant discrepancy from the expected. As a result, the child may be misidentified as having a language disorder because he or she is not proficient in either the primary language (L1) or the second language (L2). The perception of language loss also occurs when the child is exposed to more academically based material and enriched vocabulary in L2 at school while being limited in vocabulary development and exposure in L1, the language used in the home. The child's facility with more advanced forms of language, including reading and writing in L2, will progress while he or she will either lose L1 or not continue its development. It is important that children learning English as a second language continue to use their first language so that concepts and communication in the home will continue to develop.

When making decisions about a child's language status it is important to determine his or her language history as well as language proficiency in both languages (i.e., his or her ability to comprehend and produce language). Assessment of language proficiency must consider the cognitive level of the material and the context-embeddedness or amount of contextual support available for understanding the material or activity (Cummins, 1984). A child learning a second language may take 2–3 years to achieve social proficiency in Basic Interpersonal Communication Skills (BICS) in the second language, including vocabulary, morphology, and syntax to make his or her needs known, share information, and repeat and paraphrase information. It may take 5–7 years to obtain the Cognitive Academic Language Proficiency (CALP) to be able to use language to analyze, synthesize, and evaluate information in the academic curriculum. The failure to recognize the true cognitive language proficiency of students learning English as a second language is particularly evident at the secondary level when students who have basic communicative ability are expected to analyze, synthesize, and critique cognitively difficult academic material. Because the students may have the basic communication skills, their difficulty with higher-level language functions may go unrecognized, leading to frustration and inability to cope with the language demands of the secondary school. This may contribute to the failure of 42 percent of Hispanics in the United States to complete high school (versus 11 percent of non-Hispanics) (Langdon & Cheng, 1992).

Mercer (1987) and Damico, Oller, and Storey (1983) have suggested indicators of learning disabilities that are also behavioral characteristics of students in the process of learning English as a second language. There may be (1) a discrepancy between verbal and performance measures on intelligence tests, (2) academic learning difficulty, particularly with language and abstract concepts required in upper elementary and secondary grades, (3) an inability to perceive and organize information when such organization is based on different experiences and different linguistic backgrounds, (4) social and emotional problems related to frustration with the inability to communicate effectively and to function in the new culture, (5) attention and memory problems primarily because they have fewer and different experiences to which to relate new information, and/or (6) the appearance of hyperactivity or inattentiveness because they have little prior knowledge or experience on which to base information being presented.

Nonlinguistic behaviors of second-language learners or culturally and linguistically diverse (CLD) students may also contribute to mistaken identification of language disorders. Cultural differences in the use of eye-contact behaviors often contribute to identification of language disorder, particularly in young children. The use of sustained eye gaze by African Americans, Asian-Pacific Islanders, Hispanics, and Native American families differs from eye contact among Caucasians. For example, African-American children use indirect eye contact during listening and more direct eye contact when speaking (Terrell & Terrell, 1993). Among Hispanics, sustained eye contact may be interpreted as a sign of disrespect and a challenge to authority (Kayser, 1993). Young Asians do not sustain eye contact with adults or superiors (Cheng, 1993).

Delays in responding to questions also contribute to incorrect identification of language disability. The use of silence or latency between responses is culturally determined. For example, among African Americans, silence denotes refutation of an accusation. Among Native Americans silence is a culturally governed practice that can indicate respect or thoughtful consideration of what was just said (Harris, 1993). Asians consider those who speak quietly and slowly to be well mannered, lucid, and stable (Cheng, 1993).

Hoover and Collier (1985) have identified several sociocultural considerations when referring CLD children for special education. CLD children frequently do not respond when spoken to and/or prefer to be alone. Some students, when learning a second language, go through a silent period of three to six months during which they listen to the language they are learning. This may be a natural and normal stage of second-language acquisition as the child adapts to a new culture. This is particularly true among Hispanic, Native American, and some Asian cultures, where the children are encouraged to observe and be silent until they are competent to participate. CLD students are sometimes perceived as being disorganized, lacking responsibility, arriving late, wasting time, and having difficulty changing activities. These behaviors can be explained by cultural differences in the perception of time across cultures, difficulty in adapting to a new culture, confusion over locus of control, and/or resistance to change. Language difficulty may contribute to the failure to understand directions, especially those that are given indirectly or with more advanced syntactic structures.

CLD children may also exhibit behaviors such a talking out in class, short attention span, fighting, impulsive behavior, inappropriate laughter or giggling, and not following class rules. These behaviors may have been appropriate in the child's culture or they may in fact indicate true difficulty with language. The particular behavior should be investigated from the point of view of the child's culture and language use before it is determined to be an indication of a disorder.

Normal Language Development and Language Disorders

The identification of language disorders in CLD is difficult because the children are in the process of developing language with features different from those of Standard American English (SAE). Most studies of language acquisition has involved SAE (Brown, 1973; Bloom & Lahey, 1978) Much is known about linguistic features and the development of language by speakers of African-American English and Hispanic-English, although the studies vary in manner of data collection, age, class, language history of the subjects, method of study, and effects of bilingualism and bidialectalism. Little is known about language acquisition in other languages.

Language Development versus Disorders in Hispanic Children

Morphological Development and Disorders

The age of acquisition of Spanish morphological forms has been studied by Merino (1982; 1992), Gudeman (1981), Echevarrìa (1975), and Keller (1976). In spite of using different methods of investigation and different criteria for acceptance as having been acquired, the age of acquisition of various forms across the studies is only 1–2 years at the most. The studies indicate that children learning Spanish acquire an understanding of Spanish morphological forms at ages similar to those of children learning English morphology.

In general, specific grammatical features in Spanish are mastered earlier than others. By the age of 2 years correct inflection for singular forms for all persons is developed. (Gonzàlez, 1983). Present progressive, plurals, and past tense verbs are mastered before passives, subjunctives, and indirect objects. Similar to children learning English, children learning Spanish develop the use of copulative verbs (e.g., ser/estar: she is), singular forms for nouns (e.g., gata: cat; rana: frog), plural inflection (e.g., gato/gatos: cat/cats), and first- and second-person pronouns by the age of 2–5 years. Before age 3 they usually have developed present progressive (e.g., esta saltando: he/she is jumping; yo estoy hablando: I am speaking), present indicative (e.g., yo hablo: I speak); simple preterite (e.g., yo hablé: I spoke), direct imperative (e.g., mira: look), singular object pronouns (e.g., el/ella; la/lo), third-person subject pronouns, and plural clitic pronouns (e.g., los/las/les).

Before entry to school children learning Spanish have developed more complex forms involving tense and mood similar to children learning English. These later forms include the past progressive (e.g., yo hablaba: I was speaking), compound preterite (e.g., yo habla hablado: I had spoken), and irregular past tense (e.g., la niña puso eso: The little girl put that).

Because of several differences in expression in mood and aspect in Spanish, it is difficult to make a strict age by age comparison in all aspects of morphological acquisition between Spanish and English. For example, gender in noun adjectives is marked in Spanish (Un niño cortés, una niña cortés: a polite boy, a polite girl), but not in English.

Hispanic children learning English as a second language frequently have difficulty with the grammatical forms of English shown in Table 10-1.

Identifying Morphological Disorders in Hispanic Children

Ambert (1986) and Kayser (1989; 1990) described the types of syntactic problems occurring in Spanish-speaking children with language disorders. As with children learning English, the development of verb tense and mood is particularly difficult for children with language disorders learning Spanish. The children omitted articles, pronouns, prepositions, copulas *ser* and *estar,* auxiliary *estar,* reflexive pronouns, plural endings, and conjunctions. They used incorrect word order, had difficulty with noun-verb and article-noun agreement, and confused verb tenses. They used inappropriate labels for objects, actions, and persons. They used circumlocution and had word retrieval difficulties. They did not retell stories or narrate personal experiences at a level expected for their age. They could neither correct grammatical errors in a sentence presented to them nor solve problems. In other words, the

TABLE 10-1   Morphological Contrasts between SAE and Hispanic English

	SAE	Hispanic-English
Possession	postnoun modifier	-'s
	hat of my brother	my brother's hat
Plural	mark nonobligatory	-s
	The boy are here	The boys are here
Regular past	mark nonobligatory	-ed
	I walk yesterday	I walked yesterday
3rd pers. reg.	mark nonobligatory	-s
	He run fast	He runs fast
Negation	No before verb	auxiliary+not+verb
	He no eat	He does not eat
Questions	no noun-verb inversion	Noun-verb inversion
	Carlos is going?	Is Carlos going?

Adapted from Shipley & McAfee 1992; Owens, 1992; Kayser, 1993.

children learning Spanish exhibited the same types of difficulties with language as do children learning English.

Spanish Phonological Development and Disorders

Spanish phonology has 18 consonants, 4 semivowels, and 5 vowels (compared to 24 consonants, 3 semivowels, and 12–14 vowels in English). English consonants not present in Spanish include /v/, /th/, and /sh/. Whereas English has only the retroflex /r/, Spanish has a trill /r/ and a flap /rr/ in addition to consonants ñ, and /x/, which are not present in English. In addition, many of the Spanish consonants are unaspirated, giving a perceptually different production of certain consonants (such as *paper* versus *papel*). English vowels not present in Spanish include /I/ e, æ/, and /o/.

Children who speak Spanish have some difficulty learning English as a second language and may produce some English sounds differently from monolingual English speakers because of the similarities and contrasts of the two languages. For example, since there is no /th/ or /v/ in Spanish, these sounds are difficult for many children learning to speak English. Also, although many consonant sounds are similar, the consonants are not all produced in the same way. The /t/, for example, is aspirated in English, but it is unaspirated in Spanish. Moreover, in Spanish, /t/ is dental, while in English it is alveolar. While these differences are subtle, they add to the perception of language difference when Spanish speakers produce English words and may be mistakenly classified as a disorder.

Determination of the normalcy of the development of phonology in children learning Spanish is difficult because of the number of dialects within the Spanish language and the differences in criteria used to determine the normal developmental stages. However, most researchers (Acevedo, 1989; Eblen, 1982; Linares, 1982; Jimenez, 1987) agree that by the age of 4, children learning Spanish have mastered all sounds except the liquids /j/, /l/, /ch/ /s/, /rr/, and sometimes /ñ/, and of these /j/ and /l/ were acquired by age 4½. By the age of 6, all of these later developing phonemes were mastered.

The primary influences of Spanish on children learning English as a second language are shown in Table 10-2.

It is difficult for monolingual-English speakers to identify phonological errors in children speaking Spanish because of the interactive effects of development and language differences. According to Ambert (1986) and Hodson, Becker, Diamond, and Mesa (1989), unintelligible Spanish-speaking 4-year-olds make the same types of errors in Spanish that unintelligible English-speaking children commonly make: omitting, distorting, reversing the order or sounds in words and shortening the length of words (i.e., coalescence) involving /s/, /l/, /r/, /rr/, namely:

- reduction of consonant sequences, such as /epexo/ espejo (equivalent to /poon/ for spoon)
- liquid deviation /ádbol/ for árbol (similar to wug/rug)
- stidency deletion as /lápi for lápiz equivalent to /oap for soap

Normal Language Acquisition versus Disorders in AAE

African-American English (AAE) is the dialect of English spoken by approximately 80 percent of lower- or working-class African American families (Ratusnik & Koenigsknecht, 1975; Dillard, 1972). It reflects the complex social history of Africans in the United States and patterns of migration of African Americans from the rural south to the urban north. The major contrasts between SAE and AAE occur in morphology, syntax, pragmatics, and nonlinguistic features of language.

TABLE 10-2   Major Contrasts between English and Spanish Phonology

English	Spanish-Influenced English
/th/ (thumb)	/t/ (timb)
/th/ (this)	/d/ (den)
/z/ (zipper)	/s/ (sipper)
/sh/ (shoe)	/ch/ (chew)
/v/ (vacuum)	/b/ (bacuum)
/j/ (jump)	/y/ (yump)
/st/ (stove)	/est/ (estove)
devoicing of final consonants g, v, d, b, s → k, f, t, p, s	
Vowels: i, I, e, æ, ɛ, and a	

Source: Kayser, 1993; R. P. Stockwell, & J. D. Bowen. *The Sounds of English and Spanish.* Chicago: The University of Chicago Press, 1965.

Morphosyntactic Development and Disorders in AAE

The morphosyntactic development of children up to the age of 3 years who speak AAE is similar to that of children who use SAE, including the development of MLU (Blake, 1984; Stockman, 1986). Their morphosyntactic development is well advanced by 18 months of age when the use of one- and two-word utterances can be observed (Steffersen, 1974; Stockman & Vaughn-Cooke, 1992; Blake, 1984). Most of the features of AAE involve morphological features that are acquired in the same pattern as children learning SAE in Brown's stage II and beyond, such as plural, possessive, past tense, and third-person singular (Stockman, 1986; Blake, 1984; Steffersen, 1974; Reveron, 1978; Cole, 1980). The morphological features of AAE involving tense, mood and aspect markers of the verb phrase, negation, and other morphological features develop in the later preschool years. At the age of 3, well-formed multiword constructions, simple declaratives, and questions with subject, verb, and object complements are well established, with a few complex utterances also appearing (Stockman, 1986). Simple elaborated sentences with embedded object complements, negative sentences, and the formation of tag questions predominate at 3 and 4 years of age (Stockman, 1986). As the children develop through the preschool years, a variety of complex sentences and complex semantic relations are used, including coordinated, subordinate, and relative clause sentences, and complex *wh-* question forms (Craig & Washington, 1994; 1995)

The features that contrast AAE and SAE involve the later developing morphological forms. There is a marked increase in the use of AAE variants (e.g., multiple negation) by children acquiring AAE between the ages of 3 and 5 years, with social-class differences becoming most pronounced after the age of 4 years (Kovac, 1980; Reveron, 1978; Stockman, 1986; Craig and Washington, 1994). AAE forms not used until after 5 years include use of "at" in questions (where my shoes at); "go" copula (there go my shoes); distributive "be"; first-person future; embedded questions; past tense copula; present copula; and second-person pronoun. Some AAE features such as habitual "be" (She be working) and the use of "what" (He the one what ate it) in embedded clauses develop at a much later age than others (Cole, 1980). Among the later emerging contrastive AAE forms are the use of *had* to mark the simple past (then we *had* went outside); the use of *steady* as an intensified continuative marker ("he be *steady* steppin' in them number nines"); and the use of *come* to express indignation about an event or action ("He *come* walking in here like he owned the place").

The use of some AAE verb forms are not obligatory in all contexts. The copula, for example is obligatory in noncontractible morphemes (e.g., yes, he is), but is nonobligatory in contractible morphemes (e.g., John a boy). (Wyatt, 1991; Labov, 1972; Steffersen, 1974, Seymour, 1995). Some forms of AAE do not occur in SAE, such as the use of the syntactic devise known as aspect that allows the speaker of AAE to express a habitual or continuing state (e.g., he be working) in contrast to a temporary condition (e.g., he working). Because aspect does not exist in SAE, it is usually not on language tests. An AAE speaker who omits the "be" would be penalized on tests administered only in SAE. Because there is no information on the development of aspect in AAE speakers, it is not possible to determine whether a child who does not make this distinction is developing language normally in AAE.

TABLE 10-3   Major Morphological Contrasts between SAE and AAE

	AAE	SAE
Possession	Nonobligatory -'s	Obligatory -'s
	Get Mary hat	Get Mary's hat
	It be Mary's	It is Mary's
Plural	Nonobligatory -s	Obligatory -s
	She got six hat	She has six hats
Reg. past -ed	Nonobligatory	Obligatory
	I walk yesterday	I walked yesterday
3rd pers. reg.	Nonobligatory	Obligatory
	She walk	She walks
Copula	Nonobligatory	Obligatory
	She sick	She is sick
Habitual	Marked with "be"	Nonuse of 'be'
	He be working	He's working now
Negation	Triple negative	Single negative
	Nobody don't never	No one ever come

Adapted from Fasold & Wolfram, 1978; Wolfram & Fasold, 1974.

Semantic and Pragmatic Development and Disorders in AAE

AAE children between the ages of 2 and 18 months develop communicative intent and semantic categories that have been described for children acquiring other dialects with the number of functions increasing with age (i.e., informative, requestive, regulative, imaginative, affective, participative and attentive functions) (Bridgeforth, 1984; Blake, 1984; Stockman, 1986). The similarity in development of linguistic functions continues through the preschool years (Davis, Williams & Vaughn-Cooke (1992–1993; Vaughn-Cooke & Wright-Harp, 1992).

It can be expected that young CLD children will imitate, ask questions, express their needs verbally and nonverbally, answer questions, and be interested in stories and tales. However, according to Heath (1982, 1983b, 1986, 1989) in Hispanic and African-American families, storybooks and other forms of children's literature are often absent. Although stories or tales are told, comprehension is not negotiated. CLD children may be expected to engage in conversations with peers and give accounts of events of the day. Recounts of past experiences are rare among children from working-class Hispanic, African-American, and Asian families. Event casts are begun early in Asian families, but are rare in Hispanic and African-American families. Sharing picture books and reading books are usually common in middle-class Middle Eastern families (Lynch & Hanson, 1992).

Preferences for narrative style and for organization are also by-products of cultural and individual differences reflecting experience with listening and telling stories, general world knowledge, interactional styles of both speaker and listeners, and the use of paralinguistic conventions. Topic-centered narratives used by middle-class children of all racial/ethnic groups are linear around a single topic or a series of closely related topics with no major shift in perspective, thematic focus, or temporal orientation (Campbell, 1994; Gomperz, 1982; Gutierrez-Clellen & Quinn, Gutierrez-Clellen, Peña, & Quinn, 1995; 1993; Heath, 1986).

AA children frequently prefer to use topic-associated narrative style in which the narrative easily flows from one topic to another. Their stories are circular, consisting of a series of segments implicitly linked to topic with no explicit theme, less chronicity, and few formulaic openings or closings (Gee, 1989; Michaels, 1981). Listeners not accustomed to the narrative style of AA children may have difficulty identifying the child's topic or may assume that the child is unable to maintain topic. Questions addressed to the child may be mistimed, interrupting his or her train of thought. As a result the child may be perceived as having an expressive language disorder, when he or she is actually reacting to or coping with interruptions in narrative style. Narrative styles also affect the child's writing and thus his or her performance in school.

Phonologic Development and Disorders in AAE

Because SAE and AAE are dialects of the same language, several features, such as initial consonants (except /v/), are noncontrastive. The early phoneme development of speakers of AAE does not differ from that of speakers of SAE. At 36 months, the conversational speech of African-American children contains the same minimal core of initial consonants expected of speakers of standard English (e.g., /n,m,b,p,d,t,g,k,f,s,h,w,j/) (Seymour & Ralabate, 1985; Seymour & Seymour, 1981; Steffersen, 1974).

The features that contrast between AAE and SAE in the medial and final positions of words—final consonant deletion, final consonant cluster reduction, unstressed syllable deletion, and interdental fricative substitution (e.g., /th/ and /v/)—normally develop after the age of 5 years. Thus, the consonantal features that contrast AAE and SAE are not evident until after age 5 (Seymour & Seymour, 1981; Vaughn-Cooke, 1986; Haynes & Moran, 1989; Wolfram & Fasold, 1974; Stockman, 1991; Moran, 1993, Rickford, in press; Stockman & Settle, 1991; Stockman, 1995).

Little is known about the development of final consonants in speakers of AAE. Although the final consonant deletion process is reported to disappear in mainstream English speakers by the age of 3 years, it appears to continue in young AAE speakers, with the deletion or weakening of certain voiced stops /b/, /d/, and /g/ and some fricatives (/s/, /v/, and /th/) persisting until at least third grade (Seymour & Seymour, 1981; Haynes & Moran, 1989).

Standard articulation tests vary in the number of dialect-sensitive items included and thus have limited usefulness in determining African-American children's performance (Cole & Taylor, 1990; Washington and Craig, 1992). According to Bleile & Wallach (1992), the features that do not contrast between AAE and SAE are useful in distinguishing between normal and disordered AAE. These features include:

- the use of more than one or two stop errors
- initial word position errors
- glide errors in children over 4
- more than a few cluster errors
- fricative errors other than /Θ/

Assessment of Language in CLD Children

Using Norm-Referenced Standardized Tests with CLD Children

Just as language is a cultural phenomenon, the assessment of language abilities is in a cultural phenomenon. While evaluators attempt to use culture-free tests to avoid bias for or against certain cultures, such tests are rare and are difficult to develop for practical use. Systematic procedures to avoid clear cases of cultural bias in tests are poorly understood and have questionable reliability because cultural bias is considerable more subtle than is usually understood (Scriven, 1991).

Court decisions such as Diana v. State Board of Education (1970), Lau v. Nichols (1974), and Martin Luther King School Children v. Ann Arbor School District (1978) led to the Bilingual Education Act of 1976 (Public Law 95-561, 1976) and to the nondiscriminatory assessment provisions in PL 94-142 (1977) and its subsequent revisions under PL 99-457 (renamed Individuals with Disabilities Education Act, or IDEA), which require that all tests and other evaluation materials be provided and administered in the child's native language or other mode of communication unless it is clearly not feasible to do so. Evaluators must make every effort to assess children in their native language and clearly document efforts to do so. Assessment of the language skills of CLD children should enable the evaluator to collect assessment data through behavioral descriptions of the child's language skills particular to his or her indigenous culture and particular language or dialect.

Many CLD children are placed in special education because they do not do well on standardized norm-referenced tests presented in Standard American English. Language disorders involve a significant discrepancy in language skills from that expected for a child's age or developmental level. The reference to a discrepancy implies the comparison of the child's developmental level to normative data or levels expected by the general population. Any difference in the culture of the child from the culture on which norms were developed limits its usefulness for the assessment of language disorders.

Clinical decisions made on the basis of responses to tests whose norming populations are inappropriate are discriminatory. There are few, if any, standardized language tests that are nonbiased or appropriately normed for use with bidialectal or bilingual children. Because most commonly used speech-language tests do not include a representative sample of CLD children in the standardization sample, the administration, use, scoring, and interpretation of tests standardized on mainstream American English speakers is not appropriate for the language assessment of CLD children. Even when large numbers of CLD children are included in the standardization sample, there is no assurance that the culture or linguistic background of the particular child being tested has been included in the sample. If the test was standardized on northeastern urban African Americans, for example, that test is not necessarily appropriate for southern rural African Americans, Hispanics, or other cultural or linguistic groups.

Weddington (1987) made suggestions for using standardized tests with minority children. They include alteration of the time limits for the test, rewording of instructions, additional practice items, determining the appropriateness of the content and the vocabulary and the pictured items or objects, starting below the standard basal and testing beyond the standard ceiling, translating or interpreting items when the translation can be done in one or two words, and accepting as correct responses that are appropriate for the client's language or dialect. It is also important to use the widest range of the confidence interval possible to neutralize any variation in the development of features across various dialects. When needed modifications are made, the assessment will provide information about what the child can do, rather than what he or she cannot do. Such information will be useful in interpreting the results of the test.

Caution should be taken to describe the child's performance on each item or subtest and to delineate any alterations that were made in the procedure. Because the test was modified, the normative data for scoring should not be used. It is difficult to determine whether modifications or translations of a test are similar in complexity of content to the original version of the test. Alteration of tests and testing procedures cannot account for nonverbal cultural differences in the testing situation itself, such as timed responding or forced-choice responding. (Westby, 1994; Damico, 1991).

Several standardized tests have been developed specifically for CLD children and there are also specific scoring procedures for speakers of specific dialects of English. Caution should be taken in the use of these tests as well. Different results can be obtained depending on the child's language history, which may give an incorrect indication of language disability. The test may have been developed for a different dialect or cultural experience from that of the child. Although the dialects of Spanish are mutually intelligible, discrete differences in pronunciation and vocabulary may penalize a child who is still in the language-learning or second-language-learning process. Interpretation or translation of the tests is also not appropriate because the experience level of the child may not be the same as children in the normative sample and there may not be a developmentally appropriate translation. Translation violates the standardization of the test and thus makes use of the normative data inappropriate.

CLD children have been found to perform better on nonverbal tests (Hamayan & Damico, 1991). Although nonverbal tests do not require verbal ability, there are cultural variables that affect the child's performance on these tests as well. Nonverbal aspects of testing include the perception and use of time, display learning, competitiveness, and sociolinguistic dimensions such as cross-racial relationships between the child and the tester (Westby, 1994). Verbal aspects of testing include the various functions of language, differences in testing experiences, differences in the child's ability to engage in discourse or other language tasks such as cloze sentences and sentence completion tasks, and responding to direct and inferential questions. In addition, the child may not have been exposed to the vocabulary or content of the test. Each of these nonverbal and verbal variables can affect the results of the assessment, particularly when standardized or formal tests are used. Such tests are thus limited in their usefulness because it is difficult to determine whether the child's language ability was appropriately assessed separate from his or her ability to deal with the inappropriate assessment instrument and/or procedure.

Vaughn-Cooke (1983) and Musselwhite (1983) have posed several questions that are useful for evaluating the assessment instruments and procedures for use with CLD children:

1. Can the procedure account for verbal and nonverbal cultural and linguistic variations?
2. Will the sociological assumptions underlying the social occasion of testing and the particular elicitation techniques influence the results of the test?
3. Are the assumptions about language and communication that underlie the test culturally valid?
4. What is the client's relationship to the norming population?
5. What is the client's experience with the content area of the test? Has the client had an opportunity to learn the content?
6. Does the procedure include a culturally based analysis of a spontaneous speech sample?
7. Does the procedure allow the reliable determination of whether the child's language system is developing normally? Does the procedure permit an analysis of how the client is functioning within his own linguistic or dialectal community?
8. Can the test distinguish between those differences that can be attributed to dialect or cultural differences? Can the results of the test be adjusted to account for cultural or linguistic differences? Would the test be able to distinguish those children with a true language disorder from those that use the language or dialect of their indigenous community?
9. Can the procedure provide an adequate description of the child's language proficiency?
10. Do the results of the test provide principled guidelines for culturally based recommendations?

Using Criterion-Referenced Assessment with CLD Children

Criterion-referenced assessment is more appropriate for determining the nature of a language disability in young CLD children since it allows a description of the child's functioning on specific independently defined criteria rather than a comparison against a group-established norm. The assessment results are thus interpreted by comparison with predetermined performance criteria rather than by comparison with the scores of a reference group as in norm-referenced tests (Scriven, 1991). Criterion-referenced assessment has limitations in defining the criteria that should be used for CLD children; however, it is superior to norm-referenced assessment when the particular culture, linguistic background, and life experiences of the child are considered. Because criterion-referenced tests may also be standardized, the same cautions given for standardized norm-referenced tests must be made.

Criterion-referenced assessment should include a family-centered ethnographic interview and a speech-sample analysis. Through the triangulation of cultural, linguistic, and experiential factors, the ethnographic interview increases the validity of assessment data and reduces potential biases, because data collected is filtered through the client's culture rather than through the culture of the mainstream. It looks at the larger sociocultural context in which communication takes place and how language is used within a particular culture to share knowledge and to establish order (Crego and Cole, 1991; Cheng, 1990).

The family-centered ethnographic interview allows the evaluator to determine the cultural and environmental influences on the development of language in the home as well as the dimensions of communicative competence important to the family and the culture (Westby, 1990). As shown in Table 10-4, the ethnographic interview should address issues involving the child's communication partners, the usual mode of communication used by the child and used in the home, and the conversational rules and interaction patterns used by the family.

TABLE 10-4 Guidelines for Family-Centered Ethnographic Interview

- What language(s) do parents use in speaking to the child?
- What language(s) do the parents use in speaking to each other?
- What language does the child use with adults? Age peers?
- Does the child initiate conversation at home?
- Does the child participate in conversations? With whom?
- Does the child talk more or less in conversations with particular people? In particular settings? On particular topics?
- How often does the child interact with adults? Age peers?
- What is the parent's perception of the child's language ability?
- Do family members have difficulty understanding the child?
- What role do family members play in the development of language?
- How does the family view their role in intervening with their child?

Adapted from Paul, 1995; Wayman, Lynch, & Hanson, 1990; Mattes & Omark, 1984.

The collection of a language sample should be a central part of the language and communication of a CLD child. The language sample should be collected in multiple contexts with multiple interactants with the differences in language and interaction being recorded (see Table 10-5). The language samples should be collected in environments that are culturally appropriate to the child, involving people with whom the child usually communicates, including parents, age peers, and siblings. Cheng (1991) suggests collecting the language sample using several different tasks, including relating past experiences, describing objects, describing pictures, and retelling culturally familiar stories. The sample should be analyzed using criteria based on the phonology, syntax, semantics, morphology, and pragmatic rules of the child's language and culture. Analysis should consider normal development and use within the child's language and dialect and within the particular family unit.

The following criteria can be used as a guide in determining the existence of a language disorder in a CLD child when used with the parameters established for a particular culture or linguistic environment (Mattes & Omark, 1991; Kayser, 1990):

- Rarely initiates verbal interactions or activities with peers or family members
- Does not respond verbally when verbal interactions are initiated by peers or family members

- Has difficulty learning language at the normal rate even with special assistance
- Has a smaller vocabulary than expected for age
- Uses shorter, less complex sentences than expected for age
- Has difficulty communicating with parents and cultural and linguistic age peers
- Relies heavily on gestures and nonverbal means to communicate
- Needs repetition and rephrasing of instructions
- Is inordinately slow in responding to questions (in relation to cultural peers)
- Has difficulty with the noncontrastive elements of morphology and/or phonology
- Peers rarely initiate verbal interactions with the child or use a notably lower level of verbal communication when communicating with the child
- Peers have difficulty understanding the child's verbal and/or nonverbal communication
- Does not attempt to repair communication failures
- Does not comment on own actions or the actions of others or express feelings
- Does not take turns or maintain topic during conversations with peers
- Does not ask for information or request clarification
- Uses numerous false starts and self-interruptions or revisions
- Makes frequent use of expressions such as "it," "thing," or "this/that" without proper reference
- Does not learn new concepts or vocabulary presented in a variety of modes or forgets material assumed to be learnedLanguage Intervention with CLD Children

TABLE 10-5   Ethnographic Assessment Guidelines

1. Observe the child over time in multiple contexts with multiple communication partners.
2. Interview members of the family network to collect data regarding the child's language skills in the home environment.
3. Interact with the child, being sensitive to his or her need to create meaning based on his or her frame of reference and life experiences.
4. Describe the client's use of language during genuine communication in a naturalistic environment with low anxiety and high motivation.
5. Describe the child's use of language in both high-contextualized and low-contextualized material.
6. Collect narrative samples using wordless books, pictures, and other materials with low-cognitive demand.

Language Intervention with CLD Children

Models for Language Intervention with CLD Children

Providing appropriate clinical services for CLD children who have language disorders is not an easy matter because of the tremendous diversity in language history, language skills, and life experiences that exist among the children. The continuum of proficiency in English extends to include children who are English proficient and those who are limited in both

English and their primary language (ASHA, 1985). Decisions will have to be made about the proper language for education and treatment of a Limited English Proficiency (LEP) child who has a true disability. Should instruction be in the language of the home or in the language most appropriate for school? Current literature (Hamayan, 1992; Wong-Fillmore, 1991a) stresses the need to develop a firm language base in the child's first language, usually the language of the home before teaching a second language. This will allow the parents to communicate with the child and to assist in the language development process. Conflict arises when the parents wish to have the child taught in the language of the school (i.e., English) before a firm base in the first language is achieved. Ripich & Creaghead (1995) provide an inventory for assistance with the language decision that addresses home language and community/school language issues, which may be helpful in determining the best direction for the individual child.

As shown in Table 10-6, CLD children fall into four distinct groups, ranging from those with normal language ability and normal opportunity to learn language to those with language disability and limited opportunity to learn language.

CLD children from language-rich homes (Group A) may have normal language ability in their primary language or dialect. If they are from homes where English is not spoken, they may not immediately have the language skills to cope with the demands of the academic curriculum upon entry to school or preschool. While they do not have a language disorder, they perform significantly below their age expectation. These children can be expected to do well in the preschool and academic setting without special education assistance. For these children, regular education or bilingual education is appropriate. If necessary, the services of an ESL teacher or other supports may be helpful to help the child adjust to the language of instruction.

Some other children (Group B) perform below age expectation because they have had limited exposure or opportunity to learn language concepts and vocabulary in an enriched environment. This may be a result of their life experiences rather than the result of a true inability to learn language. While they perform poorly on norm-referenced tests, they do

TABLE 10-6   Models for Language Intervention

	Enriched environment	Poor Environment
Normal	A No special Services	B Language-rich regular program
Disordered	C Speech-language pathology	D Speech-language pathology Language-rich special education

not have a true language disorder. They are likely to do well in the academic setting if they are given increased opportunities to enhance their language skills through language-enriched programs and the services of an ESL teacher or bilingual education, if appropriate. Curriculum modifications may be necessary to ensure that the child has the language concepts to understand the curriculum and to aid in motivation. Because the underlying language learning ability of these children is intact, it is not appropriate for them to be placed in special education programs or to be identified as disabled.

A third group of students (Group C) may have had adequate life experiences and stimulation to prepare for the academic environment, and they may have had adequate exposure to language and to English, but they have not developed language adequately. These students may have an underlying language disability that prevents them from learning language. If they are learning English as a second language, the language disability manifests itself in both their native language as well as in the inability to learn English. Such children require special services, including speech-language pathology according to their specific needs. Depending on the extent of their disability, they may be appropriately served in a regular educational or home-based program supplemented by special speech-language services. If a language other than English is the language of the home, the child should be provided education in the home language in order to provide the child with a firm basis for learning and using language to communicate within the family unit.

A fourth group of children (Group D) has even greater difficulty since in addition to a true language disability, the children's life experiences have been limited. These children will require extensive specialized language enrichment programs including speech-language pathology services. Intervention should be in the language of the home to provide the child with a firm basis in language for communication and socialization within the family unit.

Culturally Appropriate Language Intervention

Language intervention with CLD children should be culturally appropriate and should focus on the language needs of the child. Emphasis should be placed on teaching function and use of language before form, and on semantics or meanings appropriate for the child's academic environment before form. Intervention in syntax, morphology, and phonology should focus on the noncontrastive elements that are in need of development before elements that are contrastive between the languages.

In creating a culturally appropriate intervention process the clinician should establish a collaborative relationship with the family to become familiar with the concerns, priorities, and resources of the family. Recognize that there are cultural differences in the expectations of the family in the extent of their involvement in the intervention program of the child. Also recognize that there are cultural differences in the family's understanding of the nature of and intervention for language disabilities. In developing intervention plans it is important to incorporate practices that are culturally comfortable for the family, and to involve those members of the family that are important to the child. Intervention goals, objectives, or outcomes that are developed should be consistent with the family's concerns, priorities, and needs.

Intervention materials should be based on materials and experiences that are familiar to the child's life experiences. Concepts of family, housing, foods, food preparation, arts, music, dress, and religious practices should begin with the child's experiences and then expand to include new experiences. The following guidelines are suggested for successful intervention:

1. View each clinical encounter as a socially situated communicative event that is subject to the cultural rules of both the clinician and the client that govern such events.
2. Present clear explanations of objectives, goals, and expected outcomes using language that the child and family can understand.
3. Adapt materials and experiences to the client's individual needs, including material from the child's culture into the lessons.
4. Preview and review lessons to determine whether the materials, concepts, and vocabulary are culturally and linguistically appropriate. Review the lesson to determine if the child's responses or failure to learn could be explained by cultural or linguistic conflicts. Determine ways to modify future materials to eliminate sources of conflict.
5. Incorporate content from the child's culture into lessons while helping the child to make transitions to new experiences expected in school or new environments.
6. Present material using the timing and rhythm appropriate for the culture. Asian and Native American clients expect a quiet, slower pace with more time for responding than do children from mainstream cultures.
7. Provide a variety of clinical conditions with opportunities to respond in different modes and communicative functions. Clients may learn differently under differing clinical conditions because of their cultural and language backgrounds.
8. Use speech and language appropriate to the client's level of comprehension. Repeat and rephrase instructions and language models to increase the likelihood that the child comprehends.
9. Encourage, praise, and reinforce all verbal and nonverbal communication attempts. Expect the use of the home dialect or language.
10. Use small group sessions that encourage supportive cooperative interactions, as is the custom in many cultures. Same-gender grouping may be most appropriate for some cultures.

Using Interpreters in Assessment and Intervention

When the SLP does not have native or near native proficiency in the language of the client or the family, the assessment can be assisted by the use of interpreters (ASHA, 1985). Ideally the interpreter should be a paraprofessional trained in speech and language development and disabilities or a person trained to work with children and families. The interpreters should be familiar with the language, dialect, and culture of the child and family. Interpreters are sometimes available in the community through cultural resource centers or local language institutes. With the family's permission, interpreters could also be persons from the family who are more proficient in English. Care should be taken to assure the family that the interpreter will be neutral and will regard their information as confidential.

In working with an interpreter the SLP should prepare the interpreter concerning the nature of the questions to be asked so that the appropriate professional terminology or reasonable translations can be made, so that the cultural appropriateness or inappropriateness of any questions or materials can be determined in advance, and so that the interpreter can be instructed to be cautious of verbal and nonverbal cues that may be misunderstood and thus affect the interaction. After the session, the SLP should debrief the interpreter to determine if there were any nonverbal items that were particularly relevant to the session (Medina, 1982).

Conclusion

The outcome of more than two decades of research on the acquisition of language and language disorders has increased understanding language skills of CLD children. More recent and ongoing research has indicated the need for more careful investigation of the linguistic and situational constraints that contrast the normal acquisition and use of features from acquisition and use of language so that proper clinical decisions can be made.

Study Questions

1. What is the responsibility of the monolingual English speech-language pathologist who must provide speech services to a monolingual Spanish-speaking child?
2. What resources can the speech-language pathologist use to assist with the provision of speech-language services to the culturally and linguistically different child with a language disorder?
3. What academic areas will be most difficult for the preschool child, the lower elementary school child, and the intermediate-level child with limited English proficiency?
4. How can the speech-language pathologist determine the presence of a language disorder in a culturally and linguistically different child?
5. What suggestions can be made to the classroom teacher to assist a culturally and linguistically different child with a language disorder in the classroom?

Suggested Reading

Adler, S. (1993). *Multicultural communication skills in the classroom.* Boston: Allyn & Bacon.

American Speech-Language Hearing Association (1983). Position paper on social dialects. *Asha, 25* (9), 23–24.

American Speech-Language Hearing Association. (1985, June). Clinical management of communicatively handicapped minority language populations. *Asha, 27* (6), 29–32.

Battle, D. E. (Ed.). (1993) *Communication disorders in multicultural populations.* Newton, MA: Butterworth-Heinemann.

Cheng, L. L. (1993). *Assessing Asian language performance.* Oceanside, CA: Academic Communication Associates.

Cheng, L. L. (1995). *Integrating language and learning for inclusion: An Asian-Pacific focus.* San Diego: Singular.

Kayser, H. (1995). *Bilingual speech-language pathology.* San Diego: Singular.

Langdon, H. W. (1992). *Hispanic children and adults with communication disorders: Assessment and intervention.* Gaithersburg, MD: Aspen Publication.

References

Acevedo, M. (1989, November). Typical speech misarticulations of Mexican-American preschoolers. Paper presented at the annual meeting of the American-Speech-Language-Hearing Association, St. Louis.

Ambert, A. (1986) Identifying language disorders in Spanish speakers. In A. C. Willig & H. F. Greenberg (Eds.), *Bilingualism and learning disabilities* (pp. 15–33). New York: American Library Publishing.

American Speech-Language-Hearing Association. (1983). Position paper on social dialects. *Asha,* 25(9), 23–24.

American Speech-Language-Hearing Association. (1985). Clinical management of communicatively handicapped minority language populations. *Asha,* 27(6), 29–32.

American Speech-Language-Hearing Association. (1993). Definitions of communication disorders and variations. *Asha,* 35, (Suppl.10), 40–41.

American Speech-Language-Hearing Association. (1991). Did you know? *Perspectives,* 12(2), 11.

Anderson, N., & Battle, D. (1993). Cultural diversity in the development of language. In D. Battle, *Communication disorders in multicultural populations* (pp. 158–187). Newton, MA: Butterworth-Heinemann.

Blake, I. (1984). Language development in working-class black children: An examination of form, content and use. Doctoral dissertation, Columbia University, New York.

Bleile, K., & Wallach, H. (1992). A sociolinguistic investigation of the speech of African American preschoolers. *American Journal of Speech Language Pathology,* 1(2), 54–62.

Bloom, M., & Lahey, M. (1978). *Language development and disorders.* New York: Wiley.

Bridgeforth, C. (1984). The development of language functions among black children from working class families. Paper presented at the presession of the 35th Annual Georgetown University Round Table on Language and Linguistics, Washington, DC.

Brown, R. (1973). *A first language, the early stages.* Cambridge, MA: Harvard University Press.

Campbell, L. (1994). Discourse diversity and black English vernacular. In D. Ripich & N. Creaghead, *School discourse problems* (pp. 93–131). San Diego: Singular Publishing.

Cheng, L. L. (1990). Identification of communicative disorders in Asian-Pacific students. *Journal of Childhood Communication Disorders,* 13(1), 113–119.

Cheng, L. L. (1991). *Assessing Asian language performance* (2nd ed). Oceanside, CA.: Academic Communication Associates

Cheng, L. L. (1993). In D. Battle (Ed.). *Communication disorders in multicultural populations* (pp. 38–77). Newton, MA: Butterworth-Heinemann.

Cheng, L. L. (1995). *Integrating language and learning for inclusion: An Asian-Pacific focus.* San Diego: Singular.

Cole, L. (1980). A developmental analysis of social dialect features in the spontaneous language of preschool Black children. Doctoral dissertation, Northwestern University, Evanston, IL.

Cole P., & Taylor, O. (1990) Performance of working-class African-American children on three tests of articulation. *Language, Speech, and Hearing Services in schools,* 24, 161–166.

Craig, H., & Washington, J. (1994). The complex syntax skills of poor, urban, African American preschoolers at school entry. *Language, Speech, and Hearing Services in Schools,* 25(2), 181–190.

Craig H., & Washington, J. A. (1995). African-American English and linguistic complexity in preschool discourse: A second look. *Language, Speech, and Hearing Services in Schools,* 26(1), 87–93.

Crego, M., & Cole, E. (1991). Using ethnography to bring children's communicative and cultural words into focus. In T. M. Gallagher (Ed.), *Pragmatics of language: Clinical practice issues* (pp. 99–132). San Diego: Singular.

Cummins, J. (1984). *Bilingualism and special education.* San Diego: College-Hill Press.

Damico, J. (1991) Descriptive assessment of communicative ability. In E. V. Hamayan & J. S. Damico (Eds.), *Limiting Bias in the Assessment of bilingual students.* Austin, TX: Pro-Ed.

Damico, J. S., Oller, J. W., & Storey, M. E. (1983). The diagnosis of language disorders in bilingual children: Surface-oriented and pragmatic criteria. *Journal of Speech and Hearing Disorders,* 46, 385–394.

Davis, P., Williams, J., & Vaughn-Cooke, F. (1992–1993). A comparison of lexical development in a child with normal language development and in a child with language delay. *National Student*

Speech Language Hearing Association Journal, 20, 63–77.

Diana v. State Board of Education, C. A. 70 RFT (N. D. Cal., Feb. 3, 1970).

Dillard, J. (1972). *Black English: Its History and Usage.* New York: Random House.

Doyle, A., Champagne, M., & Seglowitz, N. (1978). Some issues in the assessment of linguistic consequences of early bilingualism. In. M. Paradis (Ed.), *Aspects of bilingualism.* Columbia, SC: Hornbeam Press.

Dulay H., & Burt, M. K. (1974). Natural sequences in child second language acquisition. *Language Learning,* 24, 37–53.

Dulay, H., Hernàndez-Chàvez, E., & Burt, M. K. (1978). The process of becoming bilingual. In S. Singh & L. Lynch (Eds.) *Diagnostic procedures in hearing, language and speech* (pp. 305–326). Baltimore: University Park Press.

Eblen, R. E. (1982). A study of the acquisition of fricatives by 3 year old children learning Mexican-Spanish. *Language and Speech,* 25, 201–220.

Echeverrìa, M. (1975). Late stages in the acquisition of Spanish syntax. Doctoral dissertation. University of Washington, Seattle.

Farran, D. (1982). Mother-child interaction, language development and the school performance of poverty children. In L. Feagans & D. Farran. *The language of children reared in poverty: Implications for evaluation and intervention.* New York: Academic Press.

Fasold, R. W., & Wolfram, W. (1978). Some linguistic features of Negro dialect. In P. Stoller (Ed.) *Black American English* (pp. 49–83). New York: Delta.

Gee, J. P. (1989). Two styles of narrative construction and their linguistic and educational implications. *Discourse Processes,* 12, 287–307.

Gomperz, J. (1982). *Discourse strategies.* New York: Cambridge University Press.

Gonzàles, G. (1983). Expressing time through verb tenses and temporal expression in Spanish: Age 2.0–4.6. *NABE Journal,* 7, 69–82.

Gudeman, R. H. (1981). Learning Spanish: A cross-sectional study of the imitation, comprehension and production of Spanish grammatical forms by rural Panamanians. Doctoral dissertation, University of Minnesota, Minneapolis.

Gutierrez-Clellen, V., Peña, E., & Quinn, R. (1995). Accommodating cultural differences in narrative style: A multicultural perspective. *Topics in Language Disorders,* 15(4), 54–67.

Gutierrez-Clellen, V., & Quinn, R. (1993). Assessing narratives of children from diverse cultural/linguistic groups. *Language, Speech, and Hearing Services in Schools,* 24(1), 2–9.

Hamayan, E. (1992, September). Meeting the challenge of cultural and linguistic diversity in the schools: Best practices in language intervention. Paper presented at the Broward County Exceptional Student Education Inservice, Ft. Lauderdale, FL.

Hamayan, E. V., & Damico, J. S. (1991). *Limiting bias in the assessment of bilingual students.* Austin, TX: Pro-Ed.

Harris, G. (1993). American Indian cultures: A lesson in diversity. In D. Battle (Ed.), *Communication disorders in multicultural populations* (pp. 78–113). Newton, MA: Butterworth-Heinemann.

Haynes, W. O., & Moran, M. (1989). A cross-sectional developmental study of final consonant production in Southern Black children from preschool to third grade. *Language, Speech, and Hearing Services in Schools,* 21(4), 400–406.

Haynes, W. O., & Shulman, B. B. (1994). *Communication development: Foundations, processes, and clinical applications.* Englewood Cliffs, NJ: Prentice Hall.

Heath, S. B. (1982). What no bedtime story means: Narrative skills at home and school. *Language and Society,* 11, 49–76.

Heath, S. B. (1983a). *Ways with words: Language, life, and work in communities and classrooms.* New York: Cambridge University Press.

Heath, S. B. (1983b). Sociocultural contexts of language development. In *Beyond Language.* Los Angeles: Evaluation, Dissemination and Assessment Center.

Heath, S. B. (1986). Taking a cross cultural look at narratives. *Topics in Language Disorders,* 7(1), 84–89.

Heath, S. B. (1989, February). Oral and literate traditions among Black Americans living in poverty. *American Psychologist,* 367–373.

Hodson, B., Becker, M., Diamond, F., & Meza, P. (1989). Phonological analysis of unintelligible children's utterances: English and Spanish. In *Occasional papers on linguistics: The uses of phonology.* Carbondale: Southern Illinois University Press.

Hoover, J. J., & Collier, C. (1985). Referring culturally different children: Sociocultural considerations. *Academic Therapy, 20*(4), 503–509.

Jimenez, B. C. (1987). Acquisition of Spanish consonants in children aged 3–5 years. *Language, Speech, and Hearing Services in Schools, 18*(4), 357–363.

Kayser, H. (1989). Speech and language assessment of Spanish-English speaking children. *Language, Speech, and Hearing Services in Schools, 20,* 226–244.

Kayser, H. (1990). Social communicative behaviors of language-disordered Mexican-American students. *Child Language Teaching Therapy, 6*(3), 255–269.

Kayser, H. (1993). Hispanic cultures. In D. Battle (Ed.), *Communication disorders in multicultural populations* (pp.114–157). Newton, MA: Butterworth-Heinemann.

Keller, G. (1976). Acquisition of the English and Spanish passive voices among bilingual children. In G. D. Keller, R. V. Teschner, & S. Viera (Eds.), *Bilingualism in the bicentennial and beyond* (pp. 161–168). New York: Bilingual Press.

Kovac, C. (1980). Children's acquisition of variable features. Doctoral dissertation, Georgetown University, Washington, DC.

Labov, W. (1972). *Language in the inner city.* Philadelphia: University of Pennsylvania Press.

Langdon, H. W., & Cheng, L. (Eds.). (1992). *Hispanic children and adults with communication disorders: Assessment and intervention.* Gaithersburg, MD: Aspen Publication.

Lau v. Nichols, 411 U.S. 563 (1974).

Linares, T. A. (1982). Articulation skills of Spanish-speaking children. In *Ethnoperspectives in Bilingual Education Series Vol III: Bilingual Education Technology* (pp. 363–387), Ypsilanti, Michigan.

Lynch, E. W., & Hanson, M. J. (1993). *Developing cross-cultural competence: A guide for working with young children and their families.* Baltimore: Paul D. Brookes.

Marge, M. (1993). Disability prevention: Are we ready for the challenge? *Asha, 35,* 42–44.

Martin Luther King Junior Elementary School Children et al. v. Ann Arbor School District Board, Civil Action No. 7–71861, 451 F. Supp. 1324 (1978), 463 F. Supp. 1027 (1978) and 473 F. Supp. 1371 (1979) (Detroit, July 12, 1979).

Mattes, L. J., & Omark, D. R. (1991). *Speech and language assessment for the bilingual handicapped* (2nd ed.) San Diego: College-Hill Press.

Medina, V. (1982). *Interpretation and translation in bilingual B.A.S.A.* San Diego: Superintendent of Schools, Department of Education, San Diego County.

Mercer, C. D. (1987). *Students with learning disabilities* (3rd ed.). New York: Merrill.

Merino, B. J. (1982, October–November). Language development in Spanish as a first language: Implications of assessment. Paper presented at the National Conference on the Exceptional Bilingual Child, Phoenix, AZ.

Merino, B. J. (1992). Acquisition of syntactic and phonological features in Spanish. In H. W. Langdon & L. L. Cheng (Eds.) *Hispanic children and adults with communication disorders* (pp. 57–98). Gaithersburg, MD: Aspen.

Michaels, S. (1981). "Sharing time": Children's narrative styles and differential access to literacy. *Language in Society, 10,* 423–442.

Moran, M. (1993). Final consonant deletion in African American children speaking Black English: A closer look. *Language, Speech, and Hearing Services in Schools, 24,* 161–166.

Musselwhite, C. (1983). Pluralistic assessment in speech-language pathology: Use of dual norms in the placement process. *Language, Speech and Hearing Services in Schools, 14,* 29–37.

National Deafness and Other Communication Disorders Advisory Board. (1991). *Research in Human Communication.* NIH Publication No. 92–3317). Annual Report. Bethesda, MD: National Institutes of Health.

Office of Scientific and Health Reports. (1988). Developmental speech and language disorders: Hope through research (NIH Publication No. Pamphlet 88–2757). Bethesda, MD: National Institutes of Neurological and Communicative Disorders and Stroke.

Owens, R. (1992). *Language disorders: A functional approach to assessment and intervention.* New York: Merrill.

Owens, R. (1996). *Language development: An introduction.* Boston: Allyn & Bacon.

Paul, R. (1995). *Language disorders from infancy through adolescence: Assessment and Intervention.* St. Louis: Mosby-Yearbook.

Public Law 94–142. The Education of All Handicapped Children Act of 1975, 20 USC 1401. *Federal Register,* 42(86), May 4, 1977.

Public Law 95–561. The Bilingual Education Act (Title VII of the Elementary and Secondary Education Act of 1965).

Ratusnik, D., & Koenigsknecht, R. (1975). Influence of certain clinical variables on Black preschoolers' nonstandard phonological and grammatical performance. *Journal of Communication Disorders,* 8, 281–297.

Reveron, W. (1978). The acquisition of variable features. Doctoral dissertation, Ohio State University, Columbus.

Rickford J. R. (in press). Regional and Social Variation. In S. L. McKay & N. H. Hornberger (Eds.). *Sociolinguistics and Language Teaching.* Oxford: Oxford University Press.

Ripich, D., & Creaghead, N. (1995). *School discourse problems* (2nd ed.). San Diego: Singular Publishing.

Saville-Troike, M. (1986). Anthropological considerations in the study of communication. In O. Taylor (Ed.), *Nature of communication disorders in culturally and linguistically diverse populations* (pp. 47–72). San Diego: College-Hill Press.

Scriven, M. (1991). *Evaluation thesaurus* (4th ed.). New York: Sage Publications.

Seymour, H. (1995, November). *Theory and practice in evaluating child African-American English.* Paper presented to meeting of the American Speech-Language-Hearing Convention, Orlando, FL.

Seymour, H., & Ralabate, P. (1985). The acquisition of a phonological feature of Black English. *Journal of Communication Disorders,* 18, 139–148.

Seymour, H., & Seymour, C. (1981). Black English and Standard English contrasts in consonantal development of four- and five-year old children. *Journal of Speech and Hearing Disorders,* 46, 274–280.

Shipley, K. G., & McAfee, J. G. (1992). *Assessment in speech-language pathology: A resource manual.* San Diego: Singular Publishing.

Steffersen, M. (1974). The acquisition of Black English. Doctoral dissertation, University of Illinois, Evanston.

Stockman, I. (1986). Language acquisition in culturally diverse populations: The black child as a case study. In O. Taylor (Ed.), *Nature of communication disorders in culturally and linguistically diverse*

populations (pp. 117–155). San Diego: College-Hill Press.

Stockman, I. (1991, November). *Constraints on final consonant deletion in Black English.* Paper presented to the meeting of the American Speech-Language-Hearing Association, Atlanta.

Stockman, I. (1993). Variable word initial and medial consonants relationships in children's speech sound articulation. *Perceptual and Motor Skills,* 76, 675–689.

Stockman, I. (1995, November). Early morphosyntactic patterns of African-American children. Paper presented to the meeting of the American Speech-Language-Hearing Association, Orlando, FL.

Stockman, I., & Settle, M. S. (1991, November). Initial consonants in young Black children's conversational speech. Paper presented to the meeting of the American Speech-Language-Hearing Association, Atlanta.

Stockman I., & Vaughn-Cooke, F. (1992). Lexical elaboration in children's locative action expressions. *Child Development,* 63, 1104–1125.

Taylor, O. (1986). *Nature of communication disorders in culturally and linguistically diverse populations.* San Diego: College-Hill.

Taylor, O. (in press). Clinical practice as a social occasion. In L. Cole & V. Deal (Eds.) *Communication disorders in multicultural populations.* Rockville, MD: American Speech-Language-Hearing Association.

Taylor, O., & Clarke, M. G. (1994). Culture and communication disorders: A theoretical framework. *Seminars in Speech and Language,* 15(2), 103–113.

Terrell, S., & Terrell, F. (1993). African-American cultures. In D. E. Battle (Ed.) *Communication disorders in multicultural populations* (pp. 3–37). Newton, MA: Butterworth-Heinemann.

U.S. Bureau of the Census. (1990). Statistical Abstract of the United States: 1990. 110th Ed. Washington, DC: United States Department of Commerce.

U.S. Bureau of the Census. (1993). *Household and family characteristics: March 1993.* Current population report series P-20. Washington, DC: U.S. Government Printing Office.

U.S. Department of Education. (1994). To assure the free appropriate public education of all Americans: Sixteenth annual report to Congress on the implementation of The Individuals with Disabilities Education Act (ED/OSERS Publication No. 065–000–00700–2). Washington, DC: U.S. Government Printing Office.

Vaughn-Cooke, F. (1983). Improving language assessment in minority children. *Asha,* 9, 29–34.

Vaughn-Cooke, F. (1986). Lexical diffusion: Evidence from a decreolizing variety of Black English. In M. Montgomery & G. Bailey (Eds.). *Language variety in the South* (pp. 111–130). Tuscaloosa: University of Alabama Press.

Vaughn-Cooke, F., & Wright-Harp, W. (1992). *Lexical development in working-class Black children.* National Institutes of Health grant #RR08005–23.

Washington, J., & Craig, H. (1992). Articulation test performance of low-income, African-American preschoolers with communication impairments. *Language, Speech, and Hearing Services in Schools,* 23, 245–252.

Wayman, K. I., Lynch, E. W., & Hanson, M. J. (1990). Home-based early childhood services: Cultural sensitivity in a family systems approach. *Topics in Early Childhood Special Education,* 10, 65–66.

Weddington, G. (1987). Guidelines for the use of standardized tests with minority children. In L. Cole and V. Deal (Eds.), *Communication disorders in multicultural populations* (pp. 21–22). Rockville, MD: American Speech-Language-Hearing Association.

Westby, C. (1990). Ethnographic interviewing. *Journal of Childhood Communication Disorders,* 13(1), 110–118.

Westby, C. (1994). Multicultural issues. In J. B. Tomblin, H. L. Morris, & D. C. Spriestersbach, *Diagnosis in Speech-Language Pathology.* San Diego: Singular.

Wolfram, W., & Fasold, R. (1974). *The study of social dialects in American English.* Englewood Cliffs, NJ: Prentice Hall.

Wong-Fillmore, L. (1991a). Second language learning in children: A model of language learning in social context. In E. Bialystok (Ed.), *Language processing in bilingual children.* (pp. 49–69). Cambridge: Cambridge University Press.

Wong-Fillmore, L., (1991b). When learning a second language means losing the first. *Early Childhood Research Quarterly,* 6, 323–346.

Wyatt, T. (1991). Linguistic constraints on copula production in Black English child speech. Dissertation. University of Massachusetts, Amherst.

Part **III**

Language Disorders and Special Populations

Chapter 11

Understanding Learning
Disabilities

PEARL L. SEIDENBERG
Long Island University

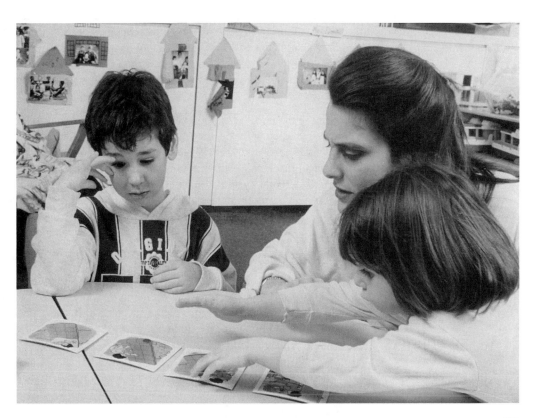

The Concept of Learning Disabilities

Historical Origins

Learning disabilities is the most recent classification to be included as a category of disability. Since the term was introduced, its use has become widespread in education, but many educators still remain unsure about the nature of this category. Currently, the learning disability field still includes concepts such as perceptual-motor problems, hyperactivity, minimal brain damage, and psychoneurological disorders that have their roots in the origins of the field. The struggle to understand and define learning disabilities has characterized the field since its inception.

Lerner (1981) and Wiederholt (1974) divided the history of learning disabilities into four distinct phases:

1. *Foundation* phase (about 1800–1930), a period devoted to scientific investigation of brain function
2. *Transition phase* (about 1930–1960), during which it was assumed that children who were not learning possessed brain function deficits resulting in disordered behaviors; professionals (Cruickshank, Bentzen, Razburg, & Tannhauser, 1961; Orton, 1937; Strauss & Lehtinen, 1947) began to develop assessment and treatment methods for these children
3. *Integration phase* (about 1960–1980), a period characterized by increased interest in learning disabilities with a subsequent increase in school programs for the learning disabled and research into assessment practices and teaching methods
4. *Contemporary phase* (1980 to the present), in which the direction is toward widening the definition of individuals served and the integration of services provided across school programs

One of the first to propose the term *learning disability* was Samuel Kirk (1963), who used it to describe a group of children with specific learning deficits. He stated that a learning disability refers to a retardation, disorder, or delayed development in one or more of the processes of speech, language, reading, spelling, writing, or arithmetic. The learning disability results from a possible cerebral dysfunction and/or emotional or behavioral disturbance, not from mental retardation, sensory deprivation, or cultural or instructional factors. Kirk explained that these disabilities refer to a discrepancy between the child's achievement and apparent capacity to learn as indicated by aptitude tests, verbal understanding, and arithmetic computational skills.

Although the concept covered diverse learning deficits, the term established a frame of reference for thinking about a child with specific learning disorders. The term avoided placing the blame for failure to learn solely on dysfunctions within the child who was assumed to have more intellectual ability than the child who is mentally retarded. Because the term did not specify a cause (i.e., minimal brain dysfunction or brain damage), it focused attention on the educational problems that the child faces and laid the framework for educational decision making and special education services.

In 1963, when the Association for Children with Learning Disabilities (ACLD) was formed, the term *learning disability* was adopted as a substitute term for such etiological labels as *brain-injured* and *perceptually handicapped.* In 1969, the following definition was presented to Congress by the National Advisory Committee on Handicapped Children:

> *The term "Children with specific learning disabilities" means those children who have a disorder in one or more of the basic psychological processes involved in understanding or in using language, spoken or written, which disorder may manifest itself in an imperfect ability to listen, think, speak, read, write, spell or do mathematical calculations. Such disorders include such conditions as perceptual handicaps, brain injury, minimal brain dysfunction, dyslexia and developmental aphasia. The term does not include children who have learning problems which are primarily the result of visual, hearing or motor handicaps, of mental retardation, of emotional disturbance, or of environmental, cultural or economic disadvantage. (Federal Register, U.S. Office of Education, 1977)*

This definition served as the basis of the 1969 Learning Disabilities Act and later, in 1975, was included in the Education for All Handicapped Children Act, Public Law 94-142.

In 1981, the National Joint Committee on Learning Disabilities revised the definition (Hammill, Leiger, McNutt, & Larsen, 1981) and agreed on the following:

> *Learning disability is a generic term that refers to a heterogeneous group of disorders manifested by significant difficulties in the acquisition and use of listening, speaking, reading, writing, reasoning, or mathematical abilities. These disorders are intrinsic to the individual and are presumed to be due to central nervous system dysfunction. Even though a learning disability may occur concomitantly with other handicapping conditions or environmental influences, it is not the direct result of those conditions or influences. (p. 336)*

This definition has been accepted by the Council for Learning Disabilities, the International Reading Association, the Division for Children with Communication Disorders, the Orton Society, and the American Speech-Language-Hearing Association.

The most basic and important difference from the definition included in Public Law 94-142 is the elimination of the phrase "basic psychological processes." The joint committee agreed that the original purpose of the statement, which was to emphasize the *intrinsic* nature of learning disabilities, had been confounded by the controversy that resulted from the association of the term with the perceptual-motor and specific abilities training models that were in use at the time the original definition was adopted. Currently, explanations of the kinds of *cognitive, metacognitive,* and *ability* deficits that characterize the nature of the intrinsic disorders of the learning disabled population are based on linguistic science and information-processing theory.

Defining Learning Disabilities

Because human behavior and learning are complex, learning disabilities may be difficult to define; but they are usually readily identifiable and distinguishable from other disabilities.

Although professionals may be unable to agree on a single definition, in practice most do not deny the validity of the condition.

The term is used to describe children and adolescents who are not learning at an expected rate despite the fact that they have experienced traditionally adequate instructional programs. The term *learning disability* does not identify a specific dysfunction or a syndrome of dysfunctions. The decision to describe a child as learning disabled is made by eliminating other causes of school failure such as emotional disturbance, mental retardation, or environmental or cultural disadvantage. The label encompasses a heterogeneous group of learners with diverse characteristics, who have common problems with learning and who do not present a clearly identifiable reason for their learning deficits. Although the label is descriptive rather than diagnostic and does not denote a specific etiology or a specific cluster of characteristics, there are a number of behavioral characteristics that are often attributed to children with learning disabilities.

Characteristics of Children with Learning Disabilities

Although the characteristics associated with learning disability are not likely to be present in all or even many learning disabled children, the behavioral characteristics are useful for helping us to understand the category. The following nine characteristics arc mentioned most frequently:

1. *Hyperactivity*—inappropriate excessive motor activity such as tapping of finger or foot, jumping out of seat, or skipping from task to task
2. *Attention deficits*—distracted by irrelevant stimuli or perseveration, or attention becomes fixed upon a single task or behavior that is repeated over and over
3. *Motor deficits*—general coordination problems resulting in awkward or clumsy movements
4. *Perceptual-motor deficits*—difficulty in integrating a visual or auditory stimulus with a motor response
5. *Language deficits*—delays in speech and difficulty in understanding and/or formulating spoken language
6. *Impulsivity*—lack of reflective behavior
7. *Cognitive deficits*—deficits in memory and concept formation
8. *Orientation deficits*—poorly developed spatial or temporal concepts
9. *Specific learning deficits*—problems in acquiring reading, writing, or arithmetic skills

These behavioral characteristics, for the most part, are *process*-oriented, as opposed to *effect*-oriented. That is, they focus on deficit behaviors exhibited by children with learning problems. In contrast, the identification of the effects of the learning deficits (e.g., deficits in verbal or written language development) directs attention to the child's deficiencies in level of performance or skill acquisition in academic areas. These effect-oriented characteristics are the only performance indicators that are useful in helping to develop appropriate educational interventions.

Attention-Deficit Hyperactivity (ADHD) and Learning Disabilities

Controversy continues to surround the relationship between the diagnostic classification of attention-deficit hyperactivity disorder (ADHD) and learning disabilities. Historically, there have been significant changes in the diagnostic criteria that were intended to separate ADHD and learning disabilities. The current Diagnostic and Statistical Manual—DSM—IV—of the American Psychiatric Association (APA, 1994) continues to categorize learning disabilities as Specific Developmental Disabilities, while attention deficit disorders are categorized as Disruptive Disorders of Children. At the same time, recent clarification of the status of ADHD as a handicapping condition by the United States Department of Education (DOE) recognized that ADHD could co-occur with other handicapping conditions and result in learning problems. However, the DOE did not believe that ADHD needed to be added as a separate disability category, indicating that children with ADHD are eligible for services under the category of learning disabled or emotionally disturbed if they satisfy the specific category criteria (Davila, Williams, & MacDonald, 1991).

Research has consistently demonstrated that learning disabilities involve a number of components, such as cognitive, attentional, and behavioral deficits and including hyperactivity and impulsivity among some students (Hiebert, Wong, & Hunter, 1982; Kavale & Nye, 1985; McKinney & Reagans, 1983, 1984; Walker, 1985; Williams, Gridley, & Fitzhugh-Bell, 1992).

At the same time, a number of studies have shown that children diagnosed as ADHD experience significant academic achievement problems (August & Garfinkel, 1990; Barkley, Fischer, Edelbrock, & Smallish, 1990; McGee, Williams, Moffett, & Anderson, 1989). However, it is still not clear whether academic failure in children with ADHD is related to attention/impulsivity, cognitive deficits (learning disabilities), or a combination of both (Biederman, Newcorn, & Sprich, 1991).

While the results of a large number of studies suggest a relationship between LD and ADHD, the underlying nature of the relationship has not, as yet, been clearly defined (Cantwell & Baker, 1991; Epstein, Shaywitz, Shaywitz, & Woolston, 1991; Shaywitz & Shaywitz, 1991). It has been suggested that the co-occurrence of LD and ADHD in subgroups of each of these populations is likely to be the result of differences in underlying neurological functioning that result in common cognitive deficits (Epstein et al., 1991; Shaywitz & Shaywitz, 1991). Based on evidence of underlying neurological dysfunction, it has been suggested that subgroups of both LD and ADHD children may present with attentional problems (August & Garfinkel, 1990; Fleisher, Soodak, & Jelin, 1984; Levine, Busch, & Aufsieser, 1982). In addition, the presence of a language disorder appears to characterize both LD and ADHD children. For children with learning disabilities, language deficits appear to be a major underlying problem for many learning-impaired children (Catts, 1991; Gibbs & Cooper, 1989; Newhoff, 1990; Paul, 1992). Similarly, many children diagnosed with attention deficit disorders demonstrate some type of language disorder (Baker & Cantwell, 1990; Neitman, Hood, & Inglis, 1990; Cohen, Devine, & Meloche-Kelly, 1989). Because of these findings, it has been suggested that linguistic development may represent the key element that underlies the relationships between some LD and ADHD children at a cognitive level and the resultant academic achievement problems demonstrated by these children (August & Garfinkel, 1990).

At the same time, because of the paucity of evidence that specifies the educations characteristics or needs of students with ADHD without the complications imposed by other co-existing conditions such as learning disabilities, educational interventions for this population should address the co-occurring learning disabilities and/or language deficits before any other accommodations are provided (Zentall, 1993).

An Information-Processing Perspective

Current characterizations of the intrinsic disorders manifested in learning disabled children's ability deficits are based on information-processing theory. Attention has shifted from an interest in identifying and remediating discrete, underlying, processing ability deficits to a focus on the inefficient, or maladaptive, information-processing skills of learning disabled children. An information-processing orientation provides a way to understand performances in more complex, higher order cognitive and linguistic tasks such as reading and writing. This perspective provides for useful conceptualizations of the cognitive processes (such as coding, comparing, storing, and retrieving) that underlie observable performance. Learning failure is viewed in terms of deficiencies in underlying cognitive processes (Torgesen, 1986; Swanson, 1989).

Psychological Processes

For some time, learning disabilities were considered to be the result of various types of specific underlying ability deficits. Historically, the research in learning disabilities centered on various psychological processing tasks involving attention, perception, and memory. Comparisons were made between learning disabled and nonlearning disabled students. These tasks were considered to be measures of underlying cognitive abilities and were used to assess separate discrete functions (i.e., visual closure, visual and/or auditory figure-ground differentiation, auditory discrimination, visual and/or auditory memory, etc.). Because early theorists contended that these factors had to be adequately developed before learning could occur, training programs and materials were designed to remediate specific processing deficits (Frostig, 1968; Kephart, 1971; Kirk & Kirk, 1972).

An assumption underlying the specific abilities deficit model was that the areas were distinct from each other and that their component parts could be identified and assessed. Therefore, each system could be measured independently. The interactive nature of the processes of perception, attention, and memory was not considered. Also, the role of the learner in cognitive processing was not viewed as an active one, and thus confounding variables such as meaningfulness of material or organizational abilities were not taken into consideration. The passive view of the child led to the belief that what was to be attended to, perceived, or memorized was "out there." Modification of the demands of tasks rather than attempts to influence the child's approach to a problem was emphasized.

From an information-processing perspective, perception, attention, and memory are considered interactive cognitive processes whose functioning reflects the influence and control of higher order, integrated, goal-directed cognitive structures (Anderson, 1975). We develop control mechanisms, "a plan to execute a plan" (Miller, Galanter, & Pribam, 1960), which organize and direct the lower order processes. Therefore, the learning difficulties experienced by some otherwise normally developing children have come to be recognized as related to the higher order cognitive controls, or strategies, that regulate attention, perception, and memory. This strategy-oriented view of learning disabilities focuses on cognitive processes that are modifiable by instruction rather than on separate, more elementary processing differences or deficits (Swanson, 1991).

The most important and useful feature of information-processing theory is that it enhances our understanding of the problems of children with learning disabilities. A much more complex picture of the learning process is emerging that focuses attention on the strategies a child uses in approaching learning tasks and suggests very different educational interventions.

The Information-Processing Model

In 1969, Chalfont and Scheffelin described learning disabilities as problems involving deviation in the ability to process information and as an inefficiency in the reception, analysis, synthesis, and symbolic use of information. Since then, information-processing concepts have provided a useful framework for understanding learning disabilities.

The conceptual model arising from information-processing theory enables us to describe systematically the way students who exhibit learning deficits process information. Cognitive psychology, or information-processing psychology, deals with the study of mental processes and begins with the idea that we have the innate capacity to make sense of our experiences. We pick up information, organize it, retain it, and retrieve it. We can call upon previously stored information to help us in managing new information. The fact that we make sense of our experience, even though nothing ever happens to us in exactly the same way twice, must mean that we are organized in some systematic way (Farnham-Diggory, 1980). Figure 11-1 is an example of an information-processing model.

Auditory, visual, and tactile stimuli (sensory data) are transmitted to the central-processing mechanism (brain) where they are analyzed, integrated, and stored. The behavioral responses of the individual serve as an additional input source (feedback) for correcting or further modifying the responses. The input is always into a dynamic, orga-

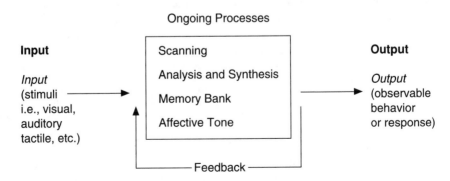

FIGURE 11-1   Information-processing model.

nized, interactive system. Behavioral responses are determined not only by the actual stimulus but also by the ongoing programs, the result of past experiences that are already stored in the system.

Modern information-processing theory suggests that individuals may differ from one another cognitively in two broad areas. First, they may differ in the basic structure of their information-processing systems. These structural, or architectural (Campione & Brown, 1978), features are the elements of the system that operate outside of the conscious control of the individual. Such things as capacity of short-term memory, duration of memory traces, and speed of operations of various processes are all part of the structure of the system.

Second, individual differences can be the result of differences in information and skills that are *learned* as a result of experience. These are the content of long-term memory (i.e., programs already in the system) and are made up of general organized knowledge of the world (i.e., hierarchical semantic structures), habitual ways of thinking (i.e., concrete versus abstract), and rules and strategies that guide performance and adaptation to tasks. The content of long-term memory and the functional features of the system are modifiable by instruction and are under our conscious control (Torgesen, 1982).

The distinction between structural and functional areas of cognitive performance made by information-processing theorists has led to new ways of thinking about the cognitive system of individuals with learning disabilities. Traditionally, learning disabled children's academic problems and poor performance on experimental tasks were explained in terms of specific ability deficits necessary for normal processing of information. A large number of disabilities such as perceptual-motor deficits, intermodel integration deficits, and psycholinguistic processing problems were considered to be relatively enduring cognitive deficits that restricted information processing. In information-processing terms, these earlier explanations claimed that all problems with learning were due to differences in the structural features of the system.

Concepts derived from information-processing theory have greater explanatory power. They provide a framework for analyzing learning deficits that differentiates between the structural and the functional elements of the system, that is, between the system and the programs that use the system. In the child who is learning disabled, some information-processing components are not operating effectively for certain tasks. Therefore, the primary problem appears to be one of programming, and although there may also be some system defects, we can search for ways to develop programs that will compensate for them. A major assumption that underlies the information-processing view is that the rules and specific strategies used by children with learning disabilities do not appear to be appropriate to their intellectual ability. They appear to have knowledge that they are unable to access under certain conditions, to have strategies that they fail to use, or to have not learned when to select particular strategies.

To account for the poor task performance of students with learning disabilities, researchers have generated a number of information-processing models that focus on isolating specific processing deficits involving metacognitive and metalinguistic variables, such as a verbal processing deficit (Vellutino, 1977), a phonological recoding deficit (Shankweiler, Liberman, Mark, Fowler, & Fischer, 1979), a rehearsal deficiency (Bauer, 1977), a selective attention deficit (Hallahan & Reeves, 1980), and a memory deficit (Mastropieri, Scruggs, & Levin, 1985; Scruggs, Mastropieri, & Levin, 1987).

In addition, more general metacognitive models have been proposed that focus on higher order cognitive processing problems involving mechanisms such as the regulation or coordination of mental activities (e.g., general control processes involved in the planful consideration, selection, execution, and evaluation of strategies) as well as the relation of affective belief systems (e.g., appropriate attributions of performance outcomes) to strategic processing (Borkowski, Johnston, & Reid, 1987; Borkowski & Kurtz, 1987; Swanson, 1988, 1989).

Based on these more global metacognitive models, a number of studies support the notion that students with learning disabilities have difficulty in modifying or transforming simple strategies into the more complex, efficient procedures needed to meet the requirements of many academic tasks (Swanson, 1988; Swanson & Cooney, 1985; Swanson & Rhine, 1985). The higher order cognitive processing problems are undoubtedly influenced by specific strategic processing deficits and dysfunctional belief systems (outlined earlier), which probably become more pervasive over time in their influence on academic performance. At the same time, a considerable body of evidence shows that training students with learning disabilities to use more efficient task-specific cognitive strategies improves their performance on many school-related tasks (Deshler, Schumaker, & Lenz, 1984; Ellis & Lenz, 1987; Ryan, Weed, & Short, 1986; Schunk & Cox, 1986; Wong, 1985).

The metacognitive and metalinguistic variables generated by these diverse information-processing models have important implications for our understanding of the three major areas of learning disabilities: (a) deficiencies in oral language, (b) deficiencies in cognitive abilities, and (c) deficiencies in written language.

Major Areas of Learning Disabilities

Deficits in Oral Language

Failure to develop adequate verbal language skills results in subsequent failure in many other areas of learning. It is important to understand the interdependencies of language disorders and learning disabilities. For many decades, the field of learning disabilities generally did not emphasize the role of language processes. Because of the origins of the field, an interest in perceptual-motor functioning and other nonverbal tasks dominated both the literature and educational programs. It was not until the 1970s that researchers began to investigate the relationship between deficits in oral language and learning disabilities.

Currently, many researchers believe that language deficits are implicated in learning disabilities (Catts & Kamhi, 1986; Liberman, 1983; Shankweiler et al., 1979; Vellutino, 1977). They propose that these deficits have an impact on reading ability and academic success. Following is a brief overview of the language problems representative of children with learning disabilities. The reader is referred to Wiig and Semel (1976, 1984) and Wallach and Butler (1984) for a more comprehensive treatment of this topic.

Preschool Language Deficits.   Preschool children who exhibit language deficits or delays are generally at risk for later school failure. Early language disorders are demonstrated in a number of areas. At-risk children frequently show no interest in verbal activities, are unable to follow a story line, and do not enjoy being read to. Although nouns, verbs, and most prepositions are understood, these children may have word retrieval difficulties or difficulty in following a series of oral directions. There is often a sustained delay in speech and language development, and syntax may be primitive with incidence of inadequate morphological pattern acquisition. Overall verbal concept development may be slow, and the children are often still unable to name colors, letters, or days of the week when they enter school.

In a comprehensive review of the research regarding young children with language impairments, Leonard (1979) presented a description of at-risk children's linguistic problems. In general, the language skills of preschoolers with language delays are similar to those of younger, normally developing children. Syntactically, the structures used by both groups of children seem to be the same, although at-risk children appear to use them less frequently and in more limited contexts. The size of their vocabulary and the length of their utterances (MLU) also resemble those of younger children. Similar findings relate to the areas of pragmatics and phonology. There is evidence of greater delays in the language impaired child's use of the pragmatic and phonological features of language.

Because inadequate language development is often the precursor to learning problems during the school years, there is an urgent need for early identification of children who show developmental language delays. As discussed in earlier chapters, the recognition of the importance of early identification and intervention programs for infants and toddlers at risk for developmental delays and preschoolers with disabilities spurred passage of the Education of Handicapped Children Act Amendments of 1986 (PL 99-457). It is well established that early intervention can prevent later learning problems from developing and can offset the negative emotional consequences of school failure (Majsterek & Ellenwood, 1990).

Language Deficits of the School-Age Child.   Many children with learning disabilities exhibit a number of language deficits that affect both language comprehension and production. The linguistic demands of a classroom require a level of abstractness and complexity much greater than that needed for ordinary social communicative competence. The mismatch between the linguistic demands of instructional language and the poor linguistic abilities of many children with learning disabilities may account in part for the hyperactive, impulsive behaviors and attentional deficits often attributed to these children.

Generally, language impaired, learning disabled children have difficulty understanding *wh-* questions and processing and using pronouns and possessives. Other aspects of syntax that often cause difficulty are the passive construction, negative constructions, relative clauses, negations, contractions, and adjective transformations (Vogel, 1975; Wiig & Semel, 1973, 1974, 1975). There is evidence of reduced mastery of the grammatical inflections for adjectives, verb tense markers, and possession (Vogel, 1975; Wiig, Semel, & Crouse, 1973). Specific difficulty with verb tense markers was found primarily in irregular past tense forms (Moran & Bryne, 1977) and with more complex grammatical structures (Edwards & Kallail, 1977).

Linguistic concepts expressing comparative, spatial, and temporal relationships are also problems for children with learning disabilities. Wiig and Semel (1976) have demonstrated that the ability to process these structures follows a developmental course, with comparative relations being easiest, followed in difficulty by temporal and spatial relationships. It is important to note that not all children who have learning disabilities will have the same difficulties with the same linguistic concepts.

An extensive description of areas of possible difficulty with different form classes, including nouns, verbs, adjectives, adverbs, and prepositions, was provided by Wiig and Semel (1984). The authors related many of the linguistic problems to more primary cognitive difficulties. They suggested that if relationships are not accurately perceived by children in their interactions with their environment, they will not be able to comprehend these relationships when they are coded linguistically. In addition, they believed that a child who has difficulty in generalizing and has a tendency toward concreteness will maintain narrower word meanings and have problems processing sentences containing multiple-meaning words and figurative language. It has been shown that elementary-age students with learning disabilities do have difficulty understanding metaphoric language when compared with their nonlearning disabled peers. It appears that, although many learning disabled children have the requisite cognitive strategies for understanding metaphors (e.g., generating and comparing semantic attributes), they fail to spontaneously access and apply them when they should (Seidenberg & Bernstein, 1986, 1988).

In development of their semantic system, children with and without learning disabilities generally have been found to perform equally well in tasks of receptive vocabulary (Wiig & Semel, 1973; Vogel, 1975). However, children with learning disabilities exhibit word-finding difficulties (Denckla & Rudel, 1976; Johnson & Myklebust, 1967; Kail & Leonard, 1986) and semantic memory deficits (Baker, Ceci, & Hermann, 1987). They also demonstrate specific deficits in rapid naming tasks, naming pictures, naming opposites, and giving word definitions (Wiig & Semel, 1976).

The primary productive syntactic language problems evidenced by children with learning disabilities appear to be a delay in the acquisition of basic operations such as negative, interrogative, or passive transformations. In sentence repetition tasks, these children appear to maintain the basic meaning or semantic relations of a sentence without difficulty, but they repeat the sentence in a reduced fashion (Menyuk & Looney, 1972). In general, children with learning disabilities appear to be performing similarly to younger, normally developing children in this area.

Generally, the phonological problems of children with language impairments are more complex than the problems exhibited by children with only an articulation disorder. The problems appear to be related to morpho-syntactic delays as well as to the ability to accurately carry out the complex motor programs of speech (Berry, 1980). Often, the language learning disabled child evidences inconsistencies in sound production. Sounds may be produced accurately in a simple sentence, but when the sentences become longer and more complex, production difficulties become evident. The child with language delays appears more vulnerable to the syntactic demands of more complex structures, in which requirements of motor patterning and idea formulation appear to create organizational problems and subsequent problems in speech production (Catts, 1986; Lieberman, Meskill, Chatillon, & Schupack, 1985).

Finally, children with learning disabilities may have deficits in pragmatics, the understanding of the rules governing the use of language in social contexts. In a review of a series of studies dealing with pragmatic competence, Bryan (1981) presented an overview of these deficits. In general, the children with learning disabilities did *not* differ from nondisabled children in conversational turn-taking or in referential communicative competence when a required response was unambiguous. However, when a situation was ambiguous or socially complex, the performance of the two groups differed. In these situations, children with learning disabilities have difficulty with such pragmatic skills as asking questions, responding to inadequate messages, disagreeing, supporting an argument, and sustaining or monitoring a conversation. The studies also indicated that the relationships among syntactic-semantic knowledge, social knowledge, and development of communicative competence are interactive and complex and may be dependent upon the development of both linguistic skills and cognitive abilities.

Deficits in Cognitive Abilities

Any attempt to understand the performance of learning disabled children in academic learning must consider the interaction of language and thought and the cognitive correlates of such an interaction. In processing written language, the learner is confronted with a combination of both abstract concepts and complex language. Without adequate development in both language and cognitive strategies for processing information, a serious mismatch between the child's ability and the academic task demands can result. The cognitive functions of perception, attention, and memory are related to each other, as well as to the acquisition of language. Understanding the nature of these interactions in the processing of verbally encoded information contributes to our understanding of the problems experienced by many children with learning disabilities.

According to current theory in cognitive psychology, perception, attention, and memory are interactive processes that reconstruct, organize, and internalize information. Cognitive development is continually emerging through stages of newly acquired strategies for actively processing environmental information. The child becomes increasingly able to attend selectively to critical attributes during perception and to hold more than one aspect of perceived information in memory simultaneously to perform cognitively on that information. As age increases, memory abilities are enhanced by the use of categorization and verbal rehearsal strategies (Ring, 1976). Similarly, with maturation, children develop increased ability to focus attention on the relevant aspects of learning tasks and to diminish attention to incidental stimuli (Hallahan & Sapona, 1984; Tarver, Hallahan, Kaufman, & Ball, 1976).

Memory, attention, and perception interact and are interdependent. The individual actively analyzes and processes information by developing strategies that tap previously stored information acquired through past experience and organizational structures. Also, there appears to be a reciprocal relationship between language development and the development of cognitive abilities. This interactive nature of the relationship is viewed within the broader framework of the child's overall ability to organize, plan, monitor, and integrate information. The view that is generally held is that the development of cognitive strategies complements linguistic development in a way that facilitates the processing of verbally encoded information. Also, increased linguistic abilities contribute to the development of a number of cognitive functions such as memory and attention.

For example, many children who have learning disabilities exhibit deficits in short-term memory of verbal information (Cohen, 1982; Jorm, 1983; Torgesen, 1985), resulting from difficulties in the use of such elaborative encoding strategies as verbal grouping and verbal rehearsal (e.g., repeating information to oneself to encourage recall). These difficulties appear to reduce the effectiveness of attention and memory in processing information. At the same time, children with learning disabilities exhibit inadequate use of the organizational structure of syntax and of category clustering of verbal material, and these deficits also appear to be related to problems in processing verbal material (Bauer, 1977; Gelheiser, 1984; Hallahan, Gajar, Cohen, & Tarver, 1978; Kamhi & Koenig, 1985; Pressley, Borkowski, & O'Sullivan, 1984; Torgesen, 1978).

In a number of previously reported studies, the performance of children with learning disabilities improved after they were taught to use selected processing strategies. These observed changes in behavior have led to the conclusion that children with learning disabilities have more ability than can be presumed from their performance. Some of their learning deficits are not due to an inability to acquire effective cognitive strategies, but to other factors that interfere with their development. One factor that appears to result in poor performance is that many children with learning disabilities tend to lack motivation and are thus characterized as inactive learners (Torgesen & Licht, 1983). It has been suggested that this passive approach to learning is the result of the children's tendency *not* to link performance outcomes to their own efforts or abilities; that is, they often regard what happens to them as unrelated to what they themselves do. It has been proposed that this view of themselves and the learning environment may prevent children with learning disabilities from actively using appropriate cognitive strategies (Butkowsky & Willows, 1980; Hallahan et al., 1978; Johnston & Winograd, 1985; Kurtz & Borkowski, 1984; Licht, 1984; Winograd & Niquette, 1988).

Some aspects of the relationship between cognition and language have yet to be examined; however, many of the behaviors reported in learning disabled children appear to support a hypothesis of a delay in cognitive development. Their cognitive development indicates deficits in the use of higher order cognitive strategies such as (a) simultaneous processing of perceptual information, (b) development of organizational structures that encode larger amounts of information, and (c) use of verbal strategies to facilitate storage and retrieval of information. Because of the importance of these higher order cognitive and linguistic variables for academic learning (e.g., metacognitive and metalinguistic abilities), they are discussed in some detail in the following section.

Deficits in Reading and Writing

The largest subgroup among the learning disabled population are those children and adolescents identified as having deficits associated with learning to read and write (Stanovich, 1986). Children with disorders in the comprehension or formulation of written language appear to process information differently than nonlearning disabled children. Often they fail to use effective strategies in interacting with written material and show deficits in their performance of reading and writing tasks.

Reading Deficits.   Although most children learn to read as effortlessly as they learn to speak, regardless of the method used to teach them, a small proportion of children with no clearly identifiable intellectual, physical, or social disabilities, find it extremely difficult to learn to read or write. For these children, learning to read is a formidable task. Those who are responsible for teaching these children find the task equally difficult. However, current theoretical advances in the cognitive and linguistic sciences provide some new approaches to this problem. Insights derived from a developmental cognitive-linguistic perspective emphasize the complex, interactive nature of the reading process and provide an additional dimension for understanding the nature of reading disabilities.

This perspective assumes that there are critical age-related cognitive and linguistic characteristics that interact with reading instruction and result in an inability to acquire specific reading skills. It is believed that the learner's cognitive-linguistic abilities set the parameters for the child's information-processing capacities. These underlying information-processing capabilities are important for learning to read and are reflected in a student's specific reading behaviors. Because reading disability is *not* a unitary phenomenon, the actual causes of difficulties in learning to read vary. There can be various points of breakdown for different learners in the learning-to-read process. Deficits in the learner's underlying information-processing capacities relative to the skills being taught contribute to these breakdowns.

Efficient reading requires the acquisition and integration of different skills at different points in the process. The acquisition of these skills is dependent on the integrative functioning of cognitive abilities (i.e., perception, attention, and memory) and their interface with linguistic variables. Therefore, the concept of reading disability can be understood only within a developmental context that considers what learners bring to the task of learning to read and how it affects reading efficiency.

Defining the Reading Process.   Reading may be broadly defined as a communication process in that it involves the ability to respond to written language. It is a process of obtaining meaning and is currently categorized not as a perceptual act, but as a language-based activity. Goodman (1973) described reading as a "psycholinguistic guessing game" in which the reader samples only a minimal amount of the visual information, relying heavily on the redundancy of language (i.e., phonology, semantics, and syntax) to predict structures. As the reader processes the subsequent language, these predictions are tested against the semantic content and are confirmed. Reading is viewed as a constructive process in which the reader's knowledge about the language and the world (i.e., past experience) interact with the textual information (Anderson, Spiro, & Montague, 1977).

To bridge the gap from print to meaning, the reader must engage a number of subprocesses that involve auditory and visual perceptual abilities, cognitive abilities (i.e., attention, memory, organization), language knowledge, and past experiences. Reading performance can be viewed as a product of the reader's cognitive and linguistic abilities, prior knowledge, and mastery of specific reading skills (see Figure 11-2). Reading performance reflects the interaction of these diverse factors, each of which contributes collectively to the reading process and, therefore, to observable reading behaviors.

Although reading may start with print and the specific skills taught in reading instruction, the level of reading efficiency demonstrated at any given point in the learning-to-read process is linked to the reader's information-processing capabilities within the different components of the model. Reading performance reflects the knowledge and competencies available to the learner and how these are activated and coordinated during the reading process.

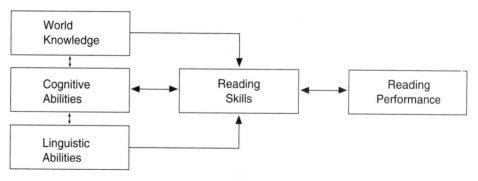

FIGURE 11-2 Interactive model of reading performance.

Deficits in Verbal Processing. The possibility of verbal deficiencies in poor readers is currently receiving greater attention than it has in past years. There is an emerging consensus about the importance of a variety of linguistic or language-based skills in explaining reading disabilities (Catts & Kamhi, 1986; Stanovich, 1986; Vellutino, 1979).

Because reading achievement necessitates the efficient use of all of the learner's cognitive and linguistic abilities, deficits in linguistic functioning have impact on both initial reading skill acquisition and on the later stages of the learning-to-read process. One theory suggests that many children with reading disabilities have deficits in processing the phonological aspects of language (Catts, 1986; Liberman, 1983; Torgesen, 1985; Torgesen, Wagner, Simmons & Laughon, 1990; Wagner, 1986).

Difficulty in acquiring beginning reading skills has been linked with deficits in phonological processing. For example, Vellutino (1979) maintained that the apparent visual-perceptual problems (i.e., word identification) encountered by beginning readers are, in fact, associated with problems in verbal mediation and/or phonological deficits. He contended that many of the errors implicated in reading disability can be understood as linguistic intrusion errors rather than as deficits in visual perception. Thus, when poor readers call a *b* a *d* or substitute *was* for *saw*, it is not because they are processing the visual information inaccurately, it is because they have difficulty in correctly naming the letter or word. Similarly, he suggested that awareness of the phonological structure of spoken language is important for the acquisition of word-decoding skills. Success in beginning reading, specifically in code acquisition (e.g., learning sound-symbol relationships), requires that learners have the ability to segment words at the phonemic level and to associate the separate phonemes with their counterparts in print. Poor readers appear to lack the phonological segmentation ability and, therefore, have difficulty in phonemic decoding and in developing phoneme-grapheme correspondences.

A number of other researchers support the idea that poor readers are less adequate than better readers in phonological segmentation ability and in both short- and long-term memory for verbal material. These difficulties have been linked to (a) a lack of phonological awareness, (b) problems in encoding verbal stimuli phonologically, and (c) deficits in retrieving phonological information from memory.

In studies of phonological segmentation ability, poor readers performed less well on phoneme and syllable segmentation tasks and on tasks involving rhyming and alliteration than good readers (Bryant & Bradley, 1981; Fox & Routh, 1980; Liberman, Shankweiler, Fisher, & Carter, 1974; Lieberman et al., 1985; Treiman & Baron, 1981; Vellutino & Scanlon, 1979; Williams, 1984b). Research indicating that poor readers exhibit deficits in short-term memory of verbal information have attributed the deficits to difficulties in using phonologically based codes to store verbal information (Catts, 1986; Perfetti & Lesgold, 1979; Ring, 1976; Torgesen, 1985; Torgesen, Rashotti, Greenstein, & Portes, 1991).

Another aspect of the phonological processing deficits of children with reading disabilities is inadequacy associated with deficits in the basic naming and labeling of verbal stimuli and in word retrieval (Blackman, 1984; Ceci, 1982; Denckla & Rudel, 1976; Perfetti & Hogaboam, 1975; Torgesen & Houck, 1980). It has been proposed that these naming and retrieval deficits are due to difficulties children have in accessing the phonological representations of words from their lexicons (Catts, 1986; Ellis, 1981).

A number of additional studies implicate other aspects of linguistic functioning in reader group differences in the development of reading comprehension abilities. These studies indicate that poor readers are not as proficient as better readers at understanding syntactically complex sentences (Brittain, 1970; Hook & Johnson, 1978; Vogel, 1975), at comprehending and using inflectional morphology (Berko, 1958; Bougere, 1969), at using syntactic constraints to assist in word identification (Samuels, Begg, & Chen, 1976; Steiner, Werner, & Cromer, 1971), in lexical development (Jansky & deHirsh, 1972; Vellutino, 1979), and at using knowledge of text or story structure (Englert & Raphael, 1988; Short & Ryan, 1984; Vallecorsa & Garriss, 1990; Williams, 1984a; Winograd, 1984, Wong, Wong, Perry, & Sawatsky, 1986).

Deficits in Metacognitive and Metalinguistic Abilities.   In addition to linguistic competence, efficient reading requires a more comprehensive awareness of cognitive and linguistic functioning. Metacognition, for example, is the ability to deal abstractly with one's own thought processes in comprehension and reasoning tasks and to identify and regulate the use of appropriate strategies (Brown, 1978; Flavell, 1978). Similarly, metalinguistic skills involve linguistic awareness, which is the ability to consciously reflect on the nature and discrete properties of language. In general, metalinguistic abilities interact with and reflect general cognitive and metacognitive abilities at different points in development (van Kleeck, 1984). Deficits in metalinguistic and/or metacognitive knowledge appear to be important factors that affect the acquisition of effective reading skills among poor readers.

It has been proposed that the development of reading skills requires a level of linguistic awareness above that required for the development and use of spoken language (Seidenberg, 1982). Many children who have learning disabilities appear to have deficits not solely in their verbal language systems but also in their metalinguistic abilities. For example, the phonological processing abilities outlined earlier that are required for the acquisition of phonics skills in beginning reading involve metalinguistic awareness, and there are developmental differences in children's ability to analyze and differentiate the phonemes in words (Cazden, 1972). The ability to make explicit judgments about the properties of language—that is, to analyze words, blend word parts, and reconstruct words—requires metalinguistic skills (Kamhi & Koenig, 1985). Similarly, the ability to recognize the syntactic structures in written text, to understand the relatedness among sentences in connected discourse, and to consider pertinent contextual information—that is, the ability to resolve contextual ambiguities—involves metalinguistic skills that are related to problems in reading comprehension. Many poor readers appear to have deficits in the ability to grasp grammatical structure and abstract meaning from larger contexts (Denner, 1970). Some poor readers are unable to segment texts into meaningful units and are, therefore, unable to attend to the focal or propositional information (Fleisher, Jenkins, & Pany, 1979). Poor readers also appear to have deficits in the metalinguistic awareness and cognitive strategies needed for monitoring and repairing comprehension failures due to textual inadequacies or inconsistencies (e.g., analogies, absurdities, anaphoric usage, figurative language, and idioms; see Chan, Cole, & Barfett, 1987; Seidenberg & Bernstein, 1988).

Research on metacognitive differences between good and poor readers indicates that less skilled readers appear to be unaware of their own failures to comprehend (Bos & Filip, 1984; Garner & Reis, 1981; Markman, 1977; Wong et al., 1986; Wong & Jones, 1982) and do not access or use effective comprehension-monitoring or repair strategies. In general, poor readers appear to be less able to evaluate task difficulty and to identify appropriate reading or studying strategies (Bransford, Stein, Shelton, & Owings, 1980; McGee, 1982; Paris & Meyers, 1981; Rinehart, Stahl, & Erickson, 1986; Schumaker, Deshler, Alley, Warner, & Denton, 1984). They are also characterized as overreliant on ineffective or inappropriate reading comprehension strategies. Poor readers continue to use inappropriate bottom-up strategies (word-decoding strategies) that affect comprehension, or inappropriate top-down strategies (conceptual strategies based on prior knowledge) that interfere with accurate word recognition (Pearson & Spiro, 1980). Additionally, poor readers tend not to use effective strategies for integrating word and sentence meanings, for extracting important information from the text, for drawing inferences, and for integrating background knowledge with the text (Golinkoff, 1976; Jenkins, Heliotis, Stein, & Haynes, 1987; Williams, 1984a; Winograd, 1984; Wong, 1978).

Writing Deficits. Generally, the student with learning disabilities involving either verbal language skills or reading skills will also experience difficulties in the acquisition of writing skills. Research indicates that writing skills are among the best correlates of reading, and that a strong relationship exists among reading, the receptive aspect of written language, and almost all other aspects of written language (Hammill & McNutt, 1981). Writing is a highly complex, interactive process that builds on pre-existing cognitive and linguistic structures. It is the final and most formal aspect of language that has to be learned. Writing disorders can be understood only within a multiple framework encompassing knowledge of what the writer must bring to the task (i.e., underlying cognitive and linguistic abilities) and knowledge of the nature of the writing task itself.

There are two major categories of problems associated with writing disorders: (a) those due to deficits in underlying cognitive or linguistic processes required for writing and (b) those due to the nature of the complex components inherent in writing activities and their interaction with underlying abilities. Written language facility involves a number of component skills including handwriting, spelling, punctuation, capitalization, vocabulary, syntax, and the formulation and organization of ideas. Typically, students with learning disabilities have difficulty in more than one aspect of written language. Therefore, it is important to understand the development of these component skills and their relationship to proficiency in written language.

Acquisition of Written Language Skills.   The abilities to read and write follow developmentally the abilities to listen and speak. Myklebust (1965, 1978) described the hierarchical process of language acquisition as developing through auditory receptive, auditory expressive, visual receptive, and visual expressive forms. He maintained that the development of abilities in the language hierarchy relies on the initial intactness of the oral language capacity. If there are significant verbal language problems, then all capacities above this level will be affected. The many cognitive and linguistic abilities outlined earlier underlie basic oral language capacities. Therefore, those aspects of functioning that affect the verbal language system will also affect writing performance.

However, the ability to write requires an additional kind of analysis beyond that required for verbal language. Writing is a form of representation that is further from the reality it represents than is spoken language. Vygotsky (1962) referred to writing as a "second order symbol system." Writing does not represent experience directly but represents a previously acquired linguistic code, a system of arbitrary signs, by means of a new system. Vygotsky concluded that writing is highly abstract compared with the immediacy of spoken language. Although written language is similar to verbal language in thought and imagery, its structure and mode of functioning differ.

Because of the complexity of writing, underlying processing capacities of attention and memory as well as higher levels of cognitive functioning need to be adapted and used in unique ways. For example, children must acquire the linguistic awareness that enables them to use effectively the syntactic and semantic aspects of language in writing. A writing task demands an awareness and control of linguistic processes that are different by nature and medium from speech. The conventions of writing have their own discourse rules that demand more formal use of complete syntactic conventions, such as connectives and embedded clauses, than those required for speech. There is also a demand for more cohesiveness, less redundancy, and fewer examples or illustrations.

Children need to develop metacognitive skills so that they are capable of monitoring their own production, evaluating what they are writing in light of their purpose, taking perspective into account, and using an expanded knowledge base. Finally, they need to develop a concept of text, an understanding of the way that coherence or unity is achieved in written language. Children need to acquire the concept of a story (as well as of other genres) that they will bring to the writing task. It is this concept of text structure that appears to support organization and memory during the writing activity (Applebee, 1978; Englert & Raphael, 1988; Thomas, Englert, & Gregg, 1987).

Before they can write, children must be able to perform the motor act of writing and must have attained a level of proficiency in spelling. Handwriting is a graphomotor skill and is primarily dependent upon visual-perceptual ability, visual memory, and eye-hand coordination. Johnson and Myklebust (1967) termed the inability to learn the appropriate motor behaviors for writing as **dysgraphia.** Severe deficits in handwriting may include the inability to maintain an appropriate pencil grasp. Less severe problems may result in handwriting that is poorly spaced, awkward, or immature. Handwriting difficulties may be only one manifestation of more generalized difficulties in the performance of motor activities (e.g., catching or throwing a ball, buttoning a coat, or following a pattern or sequence of movements).

Handwriting difficulties also may be affected by the rate of performance. In order for writing to be efficient, it must be performed at a rate appropriate for the task. Although a child's handwriting may appear adequate, it may have been produced slowly and with difficulty. Such problems result from a lack of automatic motor patterns for letter formation or from slowness in processing and organizing information for the writing task.

Another of the skills necessary for writing is the ability to recall the spelling of words. Cici (1980) outlined some of the underlying abilities necessary for children to learn to spell words. The abilities to articulate the word correctly, to recall the spoken pattern (i.e., the auditory sequence of the phonemes or syllables), and to recall the visual letter sequences are necessary for learning to spell. Also, children must be able to recall the motor pattern for writing a word and to execute the plan for the motor act. Because the complex nature of the writing task requires the simultaneous use of semantic, syntactic, and graphophonic information, trying to satisfy all of these constraints at one time makes writing difficult.

Disorders in Written Language.   Because the complexity of the writing task involves the integration of linguistic, cognitive, and motoric activities, writing presents a major problem for many students with learning disabilities. Lerner (1981) suggested that poor facility in expressing thoughts through written language is the most prevalent disorder in the acquisition of communication skills. Students who have responded well to remediation in spoken language or reading instruction during the elementary grades often continue to have difficulties with written expressive language. Among the learning disabled population, written language disorders often persist into adolescence and adulthood (Blalock, 1981; Isaacson, 1987; Johnson, Blalock, & Nesbitt, 1978; Moran, Schumaker, & Vetter, 1981).

Children with learning disabilities often continue to have spelling difficulties even after they have learned to read. Some adolescents who exhibit severe spelling deficits may also show subtle verbal language deficits, including problems in word retrieval and phonological segmentation ability (Gerber, 1984, 1986).

Wiig and Semel (1976) reported that in writing tasks, students with learning disabilities frequently omit words, confuse word order, use incorrect verbs and pronouns, use incorrect word endings, and leave out punctuation. They also indicated that, at the syntactic level, children with learning disabilities frequently produce agrammatical sentences in which elements of several transformations are combined or reversed. Learning disabled children have been found to score significantly lower on indices of syntax, vocabulary, and ideation when their writing samples are compared with those of nondisabled peers (Blair & Crump, 1984; Gregg, 1983; Myklebust, 1973; Norris & Crump, 1982). Research documents the organizational deficiencies of learning disabled students in story narrative writing skills and in generating expository compositions (Nodine, Barenbaum, & Newcomer, 1985; Thomas et al., 1987). Typically, individuals with learning disabilities approach both narrative and informational writing as an associative or linear process in which any separate idea associatively stimulates subsequent unrelated ideas. These students show no awareness or use of an overall organizational plan that restricts the generation of ideas or that ties each idea back to a major proposition or theme (Englert & Thomas, 1987). Students with learning disabilities also show significant mechanical writing skills deficits on measures of spelling, grammatical correctness, capitalization, and punctuation. In addition, their written language performance on these factors becomes more discrepant as grade level increases (Gerber, 1984; Poplin, Gray, Larsen, Banikowski, & Mehring, 1980).

Although reading and writing make different demands on underlying linguistic and cognitive capabilities, the skills needed for conveying meaning in writing are clearly interrelated with the skills necessary for extracting meaning from reading. For example, as already indicated, the reading and writing performance of students with learning disabilities suggests that they approach both tasks without sensitivity to the overall organizational pattern of the text (e.g., story schema or expository text structure type). They therefore fail to recognize the organizational pattern in written materials and neglect to use it to construct meaning while reading or writing. Because these students do not link the ideas in text into groupings of related ideas, they recall or they generate only isolated pieces of information (Raphael & Englert, 1990; Seidenberg, 1989). The interrelated, reciprocal relationship inherent in reading and writing activities and the positive influence of this relationship on the development of both processes cannot be overemphasized. It assumes special significance in our understanding of the nature of the learning disabilities associated with written language.

Assessment of Learning Disabilities

The measurement of a student's psychoeducational abilities and skills has historically been a major theme in the development and delivery of special education programs and services. Assessment, the collection and interpretation of relevant data, is a supporting activity for all subsequent decision-making activities. Before the need for a special education program or the instructional focus of the educational program can be determined for a student suspected of having a learning disability, a comprehensive functional assessment must be done.

Functional assessment and testing are not the same. Assessment involves far more than the administration of a group of tests. When we assess students, we have to consider the way they perform a variety of tasks in a variety of settings or contexts (e.g., the child with a short attention span for reading instruction but not for model plane building), the meaning of their performance in terms of their total functioning (e.g., the child's short attention span is directly related to the task demand—reading versus model plane building), and explanations for their performance (e.g., the nature of the reading instructional program may be inappropriate for the child's information-processing capacities). Assessment is always an evaluative, interpretive appraisal of performance that provides information to teachers and other school-based personnel, allowing them to make effective educational decisions for children.

Comprehensive Evaluation

A single set of indicators cannot be used to decide that a child is learning disabled because there are different causes for and, therefore, different types of learning disability. Therefore, a careful clinical description of the individual child is of primary importance in making an appropriate identification. Assessment of children suspected of having learning disabilities must be flexible and responsive to the individual differences exhibited by these children.

Because of the heterogeneity of the learning disabled population, the regulations of Public Law 94-142 mandate that a comprehensive evaluation be done by a multidisciplinary team. For the assessment of children suspected of having specific learning disabilities, the regulations (Section 12 la. 540) explicitly state that the team must be made up of

- A person knowledgeable in the area of the suspected disability
- The child's classroom teacher, or, if the child does not have a classroom teacher, a teacher qualified to teach the child
- At least one additional specialist such as a psychologist, a speech-language pathologist, or a remedial reading specialist, qualified to administer individual diagnostic assessments

Because of the interactive relationship between language disability and learning disability for many students, competent assessment requires a comprehensive evaluation that includes findings from both of these disciplines as well as from other disciplines (i.e., physician, psychologist, reading specialist, regular teacher, etc.). It is very important to the overall identification of specific learning disabilities that the team's assessment approach reflect a multidimensional model, taking into account factors ranging from the purposes of assessment to a broad-based conceptualization of the nature of learning.

The Assessment Model

Assessment is undertaken to determine if special education is warranted and, if so, to determine the nature of the student's special educational needs. To make these decisions, a systematic approach to the organization and interpretation of evaluation data must be used. Testing information must identify meaningful patterns of functioning and provide data that are relevant for learning.

An information-processing model is one of the most fruitful approaches to understanding learning disabilities. Such a model accommodates the major concerns and problems areas in learning, including the cognitive and linguistic processes necessary for the acquisition of academic skills. Also, aspects of information-processing theory serve as the foundation for an important component of intervention that must address and integrate both the process-oriented data (e.g., cognitive, linguistic) and the content-oriented data (e.g., component skills needed for acquisition of reading and writing).

There is always a potential for bias in assessment, and it can affect both the descriptive and programmatic phases of assessment. Diverse professionals involved in the assessment process are generally influenced by the knowledge base in their respective disciplines and look for what they understand to be important aspects of learning and behavior. The adoption of a comprehensive assessment model can clarify the interrelationships among disciplines and improve current practice in evaluating and developing programming for the student with a learning disability.

The translation of a comprehensive assessment model into strategies for obtaining information relevant for identification and educational planning places considerable demands upon the multidisciplinary team. It requires that team members have a strong foundation of knowledge pertaining to both the process-oriented and the content-oriented aspects, and skills in translating these factors into specific assessment techniques. Team decision making requires that members have a sound knowledge base, the ability to recognize interactive patterns, and a firm understanding of how a particular testing paradigm affects the interpretation of test results. The assessment of learning disabilities, therefore, must have a sound theoretical base, and the team members must be informed specialists who have kept up with current research in their own and related fields.

Assessment for Identification

Until we refine our understanding of what constitutes a learning disability, the decision to classify a child as learning disabled is made on the basis of a discrepancy between expected and attained achievement and by the progressive exclusion of other causes for the learning deficits. The professional expertise of the multidisciplinary team is of critical importance, and the basis for making the decision must be carefully documented. Assessment to determine eligibility for special education obtains objective descriptions of a child's cognitive, linguistic, and social/emotional status as well as descriptions of educational performance.

In general, formal tests—tests that are norm-referenced or standardized—are used extensively for screening and identification purposes. A child suspected of having learning disabilities should be measured in each of the domains (cognitive, linguistic, and social/emotional). Although the cognitive domain can be defined in many different ways, in practice it almost always refers to the measurement of intelligence, The Wechsler Intelligence Scale for Children—Revised (WISC—R) (Wechsler, 1974) is used most often and is related to and predictive of academic success. With the learning disabled child, the intelligence test is used to establish that the child is functioning intellectually within the normal range. Data from the test can also provide information on the underlying abilities that constitute intelligence. Extensive scatter or unevenness within the profile of cognitive abilities may provide insight into the child's information-processing abilities. Skilled clinical analysis of the data can provide information that can be useful in the development of an intervention program.

As is the case of cognitive assessment, formal measurement in the social/emotional domain is used to provide identification information and to rule out severe emotional disturbances as the primary cause of the learning deficits. A language assessment determines whether the child has difficulties in processing linguistically encoded information. Many children with learning disabilities have language problems that impact directly on their academic learning.

Formal measures of academic achievement are used to provide information on the difference between actual achievement and estimated potential in order to implement the identification procedures outlined in the federal rules and regulations. For the most part, the learning disabilities classification has not been operationally defined and still remains largely a matter of clinical judgment, underscoring the importance of team decision making.

Assessment for Instructional Programming

The Individualized Education Program.   In order to ensure that a child with a disability receives appropriate services that are based on planned educational goals and activities determined by the child's parents and school-based personnel, an individual Education Program (IEP) is included as a key component of Public Law 94-142. The team decision-making process described earlier is an important component of the law and is also built into the IEP process.

The specific demands of the IEP require that collected data be organized and analyzed systematically. Therefore, it is important that information be collected methodically, organized in an interpretable way, and analyzed for instructional implications. The formal tests that are administered for identification represent only the starting point in the IEP process and generally will be useful only for the most basic aspects of instructional planning. Informal assessment procedures are often the necessary bridge between formal procedures and the instructional program. Data derived from informal measures can be readily used in the construction of the IEP.

Formal measures have serious limitations in terms of generating data to explain underlying systems or in providing directly relevant intervention alternatives. Informal measures are often more descriptive and relevant to the individual and are useful in educational planning for children with learning disabilities, where an understanding of individual differences is critical to effective intervention. Informal assessment approaches assess behavior in more natural contexts (i.e., classroom observations) and in the specific curriculum content of the classroom (e.g., criterion-referenced tests, teacher-made tests, etc.). Informal assessment, which generates both qualitative and quantitative data, corresponds more closely to actual behavior. The data and conclusions are specific, representative, and relevant. Informal assessment data can be directly translated into an intervention program more closely tied to meaningful goals, strategies, and activities based on the content of the regular curriculum, the context of the classroom, and the performance patterns of the child.

Quantitative and Qualitative Data.   Although formal measures are used primarily to provide identification information rather than instructional programming information, both quantitative and qualitative data can result from the administration of a formal test. **Quantitative data** refers to the actual scores achieved on the test. Examples of quantitative data are statements such as "James scored at the 83 percentile on the Comprehension subtest of the Stanford Diagnostic Reading Test" or "Robin earned a scaled score of 12 on the Picture Completion subtest of the Wechsler Intelligence Scale for Children—Revised."

Qualitative data consists of (a) observations made while a child is being tested (e.g., child's response characteristics such as frustration tolerance, self-directive behavior, and risk-taking) and (b) systematic analysis of the child's performance in order to understand *how* the child achieved the score (e.g., item analysis). In assessment, the nature of the child's errors is often more important than knowing the child's score. For example, on the measure of reading comprehension ability, James may have performed best on factual questions while demonstrating a weakness in the ability to respond to questions requiring inferential reasoning. And, although Robin was able to score in the above-average range on the Picture Completion subtest of the WISC—R, some of her word choices indicated word-retrieval difficulties: She pointed to the "nostril" and said "ear," substituted "the things you pull on" for "knobs," and said, "the thing over here on the door" for "hinge" and so on. When tests are used in assessment, the score earned by a child is often the *least* relevant piece of information for instructional planning.

Capacity versus Strategy Deficits.   In clinical assessment, a distinction should always be made between underlying abilities and performance. Performance on a task involves the availability of four aspects of cognitive functioning: (a) underlying abilities (i.e., perception, attention, memory), (b) acquired knowledge (i.e., language skills, knowledge of the world in general based on past experience), (c) strategies (i.e., activities undertaken to achieve specific objectives), and (d) metacognition (i.e., awareness of one's own thought processes and the executive functions necessary to regulate the use of basic abilities, knowledge, and strategies).

The purpose of assessment is to measure not only acquired knowledge and how it is used, but also what the child is capable of learning. A child may have the underlying abilities but not an appropriate strategy for effectively acquiring, accessing, or applying knowledge. For example, a child with a learning disability may have the underlying ability or capacity to store verbal information in short-term memory but may not have an effective verbal rehearsal or category clustering strategy for coding the information for storage and retrieval. On the other hand, word-retrieval difficulties may be implicated in short-term memory deficits, in that the child may not have readily accessible high-quality verbal memory codes to represent information in short-term memory. Some children who have learning disabilities appear to have poorer access to a phonetic code or access to a degraded phonetic representation on memory span tasks (Shankweiler et al., 1979). Similarly, reduced language performance does not always indicate that a child does not have adequate knowledge of the linguistic system. Knowledge of the language system may be intact, and reduced language the result of memory processing constraints or situational constraints (Ervin-Tripp, 1971; Slobin, 1971). Performance characteristics in response to specific tasks do not always clearly reflect specific underlying systems; therefore, data available from testing alone cannot always be taken as evidence of underlying ability and/or knowledge deficits.

Assessment that focuses on quantitative data deals only with the products of underlying systems (e.g., the observable responses). Such assessment is more restrictive in determining educational goals than assessment that also measures the patterns of functioning that reflect underlying systems. Patterns of performance that more fully describe the nature of the individual's difficulties are important aspects of a comprehensive assessment and guide the development of effective educational goals and strategies.

Planning Assessment for Intervention.   For planning educational interventions, two levels of assessment must be considered and, integrated: the content-oriented level and the process-oriented level. At the level of content, assessment must determine what academic abilities or skills the child has already learned and what aspects still remain to be learned. The second level of assessment relates to *how* academic skills are learned, the underlying cognitive or linguistic processes relevant to the acquisition of academic skills. Information obtained from such a broadened perspective may not indicate which specific areas require intervention, but it provides considerable insight into patterns of performance, the child's readiness for structured intervention in academic areas, and appropriate strategies for either intervention or compensatory techniques.

In order to integrate the content-oriented and process-oriented approaches, the assessment process must be based on identification of the component skills that underlie performance of a specific academic task (e.g., reading, writing, etc.) and the subsequent development of specific procedures to assess the prerequisite skills and underlying processes required to learn these component skills. For the assessment of specific reading disability, the reading battery should be based on knowledge of the reading acquisition process (e.g., knowledge of letter-sound correspondences, automatization of word recognition skills, comprehension skills, etc.); the cognitive battery should be based on an analysis of the cognitive and metacognitive processes relevant to learning to read (e.g., short-term verbal memory, phonemic segmentation ability, etc.); and the language battery should be based on an analysis of the language acquisition process relevant to the acquisition of reading skills (e.g., understanding sentences and paragraphs, morphophonemic processing, etc.). With this data, the team members can make relevant decisions concerning the *why, what,* and *how* of intervention. The summary of a case history included later in this chapter illustrates how members of an evaluation team can integrate assessment data to make relevant decisions about the educational needs of a student who is language learning disabled.

Because a more complex picture of learning problems has emerged based on linguistic science and information-processing models of learning, assessment of a learning disabled child requires a multifaceted approach. An effective, interactive team approach to assessment provides the initial foundation for determining the need and nature of an intervention program.

The Intervention Program

Intervention, as well as assessment, requires a multidimensional approach. Decisions to intervene must be made jointly, and interventions must be well planned, integrated, and carefully monitored. The specialists and regular classroom teachers who work with children who have learning disabilities will, to a great extent, be faced with a series of individual problems, and the goal will be to capitalize on the strengths and minimize the limitations of the individual in the interactive learning environment. Learning disabilities are usually identified after children enter school and encounter academic failure. Intervention procedures must take into account the continuing educational demands upon the child despite cognitive and/or linguistic deficits. In addition to providing specialized instruction, the specialists working with the child, in collaboration with the regular teacher, must develop procedures that will ameliorate some of the child's problems by modifying the failure-producing aspects of the regular classroom learning environments (e.g., language of the classroom and task demands of the curriculum).

Also, it is important to maximize intervention efforts by integrating planning and implementation across disciplines. Intervention should be an integrated, comprehensive set of activities involving systematic ongoing implementation and evaluation. Specialized content and procedures, including remedial techniques, should be reconceptualized to focus on intervention both within a specific discipline and across disciplines. A generic understanding of intervention planning and implementation across disciplines helps to clarify the interrelationships among disciplines, expands the range of options available, and improves current practice in the delivery of specialized instruction for the learning disabled.

Some of the factors basic to all interventions include the following:

- *Content match.* The information and tasks must not be too different from the child's current knowledge base and way of understanding and learning.
- *Sequence.* Instruction must be sequentially ordered to correspond to the sequence of information needed by the child.
- *Pace.* Instruction must provide for practice, repetition, and overlearning of information that needs to be accessed automatically.
- *Structure.* Intervention components should be taught within and across disciplines and should correspond with the demands of the regular curriculum content.
- *Motivation.* Interventions need to accommodate interests, attitudes, and learning style. Activities that are reinforced will be continued, and immediate feedback will support the maintenance of attention.

The Transdisciplinary Approach.   Practitioners should have a comprehensive and generic understanding of intervention planning and implementation across disciplines. This understanding requires a sound grounding in the fundamentals and interrelationships of the diverse disciplines involved in the diagnostic-instructional process. Educational interventions undertaken on behalf of the learning disabled are often arbitrary and fragmented. We are only beginning to understand the developmental and behavioral characteristics of individuals with learning disabilities. Potential interventions based on linguistic science and information-processing models of learning are emerging. They strongly suggest the need for a holistic, integrated, transdisciplinary approach to educational planning. The complex interactive nature of cognitive and linguistic processes and academic learning indicates the need for a broad-based, multidimensional approach to the development of an educational program for the learning disabled child. This approach should focus on the commonalities in intervention efforts and the interrelatedness of instructional goals and objectives across diverse disciplines.

With specific reference to the student who has a language learning disability, the interactive nature of underlying information-processing abilities and academic learning has specific implications for the development of interrelated educational goals, objectives, and activities. Integration of instruction across diverse disciplines can enhance both the compensatory and remedial aspects of instruction for the student with a language learning disability.

Compensatory aspects of instruction can be addressed by the language specialist, who can make recommendations for modifications in both the style and structure of the language of the classroom. There are aspects of language processing that are applicable to the educational management of the child whose processing abilities have not developed optimally. Instructional personnel could be guided to simplify the language of instruction by using shorter, less complex sentences and by making longer pauses and more frequent restatements of information. Knowledge of more specific aspects of language processing is also important. As an example, instructional personnel should be aware that formulating oral or written instructions or directions in the affirmative, whenever possible, rather than in the negative will reduce language-processing difficulties. Also, because implicit negatives such as *different* (i.e., not the same), *absent* (i.e., not present), and *except* (i.e., not all) are processed in the same way as explicit negatives, these will be equally difficult for some children.

Similarly, the integration of remedial aspects of instruction can increase the impact of educational planning for the student with a language learning disability. An assessment model that identifies the interactive cognitive and/or linguistic correlates of reading skill acquisition at both the initial and transitional stages of reading instruction has implications for the integration of instruction. For example, at the initial stages of reading instruction, phonemic segmentation skills are critical in learning to use phonic cues (i.e., to make use of letter-sound correspondences) to help in identifying the words represented by a sequence of letters. Many children with learning disabilities have trouble learning to use phonic cues because they do not recognize that words can be segmented into syllables and syllables into distinct phonemes, and that phonemic segmentation is represented graphically by the use of specific letters placed in sequence. Assessment and subsequent remedial training of phonemic segmentation skills could be jointly undertaken by both the language and learning disabilities specialists. Also, modifications in the method of teaching initial reading need to be made for the child with poor segmentation skills. An instructional procedure that places less initial emphasis on phonic skills (e.g., a word-family or structural analysis approach) should be used for the teaching of word recognition skills.

Also, many elements of whole-language instruction should be considered for use with students with learning disabilities. This instructional approach derives from the belief that children can acquire spoken literacy in much the same way that they acquire language and emphasizes the wholeness of reading and writing. Because whole-language practices include daily writing and the reading of authentic literature (e.g., trade books), this emphasis on the inherent reciprocity and interdependence of reading and writing maximizes learning of literacy skills for students. However, explicitly instruction that promotes facility in word recognition is vitally important for efficient reading, especially for beginning readers who are likely to be at risk for reading failure (Mather, 1992; Pressley & Rankin, 1994; Stanovich, 1991; Vellutino & Scanlon, 1991). Therefore, current research appears to support a balanced approach to initial reading instruction (Vellutino, 1991; Pressley, Rankin, Gaskins, Brown, & El-Dinary, 1995; Sawyer, 1991). For students who have difficulty in making progress primarily though immersion in a language-rich environment, explicit code-based instruction should be integrated with the reading of whole authentic texts and student journal writing. The assimilation of skill instruction into a meaningful classroom enables children to learn that the ultimate goal of all reading instruction is to enhance their ability to derive meaning from text.

Similar interrelated educational goals and activities can be identified at the transitional stage of reading acquisition. The syntactic language problems evidenced by a student with a language learning disability will also be reflected in various reading behaviors such as understanding syntactically complex sentences or using syntactic constraints to assist in word identification. Remedial training to intensify awareness of the syntactic structure of complex sentences by manipulating clausal units would be a valid transdisciplinary activity that could be integrated into language, reading, and writing instruction. For example, the learning disabled student's linguistic skills and linguistic awareness can be improved by training in sentence expansion and in sentence combining and/or sentence decombining exercises (Norris & Crump, 1982; Seidenberg, 1982; Wallach & Wallach, 1976).

Because the semantic processing problems of many students with language learning disabilities also affect reading comprehension and content learning, an integrated instructional approach focusing on the structure and process of semantic memory can ameliorate some of their learning problems. Transdisciplinary training in the use of more effective word elaboration strategies (e.g., classifying and categorizing) as well as in the use of strategies for analyzing semantic features of concepts, such as semantic mapping or webbing (e.g., explicating the relationships among superordinate, coordinate, and subordinate concepts), can enhance both content learning and text comprehension (Anders & Bos, 1986; Bos, Anders, Filip, & Jaffe, 1989; Mastropieri et al., 1987).

Additionally, it is important that practitioners develop comprehensive intervention programs that incorporate instructional sequences that explicitly teach critical metacognitive strategies to students with learning disabilities (Seidenberg, 1991). Currently, strategy deficit models of learning disabilities are the most prevalent theoretical orientation shaping both intervention research and practice for this population (Scruggs, 1991). As indicated earlier, a considerable body of literature supports the notion that many children with learning disabilities; are inactive learners who fail to spontaneously access or use effective cognitive strategies for solving academic problems. These students tend not to believe in their own efforts or abilities and have an inadequate understanding of the cognitive strategies available for successful performance on academic tasks (Borkowski, Weyhing, & Carr, 1988; Torgesen, 1986). Therefore, students with learning disabilities frequently require direct instruction in those strategic processing skills that nonlearning disabled students acquire and apply automatically (Harris, 1990; Harris & Pressley, 1991).

Also, interventions derived from an information-processing perspective emphasize specific instruction and practice on component reading and writing skills in contrast to practice in general language or problem-solving skills in a context outside of reading and writing tasks. Information-processing research supports the context-bound nature of strategic processing skills for many academic tasks (Paris & Oka, 1989; Siegler, 1983; Stanovich, 1986; Vellutino, 1979). There is evidence that training students with learning disabilities to use task-specific cognitive strategies improves their performance particularly on complex reading and writing tasks that have high information-processing demands (Swanson, 1991).

Students with learning disabilities who have been taught metacognitive strategies have shown improved performance in a variety of tasks, including the self-monitoring of on-task behavior (Kneedler & Hallahan, 1981), the detection of contextual inconsistencies (Capelli & Markman, 1982), comprehension monitoring (Wong & Jones, 1982; Palincsar & Brown, 1986), improvement of spelling ability (Gerber, 1986; Wong, 1986), and awareness and use of text organization for improved comprehension and composing skills (Englert, Raphael, Anderson, Gregg, & Anthony, 1989; Englert & Raphael, 1988; Grahm & Harris, 1988; Welch, 1992; Wong & Wilson, 1984).

The instructional principles derived from the intervention research highlight the importance of interactive dialogues and the modeling of strategic activities as well as the scaffolding of instruction around domain-specific content knowledge and strategic knowledge (e.g., the associated task-specific cognitive strategies). Effective instructional interventions for complex academic tasks share a number of features, including:

1. Heightening the learner's awareness of the demands of a task
2. Instructing the learner in the appropriate strategies to facilitate successful task completion
3. Explicit modeling of the use of the strategies
4. Providing guided practice and feedback regarding the application of the strategies
5. Providing instruction for generalized use of the strategies

Table 11-1 provides an example of an instructional sequence for teaching the strategic processing skills needed for successful performance of a complex academic task. Interventions based on an information-processing perspective that directly address students' academic deficits and incorporate an instructional technology focusing on the interactive nature of the teaching-learning process appear to hold the most promise for enabling students with learning disabilities to become more successful learners.

Therefore, practitioners need to enlarge the scope of their instructional practices by gaining a better understanding of the role that metacognitive factors play in the learning needs of the learning disabled population. At the same time practitioners must integrate

TABLE 11-1 Teaching a Cognitive Strategy for a Complex Academic Task

Step 1:   *Introduction of Strategy and Performance Review*
The teacher explains the strategy, and students and teacher review the students' current level of performance (e.g., pretest outcomes).

Step 2:   *Relevance of the Strategy*
The teacher explains why the strategy should be learned, and students and teacher generate examples of strategy application.

Step 3:   *Strategy Description*
The teacher describes how to use the strategy and provides the students with a "helpsheet" listing the steps.

Step 4:   *Modeling the Strategy*
The teacher models the use of the strategy, demonstrating aloud the thinking process underlying the separate steps. As a group, the teacher and students model and rehearse the use of the strategy.

Step 5:   *When to Use the Strategy*
The teacher explains the conditions for use of the strategy.

Step 6:   *Practice in Controlled Material*
The students apply the strategy to controlled practice material while the teacher provides prompts and corrective feedback as necessary.

Step 7:   *Evaluation of Strategy Use*
The teacher shows student a method for evaluating the use of the strategy.

Step 8:   *Strategy Generalization*
The students apply the strategy to complete assignments required in regular content area classrooms.

From: P. L. Seidenberg, Cognitive and academic instructional intervention for learning disabled adolescents, *Topics in Language Disorders,* 8, No. 3, p. 65, reprinted with permission of Aspen Publishers, Inc. © 1988.

their efforts in order to maximize the impact of the intervention program and to avoid unnecessary confusion for students with learning disabilities. The learning activities provided in different settings must be coordinated so that the student perceives an organized, connected pattern of related activities.

The need to integrate intervention efforts underlies the mandate of Public Law 94-142. Educators need to assume new collaborative roles and responsibilities to meet this challenge and to fulfill the promise of meeting the special educational needs of students with learning disabilities.

Case Study

The following summary of a case history for Robert, a first grader, illustrates how members of a multidisciplinary team identify a child as learning disabled. The screening team, comprised of professionals from diverse disciplines, meets at the time of initial referral and, based on the nature of the referral information, develops a plan to guide the assessment process. Wherever possible, they see the child jointly in order to avoid miscommunication based on different disciplinary outlooks. The professionals (school psychologist, learning disability specialist, language specialist, etc.) involved in the evaluation process discuss their findings, and the final report reflects the conclusions of each team member.

Identification Information

Name: Robert G.	Birthdate: July 10, 1988
Age: 6 yrs. 6 mos.	School Placement: Windmere Elementary School
Grade: First	Date of Report: January 15, 1995

Reason for Referral

At the request of his classroom teacher and with the written consent of his parents, Robert was referred for a psychoeducational evaluation. Robert is reported to be having difficulty learning to read and write. The teacher reports that he exhibits written reversals, transposition of letters, and poor phonic decoding skills. The teacher also states that Robert's difficulties appear to be associated with distractibility, confusions in directionality and sequencing, and poor ability to process auditory information. An evaluation is being done to better understand Robert's current functional ability and to assist in educational planning.

Summary of Behavioral Observations

Robert is a sturdy, well-built youngster. He appears active and alert and was not overly apprehensive during the initial testing session. Robert speaks in well-organized sentences that are logical and easy to follow, and his vocabulary appears to be within normal limits. He exhibits some articulation difficulties. Robert was able to work steadily and persistently on many of the tasks presented. However, there were also tasks on which he performed poorly or was completely unable to perform, and restlessness and increased distractibility were observable at these times.

Summary of Background Information
Birth and developmental milestones for Robert are described as "normal." Robert's health history indicates hospitalization for a myringotomy just prior to school entrance. He also experiences an allergic reaction to milk and milk products. He still has a recurrent hearing problem, and his most recent audiological examination again detected fluid in the middle ear. This may account, in part, for his articulation problems.

Summary of Assessment Procedures
Tests administered include:

1. *Wechsler Intelligence Scale for Children—Revised* (WISC—III)
   Verbal IQ   115
   Performance IQ   105
   Full Scale IQ   112

   Verbal Scaled Score
   Information   10
   Similarities   15
   Arithmetic   11
   Vocabulary   14
   Comprehension   13
   (Digit Span)   (9)

   Performance Scaled Score
   Picture Completion   13
   Picture Arrangement   9
   Block Design   9
   Object Assembly   15
   Coding   8
2. *Bender Visual-Motor Gestalt Test* (Initial and Recall)
3. *Human Figure Drawing*
4. *Wepman Auditory Discrimination Test*
5. *Clinical Evaluation of Language Functions* (CELF-R)
   Recalling Sentences
   Formulating Sentences
   Semantic Relationships
   Oral Directions
6. *Key Math Diagnostic Arithmetic Test*
7. *Metropolitan Reading Test—Level II* (Form P)
   Beginning Consonants
   Sound-letter Correspondence
   Visual Matching
   Listening

In addition to the formal test, Robert was asked to copy numbers, letters, and words. He also completed a trial reading lesson using a language-experience approach. He dictated a brief story and then was asked to read his story to the examiner. Robert also identified a word in his own story that he wanted to learn to read and write. A multisensory approach was used successfully to teach word recognition and spelling skills.

Summary of Test Results

Robert's scores on the WISC III indicate that he is functioning intellectually in the high average range. However, there are variations in the subtest scores ranging from below average to superior.

Robert's fund of information was average, with failures on comparatively easy items and successes on more difficult ones. Verbal fluency appeared to interfere with performance on this task, and he would comment, "I know the name but I forget," or "I can't think of the name of it." At the same time, expressive vocabulary was in the superior range, and he was able to make excellent responses when he was not limited to retrieving a specific word from memory but could make semantic substitutions.

Abstract verbal reasoning (similarities) and judgment, common sense, and reality testing (comprehension) were all in the high average range. The quality of his responses indicated good ability to make abstractions and understand superordinate classification. His ability to do in-the-head arithmetic was above average, and his lowest score was on the Digit Span subtest, which was below average. He was able to repeat up to five digits forward but was unable to repeat more than two digits backward without reversing the order of presentation.

On the performance tasks, Robert's highest score (very superior on Object Assembly) reflected an ability to organize and work toward a concrete goal. His visual memory, necessary for recognition of essential details, was also above average. On the remaining tasks, such as replicating designs of blocks and sequencing a series of pictures in a logical order, he scored below average. His lowest score was for the transposition of symbols within a time limit (Coding) and was in the defective range. Robert appears to have visual-motor coordination difficulties. He is also experiencing problems with more integrative visual skills, such as sequencing, directionality, and perception of spatially defined complex stimuli (e.g., block designs). On the other hand, Robert's figure drawing was age appropriate and indicated the ability to integrate and organize the spatial details.

Robert's performance on the Bender-Gestalt, an assessment of his own response to his perceptual organization of visual information, also indicated difficulty in integration of details and organization of spatially defined stimuli. Problems with integrative skills were evidenced in his loss of angulation and difficulties in maintaining the overall structure of shapes. He has difficulty in reproducing details and in storing visual information. His visual memory for designs indicates that he was able to recall only two of the Bender designs after the initial copying task. Also, there is evidence of slowness of response to graphomotor tasks, not only on the Coding subtest of the WISC–R but also in his handwriting.

Robert's performance on a number of formal and informal language-processing measures showed an inconsistent response pattern similar to his intelligence test profile. Informal observation of his language skills indicated that he is able to understand everyday conversation and to express is ideas in age-appropriate syntax. On the Wepman Auditory Discrimination Test, Robert was able to differentiate the phonemic likenesses and differences in word pairs. However, he has articulation difficulties that appear to be persistent and systematic. Further assessment is indicated in this area. On the recalling sentences subtest of the Clinical Evaluation of Language Function (CELF–R), Robert performed well above age expectancy (fifth-grade level). However, on the sentence formulation test of the CELF–R Robert performed at only the beginning first-grade level. He performed well above age expectancy on the sentence repetition task fifth-grade level) but at only the beginning first-grade level for a task requiring the formulation of sentences (e.g., "Make a sentence with the word *car*"). His performance was age appropriate for a task tapping his understanding of semantic relationships. However, he had difficulty in retaining a series of oral directions in short-term memory and executing them. Robert attempted to use verbal rehearsal strategy to facilitate recall, but because his phonological reproduction and verbal fluency are faulty, rehearsal is also impaired.

Robert's performance on the Metropolitan Readiness subtests was slightly better for a task requiring the matching of beginning sounds (60th percentile) than it was for the other subtests administered (50th percentile). In making sound-letter correspondences, both initial consonant and consonant blend inaccuracies were noted. He was not able to match the letters *c, g, d, pl, tr, gr,* and *cl* to their phonemic counterparts in words (*cat, goat,* etc.). However, on the visual matching subtest, Robert was able to match all of the letter sequences accurately and encountered difficulty only with the letterlike shapes or designs. His performance on the listening subtest indicates good ability to integrate and draw inferences when information is presented orally but poor comprehension of comparative relationships (*taller, bigger,* etc.).

On the Key Math Diagnostic Test, Robert scored at an overall grade equivalent of 1.5. His understanding of the number system was at a 2.5 grade level, and his numerical reasoning and ability to solve simple one-step story problems was at a 2.0 grade level. His ability to perform written, single-digit addition and subtraction computations was at a 1.6 grade level. He had difficulty with money problems (e.g., coin values), but he can recognize and apply common units of measurement (e.g., ruler, thermometer) and units of time (e.g., clock, calendar). Robert was able to write the numbers from 1 to 10, but there were still some directional confusions noted (e.g., 6, 9, and 10) that are not inappropriate for a beginning first-grader. Although his graphomotor responses are slow and labored, he can copy letters and numbers accurately.

Summary of Conclusions
Robert appears to be a child of above-average intelligence with indications for better potential. He would be expected to function in academic areas at or above his grade placement. At this time, he is impeded academically by specific learning deficits in oral language, reading, and writing. His uneven performance patterns indicate that he is experiencing difficulties in those areas involving expressive language abilities (e.g., speech production, verbal fluency, and sentence formulation), auditory and visual sequential

memory, spatial concepts, and visual-motor integration. He also exhibits fatigue and distractibility, especially when tasks are hard or frustrating. His arithmetic concepts and ability to do in-the-head arithmetic are excellent, but he is not doing as well as most of the other children in his grade in the acquisition of reading and writing skills. The evaluation data indicate that Robert will not acquire reading and writing skills consistent with expectations without special education and related services, and, therefore, the classification of *learning disabled* is indicated.

Summary of Recommendations
Robert's oral expressive language deficits are implicated in his learning difficulties and indicate the need for further assessment by the speech-language pathologist. In-depth testing of Robert's receptive and expressive language skills is recommended, including a phonological, semantic, syntactic, and pragmatic analysis of a language sample. The content of an appropriate language intervention program for Robert will depend on the results of the language assessment.

A traditional synthetic phonics approach to initial reading instruction would not be appropriate for Robert at this time. Although he uses immediate rehearsal to recreate a discrete phoneme (sound), the phonological reproduction is inaccurate, resulting in impaired or inconsistent recall of phonemes and phonemic patterns. In order to utilize his cognitive and linguistic strengths, a language-experience approach, in which he dictates and then reads his own stories, could be used as an effective approach to initial reading instruction. He would also profit from a more integrative approach for the acquisition of word analysis or decoding skills for word recognition and spelling. Any method that integrates the visual-tactile and auditory aspects (e.g., Fernald technique) for teaching word recognition and spelling, particularly if based on the words found in his own stories, could be used successfully with Robert at this time.

Robert has difficulty in attending to oral directions. He attempts to use verbal rehearsal to facilitate recall, but his reproductions are inconsistent and inaccurate, and interfere with his retrieval of the auditory information. It is important, therefore, that his teachers speak clearly, use short sentences with simple syntax, and check periodically on the accuracy of his recall of the information. Robert could be asked to repeat directions to be sure that he recalls them accurately

Robert uses a great deal of verbal mediation; that is, he talks himself through tasks. This is an excellent strategy for him and should be encouraged. For example, he could be taught to use verbal supports or associations to focus attention on relevant directional aspects of letters or numbers and, thus, guide his graphomotor responses.

Handwriting skills will need to be taught in carefully sequenced incremental steps, and particular attention will need to be paid to establishing the fine-motor patterns needed for writing, Also, lengthy tasks requiring graphomotor responses should be adjusted for Robert's current level of functioning (workbook exercises, copying from the chalkboard, etc.). He attempts to compensate cognitively for his visual-motor difficulties. He can be successful if given adequate structure and time.

As is typical of underachieving youngsters with excellent potential, Robert is beginning to experience confusion in reconciling the apparent conflict in feedback from the important adults in his life. That is, on the one hand, that he is a capable youngster; and, on the other, that he is having difficulties in learning. He is becoming extremely frustrated and unhappy because of his uneven functioning. Therefore, it is important that the educational program planned for Robert provide him with opportunities to use his cognitive and linguistic strengths and help him to compensate for his deficit areas.

Summary

That deficits in learning are a major cause of school failure is currently well accepted, and new approaches to identification and educational planning have developed that are based on information-processing theory. Learning disabilities derive from innate disorders that alter cognitive processes. These alterations in cognitive functioning vary in type and degree of severity and, therefore, in behavioral consequences.

An understanding of the interactive nature of language and cognition contributes to our understanding of the problems in comprehension and formulation of written language experienced by many children who have learning disabilities. Both reading and writing performance reflect the knowledge and the linguistic and cognitive competencies available to the learner and how these are activated and integrated during the acquisition of reading and writing skills. In addition to disorders in verbal language, a fundamental deficit for many children with learning disabilities appears to be an inability to use effective cognitive strategies for the comprehension or production of written language.

Because of the heterogeneity of the learning disabled population, the assessment process must be flexible and responsive to individual differences. Practitioners from diverse disciplines need to collaborate in decision-making activities. A multidisciplinary approach based on a comprehensive assessment model that provides for the systematic collection, organization, and analysis of assessment data needs to be adopted. The data must adequately describe the nature of an individual's difficulties and guide the development of an effective educational program. An interactive, collaborative, team approach to assessment and intervention also provides the foundation for the integration of learning experiences and educational services for children with learning disabilities.

Study Questions

1. Identify and discuss the major components of the information-processing model. Include in the discussion the implications for understanding the perceptual, attentional, and memory deficits of the student who is learning disabled.
2. Briefly present six characteristics that may be exhibited by learning disabled students with language deficits.
3. How does the interaction of linguistic and cognitive variables affect the acquisition of reading and writing skills?

4. Outline the research findings pertaining to cognitive and/or metacognitive deficits in relation to how students with learning disabilities acquire reading skills.

5. Briefly discuss several factors that may be related to writing disabilities. Discuss some writing behaviors exhibited by students with learning disabilities.

6. Discuss the advantages and disadvantages of formal and informal assessment in the identification of students with learning disabilities.

7. What are the important characteristics of an effective intervention program for the student who is learning disabled?

8. Describe and discuss the key components of intervention programs that incorporate instruction in metacognitive strategies.

References

American Psychiatric Association. (1994). *Diagnostic and statistical manual of mental disorders* (4th ed.). Washington, DC: Author.

Anders, P. L., & Bos, C. S. (1986). Semantic feature analysis: An interactive strategy for vocabulary development and text comprehension. *Journal of Reading, 29*, 610–616.

Anderson, B. R. (1975). *Cognitive psychology.* New York: Academic Press.

Anderson, R. C., Spiro, R. J., & Montague, W. D. (1977). *Schooling and the acquisition of knowledge.* Hillsdale, NJ: Lawrence Erlbaum Associates.

Applebee, A. (1978). *The child's concept of story.* Chicago: University of Chicago Press.

August, G. J. & Garfinkel, B. D. (1990). Comorbity of ADHD among clinic-referred children. *Journal of Abnormal Child Psychology, 18*, 29–45.

Baker, J. G., Ceci, S. J., & Hermann, D. (1987). Semantic structure and processing: Implications for the learning disabled child. In H. L. Swanson (Ed.), *Memory and learning disabilities: Advances in learning and behavioral disabilities.* Greenwich, CT: JAI Press.

Baker, L., & Cantwell, D. S. (1990). The association between emotional/behavior disorders and learning disorders with speech/language disorders. *Advances in Learning and Behavioral Disabilities, 6*, 26–46.

Barkley, R. A., Fischer, M., Edelbrock, C., & Smallish, L. (1990). The adolescent outcome of hyperactive children diagnosed by research criteria: An 8-year follow-up study. *Journal of the American Academy of Child and Adolescent Psychology, 29*, 546–557.

Bauer, R. H. (1977). Memory processes in children with learning disabilities. *Journal of Experimental Child Psychology, 18*, 283–296.

Beitchman, J. H., Hood, J., & Inglis, A. (1990). Psychiatric risk in children with speech and language disorders. *Journal of Abnormal Child Psychology, 18*, 283–296.

Berko, J. (1958). The child's learning of English morphology. *Word, 14*, 150–177.

Berry, M. F. (1980). *Teaching linguistically handicapped children.* Englewood Cliffs, NJ: Prentice Hall.

Biederman, J., Newcorn, J., & Sprich, S. (1991). Comorbidity of ADHD with conduct, depressive, anxiety, and other disorders. *American Journal of Psychiatry, 148*, 564–577.

Blackman, B. (1984). Language analysis skills and early reading acquisition. In G. Wallach & K. Buder (Eds.), *Language learning disabilities in school-age children.* Baltimore: Williams & Wilkins.

Blair, T. K., & Crump, W. D. (1984). Effects of discourse made on the syntactic complexity of learning disabled students' written expression. *Learning Disability Quarterly, 17*, 19–29.

Blalock, J. (1981). Persistent problems and concerns of young adults with learning disabilities. In W. Cruickshank & A. Silvers (Eds.), *Bridges to tomorrow: The best of ACDL* (Vol. 2). Syracuse, NY: Syracuse University Press.

Borkowski, J. G., Johnston, M. D., & Reid, M. (1987). Metacognition, motivation and controlled performance. In S. Ceci (Ed.), *Handbook of cognitive, social and neurological aspects of learning dis-*

abilities. Hillsdale, NJ: Lawrence Erlbaum Associates.

Borkowski, J. G., & Kurtz, B. E. (1987). Motivation and executive control. In J. G. Borkowski and J. D. Day (Eds.), *Cognition in special children.* Norwood, NJ: Ablex.

Borkowski, J. G., Weyhing, R. S., & Carr, M. (1988). Effects of attributional retraining on strategy-based reading comprehension in learning disabled students. *Journal of Educational Psychology, 75,* 544–552.

Bos, C., Anders, P. L., Filip, D., & Jaffe, L. E. (1989). The effects of an interactive instructional strategy for enhancing learning disabled students' reading comprehension and content area learning. *Journal of Learning Disabilities, 22,* 384–390.

Bos, C. S., & Filip, D. (1984). Comprehension monitoring in learning disabled and average students. *Journal of Learning Disabilities, 17,* 229–233.

Bougere, M. (1969). Selected factors in oral language related to first grade reading performance. *Reading Research Quarterly, 5,* 31–58.

Bransford, J. D., Stein, B. S., Shelton, T. S., & Owings, R. A. (1980). Cognition and adaptation: The importance of learning to learn. In J. Harvey (Ed.), *Cognition, social behavior and the environment.* Hillsdale, NJ: Lawrence Erlbaum Associates.

Brittain, M. A. (1970). Inflectional performance and early reading achievement. *Reading Research Quarterly, 6,* 34–48.

Brown, A. L. (1978). Knowing when, where and how to remember, a problem of metacognition. In R. Glaser (Ed.), *Advances in instructional psychology.* Hillsdale, NJ: Lawrence Erlbaum Associates.

Bryan, J. H. (1981). Social behaviors of learning disabled children. In J. Gottlieb & S. Strichart (Eds.), *Developmental theory and research in learning disabilities.* Baltimore: University Park Press.

Bryant, P., & Bradley, L. (1981). Visual memory and phonological skills in reading and spelling backwardness. *Psychological Research, 43,* 193–199.

Butkowsky, I. S., & Willows, D. M. (1980). Cognitive-motivational characteristics of children varying in reading ability: Evidence for learned helplessness in poor readers. *Journal of Educational Psychology, 72,* 408–422.

Campione, J. C., & Brown, A. L. (1978). Toward a theory of intelligence. *Intelligence, 2,* 279–304.

Cantwell, D. P., & Baker, L. (1991). Association between attention deficit hyperactivity disorders and learning disorders. *Journal of Learning Disabilities, 24,* 88–95.

Capelli, C. A., & Markman, E. M. (1982). Suggestions for training comprehension monitoring. *Topics in Learning and Learning Disorders, 2,* 87–96.

Catts, H. W. (1986). Speech production/phonological deficits in reading-disordered children. *Journal of Learning Disabilities, 19,* 504–508.

Catts, H. W. (1991). Early identification of dyslexia: Evidence of a follow-up study of speech-language impaired children. *Annals of Dyslexia, 41,* 143–157.

Catts, H. W., & Kamhi, A. G. (1986). The linguistic basis of reading disorders: Implications for the speech-language pathologist. *Language, Speech and Hearing Services in Schools, 17,* 329–341.

Cazden, C. B. (1972). *Child language and education.* New York: Holt, Rinehart & Winston.

Ceci, S. J. (1982). Extracting meaning from stimuli: Automatic and purposive processing of the language-based learning disabled. *Topics in Learning and Learning Disabilities, 2,* 46–53

Chalfont, J. C., & Scheffelin, M. A. (1969). *Central processing dysfunctions in children: A review of research* (NINDS Monograph No. 9). Bethesda, MD: U.S. Department of Health, Education and Welfare.

Chan, L. K. S., Cole, P. G., & Barfett, S. (1987). Comprehension monitoring: Detection and identification of text inconsistencies by LD and normal students. *Learning Disabilities Quarterly, 10,* 114–124.

Cici, R. (1980). Written language disorders. *Bulletin of the Orton Society, 30,* 240–251.

Cohen, N. J., Davine, M., & Meloche-Kelly, M. (1989). Prevalence of unsuspected language in child psychiatric population. *Journal of American Academy of Child and Adolescent Psychiatry, 28,* 107–111.

Cohen, R. (1982). Individual differences in short-term memory. *International Review of Research in Mental Retardation, 11,* 43–77.

Connolly, A., Nachtman, W., & Pritchett, E. (1971). *Key Math Diagnostic Arithmetic Test.* Circle Pines, MN: American Guidance Services.

Cruickshank, W., Bentzen, F., Razburg, F., & Tannhauser, M. (1961). *A teaching-method for brain-*

injured and hyperactive children. Syracuse, NY: Syracuse University Press.

Davila, R. R., Williams, M. L., & MacDonald, J. T. (1991). *Clarification of policy to address the needs of children with attention deficit disorders within general and special education.* Washington, DC: United States Department of Education.

Denckla, M. B., & Rudel, R. (1976). Naming of pictured objects by dyslexic and other learning-disabled children. *Brain and Language, 39,* 1–15.

Denner, F. (1970). Representational and syntactic competence of problem readers. *Child Development, 41,* 881–887.

Deshler, D. L., Schumaker, J. B., & Lenz, B. K. (1984). Academic and cognitive interventions for LD adolescents: Part I. *Journal of Learning Disabilities, 17,* 108–117.

Edwards, H. T., & Kallail, K. J. (1977, November). *Ability of learning disabled and regular classroom adolescents to close structure and content words.* Paper presented at the national convention of the American Speech and Hearing Association, Chicago.

Ellis, E. S., & Lenz, B. K. (1987). A component analysis of effective learning strategies for LD students. *Learning Disabilities Focus, 2,* 94–107.

Ellis, N. (1981). Visual and name coding in dyslexic children. *Psychological Research, 43,* 201–219.

Englert, C. S., & Raphael, T. E. (1988). Constructing well-formed prose: Process, structure and metacognitive knowledge. *Exceptional Children, 54,* 513–520.

Englert, C. S., Raphael, T. E., Anderson, L. M., Gregg, S. L., & Anthony, H. M. (1989). Exposition: Reading, writing and metacognitive knowledge of learning disabled students. *Learning Disabilities Research, 5,* 5–24.

Englert, C. S., & Thomas, C. C. (1987). Sensitivity to text structure in reading and writing: A comparison of learning disabled and nonhandicapped students. *Learning Disability Quarterly, 10,* 93–105.

Epstein, M. A., Shaywitz, S. E., Shaywitz, B. A., & Woolston, J. L. (1991). The boundaries of attention deficit disorder. *Journal of Disabilities, 24,* 78–86.

Ervin-Tripp, S. (1971). Social backgrounds and verbal skills. In T. Moore (Ed.), *Language acquisition: Models and methods.* New York: Academic Press.

Farnam-Diggory, S. (1980). Learning disabilities: A view from cognitive science. *Journal of the American Academy of Child Psychiatry, 19,* 570–578.

Flavell, J. H. (1978). Metacognitive development. In J. M. Scandura & C. J. Brainerd (Eds.), *Structural process theories of human behavior.* Hillsdale, NJ: Lawrence Erlbaum Associates.

Fleisher, L. S., Jenkins, J. R., & Pany, D. (1979). Effects on poor readers' comprehension of training in rapid decoding. *Reading Research Quarterly, 15,* 30–48.

Fleisher, L. S., Soodak, L. C., & Jelin, M. A. (1984). Selective attention deficits in learning disabled children: Analysis of the database. *Exceptional Children, 51,* 136–141.

Fox, B., & Routh, D. K. (1980). Phonemic analysis and severe reading disability in children. *Journal of Psycholinguistic Research, 9,* 115–119.

Frostig, M. (1968). Education for children with hearing disabilities. In H. Myklebust (Ed.), *Progress in learning disabilities.* New York: Grune & Stratton.

Garner, R., & Reis, R. (1981). Monitoring and resolving comprehension obstacles. *Reading Research Quarterly, 16,* 569–582.

Gelheiser, L. M. (1984). Generalization from categorical memory tasks to prose by learning disabled adolescents. *Journal of Educational Psychology, 76,* 1128–1138.

Gerber, M. M. (1984). Investigations of the orthographic problem-solving ability in learning disabled and normally achieving students. *Learning Disability Quarterly, 7,* 157–164.

Gerber, M. M. (1986). Generalization of spelling strategies by LD students as a result of contingent imitation/modeling and mastery criteria. *Journal of Learning Disabilities, 19,* 530–537.

Gibbs, D. P., & Cooper, E. B. (1989). Prevalence of communication disorders in students with learning disabilities. *Journal of Learning Disabilities, 22,* 60–63.

Golinkoff, R. M. (1976). A comparison of reading comprehension processes in good and poor comprehenders. *Reading Research Quarterly, 11,* 623–659.

Goodman, K. S. (1973). Psycholinguistic universals in the reading process. In F. Smith (Ed.), *Psycholinguistics and reading.* New York: Holt, Rinehart & Winston.

Graham, S., & Harris, K. R. (1988). Instructional recommendations for teaching writing to exceptional students. *Exceptional Children, 54,* 506–513.

Gregg, N. (1983). College learning disabled writer: Error patterns and instructional alternatives. *Journal of Learning Disabilities, 16,* 334–338.

Hallahan, D., Gajar, A., Cohen, S., & Tarver, S. (1978). Selective attention and locus of control in learning disabled and normal children. *Journal of Learning Disabilities, 4,* 47–52.

Hallahan, D., & Reeves, R. (1980). Selective attention and distractibility. In B. Keogh (Ed.), *Advances in special education.* Greenwich, CT: JAI Press.

Hallahan, D., & Sapona, R. (1984). Self-monitoring of attention with learning disabled children: Past practice and current issues. *Annual Review of Learning Disabilities, 2,* 97–101.

Hammill, D., Leiger, J., McNutt, G., & Larsen, T. (1981). A new definition of learning disabilities. *Learning Disability Quarterly, 4,* 336–342.

Hammill, D., & McNutt, B. (1981). *Correlates of reading: The consensus of thirty years of research.* Austin, TX: Pro-Ed.

Harris, K. (1990). Developing self-regulation learners: The role of private speech and self-instructions. *Educational Psychologist, 25,* 35–50.

Harris, K., Pressley, M. (1991). The nature of cognitive strategy instruction: Interactive strategy construction. *Exceptional Children, 57,* 392–404.

Hiebert, B., Wong, B. Y., & Hunter, M. (1982). Affective influence on learning disabled adolescence. *Learning Disability Quarterly, 5,* 334–343.

Hook, P. E., & Johnson, D. J. (1978). Metalinguistic awareness and reading strategies. *Bulletin of the Orton Society, 28,* 62–78.

Isaacson, S. (1987). Effective instruction in written language. *Focus on Exceptional Children, 19,* 1–12.

Jansky, J., & deHirsh, K. (1972). *Preventing reading failure: Prediction diagnosis, intervention.* New York: Harper & Row.

Jenkins, J. J., Heliotis, J. D., Stein, M. L., & Haynes, M. C. (1987). Improving reading comprehension by using paragraph restatements. *Exceptional Children, 54,* 54–59.

Johnson, D., Blalock, J., & Nesbitt, J. (1978). Adolescents with learning disabilities: Perspectives from an educational clinic. *Learning Disability Quarterly, 1,* 24–36.

Johnson, D., & Myklebust, H. (1967). *Learning disabilities: Educational principles and practices.* New York: Grune & Stratton.

Johnston, P. H., & Winograd, P. (1985). Passive failure in reading. *Journal of Reading Behavior, 4,* 279–301.

Jorm, A. (1983). Specific reading retardation and working memory: A review. *British Journal of Psychology, 74,* 311–342.

Kail, R., & Leonard, L. B. (1986). Sources of word-finding problems in language-impaired children. In S. J. Ceci (Ed.), *Handbook of cognitive social and neuropsychological aspects of learning disabilities.* Hillsdale, NJ: Lawrence Erlbaum Associates.

Kamhi, A. G., & Koenig, L. A. (1985). Metalinguistic awareness in normal and language-disordered children. *Language, Speech, and Hearing Services in Schools, 16,* 199–210.

Kavale, K. A., & Nye, C. (1985). Parameters of LD in achievement, linguistic, neuropsychological, and social/behavioral domains. *Journal of Special Education, 19,* 443–457.

Kephart, N. (1971). *The slow learner in the classroom.* Columbus, OH: Merrill/Macmillan.

Kirk, S. A. (1963). Behavioral diagnosis and remediation of learning disabilities. *Conference on Exploration into the Problems of the Perceptually Handicapped Child.* Evanston, IL: Fund for Perceptually Handicapped Children.

Kirk, S. A., & Kirk, W. P. (1972). *Psycholinguistic learning disabilities.* Urbana: University of Illinois Press.

Kneedler, R. D., & Hallahan, D. P. (1981). Self-monitoring of on-task behavior with learning-disabled children: Current studies and future directions. *Exceptional Education Quarterly, 2,* 73–82.

Kurtz, B. E., & Borkowski, J. G. (1984). Children's metacognition: Exploring relationships among knowledge, process and motivational variables. *Journal of Experimental Child Psychology, 37,* 335–354.

Leonard, L. B. (1979). Language impairment in children. *Merrill-Palmer Quarterly, 25,* 205–232.

Lerner, J. W. (1981). *Learning disabilities* (3rd ed.). Boston: Houghton Mifflin.

Levine, M. D., Busch, B., & Aufseiser, C. (1982). The dimensions of inattention among children with school problems. *Pediatrics, 70,* 387–395.

Liberman, I. Y. (1983). A language-oriented view of reading and its disorders. In H. Myklebust (Ed.), *Progress in learning disabilities* (vol. 5). New York: Grune & Stratton.

Liberman, I. Y., Shankweiler, D., Fisher, F. W., & Carter, B. (1974). Explicit syllable and phoneme segmentation in young children. *Journal of Experimental Child Psychology,* 18, 210–212.

Licht, B. G. (1984). Cognitive-motivational factors that contribute to the achievement of learning-disabled children. *Annual Review of Learning Disabilities,* 2, 119–126.

Lieberman, P., Meskill, R. H., Chatillon, M., & Schupack, H. (1985). Phonetic speech perception deficits in dyslexia. *Journal of Speech and Hearing Research,* 28, 480–486.

Majsterek, D. J., & Ellenwood, A. (1990). Screening preschoolers for reading learning disabilities: Promising procedures. *L. D. Forum,* 16, 6–14.

Markman, E. M. (1977). Realizing that you don't understand: A preliminary investigation. *Child Development,* 48, 989–992.

Mastropieri, M. A., Scruggs, T. E., & Levin, J. R. (1987). Facilitating LD students memory for expository prose. *American Educational Research Journal,* 24, 505–519.

Mather, R. E. (1992). Whole language reading instruction for student with learning disabilities: Caught in the crossfire. *Learning Disabilities Research and Practice,* 7, 87–95.

Mattingly, J. G. (1972). Reading, the linguistic process and linguistic awareness. In J. F. Kavanaugh & J. G. Mattingly (Eds.), *Language by ear and by eye.* Cambridge: MIT Press.

McGee, L. M. (1982). Awareness of text structure: Effects on children's recall of expository text. *Reading Research Quarterly,* 17, 581–590.

McGee, R., Williams, S., Moffett, T., & Anderson, J. (1989). A comparison of 13-year-old-boys with an attention deficit and/or reading disabilities on neuropsychological measures. *Journal of Abnormal Child Psychology,* 17, 37–53.

McKinney, J. D., & Feagans, L. (1983). Adaptive classroom behavior of learning disabled students. *Journal of Learning Disabilities,* 16, 360–367.

McKinney, J. D., & Feagans, L. (1984). Academic and behavioral characteristics: Longitudinal studies of learning disabled children and average achievers. *Learning Disability Quarterly,* 7, 251–265.

Menyuk, P., & Looney, P. (1972). A problem of language disorder: Length versus structure. *Journal of Speech and Hearing Research,* 15, 264–279.

Miller, G. A., Galanter, E., & Pribam, K. (1960). *Plans and the structure of behavior.* New York: Holt, Rinehart & Winston.

Moran, M. R., & Bryne, M. C. (1977). Mastery of verb tense markers by normal and learning disabled children. *Journal of Speech and Hearing Research,* 20, 529–542.

Moran, M. R., Schumaker, J. B., & Vetter, A. F. (1981). *Teaching a paragraph organization strategy to learning disabled adolescents* (Research Rep. No. 54). Lawrence: University of Kansas Institute for Research in Learning Disabilities.

Myklebust, H. R. (1965). *Development and disorders of written language, Vol. I: The Picture Story Language Test.* New York: Grune & Stratton.

Myklebust, H. R. (1973). *Development and disorders of written language, Vol. 2: Studies of normal and exceptional children.* New York: Grune & Stratton.

Myklebust, H. R. (1978). Toward a science of dyslexiology. In H. Myklebust (Ed.), *Progress in learning disabilities* (Vol. 4). New York: Grune & Stratton.

Newhoff, M. (1990). Oral language deficits as the basis of learning disabilities. *Clinical Connection,* 4, 16–17.

Nodine, B. F. Barenbaum, E., & Newcomer, P. (1985). Story composition by learning disabled, reading disabled and normal children. *Learning Disability Quarterly,* 8, 167–181.

Norris, N. T., & Crump, W. D. (1982). Syntactic and vocabulary development in the written language of learning disabled and non-learning disabled students at four age levels. *Learning Disability Quarterly,* 5, 167–181.

Orton, S. T. (1937). *Reading, writing and speech problems in children.* New York: Norton.

Palincsar, A. S., & Brown, A. L. (1986). Interactive teaching to promote independent learning from text. *The Reading Teacher,* 39, 771–777.

Paris, S. G., & Meyers, M. (1981). Comprehension monitoring, memory and study strategies of good and poor readers. *Journal of Reading Behavior,* 13, 7–22.

Paris, S. G., & Oka, E. R. (1989). Strategies for comprehending text and coping with reading difficulties. *Learning Disability Quarterly,* 12, 32–42.

Paul, R. (1992). Language and speech disorders. In S. R. Hooper, G. W. Hynd, & R. E. Mattison (Eds.). *Developmental disorders: Diagnostic criteria and clinical assessment* (pp. 209–238). Hillsdale, NJ: Lawrence Erlbaum Associates.

Pearson, P. D., & Spiro, R. J. (1980). Toward a theory of reading instruction. *Topics in Language Disorders, 1,* 71–88.

Perfetti, C. A., & Hogaboam, T. W. (1975). The relationship between single word decoding and reading comprehension skill. *Journal of Educational Psychology, 67,* 461–469.

Perfetti, C. A., & Lesgold, A. M. (1979). Coding and comprehension in skilled reading and implications for reading instruction. In L. B. Resnick & P. A. Weaver (Eds.), *Theory and practice of early reading* (Vol. 1). Hillsdale, NJ: Lawrence Erlbaum Associates.

Poplin, M., Gray, R., Larsen, S., Banikowski, A., & Mehring, T. (1980). A comparison of components of written expression abilities in learning disabled and non-learning disabled students at three grade-levels. *Learning Disability Quarterly, 3,* 46–53.

Pressley, M., Borkowski, J. G., & O'Sullivan, J. T. (1984). Memory strategy instruction is made of this: Metamemory and durable strategy use. *Educational Psychologist, 19,* 94–107.

Pressley, M., & Rankin, J. (1994). More about whole language methods of reading instruction for students at-risk for early reading failure. *Learning Disabilities Research and Practice, 9,* 157–168.

Pressley, M., Rankin, J., Gaskins, I., Brown, R., & El-Dinary, P. (1995). Mapping the cutting edge in primary level literacy for at-risk readers. In T. E. Scruggs, and M. Mastropieri (Eds.). *Advances in Learning and Behavioral Disabilities* (pp. 47–90). Greenwich, CT: JAI Press Inc.

Raphael, T. S., & Englert, C. S. (1990). Reading and writing: Partners in constructing meaning. *The Reading Teacher, 43,* 388–400.

Rinehart, S. D., Stahl, S. A., & Erickson, L. G. (1986). Some effects of summarization training on reading and studying. *Reading Research Quarterly, 12,* 422–438.

Ring, B. C. (1976). Effects of input organization on auditory short-term memory. *Journal of Learning Disabilities, 9,* 59–63.

Ryan, E. B., Weed, K. A., & Short, E. J. (1986). Cognitive behavior modifications: Promoting active self-regulatory learning styles. In J. Torgesen & B. Wong (Eds.), *Psychological and educational perspectives on learning disabilities.* New York: Academic Press.

Samuels, S. J., Begg, G., & Chen, C. C. (1976). Comparison of word recognition speed and strategies of less skilled and more highly skilled readers. *Reading Research Quarterly, 1,* 73–86.

Sawyer, D. J. (1991). Whole language in context: Insights into the current great debate. *Topics in Language Disorders, 11,* 1–13.

Schumaker, J., Deshler, D., Alley, G., Warner, M., & Denton, P. (1984). Multipass: A learning strategy for improving reading comprehension. *Learning Disability Quarterly, 5,* 295–304.

Schunk, D. H., & Cox, P. D. (1986). Strategy training and attributional feedback with learning disabled students. *Journal of Educational Psychology, 78,* 201–209.

Scruggs, T. E. (1991). Commentary: Foundations of interaction research. In T. E. Scruggs and B. Y. L. Wong (Eds.), *Intervention research in learning disabilities.* New York: Springer-Verlag.

Scruggs, T. E., Mastropieri, M. A., & Levin, J. R. (1987). Transformational mnemonic strategies for learning disabled students. In H. L. Swanson (Ed.), *Memory and learning disabilities.* Greenwich, CT: JAI Press.

Seidenberg, P. L. (1982). Implications of schemata theory for learning disabled readers. *Journal of Learning Disabilities, 15,* 352–355.

Seidenberg, P. L. (1988). Cognitive and academic instructional intervention for learning disabled adolescents. *Topics in Language Disorders, 8,* 56–71.

Seidenberg, P. L. (1989). Relating text-processing research to reading and writing instruction for learning disabled students. *Learning Disabilities Focus, 5,* 4–12.

Seidenberg, P. L. (1991). *Reading, writing and studying strategies: An integrated curriculum.* Gaithersburg, MD: Aspen.

Seidenberg, P. L., & Bernstein, D. K. (1986). The comprehension of similies and metaphors by learning disabled and non-learning disabled children. *Language, Speech and Hearing Services in Schools, 17,* 219–229.

Seidenberg, P. L., & Bernstein, D. K. (1988). Metaphor comprehension and performance on metaphor-related language tasks: A comparison of good and poor readers. *Remedial and Special Education, 9,* 39–45.

Shankweiler, D., Liberman, I. Y., Mark, L. S., Fowler, C. A., & Fischer, F. W. (1979). The speech code and learning to read. *Journal of Experimental Psychology, 5,* 531–545.

Shaywitz, B. A., & Shaywitz, S. E. (1991). Comorbidity: A critical issue in attention deficit disorder. *Journal of Child Neurology, 6,* 13–22.

Short, E., & Ryan, E. (1984). Metacognitive differences between skilled and less skilled readers: Remediating deficits through story grammar and attribution training. *Journal of Educational Psychology, 76,* 225–235.

Siegler, R. S. (1983). Information processing approaches to development. In H. Mussen (Ed.), *Carmichael's manual of child psychology.* New York: Wiley.

Slobin, D. (1971). *Psycholinguistics.* Glenview, IL: Scott, Foresman.

Stanovich, K. E. (1986). Cognitive processes and the reading problems of learning disabled children: Evaluating the assumption of specificity. In J. K. Torgesen & B. Y. L. Wong (Eds.), *Psychological and educational perspectives in earning disabilities.* New York: Academic Press.

Stanovich, K. E. (1991). Word recognition: Changing perspectives. In R. Barr, M. L. Kamil, P. Mosenthal, & P. E. Pearson (Eds.). *Handbook of reading research* (pp. 418–452). New York: Longman.

Steiner, R., Werner, M., & Cromer, W. (1971). Comprehension training and identification of poor and good readers. *Journal of Educational Psychology, 62,* 506–513.

Strauss, A., & Lehtinen, L. (1947). *Psychopathology and education of the brain-injured child.* New York: Grune & Stratton.

Swanson, H. L. (1988). Learning disabled children's problem-solving: Identifying mental processes underlying intelligent performance. *Intelligence, 12,* 261–278.

Swanson, H. L. (1989). Central processing strategy difference in gifted, normal achieving, learning disabled and mentally retarded children. *Journal of Experimental Child Psychology, 47,* 378–397.

Swanson, H. L. (1991). Instruction derived from the strategy deficit model: Overview of principles and procedures. In T. E. Scruggs & B. Y. L. Wong

(Eds.), *Intervention research in learning disabilities.* New York: Springer-Verlag.

Swanson, H. L., & Cooney, J. (1985). Strategy transformations in learning disabled children. *Learning Disability Quarterly, 8,* 221–231.

Swanson, H. L., & Rhine, B. (1985). Strategy transformations in learning disabled children's math performance: Clues to the development of expertise. *Journal of Learning Disabilities, 18,* 596–603.

Tarver, S. G., Hallahan, D. P., Kaufman, J. M., & Ball, D. W. (1976). Verbal rehearsal and selective attention in children with learning disabilities: A developmental lag. *Journal of Experimental Child Psychology, 22,* 375–385.

Thomas, C. C., Englert, C. S., & Gregg, S. (1987). An analysis of errors and strategies in the expository writing of learning disabled students. *Remedial and Special Education, 8,* 21–30.

Torgesen, J. K. (1977). The role of nonspecific factors in the task performance of learning disabled children: A theoretical assessment. *Journal of Learning Disabilities, 10,* 27–34.

Torgesen, J. K. (1978). Performance of reading disabled children on serial memory tasks: A review. *Reading Research Quarterly, 19,* 57–87.

Torgesen, J. K. (1980). The use of efficient task strategies by learning disabled children: Conceptual and educational implication. *Journal of Learning Disabilities, 13,* 364–371.

Torgesen, J. K. (1982). The study of short-term memory in learning disabled children. In K. Gadow & I. Bialer (Eds.), *Advances in learning and behavioral disabilities* (Vol. 1). Greenwich, CT: JAI Press.

Torgesen, J. K. (1985). Memory processes in reading disabled children. *Journal of Learning Disabilities, 18,* 350–357.

Torgesen, J. K. (1986). Learning disabilities theory: Its current state and future prospects. *Journal of Learning Disabilities, 19,* 399–407.

Torgesen, J. K., & Houck, G. (1980). Processing deficiencies in learning disabled children who perform poorly on the digit span task. *Journal of Educational Psychology, 72,* 141–160.

Torgesen, J. K., & Licht, B. G. (1983). The learning disabled child as an inactive learner: Retrospect and prospects. In J. D. McKinney & L. Feagan (Eds.), *Current topics in learning disabilities* (Vol. 1). Normand, NJ: Ablex.

Torgesen, J. K., Rashotti, C. A., Greenstein, J., & Portes, P. (1991). Further studies of learning disabled children with severe performance problems on the digit span test. *Learning Disabilities Research and Practice, 6,* 134–144.

Torgesen, J. K., Wagner, R. K., Simmons, K., & Laughon, P. (1990). Identifying phonological coding problems in disabled readers. *Learning Disability Quarterly, 13,* 236–244.

Treiman, R., & Baron, J. (1981). Segmental analysis ability: Development and relation to reading ability. In G. MacKennon & T. Waller (Eds.), *Reading research: Advances in theory and practice* (Vol. 3). New York: Academic Press.

U.S. Department of Education. (1986, October). Education of handicapped children act: Amendments of 1986. *Federal Register.* Washington, DC: Department of Education.

U.S. Office of Education. (1977, December). Education of handicapped children: Assistance to states: Procedures for evaluating specific learning disabilities. *Federal Register, Part III.* Washington, DC: Department of Health, Education and Welfare.

Vallecorsa, A. L., & Garriss, E. (1990). Story composition skills of middle-grade students with learning disabilities. *Exceptional Children, 57,* 48–55.

van Kleeck, A. (1984). Metalinguistic skills: Cutting across spoken and written language and problem solving abilities. In G. P. Wallach & K. G. Butler (Eds.), *Language learning disabilities in school-age children.* Baltimore: Williams & Wilkins.

Vellutino, F. R. (1977). Alternative conceptualizations of dyslexia: Evidence in support of a verbal-deficit hypothesis. *Harvard Educational Review, 47,* 334–354.

Vellutino, F. R. (1979). *Dyslexia: Theory and research.* Cambridge: MIT Press.

Vellutino, F. R. (1991). Has basic research in reading increased our understanding of developmental reading and how to teach reading? *Psychological Science, 2,* 81–83.

Vellutino, F. R., & Scanlon, D. M. (1979, April). The effect of phonemic segmentation training and response acquisition on coding ability in poor and normal readers. Paper presented at the American Education Research Association annual meeting, San Francisco.

Vellutino, F. R., & Scanlon, D. M. (1991). The preeminence of phonologically based skills in learning to read. In S. Brady & D. Shankweiler (Eds.), *Phonological processes in literacy* (pp. 237–252). Hillsdale, NJ: Erlbaum.

Vogel, S. A. (1975). *Syntactic abilities in normal and dyslexic children.* Baltimore: University Park Press.

Vygotsky, L. S. (1962). *Thought and language.* Cambridge: MIT Press.

Wagner, R. K. (1986). Phonological processing abilities and reading: Implications for disabled readers. *Journal of Learning Disabilities, 19,* 623–630.

Walker, N. W. (1985). Impulsivity in learning disabled children, past research findings and methodological inconsistencies. *Learning Disabilities Quarterly, 8,* 85–94.

Wallach, G. P., & Butler, K. G. (1984). *Language learning disabilities in school-age children.* Baltimore: Williams & Wilkins.

Wallach, M. A., & Wallach, L. (1976). *Teaching all children to read.* Chicago: University of Chicago Press.

Wechsler, D. (1974). *Wechsler Intelligence Scale for Children—Revised* (manual). Austn, TX: Psychological Corp.

Welch, M. (1992). The PLEASE strategy: A metacognitive learning strategy for improving the paragraph writing of students with mild learning disabilities. *Learning Disability Quarterly, 15,* 119–128.

Wepman, J. M. (1973). *Wepman Auditory Discrimination Test.* Chicago: Language Research Associates.

Wiederholt, J. L. (1974). Historical perspectives in the education of the learning disabled. In L. Mann & D. Sabatino (Eds.), *The second review of special education.* Philadelphia: Journal of Special Education Press.

Wiig, E. H., & Semel, E. M. (1973). Comprehension of linguistic concepts requiring logical operations by learning disabled children. *Journal of Speech and Hearing Research, 16,* 627–636.

Wiig, E. H., & Semel, E. M. (1974). Logico-grammatical sentence comprehension by learning disabled adolescents. *Perceptual Motor Skills, 38,* 1331–1334.

Wiig, E. H., & Semel, E. M. (1975). Productive language abilities in learning disabled adolescents. *Journal of Learning Disabilities, 8,* 578–586.

Wiig, E. H., & Semel, E. M. (1976). *Language disabilities in children and adolescents.* Columbus, OH: Merrill/Macmillan.

Wiig, E. H., & Semel, E. M. (1984). *Language assessment and intervention for the learning disabled* (2nd ed.). Columbus, OH: Merrill/Macmillan.

Wiig, E. H., Semel, E. M., & Crouse, M. A. (1973). The use of English morphology by high risk and learning disabled children. *Journal of Learning Disabilities, 6,* 457–465.

Williams, D. L., Gridley, B. E., & Fitzhugh-Bell, K. (1992). Cluster analysis of children and adolescents with brain damage and learning disabilities using neuropsychological, psychoeducational, sacrobehavioral variables. *Journal of Learning Disabilities, 25,* 290–299.

Williams, J. P. (1984a). Categorization, macrostructure, and finding the main idea. *Journal of Educational Psychology, 76,* 874–879.

Williams, J. P. (1984b). Phonemic analysis and how it relates to reading. *Journal of Learning Disabilities, 17,* 240–245.

Winograd, P. (1984). Strategic difficulties in summarizing texts. *Reading Research Quarterly, 21,* 404–425.

Winograd, P., & Niquette, G. (1988). Assessing learned helplessness in poor readers. *Topics in Language Disorders, 8,* 38–55.

Wong, B. Y. L. (1978). The effects of directive cues on the organization of memory and recall in good and poor readers. *Journal of Education Research, 72,* 32–38.

Wong, B. Y. L. (1985). Metacognition and learning disabilities. In T. G. Weller, D. Forrest, & E. MacKinnon (Eds.), *Metacognition, cognition and human performance.* New York: Academic Press.

Wong, B.Y. L. (1986). A cognitive approach to teaching spelling. *Exceptional Children, 53,* 169–173.

Wong, B. Y. L., & Jones, W. (1982). Increasing metacomprehension in learning disabled and normally achieving students through self-questioning training. *Learning Disability Quarterly, 5,* 228–246.

Wong, B. Y. L., & Wilson, M. (1984). Investigating awareness of and teaching passage organization in learning disabled children. *Journal of Learning Disabilities, 17,* 477–482.

Wong, B. Y. L., Wong, R., Perry, N., & Sawatsky, D. (1986). The efficacy of a self-questioning summarization strategy for use by underachievers and learning disabled adolescents in social studies. *Learning Disabilities Focus, 2,* 20–35.

Zentall, S. (1993). Research on the educational implications of attention deficit hyperactivity disorder. *Exceptional Children, 60,* 143–153.

Chapter 12

Mental Retardation: Difference and Delay

ROBERT E. OWENS, JR.
State University of New York at Geneseo

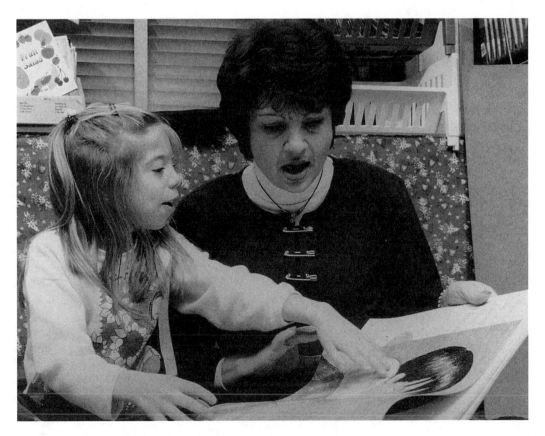

> *I wanted to make this book all about pop music, but my Dad says people will be more interested in my adventures. But I must write a bit about pop. (Hunt, 1967, p. 89)*

In *The World of Nigel Hunt: The Diary of a Mongoloid Youth,* the author expresses the interests of many other teenagers. This particular adolescent is mentally retarded. He was born with Down syndrome, a genetic disorder that is one of hundreds of identifiable causes of or factors related to mental retardation. Yet Nigel is more like his nonretarded peers than he is unlike them.

It is difficult to characterize the mentally retarded population because of its diversity. This heterogeneous population includes individuals who are totally dependent and those who are nearly independent in their daily living. We can say, however, that they develop more slowly or at a more retarded rate than the nonmentally retarded population. In addition, they are different in some ways from the nonretarded population. This characteristic can be seen in several aspects of the development of mentally retarded individuals, including language.

In this chapter, I will explore a definition of mental retardation and discuss the implications for communication and language development. I will characterize the special language problems of this population and suggest intervention techniques and programs that might be helpful for the speech-language pathologist. More specifically, I will address the following questions:

1. How can we characterize or define the mentally retarded population?
2. What are the cognitive and linguistic characteristics of the mentally retarded population? Do these characteristics reflect a difference or a delay?
3. What intervention techniques are suggested by the learning characteristics of the mentally retarded population?
4. What is the developmental intervention approach, and how is it used?
5. What behaviors should be targeted, and what techniques should be used in intervention by the speech-language pathologist?

A Definition of Mental Retardation

The American Association on Mental Deficiency (AAMD), the primary organization for professionals working with the mentally retarded population, defines mental retardation as a "significantly subaverage general intellectual functioning, existing concurrently with related limitations in two or more . . . adaptive skill areas [, and] . . . manifest[ed] before age 18" (*Mental Retardation*, 1992). To understand this definition fully, we must look at its various components.

Significantly subaverage is generally defined as an IQ of 70 or lower, but this upper limit is not inflexible and may be extended upward, depending on the reliability of the testing that helped to establish the IQ. In the entire population, the mean or average IQ is 100, but the range of normality extends from 85 to 115. This range, which is considered to be one standard deviation from the norm, contains two thirds of the population. An IQ of 70 is two standard deviations below 100, or significantly below average.

Intellectual functioning refers to the results of a standardized general intelligence test. The test should be pluralistic and culture-free and should be administered individually. The generally accepted measurement of intelligence is IQ, a ratio of mental age to chronological age. If the mental age is 10 years and the chronological age is 10 years, the relationship is 10/10 or 1, which is interpreted as an IQ of 100. In contrast, a mental age of 5 and a chronological age of 10 yields 5/10 or 0.5, which is an IQ of 50.

As stated previously, testing should be pluralistic and culture-free. A test based solely upon language abilities would be unfair to many second-language learners and to many children with learning disabilities. Intelligence testing should also include nonlinguistic abilities, such as problem solving, sensorimotor development, and social skills. Likewise, culturally biased tests would be prejudicial to many minorities. The author knows of one recent Southeast Asian immigrant classified as mentally retarded based upon an English receptive vocabulary test.

Deficits in adaptive behavior are defined by Grossman (1983) as "significant limitations in an individual's effectiveness in meeting the standards of maturation, learning, personal independence, and/or social responsibility that are expected for...age level and cultural group" (p. 11). Adaptive skills vary for different ages. During infancy and preschool years, adaptive skills include sensorimotor, speech and language, self-help, and interactional development. In middle childhood and early adolescence, the emphasis shifts to academic and reasoning skill development and to group and interpersonal relationships. Late adolescent and adult adaptive skill development relates to vocational and social responsibility. Adaptive behavior frequently correlates very positively with intelligence but not always, especially for very low IQs (Grossman, 1983). One standardized measure of adaptive behavior is AAMD's (1974) Adaptive Behavior Scale.

The period prior to age 18 is considered by many to be the **developmental period.** For those with mental retardation, development may be slow, arrested, or incomplete. The developmental rate decreases as all humans reach the late teens. Thus, young adults who are profoundly retarded may experience only moderate developmental change after age 18, although they function at a mental age of only 3 years.

The AAMD definition includes only those individuals who meet all the criteria. Children who have learning disabilities are not included because they possess normal intelligence; and elderly patients who have aphasia do not qualify because their disorder did not manifest itself during the developmental period. Although individuals with both types of disorders might function within the retarded range on some tasks, they cannot be classified as mentally retarded. Figure 12-1 illustrates the AAMD definition.

The definition does not specify causes or etiologies but emphasizes the current functioning level of the individual. In other words, it is not assumed that Down syndrome is synonymous with mental retardation. In part, the definition reflects a bias held by most professionals that functioning levels can be modified or changed, that the mentally retarded individual is a developmental being.

Prevalence and Levels of Functioning

The number of mentally retarded individuals in the United States is unknown. Estimates vary from 1 percent to 3 percent of the population, or approximately 2.5 to 7 million indi-

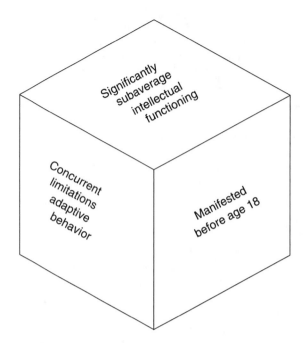

All criteria must be met in order to establish mental retardation

FIGURE 12-1   AAMD definition of mental retardation.
(Adapted from *Mental Retardation,* 1992)

viduals. Upper figures are based solely on IQ score data. Mental retardation is approximately 15 times more prevalent than blindness. Most of the approximately 125,000 retarded individuals born in the United States each year are only mildly retarded.

There are four categories of mental retardation based on IQ—mild, moderate, severe, and profound. The characteristics of each category are listed in Table 12-1.

The distribution of mental retardation within the population is not uniform. The distribution of individuals with severe and profound retardation reflects the general population. However, among the mildly and moderately retarded, there is a greater percentage of poor and minority individuals as well as a greater percentage of individuals with a family history of retardation (Birch, Richardson, Baird, Horobin, & Illsley, 1970). The disproportionately higher percentage among the poor and minority populations may reflect the environmental effects of poverty. In American culture, many minorities are found in the lower socioeconomic levels because of discriminatory practices. Also, middle-class professionals are more likely to classify lower class or minority children as retarded. Lack of proper nutrition or poor health may contribute to delayed development among the poor. In addition, because mildly mentally retarded parents are most likely to find themselves among the poor genetic influences may play a role. These adults are more likely than nonretarded adults to produce offspring with depressed cognitive functioning. This factor does not occur with the severely and profoundly retarded because very few of these individuals produce offspring.

TABLE 12-1   Categories of Mental Retardation

Category	IQ Range	% of MR Population	Characteristics
Mild	52–68	89	Usually absorbed into the community where they work and live independently
Moderate	36–51	6	Capable of learning self-care skills and working within a sheltered environment; live semi-independently, with relatives or in a community residence
Severe	20–35	3½	Capable of learning some self-care skills and are not totally dependent; often exhibit physical disabilities and deficits in speech and language
Profound	below 20	1½	Capable of learning some basic living skills but require continual care and supervision; often exhibit severe physical and/or sensory problems

Adapted from Grossman (1983).

Causes of Mental Retardation

Biological causes may be a factor for more than half of the individuals within the mentally retarded population. Many individuals whose mental retardation was previously believed to have resulted from social-environmental factors may actually exhibit a recently discovered syndrome called Fragile X (Nussvaum & Ledbetter, 1986; Wolff, Gardner, Lappen, Paccia, & Meryash, 1988). Fragile X syndrome is the most common cause of mental retardation next to down syndrome (Caron, 1994). A weakness in the female, or X, chromosome found in all humans is related to mental retardation and possibly to other learning disorders. Fragile X, a recessive trait more prevalent in males because they carry only one X chromosome is found in 1 out of every 1350 live male births and 1 out of every 2033 live female births (Webb, Bundey, Thake, & Todd, 1986). Most males with the Fragile X trait are mentally retarded, whereas only about a third of females with the trait are so affected (Caron, 1994). Language problems affect all males with Fragile X, even those whose IQs are within normal limits (Caron, 1994). Females are more likely to exhibit characteristics of a learning disability (Wolff et al., 1988).

Other biological causes may be genetic, such as Down syndrome; congenital, such as metabolic disorders or malformations of the skull and brain, or illness- or toxin-related, such as maternal rubella or lead poisoning. The correlation between severity of retardation and biological factors is very strong.

Social-environmental factors are not as easy to identify as biological factors and involve many interactive variables. Poor housing and hygiene, as well as inadequate medical care and nutrition, may contribute. Lack of prenatal care and of infant stimulation may affect the developing child more directly.

Certainly any discussion of causality offers only the grossest of estimates and must be cautiously taken for several reasons. First, certain conditions may be related to mental retardation but not be a direct causal agent. Second, individuals may have several identifiable causes or related factors. Third, the specific etiology is unknown for a significant portion of the retarded population. Known causes of mental retardation are listed in Table 12-2.

Associated Disorders

There is a higher incidence of neurological disorders among the mentally retarded population, especially that segment that is severely and profoundly involved. Approximately one third of the profoundly involved have at least two profoundly disabling disorders (Cegelka & Prehm, 1982). Two areas of note are neuromuscular disorders and emotional disorders.

Neuromuscular Disorders.   Cerebral palsy and/or epilepsy are found in a greater percentage of the mentally retarded population than in the nonretarded population. This difference is especially evident among the severely and profoundly retarded. These individuals frequently exhibit neuromuscular disorders as part of a complex of multiple disabilities.

Among the cerebral palsied population, approximately 50 percent demonstrate IQs lower than 70. Such scores may reflect a lack of sophistication by the tester or by the test. In other words, individuals with cerebral palsy may be difficult to test using standard procedures because of neuromuscular interference. Nonetheless, it seems safe to conclude that a substantial proportion of the cerebral palsied population also exhibit mental retardation.

Epilepsy affects less than 1 percent the general population. The percentage increases with decreased intelligence, and as high as 65 percent of the profoundly retarded population may exhibit seizure activity (Chaney, Eyman, & Miller, 1979). Frequent causes of epilepsy in young children are central nervous system (CNS) malformation, CNS injury from infection or accident, and CNS malfunction caused by a metabolic error.

Related neurological disorders further complicate the learning task for persons with mental retardation. The increased occurrence with decreased intelligence may also indicate an underlying organic cause for the more severe forms of retardation.

Emotional Disorders.   Mental retardation and mental illness are *not* the same, although there is a high prevalence of emotional problems within the mentally retarded population (Phillips & Williams, 1975; Russell & Tanquay, 1981). Among children with schizophrenic disturbances, it has been estimated that one third to one half exhibit prolonged or permanent functioning within the mentally retarded range. Among persons with mental retardation, behavioral disturbances are the second most frequent cause of institutionalization after intellectual deficiency (Russell & Tanquay, 1981). Emotional disorders may be of any type, and mentally retarded individuals may exhibit a full range of emotional and personality disturbances (Balthazar & Stevens, 1974, Szymanski & Tanquay, 1980). Incidence figures may be higher than has been reported because of "diagnostic overshadowing" in which the intellectual deficit may be such a salient feature that accompanying emotional disorders are overshadowed (Reiss, Levitan, & Szyszko, 1982).

Very few depressive types of psychosis are reported for the mentally retarded population (Russell & Tanquay, 1981); however, many emotional diagnoses relate to bizarre be-

TABLE 12-2   Known Causes of Mental Retardation

Type	Examples	Characteristics
Biologic		
Genetic and chromosomal	Down syndrome (Trisomy 21)	Broad head and characteristic facial features, small stature, mental retardation
	Klinefelter syndrome (sex-linked, XXY)	Feminine roundness to body, small testes, possible mental retardation
	Cri-du-chat syndrome	Catlike cry, microcephaly, mental retardation
Infectious processes	Maternal rubella	Cardiac defects, cataracts, hearing loss, microcephaly, possible mental retardation
	Congenital syphilis	Deafness, vision problems, possible epilepsy or cerebral palsy, mental retardation
Toxins and chemical agents	Fetal alcohol syndrome	Persistently deficient growth, low brain weight, facial abnormalities, cardiac defects, mental retardation
	Lead poisoning	Central nervous system and kidney damage, hyperactivity
Nutrition and metabolism	Phenylketonuria (PKU)	Reduced pigmentation, motor coordination problems, convulsions, microcephaly, mental retardation
	Tay-Sachs disease	Progressive deterioration of nervous system and vision, mental retardation, death in preschool years
	Inadequate diet	Small stature, possible mental retardation
Gestational disorders	Hydrocephalus	Enlarged head caused by increased volume of cerebral-spinal fluid, visual defects, epilepsy, mental retardation
	Cerebral malformation	Absence or underdevelopment of cerebral cortex and resultant mental retardation
	Craniofacial anomalies	Malformed skull and associated mental retardation
Complications of pregnancy and delivery	Extreme immaturity or preterm infant	Low birth weight, higher prevalence of central nervous system disorders
	Exceptionally large baby	Possible birth injury to central nervous system
	Maternal nutritional disorders	Low birth weight, higher prevalence of central nervous system disorders
Gross brain diseases	Tumors and tuberous sclerosis	Tumors in heart, seizures, tuberous "bumps" on nose and cheeks, mental retardation
	Huntington disease	Degenerative neurological functioning evidenced in progressive dementia and cerebral palsy
Social-Environmental		
Psychosocial disadvantage	Subnormal intellectual functioning in immediate family and/or impoverished environment	Functional retardation
Sensory deprivation	Maternal deprivation Prolonged isolation	Functional retardation and failure to thrive

Adapted from Grossman (1983).

haviors, especially with institutionalized populations. Some institutionalized individuals have not been prevented from evolving behavioral repertoires that include self-injurious and self-stimulatory behaviors.

Cognitive Functioning

Volumes of research have been published on the cognitive abilities of individuals with mental retardation. Still, for a number of reasons, we do not fully understand the cognitive and learning processes of this population (Cegelka & Prehm, 1982). First, the complex nature of the cognitive process necessitates research that targets very limited aspects. Therefore, there are no definitive studies of the entire process of cognitive functioning among either the retarded or nonretarded population. Second, the cognitive functioning level of retarded subjects in many studies is poorly defined. This factor can be extremely important because there seems to be a very strong link between IQ and cognitive abilities. It is difficult to draw conclusions across studies when the functioning levels of the subjects differ greatly. Finally, it is difficult to extrapolate from a limited experimental setting to the daily environments of retarded individuals.

Researchers have interpreted their data in two general ways. One interpretation holds that there are discrepancies or differences in the cognitive processing abilities of the mentally retarded population that cannot be accounted for by mental age alone (Das, Kirby, & Jarman, 1975; Detterman, 1979; Greenspan, 1979; Spitz, 1979; Stephens & McLaughlin, 1974). Individuals with mental retardation do not perform in the same manner as nonretarded peers of the same mental age. Pointing to methodological problems in many of these studies, a second group of researchers considers the mentally retarded population to develop cognitively in the same manner as the nonretarded population, but at a slower rate (Balla & Zigler, 1971; Humphreys & Parsons, 1979; Kamhi, 1981).

In general, individuals in the mentally retarded population develop many cognitive skills in a developmental sequence similar to that of the nonmentally retarded population. There are differences, however, that indicate fundamental processing differences. Some of these similarities and differences can be identified in learning processes and in memory. **Learning** is a change in behavior that results from rehearsal of the behavior to be learned. Cognitive abilities important for learning include attention, organization, transfer, and memory The variables to which an individual attends and the organization of these variables are important for memory, which in turn affects transfer or generalization to novel situations or problems. Figure 12-2 demonstrates this process schematically.

Attention.   Attention includes awareness of a learning situation and active cognitive processing. As noted in Figure 12-2, we do not attend to all stimuli. Research on attention has examined the orienting, reacting, and discriminating abilities of mentally retarded individuals. **Orientation** is the ability to sustain attention over time. In general, individuals who are mildly retarded exhibit equal or slightly greater ability to sustain attention and to orient when compared to their mental-age-matched (MA-matched) nonretarded peers (Karrer, Nelson, & Galbraith, 1979).

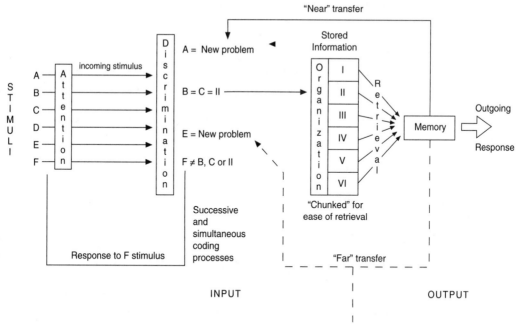

FIGURE 12-2   Schematic of major cognitive functions.

Reaction time refers to the amount of time required for an individual to respond to a stimulus. In Figure 12-2, the subject responds to stimulus F immediately. Mildly mentally retarded individuals react similarly to MA-matched nonretarded peers, but their performance is very individualistic (Krupski, 1977; Liebert & Baumeister, 1973). In part, reaction time is a function of the individual's ability to select the relevant dimensions of a task before responding. Individuals with mental retardation appear to be deficient in their abilities to scan and attend selectively.

Discrimination is the ability to identify differing stimuli from a field of similar stimuli. For example, a discrimination task might involve picking a different pitch tone from a series of pitch tones. In a more complicated task, a subject might be required to attend to several dimensions of a sample, such as color, shape, and size, at the same time. For example, in Figure 12-2, stimuli B and C are found to be similar to each other and to information already stored. In contrast, A and E are new information. In general, individuals with mental retardation exhibit difficulties identifying and maintaining attention to the relevant stimulus dimensions (Mercer & Snell, 1977; Zeaman & House, 1963, 1979). As a group, mildly and moderately retarded persons attend to fewer dimensions of a task than do the nonretarded, and these dimensions are not necessarily the salient or important ones. This deficiency reduces an individual's ability to compare new information with stored information from previous learning. In addition, it takes a longer time and more practice for persons who are mentally retarded to understand the dimensions of a task. Once a task is understood or learned, however, mentally retarded individuals can perform as well as their MA-

matched nonretarded peers (Ross & Ross, 1979). In general, mentally retarded individuals who have higher functioning abilities can learn discrimination tasks more rapidly than who have lower functioning abilities (Ellis et al., 1982). There are substantial individual differences among persons who are severely and profoundly retarded, however, and some subjects learn the tasks as well as the mildly retarded, although they may have more limited attentional capacity and may be less efficient at attention allocation (Nugent & Mosley, 1987).

In general, persons with mental retardation seem able to attend as well as their MA-matched nonretarded peers. They may be less able, however, to select the relevant information from a field. Therefore, new or relevant features of a task need to be highlighted in order to call attention to them (Meador, 1984).

Organization of Input Material.   The organization of incoming sensory information is very important for later retrieval. This organization can be demonstrated when we try to recall the name of an object. Frequently, the names of related objects will also come to mind. Therefore, we may name the washing machine by *dryer* or *refrigerator,* but rarely *spoon* or *window.* As shown in Figure 12-2, information is organized or "chunked" by category for easy retrieval. Mildly retarded and nonretarded persons exhibit similar developmental trends in the grouping of information (Stephens, 1972). In general, individuals who are mentally retarded exhibit difficulty developing categorizing strategies for organizing new material into more easily remembered "chunks" (Spitz, 1966). Because it is much more difficult to remember unrelated bits of information, any organizational deficit will hinder later recall and quickly overload memory capacity. Every reader can recognize that it is easier to recall a 10-word sentence than 10 unrelated words. If, as some propose, memory capacity is fixed, more efficient processing will require increasingly better organization (Case, 1978). In turn, better organization leaves more room for new input.

Mildly and moderately retarded individuals do not seem to rely on mediation or associative learning strategies nor to use them as efficiently as do the nonretarded. In mediating strategies, a word or symbol forms a link between two inputs. For example, a person's name might relate past experiences with feelings, life-styles, or opinions. In associative strategies, one word or symbol aids in recall of another. Common examples are "salt and _____" "black and _____" and so on. Mildly retarded individuals can use associative strategies if the two symbols are easily associated and nonabstract.

Das, Kirby, and Jarman (1979) proposed four components of information integration: input, sensory register, central processor, and output. The three processes of the central processor are simultaneous synthesis; sequential, or successive, synthesis; and regulatory activities (Cummins, 1979; Cummins & Das, 1978; Luria, 1975). Simultaneous synthesis, or coding, which takes place in the occipital-parietal region of the brain, is related to higher thought. Separate elements are synthesized into groups so that all members of the group can be retrieved simultaneously. For example, various examples of dogs are coded for the *dog* category. In sentence coding, the overall meaning, rather than the individual syntactic and phonological units, is processed. Sequential, or successive, coding is related to language form and takes place in the frontal-temporal region of the brain. Linguistic information is coded in linear fashion. Both processes are used for coding input and for planning behavior.

Obviously, these coding processes are influenced by sensory input, memory, and other intellectual processes.

Both mildly retarded and nonretarded persons exhibit simultaneous and successive coding (Jarman, 1978; Jarman & Das, 1977). There appears to be some difference in the use of this coding for the planning function, however, and the "two groups may *employ* the processes differently in solving more complex tasks" (Das et al., 1979, p. 100). Individuals with Down syndrome may even possess different coding functions. As a group, persons with Down syndrome perform more poorly than either brain-damaged individuals or other MA-matched retarded individuals on successive processing tasks. This deficiency may be an underlying cause for auditory memory and expressive language problems of the Down syndrome population (Burr & Rohr, 1978; Evans, 1977; Sommers & Starkey, 1977). The poor auditory processing and memory behavior of individuals with Down syndrome may indicate a structural difference in the processing portions of the brain (Ellis, Deacon, & Wooldridge, 1985; Lincoln, Courchesne, Kilman, & Galambos, 1985). More severely retarded persons may sustain some organic problems and, therefore, have qualitatively different neurological functioning also (Robinson & Robinson, 1976; Snart, O'Grady, & Das, 1982; Zigler, 1967).

In general, individuals with mental retardation demonstrate some organizing difficulties and thus benefit from preorganized input. Organizational deficits can hinder recall and generalization, both essential for learning.

Transfer.   Transfer, or generalization, is the ability to apply previously learned material in the solving of similar but novel problems. Although persons who are mildly retarded can be taught cognitive processing strategies, attempts to generalize these strategies have been less successful (Brown, 1978; Campione & Brown, 1977; Evans & Bilsky, 1979). The learning of more severely retarded individuals is characterized by even weaker transfer (Bricker, Heal, Bricker, Hayes, & Larsen, 1969; Ellis et al., 1982; Reid, 1980). Learning enhances performance but not generalization (Borkowski & Cavanaugh, 1979; Taylor & Turnure, 1979).

Near generalization involves only minimal changes between the training and novel, testing situations, whereas **far generalization** involves substantial changes. In Figure 12-2, Stimulus A is considered to be similar enough to stored information to qualify for near generalization. Stimulus E is less similar and thus represents far generalization. Persons who are mentally retarded have difficulties with both near and far generalization, which appear to be a function not of the similarity of the old and new tasks but of the level of awareness required to detect such similarities.

Understanding the task is essential for transfer. Individuals with mental retardation can benefit from training in all components of a task and in applying these components to new task settings (Burger, Blackman, Clark, & Reis, 1982; Butterfield & Belmont, 1978). However, explicit training does not appear to be necessary for all retarded individuals. Mildly retarded persons can gain knowledge to increase transfer solely through observation of the task (Burger, Blackman, & Clark, 1981).

The generalization deficits of retarded individuals may reflect the selection and organization problems noted previously. Generalization can be facilitated, however, if the client is helped in analyzing the similarities between old and new tasks.

Memory.   The ability to retrieve needed information that was previously learned is necessary for recall or memory. Individuals with mild and moderate retardation seem to be able to retain information within long-term memory as well as nonretarded individuals, although overall recall is slower (Belmont, 1967; Ellis, 1963; Merrill, 1985). Organizational deficits, however, may result in an overreliance on rote memory by mildly retarded persons (Spitz, 1966). In contrast, profoundly retarded individuals exhibit significant forgetting of learned behavior within only a short interval.

Short-term memory deficiencies are more evident in the retarded population (Brown, 1974; Butterfield, Wambold, & Belmont, 1973; Ellis, 1970; Gutowski & Chechile, 1987). In turn, such deficiencies may affect discrimination abilities (Lobb, 1974; Ullman, 1974). In general, short-term memory is very limited—nonretarded individuals can hold fewer than 10 entities only briefly. Retarded individuals may experience difficulty with short-term storage due to a lack of associational strategies (Gutowski & Chechile, 1987). They retain pictures better than printed words or letters (as compared with nonretarded adolescents and adults, for whom the reverse is true). Short-term memory is particularly affected by the rapid rate of forgetting found in the retarded population, especially within the first 10 seconds (Ellis et al., 1985). Increased encoding time does not normalize the rate of forgetting, indicating encoding and storage deficits (Ellis et al., 1985).

Information is retained and/or transferred to long-term memory through rehearsal or repetition. It has been reported that retarded persons do not rehearse information spontaneously (Brown, 1974; Butterfield et al., 1973; Ellis, 1970; Frank & Rabinovitch, 1974; Kellas, Ashcroft, & Johnson, 1973; Reid, 1980). They exhibit a "rehearsal deficit" (Bray, 1979). More recent studies indicate that rehearsal occurs when the retarded individual is given sufficient time (Turner & Bray, 1985).

The type of information and the stimulus mode greatly affect memory. For example, there appears to be little difference in spatial location memory for nonmentally retarded children and adults and mentally retarded adults, even those with IQs as low as 30 (Ellis, Woodley-Zanthos, & Dulaney, 1989). In contrast, adults who are mentally retarded perform much less well on free recall tasks of auditory information.

Each auditory stimulus event has a sensory, or sign, impression inherent in the event and an abstract, or symbol, representation for that event (Dance, 1967; Whatmough, 1956). The sign is meaningful but nonlinguistic. For example, the sound of a horn may signal an automobile. In contrast, the abstract representation, or word, is linguistic in nature. Memory should be better for signs because internal representation is based originally on perception. In other words, our early meaning of *doggie* is based on the perceptual attributes of the examples of *doggie* that we have encountered. The name or word *doggie* is superimposed later. Our ability to infer an entity from an auditory sign is part of our early linguistic knowledge base (Ervin-Tripp, 1973; Macnamara, 1972). Retarded school children and MA-matched nonretarded preschoolers have similar recall for signal information, but retarded children have significantly poorer recognition and recall of symbolic representations (Lamberts, 1981). There may be a link, therefore, between the reported language deficits and auditory memory deficits of the mentally retarded population (Brown, 1974; Ellis, 1970; Mittler, 1974; Rein & Kirnan, 1979).

Sentence recall probably involves reproduction of the memory episode and then editing of the text (Kintsch & van Dijk, 1978). Because individuals who are retarded make frequent word substitution errors, performance may break down in the second stage (Bilsky, Walker, & Sakales, 1983). Poor sentence recall by individuals in the retarded population may reflect poor editing skills or a breakdown in syntactic-semantic analysis, although phonological processing may be unaffected (Merrill & Mar, 1987).

Poor reading recall, on the other hand, may be related to failure to use important textual information for organization (Borkowski & Wanschura, 1974; Brown, Campione, & Murphy, 1974). Selective attention to important portions of reading passages can be taught, however, with resultant recall improvement (Luftig & Johnson, 1982).

Auditory memory deficits are particularly evident in the Down syndrome population (Marcell & Weeks, 1988). In general, "Down syndrome individuals have trouble remembering verbal-auditory material" (Marcell & Armstrong, 1982, p. 92). This difficulty may be related to **echoic memory,** "the ability to hear a sound for some time after physical stimulation has ceased" (Watkins & Watkins, 1980, p. 252). In other words, echoic memory is the ability to remember what has been heard even when it is no longer present. Echoic memory is a passive retention strategy related to immediate recall of linguistic stimuli and seems to be most efficient with the fast rates found in conversation (Hockey, 1973). Among individuals with Down syndrome, however, this echo may decay more rapidly than in the nonretarded population or at a rate at which the slower processing of the retarded cannot access it. Individuals with Down syndrome may not realize how to use such passive strategies effectively (Marcell & Armstrong, 1982). Other studies have demonstrated the generally inefficient use of memory strategies by the retarded population (Engle & Nagle, 1979). As reported previously, Down syndrome individuals have poorer successive cognitive processing than do other retarded individuals and, thus, poorer auditory sequential memory (Snart et al., 1982). Individuals with Down syndrome also exhibit difficulties in vocabulary storage and retrieval (Varnhagen, Das, & Varnhagen, 1987). These data would support the reportedly low language performance of those with Down syndrome in comparison to other retarded individuals (O'Connor & Hermelin, 1978).

In general, persons with mental retardation demonstrate poorer recall than MA-matched nonretarded peers. Not all areas are affected equally, and there is some indication that memory for spatial location is a strength that can be used to enhance learning (Nigro & Roak, 1987).

Conclusion. The mentally retarded population seems to develop cognitively in a manner similar to the nonretarded but at a slower rate. Overall, mental development of adults, as measured in Down syndrome individuals, continues well into midlife (Berry, Groeneweg, Gibson, & Brown, 1984). Some cognitive processing differences exist, however, especially in organization and memory (Das, 1972; Das et al., 1975; Semmel, Barritt, & Bennett, 1970; Stephens & McLaughlin, 1974). It is important to remember, however, that information processing differences do not explain mental retardation and may represent the cause or result, or a concurrent problem (Leonard, 1987).

Reported differences in personality and motivational functioning may reflect experiential differences (Leahy, Balla, & Zigler, 1982). In general, as the level of severity increases, wide individual differences become more apparent. With more severe retardation, cognitive functioning may be complicated by accompanying organic disorders. For persons who are mildly retarded however, IQ alone is not a particularly powerful predictor of life adjustment (McCarver & Craig, 1974; Windle, 1962). It is important to recall that individuals with mental retardation, especially those who are noninstitutionalized, exhibit integrated problem-solving abilities daily. For example, they must make decisions regarding their daily schedule, personal hygiene, nutrition, and employment. The individuals who are independent or challenged early are even more flexible problem solvers, because they have developed internal models of the mechanics of addressing problems (Levine & Langness, 1985).

Language and Communication Skills: Difference and Delay

The language behavior of the mentally retarded population is frequently one of the most problematic areas of adaptive behavior and may be the single most important characteristic of this population (Ingalls, 1978). Ultimately, language behavior will determine an individual's ability to function independently in the outside world. Although MA-matched mentally retarded and nonretarded individuals may be similar in many cognitive functions, mentally retarded individuals often exhibit difficulty with symbolic functions, including language (Kamhi, 1981).

The exact relationship of cognition and language for all humans is unknown. The relationship may be inconsistent—cognition might influence language at some phases of development and language influence cognition during other phases (Miller, Chapman, & MacKenzie, 1981). Among individuals who are mentally retarded, several patterns emerge and may vary with age, severity of retardation, and task. The most frequent patterns are as follows (Miller et al., 1981):

1. Comprehension and cognition are at similar levels, but production is below that of cognition.
2. Both comprehension and production are below the level of cognition.
3. Both comprehension and production are at the level of cognition.

As much as 50 percent of the mentally retarded population may be within the third group. It is important to note that the relationship of cognition and language, a prognostic measure often used in intervention, is not stable over time for any individual (Cole, Dale, & Mills, 1992).

Questions of difference versus delay and quality versus quantity of language and communication behaviors have been debated for decades (Kamhi & Masterson, 1989). In general, before a mental age of 10 years, the language development of the retarded population seems to follow that of the nonretarded and to differ only in the quantity of language or the length of utterances produced (Weiss, Weisz, & Bromfield, 1986). After a mental age of 10, the developmental paths seem to deviate, and the language of the two groups shows qualitative differences as well.

Such debates may turn on nonissues, given that language and cognition are not the same (Kamhi & Masterson, 1989). Nor can we assume that all aspects of language differ in a similar manner. Some areas of language and cognition overlap; others are distinct.

Studies of the language development of the retarded population suffer from a number of limitations (Kamhi & Masterson, 1989). First, the retarded population is not homogeneous and it is difficult to make generalizations. Second, results may vary with the assessment instruments used. Third, attempts to match subjects by mental age may be inappropriate given the lack of knowledge of the relationship between cognition and language.

I will attempt to examine a number of studies of language of the retarded population, threading through the mix of severity of retardation, subject matching, and level of development. The major characteristics of the language of the retarded population are listed in Table 12-3. This table is based on summarized data and on group data. Individuals or specific subgroups, especially the more severely impaired, may exhibit different behavior. Some profoundly retarded individuals will not use expressive language beyond single symbols, if at all.

TABLE 12-3   Language Characteristics of Children with Mental Retardation

Pragmatics	Gestural and intentional developmental patterns similar to those of children developing normally.
	May take less dominant conversational role.
	Poorer clarification skills than mental age-matched peers developing normally.
Semantics	More concrete word meanings.
	Slow vocabulary growth.
	More limited use of a variety of semantic units.
	Children with Down syndrome able to learn word meanings from exposure in context as well as mental age-matched peers developing normally.
Syntax/ Morphology	Length-complexity relationship similar to that of preschoolers developing normally.
	Same sequence of general sentence development as children developing normally.
	Shorter, less complex sentences with fewer subject elaborations or relative clauses than mental age-matched peers developing normally.
	Sentence word order takes precedence over word relationships.
	Reliance on less mature forms, though capable of more advanced.
	Same order of morpheme development as preschoolers developing normally.
Phonology	Phonological rules similar to those of preschoolers developing normally but reliance on less mature forms, though capable of more advanced ones.
Comprehension	Poorer receptive language skills, especially children with Down syndrome, than mental age-matched peers developing normally.
	Poorer sentence recall than mental age-matched peers.
	More reliance on context to extract meaning.

Based on Abbeduto, Davies, Solesby, & Furman (1991); Bedrosian & Prutting (1978); Bender & Carlson (1982); Bradbury & Lunzer (1972); Chapman, Kay-Raining Bird, & Schwartz (1990); Chapman, Schwartz, & Kay-Raining Bird (1988); Dever & Gardner (1970); Graham & Graham (1971); Greenwald & Leonard (1979); Ingram (1972); Kahn (1975); Kernan (1990); Klink, Gerstman, Raphael, Schlanger, & Newsome (1986); Lackner (1968); Layton & Sharifi (1979); Lobato, Barrera, & Feldman (1981); McLeavey, Toomey, & Dempsey (1982); Merrill & Bilsky (1990); Mervis (1988); Moran, Money, & Leonard (1984); Naremore & Dever (1975); Newfield (1966); Owens & MacDonald (1982); Prater (1982); Rondal, Ghiotto, Bredart, & Bachelet (1988); Rosin, Swift, Bless, & Vetter (1988); Semmel & Herzog (1966); Shriberg & Widder (1990); Vihman (1978).

Parameters of Language

Five parameters of language are generally recognized—syntax, morphology, phonology, semantics, and pragmatics. All five parameters have been examined in research studies of the language of persons who are mentally retarded.

Pragmatics.   The area of pragmatics, or language use, has generated considerable academic interest, especially in the field of retardation. Many individuals with mental retardation "are seriously and basically deficient in this area of social . . . functions" (McLean & Snyder-McLean, 1978, p. 190). Research studies have reached varying conclusions, but there is little doubt that those individuals residing in institutions for the mentally retarded demonstrate greater deficiencies in language use.

Pragmatic functions first become evident with the development of gestures. At this point, children begin to express primitive intentions, such as signaling notice, attracting attention, or making demands (Bates, Benigni, Bretherton, Camaioni, & Volterra, 1979; Dore, 1974). Both mildly and moderately retarded children with Down syndrome and nonretarded children exhibit gestures at the same level of cognitive development (Greenwald & Leonard, 1979). Both groups of children use gestures to enlist help or to gain an object and use declarative gestures to gain attention. These gestures develop in Piaget's sensorimotor Substage 4 (age 8–12 months for the nonretarded infant).

For severely retarded children, gestures do not appear until Substage 5 (Lobato, Barrera, & Feldman, 1981). The gestures of individuals with profound mental retardation primarily function to regulate behavior of others (Ogletree, Wetherby, & Westling, 1992). Initiated by the individual rather than by the conversational partner, these gestures are often performed in isolation with little vocalization.

For both the retarded and nonretarded populations, the appearance of language is strongly correlated with the cognitive functions of Substage 4 (Kahn, 1975; Lobato et al., 1981; Woodward & Stern, 1963). In general, the language of retarded and nonretarded children fulfills the functions earlier expressed in gestures. The distribution of most functions is similar for both groups of children when matched for language development level (Owens & MacDonald, 1982). Both groups of children are able to answer and to spontaneously ask questions, to reply to the comments of others, to make spontaneous declarations and demands, to name or label entities, and to imitate and spontaneously practice language.

Imitation of others and self-repetition may develop differently for individuals with Down syndrome (Owens & MacDonald, 1982; Sokolov, 1992). In general, imitation decreases for children developing normally as they begin to learn syntax. The rate of decrease is significantly less for children with Down syndrome. This difference may indicate a continued reliance on outmoded learning strategies by children with mental retardation. The child developing normally may discard inefficient strategies more readily.

At the single-word or early multiword stage, normally developing children begin to demonstrate presuppositional skills. They presuppose that their communication partners are aware of redundant or old information in a situation, and therefore label only aspects of a situation that are undergoing change or are new information. For example, the child may not name the cup on the high chair each morning but may label with the word *cup* a new cup recently received from Grandma. Toddlers with mild retardation also exhibit this behavior (Leonard, Cole, & Steckol, 1979).

Presuppositional skills may be a forerunner of several perspective-taking behaviors used in everyday communication (Ambron & Irwin, 1975), such as the ability to assume the communication partner's perceptual viewpoint in interpretation of terms such as *here* and *there* and to assess a partner's knowledge or emotional state. Mild and moderately retarded children and younger, nonretarded second graders matched for cognitive abilities exhibit similar perspective-taking behaviors (Bender & Carlson, 1982).

Other studies have reported that individuals with mental retardation are delayed in role-taking and in referential communication (Affleck, 1976; Chandler, Greenspan, & Barenboim, 1974; Hoy & McKnight, 1977; Longhurst & Berry, 1975; Volpe, 1976). These differences are not found when subjects are matched for social maturity (Blacher, 1982).

Referential communication refers to a target referent by distinguishing it from others, such as "the girl with the white dress" or "big doggie." Children with mental retardation are less able to distinguish referents for their listeners than are their MA-matched peers who are nonretarded (Brownell & Whitely, 1992). These referential skills can be taught.

Although individuals who are mentally retarded seem as adept as their MA-matched nonretarded peers in selecting the appropriate referent or subject of discussion within context, they are less skilled in requesting clarification of information when the context is uninformative (Abbeduto, Davies, Solesby, & Furman, 1991). This conclusion seems odd given the abilities of mentally retarded individuals to request clarification (Abbeduto & Rosenberg, 1980) and to use the context for referent identification (Abbeduto, Davies, & Furman, 1988). Possibly the requirements of conversation are such that the individual who is mentally retarded cannot integrate these skills when needed. An inability to seek such clarification may be critical given the report that individuals with Down syndrome have difficulty understanding sentences without a supporting extralinguistic context (Kernan, 1990).

The requirements of the conversational context may also account for the amount of verbal perseveratives found in the speech of adults with mental retardation (Rein & Kernan, 1989). Verbal perseveration is excessive talking on a topic even when inappropriate or previously addressed in the conversation. Such behavior may be used by retarded individuals to maintain the interaction or to "buy time" until they can produce a more appropriate response. The use of verbal perseveratives varies within the retarded population. Males with Fragile X syndrome have been shown to produce more perseverative, repetitive, inappropriate, and off-topic utterances than males with Down syndrome (Sudhalter, Cohen, Silverman, & Wolf-Schein, 1990; Wolf-Schein et al., 1987).

All of the preceding skills are interrelated in the conversational context. In a conversation, roles and topics change, and each partner must try to assess how much information his partner needs. In general, retarded individuals are less able to judge the nonverbal emotions of their communication partners than are MA-matched nonretarded peers, and thus are less able to respond appropriately (Marcell & Jett, 1985). The conversational role of retarded persons seems to be one of nondominance. Children with mental retardation are more likely to keep greater interpersonal distance, a possible reflection of the child's perception of little personal control (Hayes & Koch, 1977). Likewise, adults with mental retardation rarely exert dominance in a conversation even when the communication partner is a child, although these adults possess the communication skills to do so (Bedrosian & Prutting, 1978). This subservient conversational behavior is more pronounced in institutionalized populations (Prior, Minnes, Coyne, Golding, Hendy, & McGillivray, 1979) and can be noted in the case study at the end of the chapter.

Semantics.   As a group, mentally retarded individuals exhibit poorer receptive language skills than their MA-matched peers, although there are many variations among individuals (Abbeduto, Furman, & Davies, 1989). These two facts may relate to the type and severity of mental retardation, to cognitive processing, and/or to environment.

Several studies have concluded that the word meanings of the retarded population are more concrete than those of the nonretarded (Semmel & Herzog, 1966). For example, *cold* may be defined in relation to temperature but not to the psychological aspects, such as in a *cold personality.* There appears to be no difference in the quality of definition, however, as measured by the Stanford-Binet intelligence test (Papania, 1954).

Word meanings are established in a two-step process that includes a quick, general determination of meaning from the context, a process called fast mapping, and a slower evolution of meaning from use. Children with Down syndrome are as skilled as mental age-matched peers who are nonretarded in inferring novel word meanings. They are also equally skilled at producing words correctly thereafter (Chapman, Kay-Raining Bird, & Schwartz, 1990).

As might be expected, figurative language processing poses particular difficulties. Context is very important in aiding comprehension for individuals with Down syndrome (Ezell & Goldstein, 1991).

Finally, both mildly retarded individuals with Down syndrome and MA-matched nonretarded individuals display all features of verbs and noun inflections. Individuals with Down syndrome use these features less frequently (Layton and Sharifi, 1979).

Syntax.   In general, the overall sequence of development of syntactic structures is similar for the mildly retarded and the nonretarded populations; however, the rate of development is slower (Ingram, 1972; Lackner, 1968; McLeavey, Toomey, & Dempsey, 1982; Naremore & Dever, 1975). Both sentence length and complexity increase with development (Graham & Graham, 1971; Lackner, 1968). In addition, the same sentence types appear and in the same order for both groups. There is a general trend from simple declarative to negative sentences, and then interrogative to negative interrogative sentences (Lackner, 1968). Within interrogatives, the order of development is also similar (Ingram, 1972). For example, *what* and *where* types develop initially, and *when, why,* and *how* appear last.

Even at equivalent mental age levels, however, individuals with retardation appear to use shorter, less complex sentences than their nonretarded peers (McLeavey et al., 1982; Naremore & Dever, 1975). These characteristics are evident in the case study at the end of this chapter. Individuals with mild retardation use fewer complex structures, such as subject elaborations and relative clauses (Naremore & Dever, 1975). These deficiencies may reflect poorer linguistic rule generalization. Poor rule generalization does not imply an inability to learn language rules, although retarded persons seem to rely more on sequential placement than on grammatical rules (Semmel, 1967). In other words, sentence word order takes precedence over the relationships between different word classes. The result is less flexible linguistic structure. Other studies have concluded that "the types of deviations . . . suggest that mildly retarded children are rule-oriented in their approach to language" (McLeavey et al., 1982, p. 492). Even individuals with severe retardation are capable of using linguistic rules (Graham & Graham, 1971). Taken together, these findings suggest that persons with retardation learn and use linguistic rules but also rely more on primitive word-order rules than do their nonretarded language peers.

One measure of sentence complexity for initial sentence development is mean length of utterance (MLU). For both Down syndrome and nonretarded children, MLU correlates strongly with chronological age and predicts complexity and diversity of sentence development (Rondal, Ghiotto, Bredart, & Bachelet, 1988). MLU appears to be a good measure of complexity to an average of 3.5 morphemes for both groups.

Any syntactic lag noted among retarded persons may represent a dependence upon older syntactic forms for a longer time (McLeavey et al., 1982). Advanced syntactic forms are learned but used less frequently.

Finally, individuals with mental retardation exhibit poorer recall of sentences than their MA-matched peers (Merrill & Bilsky, 1990). Within the mentally retarded population, males with Fragile X syndrome appear to have more difficulty with auditory sequential memory and auditory reception than males with Down syndrome (Hagerman, Kemper, &, Hudson, 1985). This poorer performance may reflect poorer quality mental representations of the sentences to be recalled or an inability to encode the significant semantic information for a holistic, integrated memory (Merrill & Mar, 1987). Although individuals with Down syndrome seem to have recall patterns similar to those of nonretarded individuals, they have greater difficulty when there is no supporting extralinguistic context (Kernan, 1990).

Sentence recall and context utilization for individuals with mental retardation can be enhanced when the semantic relatedness of the words in a sentence is increased (Merrill & Jackson, 1992). For example, the sentence "The hunter shot the rabbit" has more relatedness across the words "The photographer chased the rabbit" and is thus easier to recall.

Morphology.   Several studies have assessed the morphological development of retarded individuals, using the Test of Children's Learning of English Morphology (Berko, 1958). This test uses nonsense words to evaluate the child's morphological skills. In general, children who are retarded performed in a manner similar to nonretarded MA-matched peers, with some minor differences (Bradbury & Lunzer, 1972; Dever & Gardner, 1970; Newfield & Schlanger, 1968).

In developmental studies, the same order of morphological acquisition has been reported for both the retarded and the nonretarded populations (Johnston & Schery, 1976; Newfield, 1966). Again the pattern of development seems to be delayed, even beyond what one might expect for mental age, but not significantly different.

Phonology.   Individuals with profound retardation vocalize less when gesturing than do individuals developing normally. These vocalizations are often nontranscribable or lacking consonants (Ogletree, Wetherby, & Westling, 1992). Infants with Down syndrome and less severe retardation babble in a fashion similar to that of chronological age-matched peers who are developing normally (Steffens, Kimbrough, Oller, Lynch, & Urbano, 1992). Over time, both groups of children produce more mature vowels and more well-formed syllables, and fewer quasi-vowel sounds and fewer marginal syllables.

The phonological characteristics of the mentally retarded population can be summarized as follows (Shriberg & Widder, 1990):

1. Articulation errors are more common than in the nonretarded population.
2. Most frequent error is deletion of consonants.
3. Errors are likely to be inconsistent.
4. Patterns are similar to those of nonretarded children or children with a functional delay.
5. Individuals with Down syndrome have perceptually and acoustically distinct prosody.

The types of errors and the level of mental retardation do not seem to be related.

A number of researchers have studied the articulation deficiencies of the mentally retarded population (Bangs, 1961; Schiefelbusch, 1963; Spradlin, 1963; Wolfensberger, Mein, & O'Connor, 1963). In general, they demonstrated that a majority of institutionalized and/or severely retarded persons exhibit articulation disorders (Yoder & Miller, 1972). Articulation, or the production of speech sounds, is not the same as the rules for sound combinations, called phonology.

In general, individuals who are mentally retarded use the same phonological processes as nonretarded children but with greater frequency (Klink, Gerstman, Raphael, Schlanger, & Newsome, 1986; Moran, Money, & Leonard, 1984). The most common phonological processes exhibited by the mentally retarded population are reduction of consonant clusters and final consonant deletion (Klink et al., 1986; Bleile & Schwartz, 1984; Oller & Seibert, 1988; Sommers, Patterson, & Wildgren, 1988; Van Borsel, 1988). When a nonretarded child cannot produce two consonants together (e.g., *stop*), the child deletes one consonant to produce a simpler version, (e.g., *top*). Final consonant deletion is usually the result of consonant-vowel (CV) syllable learning. In this process, words consist of CV or CVCV constructions. Because final consonants, such as a CVC construction, violate this process, the child may delete the final consonant. Individuals with mental retardation may exhibit much variability in their use of these processes.

Other processes are the same as those of younger, nonretarded children (Prater, 1982). Mentally retarded individuals may use these processes even when they are capable of producing the deleted or modified sound. It is possible, therefore, that these processes serve a different purpose for the retarded population than for the nonretarded (Vihman, 1978). For example, consonant deletions may reflect cognitive processing constraints in the motor assembly stage of speech production (Shriberg & Widder, 1990).

Prosody includes voice quality, phrasing, rate, and stress. Error in this area may reflect deficits in pragmatic knowledge and a lack of monitoring during conversation.

Summary.   Studies of the language of the mentally retarded population offer varying, sometimes conflicting, results. In general, however, the language abilities of retarded persons are similar to those of mental-age-matched nonretarded peers, although some differences do exist.

Several studies have indicated that language abilities among individuals with mental retardation are delayed beyond expectations based upon mental age alone, although the course of development is similar for retarded and nonretarded persons. This language delay, particularly evident among individuals with Down syndrome (Greenwald & Leonard, 1979; Mahoney, Glover, & Finger, 1981; Ryan, 1975; Share, 1975; Snyder, 1978), becomes evident soon after language acquisition begins, as the level of vocabulary development begins to lag behind cognitive development (Cardosa-Martins, Mervis, & Mervis, 1985).

Any reported differences may reflect symbol processing deficiencies within the retarded population. Therefore, in language therapy, "it seems more defensible to teach individuals how to learn, and this implies the training of underlying processes" (Ashman, 1982, p. 636).

Environmental Influences on the Language of Individuals with Mental Retardation

Individuals with mental retardation are generally found in two types of environments: home-centered or residential. The different environmental influences upon learning have been well documented (Conroy, Efthimiou, & Lemanowicz, 1982). In general, mentally retarded individuals who live in institutions have fewer adaptive skills and are more dependent. Both language and communication are adaptive behaviors. Some aspects of language may be affected differently by institutionalization (McNutt & Leri, 1979; Montague, Hutchinson, & Matson, 1975). For example, "The grammatical structure of language is apparently less affected by environment than are semantic or auditory elements" (McNutt & Leri, 1979, p. 344). In general, there is a deterioration of language abilities with extended institutionalization (Phillips & Balthazar, 1979). The adult described at the end of this chapter exhibits few conversational initiations. Her verbal behavior is mostly responsive.

Parent–Child Interaction.   Is there some special feature of the language-learning home environment of retarded children that can account for the mental age-language age gap? One theory contends that if retarded infants behave differently from nonretarded infants, the mothers of each group must respond to their infants differently. According to this theory, mother-child interaction patterns can adversely affect a child's language development.

The importance of early mother-child interaction has been increasingly recognized (Bruner, 1974–1975, 1977; Bullowa, 1979; Snow & Ferguson, 1977). Normally developing children have an established repertoire of communication skills before they speak their first words. These words usually fulfill the communicative functions already in place. The infant's communication skills develop within the interaction of mother and child (Owens, 1996).

The stress that accompanies the birth of an infant with a disability may alter the dynamics of family relations. There is an initial period of grief before a more normal relationship evolves. The sense of grief may be compounded by feelings of estrangement from an infant whose communication skills do not fulfill parental expectations (Frailberg, 1979).

Because the interactional process is one of mutual adaptation by the two partners, some researchers assume that a child with retardation will alter the mother's behavior differently than will a nonretarded infant. In addition, infants with Down syndrome may allow less time for maternal turn-taking and use less referential eye contact (Jones, 1977). Consequently, "this reduction in the quality of the dialogue of emotional expression may result in parents being less effective with such children" (Trotter, 1983, p. 20). Mothers whose children are mentally retarded must contend with ambiguous parent-child social norms and with inconsistent child behaviors (Eheart, 1982; Osofsky & O'Connell, 1972; Wolfensberger, 1967; Zigler, 1971). The situation is made more acute by a lack of information on and assistance with development (White, Watts, Barnett, Kaban, Marmor, &

Shapiro, 1973), by feelings of grief and guilt (Klaus & Kennell, 1976), and by fear of an unknown future (Kearsley, 1979). Several studies have attempted to assess the degree of modification in the interactions of mothers with their retarded children and the results of this modification.

Among children who are language delayed but who exhibit no other disability, professionals have assumed that maternal or family language patterns are a contributing factor (Bee, Van Egeren, Streissguth, Nyman, & Leckie, 1969; Brophy, 1970; Emery & Ramey, 1976). For example, mothers of language-delayed children reportedly use more directives (Cardosa-Martins, Mervis, & Mervis, 1985; Hanzlik & Stevenson, 1986; Hess & Shipman, 1965), provide fewer opportunities for their children to use language (Jones, 1972), use less referential or object-directed speech (Cardosa-Martins et al., 1985), and are less verbally responsive (Hanzlik & Stevenson, 1986; Wulbert, Inglis, Kreigsmann, & Mills, 1975). Although this maternal behavior is found in some language delay cases, it cannot be assumed that this pattern represents general maternal interaction with language delayed children who are mentally retarded.

Several researchers have studied the interaction in free-play situations between mothers and their children with Down syndrome and between mothers and their nonretarded children. Mothers of preschool children with Down syndrome and MA-matched nonretarded children both use control to support and encourage their children's play (Tannock, 1988). As a group, the mothers of the children with Down syndrome have been found to exert more verbal control, whereas the mothers of the nonretarded children are more likely to watch quietly (Tannock, 1988). The mothers of children with Down syndrome talk more to their children (Berger & Cunningham, 1983). They have been reported to initiate more topics, repeat more utterances, and take more turns (Maurer & Sherrod, 1987). In general, the children with Down syndrome are more passive and do not respond in turn as frequently. Both groups of mothers are equally responsive to their children's verbalizations.

In teaching situations, both groups of mothers have been found to be equally directive (Rondal, 1978). Possibly the mothers of Down syndrome children perceive their role as instructional, aware of their children's language learning difficulties (Davis, Stroud, & Green, 1988).

The patterns of directives used by mothers of retarded and nonretarded children are similar in their hierarchy of change over time, although the mothers of children with Down syndrome demonstrate more reluctance to change to more mature patterns such as indirect requests (Maurer & Sherrod, 1987).

In general, more active and less irritable infants receive optimum maternal responsiveness (Rheingold & Eckerman, 1975; Stevenson & Lamb, 1979). Mothers act according to their expectations of the infants' behavior and attempt to keep their infants within these expectations. Infants with Down syndrome or early medical disorders exhibit rather inactive behavior (Connor, Williamson, & Siepp, 1978; Field, 1979). Infants in intensive care nurseries are reported to have high irritability (Duhammel, Lin, Skelton, & Hantke, 1974). It might be expected, therefore, that mothers of these children would be less responsive than mothers of nondisordered infants and that lack of maternal responsiveness might result in the infant's withdrawal. However, further research is needed in this area.

Predictable and responsive infants participate more in the parent-infant interactional environment (Goldberg, 1977). At-risk infants are less predictable and less responsive

(Affleck, Allen, McGrade, & McQueeney, 1982). Nevertheless, research does not support the conclusion that mothers of mentally retarded infants are more restrictive of the infants activities and less responsive. In fact, mothers of infants with mental retardation interpret more of their children's behaviors as communicative than do mothers of nonretarded children (Yoder & Feagans, 1988). It is the mothers' attribution of meaning to the child's behavior, not just the behavior itself, that affects the mothers' responses (Harding, 1984).

In studies of the mothers of retarded children and chronological-age-matched (CA-matched) nonretarded children, the mothers of retarded children have been found to use more "primitive" forms of speech (Buium, Rynders, & Turnure, 1974; Kogan, Wimberger, & Bobbitt, 1969; Marshall, Hegrenes, & Goldstein, 1973). The unwarranted conclusion has been that these mothers are inhibiting their children's growth. We would expect children with retardation to function at a lower cognitive and language level than chronological peers. The real concern should be the appropriateness of this maternal input for the linguistic competence of the child.

Mothers of children with Down syndrome alter their linguistic input appropriately for the language level of their children. Research has shown no significant difference between the mothers of children with Down syndrome and mothers of nonretarded children in both verbal and nonverbal behaviors (Buckhalt, Rutherford, & Goldberg, 1978; Cardosa-Martins & Mervis, 1990; Rondal, 1976). As discussed in earlier chapters, mothers use motherese, a style of speaking that is characterized by short sentences, redundancy, long pauses, gesturing, and exaggerated intonation and stress patterns.

In addition, mothers of Down syndrome and nonretarded children have been found to use similar response classes (Skinner, 1957) with a few exceptions (Gutmann & Rondal, 1979). Mothers of nonretarded children use more whole and partial repetitions, as do their children. In contrast, retarded children and their mothers have been reported to use more comments and replies. In both groups, repetitions decrease and comments and replies increase with the children's increasing language abilities. In part, the more conversational style of the mothers with their retarded children may reflect the older age of these children compared to the nonretarded subjects.

Other changes accompany children's changing abilities (Petersen & Sherrod, 1982). With retarded, language delayed, and nonretarded children, mothers use language more prominently in interactions as their children's language progresses. Requests for nonverbal behavior decrease, and language-seeking utterances and verbal feedback increase. Language-seeking utterances consist of questions, requests for elaboration, labeling, and imitation. Both negative and positive feedback increase with children's increasing language abilities as mothers become more discriminating and more demanding (Petersen & Sherrod, 1982).

There are differences among these groups of mothers, however. Some researchers report a lack of rapport on the part of mothers of children with language delays and mothers of children with Down syndrome (Petersen & Sherrod, 1982). In addition, mothers of retarded children dominate the parent-child interaction more than mothers of CA-matched nonretarded children (Eheart, 1982). Mothers of retarded children are more directive and initiate interactions more frequently (Seitz & Riedel, 1974). For example, mothers of children with Down syndrome require their children to imitate more. The continued use of verbal imitation by children with Down syndrome long after such a language learning strategy has ceased to be a viable learning technique has been noted (Owens & MacDonald, 1982). If mothers foster imitation beyond a language age of approximately 30 months, it could negatively affect language development (Petersen & Sherrod, 1982). In addition, the utterances of mothers of children with mental retardation may be more noncontingent or more off-topic than those of mothers of nonretarded children (Mahoney, Fors, & Wood, 1990). These mothers incorporate fewer of their children's topics than do mothers of nonretarded children (Miller & Newhoff, 1978). Thus, the child may lack the vital extralinguistic and linguistic context needed for interpretation.

Children with mental retardation respond less frequently to their mothers' initiations (Eheart, 1982). In addition, the children initiate communication only half as often as nonretarded children. In part, this behavior may reflect the larger ratio of adult to child utterances found within these dyads (Giattinno, Pollack, & Silliman, 1978).

Staff-Client Interaction.   Several studies have reported on the lack of appropriate verbal interactions within residential settings (Prior et al., 1979; Tizard, Cooperman, Joseph, & Tizard, 1973). Tizard and colleagues found a large percentage of directives were used by the institutional staff. Such behavior is unlikely to elicit much verbal interchange. In fact, Prior and colleagues reported that mentally retarded clients were least responsive following staff directives, the most frequent staff verbal behavior. In contrast, the least frequent behavior, staff-initiated conversation, elicited the most client verbal responses. When clients did verbalize, staff personnel were equally likely to ignore the behavior as to respond with a verbal comment or reply. The most frequent staff behavior was a nonverbal agreement in the form of a head nod. Even though clients responded very little to staff instructions, such communication does provide language input. Yet, for most of the day, clients are left alone in unstructured settings. Prior and colleagues concluded that "there are features of the institutional environment which mitigate against the development of verbal communicative competence in mentally retarded persons" (p. 68).

Residence in a developmental center or community residence is likely to have its greatest effect on pragmatics. Individuals who reside in community residences are more likely to use their pragmatic skills (Van Der Gagg, 1989).

Summary.   The preceding studies indicate that, in general, individuals who are mentally retarded receive better linguistic input and more conversational opportunities within a home environment. The mother-child data are mixed, however, suggesting that although mothers adapt form and content to the linguistic competence of their retarded children, these same mothers provide primarily a responsive verbal environment. Thus, children with mental retardation initiate less communication than their nonretarded peers. After examining maternal language use, Eheart (1982) concluded that "many of the maternal skills that are important for fostering the development of social adaptability in children are less frequently demonstrated by mothers of retarded children than by mothers of nonretarded children" (p. 24).

We cannot assume, however, that differences indicate a cause for language delay. As Bellinger (1980) noted, "While many studies indicate that the language produced by mothers of language-delayed or impaired children differs from that of mothers whose children are progressing normally . . . , we cannot be sure that the atypicality of this speech is not a response to the children's language problems rather than their cause" (p. 485). Even if mothers of retarded children did provide linguistic form, content, and use styles similar to those of mothers of nonretarded children, it might not be appropriate for the special language learning needs of their retarded children.

Language and Communication Intervention

Many of the language and communication intervention techniques discussed in this text for use with other language disordered populations can also be used with retarded individuals. Some intervention methods, however, seem particularly germane for persons with mental retardation.

Our knowledge of the cognitive functioning and language processes of the mentally retarded population, although limited, suggests some principles and techniques for intervention. I will discuss these globally and then specifically address different aspects of language assessment and intervention. The breadth of this topic and the discussion of and intervention in other chapters will allow for only general discussion of the topic.

Principles of Assessment and Intervention

The characteristics of the mentally retarded population suggest some guiding principles for speech-language pathologists. Of necessity, these principles will be general. The speech-language pathologist must remember that each mentally retarded person is an individual and that individual differences such as age, level of cognitive functioning, previous training, residential environment, and learning style will alter the methods actually used. The principles are summarized in Table 12-4.

Language and Communication Intervention Methodologies

In general, training goals should be explicit with the information organized for easy learning and recall. For example, direct teaching of vocabulary words seems to be superior to more indirect training (Hanley-Maxwell, Wilcox, & Heal, 1982).

TABLE 12-4   Principles for Intervention with Clients Who Are Mentally Retarded

---

1. Highlight new or relevant material.
2. Preorganize information.
3. Train rehearsal strategies.
4. Use overlearning and repetition.
5. Train in the natural environment.
6. Begin as early as possible.
7. Follow developmental guidelines.

The clinician should consider the skills that the client brings to the task and those skills required for successful learning. To require too much in the form of new learning or transfer often hinders the client's ability to be successful. A question-probe technique can foster comprehension and help individuals with mental retardation to assess the learning that they bring to a new situation (Zetlin & Gallimore, 1983). In this technique, newly learned skills are questioned and probed continually as they are learned to ensure understanding by the client.

Some structured training is usually necessary for initial learning, and repetition of initial procedures may aid further learning of the targeted skill. It may even facilitate learning if the material is presented in the same order until a certain criterion of performance is reached.

Transfer can be facilitated by keeping the training situation as close to the everyday environment as possible. The clever clinician will use objects, persons, and events from this environment for training.

The developmental model of language intervention also works well with the individuals who are mentally retarded. Theoretically, the easiest structures are learned first by nonretarded children and, therefore, are targeted first for the retarded client.

Highlight New or Relevant Material.   Individuals who are mentally retarded are capable of attending well when they understand what they should attend to. New information, materials, or methods should be highlighted so that the client does not miss them or assume that they are unimportant. For example, new pictures on a communication board might be drawn in a different color or placed in a special area of the board. Stimuli that require certain responses or language features that govern language use should also be highlighted. For example, words such as *yesterday* and *last week* signal use of past tense. The waiter's utterance "What may I get for you?" signals an ordering response.

Attending need not be directly targeted for intervention. Improved attending has been reported as a result of augmentative communication training with severely retarded institutionalized children and adults (Abrahamsen, Romski, & Sevcik, 1989).

Generalization is enhanced by a related principle: *Train scanning of a task for relevant or similar stimuli.* Generalization is often difficult for mentally retarded individuals because they are unsure of which stimuli are relevant.

Preorganize Information.   Teachers can aid learning by pregrouping information to facilitate organization and later recall. Organization strategies such as physical conceptual arrangement, grouping, and consistent ordering can also be taught (Burger, Blackman, Holmes, & Zetlin, 1978; Evans & Bilsky, 1979; Glidden, 1977; Taylor & Turnure, 1979).

In general, persons who are mentally retarded are able to retain information better if it is organized first, and if the learning task is explained by the teacher. Mildly retarded individuals have better recall if material is grouped spatially rather than presented singly (Harris, 1982; MacMillan, 1972; Spitz, 1966). For example, a mildly retarded adult who is experiencing difficulty recalling four digits, such as 6–3–8–5, may do better if the digits are grouped in pairs to form 63 and 85. Such grouping does not seem to aid the recall of nonretarded individuals, possibly because they already employ this strategy. In conclusion, instructions and procedures should be clear, logically sequenced, and involve as many senses as possible (Pruess, Vadasy, & Fewell, 1987).

Train Rehearsal Strategies.   Mildly and moderately retarded individuals can improve their memory abilities through the training of rehearsal strategies (Brown, 1974; Burger, Blackman, & Tan, 1980; Engle & Nagle, 1979; Reid, 1980). Such rehearsal aids the transfer of learned material to long-term storage. This may be especially true for visual information such as communicative signs or gestures, the learning of which enhances associated word recall (Bowler, 1991).

Use Overlearning and Repetition.   Although rehearsal or extra training facilitates learning and recall, it does not seem to directly enhance transfer (Day & Hall, 1988). Those who receive extra training, however, subsequently need less assistance with transfer.

Train in the Natural Environment.   Although highly structured training may increase the rate of learning, especially for severely retarded individuals, such training "may well be limited to that context" (Salzberg & Villani, 1983, p. 403). In short, "it appears easier to 'establish' a rudimentary language repertoire in language-deficient children than it is to teach the spontaneous use of skills in untrained situations" (Guess, Koegh, and Sailor, 1978, p. 375). Highly structured settings offer a limited variety of communication situations. Accordingly, "the problem is how to incorporate procedures into the initial training that will actively induce generalization" (Spradlin & Siegel, 1982, p. 3). It should be recalled that individuals with mental retardation have great difficulty generalizing training to novel contexts.

Looney (1980) noted that "many teachers view language as a 45-minute period or lesson . . . yet language is an integral part of any interpersonal communication and is best learned in the natural context of those daily interactions" (p. 31). We can expect little generalization with pictures or with objects not within the natural environment (Simic & Bucher, 1980; Welch & Pear, 1979). The typically limited stimuli used in the classroom or clinic often have little relation to the natural environment. In other words, difficulties in generalization can be minimized if training occurs using familiar materials within daily activities occurring in everyday locations of the client (Gullo & Gullo, 1984; McCormick, 1986; Stowitschek, McConaughy, Peatross, Salzberg, & Lignngaris/Kraft, 1988). Most communication training approaches for moderately to severely mentally retarded individuals advocate use of the natural environment (Caro & Snell, 1989).

Language training is more functional if taught in the situations where there is actually a need for language to be used. The general result is more spontaneous usage, which in turn motivates the individual to learn more language (Rees, 1978). Wulz, Hall, and Klein (1983) concluded:

> *One of the reasons so little spontaneity has been observed with this population is that the training has not been functional. Functional training employs stimuli, responses, and consequences which are similar to those in the target environment. (p. 3)*

Natural stimuli present in the training environment become "signals" associated with the behavior trained.

Everyday routines also provide an excellent vehicle for training and facilitate generalization. Routines provide a familiar script or scaffolding that enables the client to participate more fully by freeing cognitive energy that might otherwise be used to aid participation. Children with mental retardation seem to produce more speech and more diverse vocabulary in routine situations than in other less familiar situations (Yoder & Davies, 1992).

People within the natural environment, such as parents, teachers, and aids, should be included in the training as language trainers and as clients themselves (MacDonald, Blott, Gordon, Spiegal, & Hartmann, 1974; Owens, 1982d, 1995). Further, greater involvement yields greater results: "The more parents are involved with the children's training, the more likely is the children's functioning to generalize to the home and other settings" (Miller & Miller, 1973, p. 84).

The effective use of parents as behavior change agents is well established (Baker, 1976; Heifetz, 1980). Infant stimulation programs conducted in the home by trained parents can significantly improve the functioning of retarded children (Sharav & Shlomo, 1986). Several parent variables can affect the outcome. Parent socioeconomic status, pretraining skills, and experience positively correlate with the short-term learning outcomes (Clark, Baker, & Heifetz, 1982). The relationship may explain why parent training programs traditionally neglect low socioeconomic families (Hargis & Blechman, 1979). It is my experience, however, that lower-class mothers can make positive strides with their children, because prior to training, these mothers often overlook natural teaching situations used by middle- and upper-class mothers. The successful use of higher functioning institutionalized individuals as language trainers for more severely retarded clients has also been reported (Snell, 1979). The key to success with language trainers is consideration of individual trainer differences and learning styles, and individualization of the techniques that these trainers use (Reese & Serna, 1986).

In a study with the parents of Down syndrome children, mothers assumed a manager or teacher role more often and were more responsive than fathers (Stoneman, Brody, & Abbott, 1983). Parents with some instruction were able to modify their speech to their retarded children in order to improve the children's expressive skills (Cheseldine & McConkey, 1979). Apparently, knowledge of the direction in which training should proceed is sufficient information to allow some parents spontaneously to adopt suitable teaching strategies.

The variables that control transfer of parental skills to natural settings are not fully understood (Forehand & Atkeson, 1977). Transfer increases with the similarity of the tasks and of training structure to the natural environment (Mindell & Budd, 1977; Miller & Sloan, 1976; Salzberg & Villani, 1983). Feedback from the speech-language pathologist regarding the application of newly acquired training skills is also important (Polk, Schilmoeller, Embry, Holman, & Baer, 1976; Salzberg & Villani, 1983).

Successful use of parents as language facilitators seems to depend upon three components (Salzberg & Villani, 1983). Parents must be asked to use their training skills at home, they must be specifically taught to adapt training techniques to these more informal situations, and they need to receive professional feedback.

Interactive models that train parents in general interactive strategies may result in parents becoming more responsive, less directive, and better able to model language, even months after parent training has ceased, but may have little effect on their children's development (Tannock, Girolametto, & Siegel, 1992). General strategies may result in achievement of general goals such as increased vocal turn taking, but specific skills training is needed by parents if more specific learning is expected.

The present child-parent or client-caregiver interactional pattern while nurturing may be insufficient for training. These interactions can be systematically modified. Thus, "a major task in parent training is to demonstrate to parents that, since they are the children's major language teachers, they can become more effective by incorporating language training principles in their natural interactions with their children" (MacDonald et al., 1974, p. 411). There is still no assurance that the new interactional patterns will be used in the home. Several suggestions are offered in Table 12-5 for facilitating language development in both clinical and more natural settings. Although "parents can readily acquire skills that allow them to be more effective educators of their handicapped children; . . . effective parent training requires that parental skills be evident in circumstances beyond those in which they were initially acquired" (Salzburg & Villani, 1983, p. 412). There is often little or no generalization from the structured training mode to free-play situations in the home.

Generalization doesn't just happen. The environment must be modified systematically to increase the likelihood of generalization. The skilled speech-language pathologist can train other language facilitators to use client content and developmental units in various settings and with various reinforcement conditions.

Initial Communication and Language Training

For many individuals who are mentally retarded, training begins at a presymbolic or early symbolic level. Many young retarded children will participate in infant stimulation or preschool programs. Often nonspeaking, profoundly retarded adults may also be trained at this level.

Begin as Early as Possible. Training should begin as soon as it is recognized that the child may be at risk (Mahoney & Snow, 1983). Speech-language pathologists can work with caregivers to help them fine-tune the infant-caregiver interaction to better facilitate language learning.

TABLE 12-5   Suggestions for Facilitating Language Generalization

In the natural environment:
1. Arrange environment to accomplish with language what cannot be accomplished easily in other ways.
2. Delay reinforcement and provide cues when appropriate verbal response is obvious.
3. Be responsive to communication attempts.
4. Restructure environment to create opportunities for a particular response to occur.

In the language training environment:
1. Teach language skills generalizable outside of the clinic.
2. Vary the contexts, trainers, and training materials.
3. Use the consequences that are varied and related to language use being taught.
4. Reduce density of reinforcement as performance improves.

Adapted from Spradlin and Siegel (1982).

Follow Developmental Guidelines.   There are three tenets to a normative developmental model (Haring & Bricker, 1976). First, development or change follows a developmental hierarchy. Children use single-word verbalizations, then short, multiword utterances. Second, behavioral change goes from simple to complex. Short word-order rules appear before complex syntactic systems. Finally, complex behavior results from coordination or modification of simpler responses. Thus, localization to sound is presumed to result from a coordination of less complex visual and auditory skills. It is assumed that behaviors observed in normal development can serve as a basis for training with disordered populations, especially individuals with mental retardation. Many training tools designed for the retarded population are based upon these tenets.

Professional caregivers or parents cannot teach all of the complex behaviors found among humans. Therefore, these individuals must determine which behaviors to target. Because development is rarely linear, educators must also determine the sequence of trained skills. "These two decisions are crucial considering that not all stages and sequences of normative development must be slavishly followed" (Switsky, Rotatori, Miller, & Freagon, 1979, p. 169) and that any intervention must consider the individual needs of the client.

Selection of appropriate training targets is critical. It cannot be assumed that all behaviors of the nonretarded child will be appropriate for the retarded child. Selection of content for training should be based in part upon *ecological validity* and *ultimate functioning* (Brooks & Baumeister, 1977). In other words, language training should reflect the expected functioning level and future use environment of the client.

A stage approach of language intervention specifies syntactic, morphological, phonological, semantic, and pragmatic targets to be trained at each stage (Prutting, 1979). The basic premise of this approach is that there are identifiable language features across all aspects of language that develop at about the same time. Although this may be somewhat true in initial language development, the validity of this approach may decline with increasing chronological age.

Normative development sequences probably cannot provide programming content, at least in a direct manner (Hogg, 1975). For example, nonretarded children often use the regular past ending with irregular verbs. To teach such use to retarded children might confuse them when later they are required to learn irregular past tense. Instead, "developmental language profiles should . . . serve as a guide for the emphasis of certain structures and, perhaps, the avoidance of others" (Winitz, 1983, p. 33). The clinician should be free to adapt developmental guidelines to the particular learning characteristics of each child. Thus, a developmental sequence might be modified based upon some sound educational rationale.

Overall Model.   In communication intervention with nonspeaking clients, clinicians often use a dual approach with major emphasis on establishing an initial communication system and secondary emphasis on training presymbolic skills (Figure 12-3). These two paths merge when the client begins to use symbols. Clients who do not reach this point still have a communication system even if it is limited to gestures or a generalized "request" signal.

Assessment.   The goal of assessment is to identify the client's communication behaviors and to identify the contexts, times, and individuals that affect the client's communication (Mahoney & Weller, 1980). It is assumed that all individuals communicate, that each communication occurrence offers an opportunity for reciprocity, and that the behaviors of

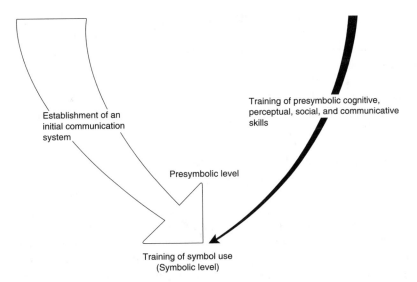

The primary presymbolic approach establishes an initial communication system, whereas the secondary approach teaches skills believed essential to symbol use. These two approaches join at the symbolic level in which the child is taught to use symbols within the context of the previously established communication system.

FIGURE 12-3   Dual intervention approach with presymbolic children.

(From R. Owens, *Language Disorders, a Functional Approach to Assessment and Intervention.* Reprinted with permission of Merrill, an imprint of Macmillan Publishing Company. Copyright © 1991 by Macmillan Publishing Company.)

each communication partner affect the other (MacDonald, 1985). In addition, the speech-language pathologist is interested in the level of presymbolic functioning and the content of communication.

For presymbolic clients, it is essential that background data be integrated with observational and testing data to form an overall image of communication characteristics. Initial information can be gathered by observation and then supplemented through interviews with the client's caregivers. The speech-language pathologist should attempt to obtain information about the following (Calculator, 1988; MacDonald, 1978; Owens & Rogerson, 1988):

1. How does the client communicate primarily?
2. Does the client demonstrate any turn-taking behaviors?
3. What situations seem to be high-communication contexts?
4. What high-interest items does the client have?
5. Do caregivers provide enough time for the client to respond? How do caregivers cue the client to respond? How do they evaluate responses?
6. Which caregivers seem to elicit the most client responses? Why?
7. Does the client seem to enjoy making sounds? Give examples. How often does the client vocalize? Which situations elicit maximum vocalization? Imitated vocalizations?

8. Which daily situations result in the most client-caregiver interaction? Describe these interactions. When do these occur daily? Are the client's responses consistent?

9. Does the client ever initiate communication? How? In what situations?

10. Does the client—

Make wants known? How?

Request help? How?

Point to things, name them, or both? Does the client look at the object and/or partner while pointing or naming?

Ask questions or seek information? How?

Indicate emotions (pain, happiness, like/dislike)? How?

Seek attention? How? What happens if attention doesn't follow?

This general information can be supplemented by specific questions related to the functioning level of the client. Several language assessment tools are available for this purpose, as listed in Table 12-6. Tests are grouped by the ages for which they are most appropriate. It is inappropriate to use an assessment tool design for infants with adults even when these adults are functioning at a presymbolic level. Infants and adults are very different and their presymbolic behaviors are manifested in very different ways. In addition, individuals with developmental delays may not exhibit strong behavioral stages found in children developing normally (Kangas & Lloyd, 1988).

The *Ages and Stages Questionnaires (ASQ)* (Bricker, Squires , & Mounts, 1995), *Caregiver Interview and Environmental Observation* (Owens, 1982a), *Infant Scale of Communication Intent* (Sacks & Young, 1982), *MacArthur Communicative Development Inventories* (Fenson, Dale, et al., 1993), Oliver (MacDonald, 1978), and *Receptive Expressive Emergent Language Scale* (REEL) (Bzock & League, 1978) are primarily questionnaire or interview format. The REEL, designed for children functioning between ages 0 and 36 months, and Infant Scale, 0–18 months, attempt to establish an approximate functional developmental age from a range of questions about communicative behaviors. *Ages and Stages* goes beyond communication to ask questions about motor, social, and problem-solving behaviors as well. The MacArthur Infant and Toddler scales ask caregivers to check gestures, words, and phrases comprehended and produced by the child. Data from such parental reports compares favorably to clinical data (Miller, Sedey, & Miolo, 1995). The Oliver uses a questionnaire format complemented by caregiver recall and actual eliciting of specific presymbolic behaviors. The *Caregiver Interview and Environmental Observation* also includes observation by the speech-language pathologist of specific communicative behavior.

The speech-language pathologist's goal is to obtain an estimate of client functioning in order to provide a more thorough assessment. In addition, such probing familiarizes the caregiver with the behaviors to be tested and taught. This familiarization is vital if caregivers are to become fully participating members in the intervention process. These tools are best used as guides for describing the client's behavior; the goal should not be to fix a developmental age.

Clients should also be observed by the caregiver and/or speech-pathologist to verify information from questionnaires and interviews and to enhance the validity of the overall assessment. Of interest are the methods used by the client to communicate and the contexts in which these behaviors occur, The *Birth to Three Developmental Scales* (Bangs & Dod-

TABLE 12-6   Assessment Proticols for Clients Functioning below Three Years

Assessment Tool	Infant–Preschool	School age–Adult
Ages and Stages Questionnaires (ASQ): A Parent-Completed Child-Monitoring System. Bricker, D., Squires, J., & Mounts, L. (1995).	X	
Assessing Linguistic Behavior (ALB). Olswang, L., Stoel-Gammon, C., Coggins, T., & Carpenter, R. (1987a).	X	
Assessment, Evaluation, and Programming Systems: AEPS Measurement for Birth to Three Years (Volume 1). Bricker, D. (1993).	X	
Birth to Three Developmental Scales. Bangs, T., & Dodson, S. (1979).	X	
Callier-Azusa Scale. Stillman, R. (1978).	X	X
Caregiver Interview and Environmental Observation. Owens, R. (1982a).	X	X
Carolina Curriculum for Infants and Toddlers with Special Needs. Johnson-Martin, N., Jens, K, Attermeier, S., & Hacker, B. (1991).	X	
A Clinical and Educational Manual for Use With the Uzgris and Hunt Scales of Infant Psychological Development. Dunst, C. (1980).	X	X
Communication and Symbolic Behavior Scales. Wetherby, A., & Prizant, B. (1993).	X	X
Comprehension of Social-Action Games in Prelinguistic Children: Levels of Participation and Effect of Adult Structure. Platt, J. & Coggins, T. (1990).	X	
Developmental Activities Screening Inventory. Fewell, R., & Langley, M. (1984).	X	
Developmental Assessment Tool. Owens, R. (1982b).	X	X
Developmental Communication Curriculum Inventory. Hanna, R., Lippert, E., & Harris, A. (1982).	X	
Diagnostic Interactional Survey. Owens, R. (1982c).	X	
Early Language Milestone Scale. Coplan, J. (1987).	X	
Environmental Communication System (ECO) MacDonald, J., and Gillette, Y. (1978).	X	
Environmental Language Inventory. MacDonald, J. (1978a).	X	X
Environmental Prelanguage Battery. Horstmeier, D., & MacDonald, J. (1978).	X	X
Evaluating Acquired Skills In Communication. Riley, A. (1984).	X	X
Family Administered Neonatal Activities. Cardone, I., & Gilkerson, L. (1989).	X	
Infant-Toddler Language Scale. Rossetti, L. (1990).	X	
Language Development Survey. Rescorla, L. (1989).	X	X
MacArthur Communicative Development Inventories. Fenson, L., Dale, P., Reznick, S., Thal, D., Bates, E., Hartung, J., Pethnick, S., & Reilly, J. (1993).	X	X
Observation of Communicative Interactions. Klein, M., & Briggs, M. (1987).	X	
Parent/Professional Preschool Performance Profile (5Ps). Variety Pre-Schooler's Workshop. (1987).	X	
Preverbal Assessment Intervention Profile. Connard, P. (1984).	X	X
Receptive Expressive Emergent Language Test. Bzock, K., & League R. (1978).	X	

son, 1979), *Caregiver Interview and Environmental Observation, Diagnostic Interactional Survey* (Owens, 1982a, c), *Ecological Communication System (ECO)* (MacDonald & Gillette, 1988), *Observation of Communicative Interactions* (Klein & Briggs, 1987), and *Parent/Professional Preschool Performance Profile (5Ps)* (Variety Pre-Schooler's Workshop, 1987) offer formats for structured collection of observational data.

Clients who communicate in a nonstandard manner will need to be observed carefully to determine the intent of such communication (Houghton, Bronicki, & Guess, 1987). For example, a client who bashes her head with her fist might be attempting to communicate. By observing the times and circumstances of this behavior, the speech-language pathologist can form hypotheses about the child's intended meaning (Robinson & Owens, 1995). Not all such behaviors contain communicative content, although consistent, predictable behaviors are likely to be meaningful. Hypotheses on the intent of such behaviors can be tested by carefully manipulating the events that precede and follow the behavior and carefully recording the effect on the behavior. For example, it might be hypothesized that head bashing before meals indicates a request for help. If aid given before or after the behavior results in nonperformance or cessation of the behavior, respectively, this may confirm the hypothesis. The speech-language pathologist is interested in the range of communication needs expressed and in the modes of communication (visual, manual, vocal, tactile) used receptively and expressively (Owens, 1995; Caro & Snell, 1989).

Formal assessment of presymbolic skills might include the content listed in Table 12-7. Skills essential to language acquisition form four categories: cognitive, perceptual, social, and communicative (McLean & Snyder-McLean, 1978; Owens, 1996). Clients using symbols, such as words, signs, pictures, or pictographs, should be evaluated for the range of semantic and illocutionary functions expressed by these symbols (Table 12-8). This can be done using both formal testing and sampling, although the latter is more valuable as a source of information.

Several formal assessment tools are available for use with presymbolic and minimally symbolic clients. These include *Assessing Linguistic Behavior* (Olswang, Stoel-Gammon, Coggins, & Carpenter, 1987b), *Carolina Curriculum for Infants and Toddlers with Special Needs* (Johnson-Martin, Jens, Attermeier, & Hacker, 1991), *Communication and Symbolic Behavior Scales* (Wetherby & Prizant, 1993), *Developmental Activities Screening Inventory* (Fewell & Langley, 1984), *Developmental Assessment Tool* (DAT) (Owens, 1982b), *Developmental Communication Curriculum Inventory* (Hanna, Lippert, & Harris, 1982), *Environmental Prelanguage Battery* (EPB) (Horstmeier & MacDonald, 1978), *Environmental Language Inventory* (ELI) (MacDonald, 1978a), and *Infant-Toddler Language Scale* (Rossetti, 1990). Many, such as the DAT and the Rossetti Scale, use data collected by a variety of methods including direct testing, observation, and parental report.

Sampling may occur in a free-play situation or in a combination of free-play and structured sampling plus imitation (MacDonald, 1978b). Usually 50 utterances, either spoken, signed, or picture-indicated, are adequate. The clinician should be interested in both the breadth and depth of semantic and illocutionary functions. Of particular interest are the nonexistence of certain functions, the low incidence of others, and the length of each function. This can be accomplished by a short, rated sample (Owens, 1982d) or by a more descriptive analysis (Wilcox & Campbell, 1983).

Early single-word and early multiword utterances are organized following word order rules based on semantics (Brown, 1973), and early prelinguistic and single-word semantic functions do exist (Greenfield & Smith, 1976). Many of these, such as recurrence and negation, seem to be based on the early object knowledge of developing children. These semantic functions can be expanded or combined into two-, three-, and four-word utterances.

Likewise, specific illocutionary acts or communicative intentions can be found in early vocalizations or single-word utterances (Dore, 1974; Owens, 1978). A language sample can be analyzed to determine the range of such functions. The speech-language pathologist should be cautioned that although these semantic and illocutionary categories represent what linguists believe children mean and intend by their early verbalizations, there is no way of knowing a child's actual meaning or intention. In addition, these categories are pre-

TABLE 12-7   Possible Presymbolic Targets

Behavior	Cognitive	Perceptual	Social	Communicative
Physical imitation—imitating behaviors of others	X		X	
Imitation with objects—using extension of self for imitation	X			
Deferred imitation—retrieving a behavior for imitation	X			
Repetitive and sequential imitation—retrieving patterns	X	X		
Object permanence—retrieving object form from memory	X			
Turn-taking—using motor imitation or eye contact in turn				X
Functional use—using objects for intended purpose in order to gain functional knowledge of meaning	X			
Means-ends—using one object or person to attain another	X		X	
Communicative gestures—displaying early intentions				X
Auditory memory—remembering sound patterns	X	X		
Word recognition—pairing names with entities				X
Vocal response—vocalizing in response to another person			X	X
Vocal turn-taking—vocalizing turns			X	X
Vocal imitation—shaping vocalizations to resemble a model		X		X
Sequencing vocal imitation—imitating vocal sequences		X		X

From: *Program for the Acquisition of Language with the Severely Impaired (PALS)* by R. Owens, 1982, San Antonio: The Psychological Corporation. Copyright 1982 by The Psychological Corporation. Adapted by permission.

TABLE 12-8   Semantic and Illocutionary Targets of Early Childhood

Functions	Examples

SEMANTIC

Nomination—naming a person or object using a single- or multiword name or a demonstrative-plus as a name.

Doggie, Choo-choo
This horsie

Location—marking spatial relationships. Utterances may contain single location words or two-word utterances containing an agent, action, or object plus a location word. The function can be demonstrated in response to *where* questions.

PARTNER: Where's doggie?
CLIENT: Chair.
Ball table, Doggie chair, Throw me,
Throw here (*X* + locative)

Negation—marking of nonexistence, rejection, and denial using single negative words or a negative followed by another word (negative + *X*).

All gone (count as a single word), Away, No milk (client drank it), All gone car (the ride is over), No

Nonexistence generally develops first and marks the absence of a once-present object.

PARTNER: Time for bed.
CLIENT: No (or No bed).

Rejection marks an attempt to prevent or to stop an event.

Stop it. No milk (pushes glass away).
PARTNER: See the bear?

Denial marks rejection of a proposition.

CLIENT: No bear.

Modification

Possession—appreciating that an object belongs to or is frequently associated with someone. Single-word utterances signal the owner's name. In two-word utterances, stress is usually on the initial word, the possessor.

Mine, My dollie, Johnnie bike (modifier + head)
Dollie (client clutches doll)

Attribution—using descriptors for properties not inherently part of the object.

Yukky, Big doggie, Little baby (modifier + head)

Recurrence—understanding that an object can reappear or an event can be reenacted.

More, More milk, 'Nuther cookie (modifier + head)

Notice—signaling that an object has appeared, an event has happened, or an attempt to gain attention.

Hi Mommy, Bye-bye, Look Jim

Action—marking an activity.

Action—single action words.
Agent + Action—two-word signal that an animate initiated an activity.
Action + Object—two-word signal that an animate or inanimate object was the recipient of action.

Jump, Eat
Mommy throw, Doggie eat, Baby sleep

Eat cookie, Throw ball

ILLOCUTIONARY

Answer—client responds to questions. The questioner's behaviors are a cue for the client's response; the response probably would not be produced without this cue. The client's responses are cognitively related to the question, although they may be incorrect.

PARTNER: (*holding doll*) What's this?
CLIENT: Baby.
PARTNER: Is this a mirror?
CLIENT: No.

Question—client asks for information or verification by addressing the other person verbally. The client's behavior is a stimulus or cue and indicates that she expects an answer. The client can ask herself questions when engaged in egocentric play.

CLIENT: (*picks up toy telephone*) Phone?
CLIENT: What this?

Functions	**Examples**
Reply—client makes meaningful response to the content of the other speaker's previous utterance, a verbal cue external to the client. The client may continue to build on the content and ignore the form of the utterance, such as responding to a word or thought in a question without answering the question. In many cases, the client will build on the content *and* respond with an appropriate form. This category does not include mere repetition.	PARTNER: Johnny, bring me the scissors. (command) CLIENT: No. PARTNER: May I have the keys? (request) CLIENT: In a minute. PARTNER: This is a cute dog. (declaration) CLIENT: My doggie.
Elicitation—client self-repeats in response to a request for repetition or clarification or in response to "Say *x*."	CLIENT: Kitty go.(declaration) PARTNER: What? CLIENT: Kitty go. PARTNER: Mary, say "ball." CLIENT: Ball.
Continuant—client signals that she is listening and wants to continue the interchange, or that she missed what was said.	Uh-huh, Okay. I see, Yes What? Huh?
Declaration—client makes a statement that is situationally related and for communication but is not in response to another speaker. The utterance is more like a commentary. Cues are internal or situational but not verbal. This category also includes situationally related phonemic exclamations.	CLIENT: (*playing game with mother and glances out*) It raining out. CLIENT: (*playing with car*) Car go up. PARTNER: This is a cute doggie. CLIENT: My doggie. (reply) He lives in a house. (declaration) PARTNER: This is a cute doggie. CLIENT: My doggie. (reply) I have kitty, too. (declaration)
Practice—client repeats or imitates in whole or part what she or another person says with no change in intonation that would indicate a change of intent. In addition, internal replay without added new information is considered practice. This category also includes counting, singing, babbling, or rhyming behaviors in which the client seems to be experimenting or rehearsing.	PARTNER: Ball. CLIENT: Ball. PARTNER: See the red ball. CLIENT: Red ball. PARTNER: See the red ball. CLIENT: See ball. (practice) Ball, ball, ball. (practice)
Perseverative responses, even if the other person interjects an utterance between them, are considered practice as long as they do not mark discrete events or objects.	
Name—client labels an object or event that is present, but the label is not in response to a question. This verbal behavior is usually accomplished by pointing or nodding.	CLIENT: (*picks up ball*) Ball. CLIENT: (*points to ball*) That ball.
Suggestion, Command, Demand, Request—The primary function of the client's utterance is to influence another person's behavior by getting that person to do something or to give the client permission. The form may be imperative, declarative, or interrogative.	CLIENT: Gimmie cookie. CLIENT: Stop that. CLIENT: Mommy. CLIENT: Throw ball. (*parent throws ball*) Throw ball. (*parent throws ball*) Throw ball.

From: *Program for the Acquisition of Language with the Severely Impaired (PALS)* by R. Owens, 1982, San Antonio: The Psychological Corporation. Copyright 1982 by The Psychological Corporation. Adapted by permission.

determined and may not accurately reflect the behavior of mentally retarded communicators (Leonard, Steckol, & Panther, 1983).

More valid results may be attained if caregivers participate with the client, and if the client uses familiar objects. Westby (1980) has suggested a play format for assessing the development of early cognitive and language abilities. Her symbolic play scale describes 10 stages of early development.

Because caregivers act as language facilitators, it is necessary for the speech-language pathologist to obtain a sample of the client-caregiver interaction. Such a sample might range from a 10-minute rated play sample (Owens, 1982d) to a more descriptive, lengthier analysis (Wilcox & Campbell, 1983). Analysis might involve the physical distance of the communicators; the use of reinforcement, responses, and cues by the caregiver; appropriate language by the caregiver for the perceived language skills of the client; turn-taking, body posture, and movement, and the termination and reengagement of the interaction (MacDonald & Gillette, 1982; Owens, 1982d; Wilcox & Campbell, 1983).

Once the initial evaluation is complete, the speech-language pathologist should know the client's interactional strategies, most frequent topics, communication partners, functioning level, and the quality of the client-caregiver interaction. Throughout the clinical intervention phase, the speech-language pathologist should test and probe in order to fine-tune training techniques.

Intervention.   The first step in training is to decide what to teach, who will teach it, and under what circumstances it will be taught. In the previous section, I suggested a number of training targets for early intervention. The participants and the circumstances are related and will significantly shape the intervention program.

It is essential in initial language programming that the natural environment of the client be included. In establishing early communication, the speech-language pathologist must enlist the aid of the client's caregivers in the intervention process.

Several models of intervention are possible using caregivers as communication facilitators. Within the instructional communication strategy model, the professional trains client responses, and the parents elicit these responses within the home (Wulz, Hall, & Klein, 1983). The components are environmental manipulation and teaching interaction. In environmental manipulation, parents restructure needs-meeting situations so that their children's needs are not anticipated but are dependent upon the children's communication behavior. Within the teaching phase, children are taught to respond to "need-to-communicate" situations. The purpose of the training is to expand the children's communication repertoire and to stimulate responding.

Home-based training should not be disruptive. The goal is not to give parents added responsibilities but rather to help them make use of teaching opportunities in daily routines—to "restructure ongoing activities" (Wulz et al., 1983, p. 6). Called **incidental teaching,** this type of training should be given primacy as an early communication training strategy (Owens, 1982d). If, for example, the parent is training object permanence, nonfloating soap and toys can be incorporated into the bathing routine. Because almost any routine can be adapted for language training, there is no need to rely solely on formal, out-of-context training modes. With children, the modality for training may be play. Play is child-centered, and the child's activity can provide the focus of training.

Training should occur in short, repetitive, daily activities in which the reinforcer is part of the activity, such as requesting another cookie at snack time (Halle, Alpert, & Anderson, 1984). The content should be meaningful in the situation and result in real consequences.

MacDonald (1978b) has relied upon environmental rules to restructure client-caregiver interactions. Once clients have learned a skill, they are required to perform that skill in order to attain desired entities or privileges. For example, if the client can sign *cookie,* the sign is required in order to get a cookie. Previously accepted pointing or whining is unacceptable. Environmental rules affect both client and caregiver behaviors.

Language stimulation techniques can also be used in the natural environment (Cheseldine & McConkey, 1979; Owens, 1982d). Ideally, such stimulation would precede slightly the client's actual level of functioning. Stimulation can take the form of motherese, discussed earlier. It is important that language trainers maintain an interactive style in order to preclude solitary nonlanguage activities common among children with mental retardation. (Smith & Hagen, 1984).

The importance of formal or structured training cannot be overlooked but should be minimized when possible (MacDonald, 1978b, 1985; Owens, 1982d). Often this training can be adapted to a play modality (Manolson, 1983). Two trainers can facilitate client responding (Richmond & Lewallen, 1983). One trainer cues the client while the second trainer models or prompts the appropriate response.

It is not always possible to train within the home. An alternative is the classroom (Brightman, Ambrose, & Baker, 1980). Within residential settings, aides, direct care staff, or foster grandparents may serve as language facilitators (Owens, McNerney, Bigler-Burke, & Lepre-Clark, 1987). Direct care staff teaching behaviors can be modified by simple praise or by feedback plus praise (Realon, Lewallen, & Wheeler, 1983).

Basic signal systems can be established using behavior chain interruption techniques (Goetz, Gee, & Sailor, 1985; Hunt, Goetz, Alwell, & Sailor, 1986; Romer & Schoenberg, 1991; Sternberg, Pegnatore, & Hill, 1983). There are two basic elements to behavior chain interruption. First, the client engages in a pleasurable activity that the trainer interrupts. Second, the client is prompted to give a communicative response, such as a touch, in order to have the activity begin again. The communicative response or signal can be modified or expanded into a more conventional gesture or sign.

Communication systems can also be initiated through the use of pictures or signs to signal a generalized request (Reichle, 1990). This procedure will be discussed in more detail under augmentative communication.

Several programs target presymbolic and early symbolic skills (Guess, Sailor, & Baer, 1976; Hanna, Lippert, & Harris, 1982; MacDonald, 1978b; MacDonald & Gillette, 1982; Miller & Yoder, 1974; Musslewhite & St. Louis, 1982; Owens, 1982d). Programs designed for less severely delayed clients, such as the Environmental Language Intervention Program (MacDonald, 1978b), may contain fewer presymbolic skills than those presented in Table 12-7. Others, such as the Program for the Acquisition of Language With the Severely Impaired (PALS) (Owens, 1982d), target more. Crais and Roberts (1991) offer a series of decision trees for presymbolic and early symbolic training. Decisions on the direction of therapy are based on the client's social interactional skills, comprehension, and imitative and spontaneous expression. Intervention suggestions are provided at each level.

In general, the younger the client, the more important such presymbolic training. With older children and adults, programming emphasizes establishing an initial communication system with less stress on presymbolic targets. Natural behaviors, such as reaching, can be modified into a requesting gesture or a point to a printed symbol (Reichle & Sigafoos, 1991).

All spontaneous vocalizations and other attempts to communicate should be encouraged and reinforced. The amount of vocalizing can be increased through reinforcement and modified into meaningful communication (Drash, Raver, Murrin, & Tudor, 1989; Poulson, 1988).

Once trained in imitation, the single word can be trained in a variety of semantic and illocutionary functions. Thus, "a single form may be used to express several functions and several forms can express a single function" (Miller & Yoder, 1974, p. 523). Single words are typically trained in response to "What's this?" but this question-naming paradigm has only limited application. Possible semantic and illocutionary training targets appear in Table 12-8. Using this table, the clinician may pair each semantic category with each of the illocutionary acts. For example, a "location-answer" response might follow the cue "Where is baby?" A "nomination-question" might consist of "Cup?" or "What?" A "location-question" might also consist of "Cup?" if the client is trying to guess the location of some small object. Within these category combinations, longer utterances may also be learned. It has been demonstrated that children continue to use combinations of the semantic rules in utterances of up to four words. After this point, learning focuses upon internal sentence re-organization, and new structures are learned.

Some developmental guidelines exist for the semantic functions. In general, the order is nomination, negation, action, objects, state or attribution, change in state or attribution, possession and location, experiencer of action, and agent (Menyuk, 1974). The first expansions are relational (Bloom, 1973; Miller & Yoder, 1974). Initial training with two-word utterances can begin with the same type of expansions. Initial two-word functions include nomination ("that _____"), recurrence ("more _____"), and nonexistence ("no _____"). Next, separate semantic classes are combined to produce utterances to indicate agent + action ("Mommy eat"), possession ("Baby cookie"), and location ("Doggie bed").

Guess, Sailor, and Baer (1976) targeted different language functions than those presented in Table 12-8. Of particular interest is their training of questions. Before asking a question, the clients must realize that they do not know something and then formulate a question in order to gain that knowledge. Knowing when we don't know something is as important as knowing how to attain the answer. Often clients are trained to ask questions with obvious answers, thus negating the need for a question.

MacDonald and Gillette (1982) have produced some interesting clinical results using a conversational paradigm almost exclusively. By modifying the behaviors of significant others in the client's environment, the clinician can affect the communication behaviors of the language-delayed client. In a similar manner, the facilitative language model of Blodgett and Miller (1981) builds conversationally upon the initial vocalizations of the client.

Augmentative Communication

Some mentally retarded individuals, particularly the more severely impaired, experience great difficulty with speech and with the use of symbols. For these nonspeaking clients, an augmentative form of communication may be necessary. Augmentative forms increase or expand the symbolic communication capabilities of these nonspeaking individuals. Common forms of augmentative communication include manual communication, communication boards, and electronic or computer-based communication. These augmentative communication forms will be discussed along with assessment and programming considerations.

Contrary to common misconception, use of augmentative communication systems does not deter further development of speech. Several studies have demonstrated that augmentative communication facilitates symbol learning (Bricker, 1972; Van Biervliet, 1977); increases verbalization of trained symbols (Burggraf, 1972); increases attention, intentional communication, and sociability (Abrahamsen et al., 1989); facilitates spontaneous verbal communication (Kahn, 1977; Konstantases, Oxman, & Webster, 1977; Reich, 1978); increases communication initiations (Harris-Vanderheiden, Brown, MacKenzie, Reinen, & Scheibel, 1975); and increases the range of meanings and communication partners (Harris, Lippert, Yoder, & Vanderheiden, 1977). Augmentative communication, however, "will not, in itself, assure effective communication" (Calculator & Luchko, 1983, p. 185). According to Shane, Lipschultz, and Shane (1982), "an augmentative communication system is not a panacea. It does not solve all of the communication problems of the non-speaking person" (p. 83).

Types of Augmentative Communication.   Augmentative communication aids can be divided into two types, aided and unaided. Aided augmentative communication uses a device such as a communication board or an electronic means of communication. Unaided systems consist of manual communication, such as gestures, signs, and fingerspelling.

Communication boards come in many different shapes and varieties. In general, boards are easy to make, portable, and very adaptable. The visual symbols used may include, from least to most symbolic, models or miniatures, pictures, drawings, Rebus symbols, Blissymbols, or letters and words. Rebus symbols are pictographic representations of concepts. Blissymbols are generally less iconic than Rebus symbols but allow for more generative language use. For example, the Rebus symbol for the word *book* is a pictograph showing simplistic details of an open book; the Blissymbol is a square with a vertical line through its center that schematically represents an open book. These encoding forms are not exclusive and may be used in combination. In general, the more iconic or "guessable" the encoding system, the easier it is to learn (Clark, 1981). In turn, the less iconic systems are more flexible and generative, allowing more adultlike representation.

The tremendous growth of computer technology is opening many new possibilities for the nonspeaking (Vanderheiden, 1982). Input systems may be similar to those used on communication boards, and output may include print, graphics, and/or prerecorded or synthesized speech. In general, there are three types of indicating methods used by clients: scanning, encoding, and direct selection. In the scanning method, the device continually scans the display of symbols. The client stops the scan on the desired symbol. With encoding, a code such as numbers or digits is used to access the computer's memory. Finally, in direct selection, the client moves a cursor or pointer to the desired symbol or may, if possible, type the message.

Accessing computers may be the most difficult problem, particularly for individuals with severe motoric involvement. Vanderheiden (1982) noted that "the major barrier for using microcomputers as communication aids is the need for custom interfacing to achieve optimum speech" (p. 139). The interface switch between the client and the microcomputer must often be modified or custom designed to the motoric abilities of an individual client. The slowness of interface use may actually negate some of the speed advantages associated with microcomputers.

There are several types of unaided sign systems from American Sign Language (ASL), which is a language of its own, to Seeing Essential English (SEE$_1$) or Signing Exact English (SEE$_2$), which closely approximate English syntax. Signed English uses signs from both systems but does not adhere as closely to English morphological rules as SEE$_1$. American Indian sign language (Amer-Ind) has also been used successfully with persons who are mentally retarded. One reason for these results may be the transparency of Amer-Ind. Transparency is the case of understanding a sign once its origin is explained. Amer-Ind is significantly more transparent than ASL (Daniloff, Lloyd, & Fristoe, 1983).

It may be advantageous for some clients to have more than one type of augmentative system. Different systems may have application in different environments. In addition, the speech-language pathologist should continue to train speech.

Evaluation. Evaluative decisions on client use of an augmentative communication system are made by a team of professionals, usually consisting of a speech-language pathologist, psychologist, physical therapist, occupational therapist, special education teacher, a client advocate such as a parent, and the client. Assessment is a continuing process which, in this case, is essential to adapt the augmentative system to the client's changing needs and abilities.

The American Speech-Language-Hearing Association (ASHA) Ad Hoc Committee on Communication Processes and Non-Speaking Persons (1980) identified three components of the assessment for augmentative communication. First, the team must assess the appropriateness of an augmentative system. Not all nonspeaking individuals are candidates for augmentative communication. For example, the abilities needed for spontaneous symbol use apply to augmentative communication as well as to verbal language (Bryen, Goldman, & Quinlisk-Gill, 1988; Goossens, 1984; Owens & House, 1984; Shane & Bashir, 1980; Silverman, 1980). The environment also must be supportive of augmentative system use (Owens & House, 1984; Shane, Lipschultz, & Shane, 1982).

The second component of an evaluation is selection of the appropriate communication mode. The team must decide which type or types of augmentative systems will be appropriate for the nonspeaking individual. Of particular importance are the motoric abilities of the client (Shane & Wilbur, 1980; Silverman, 1980). For clients who are physically disabled, "interaction must be explored in the context of the body's total movement patterns" (Bottorf & DePape, 1982, p. 60), The evaluative team is interested in the range, speed, strength, and consistency of movement. Clients with good motor skills may be candidates for manual systems, whereas those with less ability may use communication boards or electronic systems. For electronic devices, decisions should be based on a task analysis that includes the client's present skills and those behaviors needed to operate the communication aid (Coleman, Cook, & Myers, 1980).

Finally, the team must select the appropriate symbol system or systems. Questions of appropriateness relate to cognitive ability, visual acuity, and environmental receptivity (Chapman & Miller, 1980). For example, greater cognitive skills and visual discrimination abilities are needed for word use than for picture use. Pictures are generally easier to discriminate than lexigrams, which are, in turn, easier than printed words (Romski, Sevcik, Pate, & Rumbaugh, 1985). In addition, the use of a symbol system such as Blissymbols might hinder communication in a nonreceptive environment.

Intervention.   Bottorf and DePape (1982) noted that "although the tool should be selected or created carefully and on an individual basis, the focus of intervention must always be centered on increasing successful interactions" (pp. 55–56). In general, communication interactions can be fostered by adapting the augmentative system to the individual client and to the communication environment.

The creative speech-language pathologist will attempt to establish an augmentative environment around the client. The augmentative system should be available at all times, and others should be encouraged to use the system. Signs are always available, but others may not use them when talking to the client. Their use by others may facilitate client comprehension and will help the client feel less an "odd-man-out." In addition, the daily routine of the client can foster augmentative communication use. As Bottorf & DePape (1982) observed, "If an effective communication system is to be developed, intervention must take place within the context of day-to-day experiences unique to each individual" (p. 64). Lack of generalization of augmentative systems may be related to lack of knowledge and infrequent use by caregivers (Bryen & McGinley, 1991).

Selection of individualized content should reflect client routines, interests, and needs. The vocabulary selected will affect the types of interactions in which it is used (Bottorf & DePape, 1982). Fristoe and Lloyd (1980) proposed a guide to initial sign vocabulary based on ease of production and iconicity. They stressed, however, that their list is merely a guide, not a prescription. Initial vocabularies should be based upon each client's individual interests and routines, basic needs, and the recommendations of others within the environment. In addition, signs may be chosen on the basis of symmetry, taction, and iconicity. Individuals with severe retardation can learn signs more rapidly if the signs are symmetrical or contain identical hand movements, have some contact with the body (taction), and are iconic or highly representational (Kohl, 1981; Kohl, Karlan, & Heal, 1979).

Augmentative communication is not a panacea and the results are not always favorable. The average client with severe or profound mental retardation may learn to produce only four signs spontaneously after three years of training (Bryen et al., 1988). Lack of progress seems to be related to imitative training with little thought toward spontaneous use, nonmeaningful training situations, inappropriate vocabulary or augmentative system, and little environmental support by caregivers.

Finally, the environment should be modified systematically to encourage augmentative communication. Nonspeaking mentally retarded clients must be given an opportunity to use their augmentative systems. Teachers and caregivers need to be cautioned not to dominate communication. Communication partners must be patient and await client responses. Clients should also be given a choice in their daily routine and among alternative activities in order to foster active system use. Even individuals who are severely retarded can retain symbol vocabularies well over long periods of time if these symbols are used by them to control their daily environment (Romski, Sevcik, & Rumbaugh, 1985).

Summary.   Augmentative communication systems can be part of a nonspeaking individual's effective interaction system if continually evaluated and adapted to that client's communication needs. These systems "can be used to express a variety of communication functions, but only if the environment provides opportunities for meaningful use" (Shane et al., 1982, p. 83).

Language Rule Training

Once the client begins to use symbols meaningfully, training targets become the rule systems used with these symbols. The speech-language pathologist should be knowledgeable in the rules used within the five generally recognized areas of language: syntax, morphology, phonology, semantics, and pragmatics.

Children with language delays differ in their comprehension of sentences according to linguistic stage (Page & Horn, 1987). For example, children using four-word sentences or less use semantic comprehension strategies, not syntactic ones. Therefore, clinicians must be concerned with selecting the appropriate level of linguistic input in order to facilitate both comprehension and production. It is best to present examples of the language code that slightly exceed the child's expressive language skills.

Professionals frequently assume that only the adult forms of these rules are acceptable training targets. A 2-year-old who says "What Mommy eating?" is not considered to be language disordered but to be following an age-appropriate rule. Likewise, individuals with mental retardation follow rules that generally reflect their level of cognitive functioning. Luckily, these individuals have professionals to guide their language learning.

Not all child rules are appropriate for training. For example, nonretarded children develop a few irregular past tense verbs, such as *come* and *go,* before learning the *-ed* rule for regular past. Once this rule is learned, however, forms such as *went* become *goed* or *wented.* No one seriously proposes that we teach these forms to retarded individuals. On the other hand, it may be justifiable to teach "No eat peas" before "I no eat peas," followed by "I can't eat peas." Training in this sequence seems more logical than the previous example.

Evaluation.   Initial evaluation should attempt to determine which rule systems the client uses expressively and which ones she comprehends. Assessment ideally would include both formal testing and informal evaluation.

Very few formal tests were designed for and normed on the retarded population. Most commercially available tests were developed and normed on nonretarded children. Careful consideration must be given to the appropriateness of such tests and materials with older retarded clients, particularly adults. The speech-language pathologist must consider the child's motor and cognitive abilities before choosing a language test or tests. The means of responding may need to be modified for those with oral motor difficulties or those who use augmentative communication. These individuals may need more time to complete timed tests.

Test norms may also be inappropriate for clients with mental retardation. It is of little value for intervention planning to demonstrate that a retarded client is in fact delayed in language. Testing can be of more value when used to help describe the client's language features and behavior.

Existing materials can be modified and new assessment tools developed (Owings & Guvette, 1982). Many speech-language pathologists supplement formal tests with their own locally prepared instruments (Pickett & Flynn, 1983). This procedure is supported by a number of speech-language professionals (Mittler, 1976; Muma, 1978; Siegel, 1975).

According to Dever (1978), "Attempts to assess the ability to use language on the basis of responses to items on a formal test are probably a waste of time and money" (p. 19). Testing situations are artificial and generally lacking in the natural cues available in a conversation. Additional sources of information are needed. Informally collected language samples can provide valuable information. Samples can be analyzed in a number of ways. Initially, the speech-language pathologist should determine the MLU. Increasing MLU correlates with increasing complexity up to an MLU of 4.0 morphemes. Table 12-9 contains MLU values and equivalent ages.

Of the commercially available analysis methods, Miller's Assigning Structural Stage (1980) seems to be the most functional. Others, such as Developmental Sentence Scoring (Lee, 1974), result in a normative score but provide little direction for intervention. Using Miller's approach, the speech-language pathologist determines the correct percentage of use of Brown's (1973) 14 morphemes. This data, plus the MLU, suggest a developmental stage. Internal sentence analysis of noun phrase, verb phrase, and sentence type development results in assignment of the client to a stage or stages of language development.

Because the instrument informs the speech-language pathologist of the characteristics of the next stage of development, programming is relatively straightforward. Similar analysis can be performed semantically and phonologically.

Language samples may also be analyzed using less formal, more descriptive methods (Owens, 1995). The speech-language pathologist should attempt to describe all aspects of language. Pragmatic concerns, such as inappropriate communication, are difficult to measure directly but are very important for overall communication effectiveness.

TABLE 12-9 MLU and Approximate Age

MLU	Predicted Chronological Age in Months	Predicted Age in Months ± 1 S.D.
1.5	23.0	18.5–27.5
2.0	26.9	21.5–32.3
2.5	30.8	23.9–37.7
3.0	34.8	28.0–41.6
3.5	38.7	30.8–46.6
4.0	42.6	36.7–48.5
4.5	46.6	40.3–52.9
5.0	50.5	42.1–58.9
5.5	54.4	46.0–62.8
6.0	58.3	49.9–66.7

Adapted from Miller (1980).

Intervention.   Again, generalization is best ensured by use of the natural environment for language training. Caregivers can be instructed in the use of evaluative feedback and in expansion techniques. For example, caregivers can provide corrective feedback in the form of modeling of the correct production. Incomplete or primitive responses can be expanded into a more adultlike form. The conversational context should not be overlooked for the training opportunity that it provides. Generalization to spontaneous conversational use does not happen automatically for many retarded clients. Training within structured conversations familiarize the client with the situations and the contexts that govern language feature use.

The primary criterion for selecting training targets should be the usefulness to the client of the language features targeted. Targets should include those language features or behaviors that facilitate communication, such as asking questions, or that offer more communication options to the client, such as using the telephone.

It is best if the trainer does not introduce too many new items into the training task. Training cues, prompts, and materials should change gradually. Previously trained information should be used to aid new learning. For example, knowledge of the semantic categories and rules previously discussed can be used to train syntax. Agent words (*mommy, doggie*) because of their position in the utterance and their use can become subjects. Possession, previously expressed by word order, can be expanded through the training of the possessive marker (*'s*).

Miniature linguistic systems may be helpful in training word order (Bunce, Ruder, & Ruder, 1985). Table 12-10 demonstrates a miniature system matrix in which one language

TABLE 12-10   Miniature Linguistic Systems

	Cookie	Cake	Pudding	Pie	Bread
Eat	X	X	X	X	X
Bake	X				
Mix	X				
Want	X				
Give	X				

	Pet	Dog	Cat	Horse	Ferret
Feed	X	X			
Bathe		X	X		
Groom			X	X	
Walk				X	X
Brush	X				X

Verbs on one axis are combined with nouns on the other to form short phrases. Each combination taught is marked with an *X*. Rule learning will generalize to the untrained combinations.

feature occupies each axis. The child can learn a word order rule by combining words from each grouping. Good generalization has been reported with miniature systems from training of some but not all possible combinations. The *X*s in Table 12-10 identify the combinations most effective in training.

New language features can be introduced using focused stimulation in which examples of the feature are given frequently in context. For example, when introducing the present progressive verb form (verb + *-ing*) the trainer might use self-talk to describe what he is doing or parallel talk to describe what the child is doing. Repeated use in context will highlight the feature for the child and help to focus attention.

When attempting to elicit full sentences, the speech-language pathologist should be very careful to use cues that make sense pragmatically and reflect general language use. For example, the cue "What do you want?" is most likely to elicit a single-word or short-phrase response, such as "Cookie." Demanding "I want cookie" as a response is inappropriate pragmatically.

Vocabulary, often a deficit area, can also be trained within the context of daily events in which the symbols have some relevance. The use of key words or pictures can facilitate learning and ensure memory better than direct instruction (Scruggs, Mastropieri, & Levin, 1985). For example, the word *popover* contains the key word *pop;* pictures that show the word *popover* "popping" out of a toaster may aid word recall. Stories can also be used to facilitate recall of single words or series of words (Glidden & Warner, 1985).

In addition, speech-language pathologists should be aware of the special learning needs of the retarded population. Cognitive operations should be trained before linguistic skills that express those operations. For example, the client should understand reversibility of processes before learning linguistic concepts such as *before, after,* and *because.*

Clients such as those with Down syndrome may need help with successive processing skills. Simultaneous skills related to overall meaning may be employed to facilitate sequential operations.

Finally, some individuals with retardation, such as those with Down syndrome, will require additional input beyond auditory symbols. Visual and tactile input can enhance learning for these persons. The use of pictures or experiential activities might facilitate concept learning and elicit more client responses. Involvement in activity by the client results in more verbal responsiveness than involvement by the clinician or use of pictures (Cook & Seymour, 1980). Likewise, active participation by the severely retarded client becomes a cue for verbal behavior that was situationally appropriate (Spiegel, 1983).

Language Use

With higher functioning adults or teenagers with mental retardation in prevocational or vocational training programs, the focus of training should be language use. Language forms are not as critical to life success. Naturally, a minimum of language structure is required.

The main difference between occupationally and socially successful and nonsuccessful adults with retardation seems to be integration at work and in society (Reiter & Levi, 1980). Further, there is great need among individuals in the retarded population for attaining regular employment and for having nonretarded friends. One difference between the successful and unsuccessful person is found in the area of social skills, including language. Therefore, more appropriate language use may become the training target.

Some language factors, such as following directions or asking questions, may be more important than others, particularly in the work setting. Malgady, Barcher, Towner, and Davis (1979) compiled a list of maladaptive social behaviors observed by vocational training supervisors and used this list to rate mildly to severely retarded clients for employability. In general, language skills were rated as less important than acceptable verbal manners, such as not interrupting. Adults with mental retardation are less likely to be employed if their language use is inappropriate, such as being abusive, argumentative, vulgar, bossy, loud, interruptive, or irrelevant. Additional skills for training might also include conversational abilities and direction following.

These vocational-interpersonal skills can be modified through a combination of modeling, coaching, and behavior rehearsal (LaGreca, Stone, & Bell, 1983). Appropriate verbal behavior can be modeled while clients are trained in appropriate use. Rehearsal and role-playing in situations close to those of actual use can be beneficial. Social feedback in the form of praise, instruction, and reprimands has been more effective than reprimands and instruction in reducing inappropriate verbalizations (Dwinell & Connis, 1979).

Other conversational skills may also be taught. Teenagers who are mentally retarded may have particular difficulties communicating with their parents and expressing their feelings (Shepard & Marshall, 1976). Rees and Wollner (1981) have constructed a taxonomy of pragmatic abilities for teaching the conversational use of language. These abilities relate to organizing and participating in a conversation, repairing conversational errors, establishing and varying conversational roles, and producing and comprehending speech acts. As conversational partners, mentally retarded individuals should observe the rules of turn-taking and be able to introduce, sustain, and contribute to the topic of conversation. In addition, they should be able to take their communication partner's perspective and to vary their own role and informational contribution accordingly. Pragmatic abilities of those functioning at school-age or adult levels may also be assessed and trained for a range of intentions and forms of expression (Prutting & Kirchner, 1983). Normally developing peers can serve effectively as models and can elicit appropriate conversational responses (Wilkinson & Romski, 1995).

Critical social and communication skills can be taught within the classroom, home, or workplace (Stowitschek et al., 1988). Even adolescents and adults with severe retardation can be taught successfully to answer the telephone and to respond to a variety of messages and callers (Karen, Astin-Smith, & Creasy, 1985). Many mentally retarded individuals recognize the need for these conversational skills. In a "social" room in a day training program, the clients established the following rules:

- Stay on topic.
- Be quiet when others are talking.
- Listen to what you hear.
- Don't interrupt others.
- Take turns—give everyone a chance.
- Speak so others can hear you.
- Don't talk to yourself.

Summary

Within this chapter, I have explored a definition of mental retardation that considers cognitive functioning and adaptive behavior. Overall, this definition reflects empirical findings that retarded individuals are developmental beings whose behavior is characterized by delay rather than by difference. Some differences do exist, but the overall developmental picture is one of delay. This finding is also true for the language development of the retarded population. Differences are quantitative rather than qualitative.

These characteristics suggest a developmental language intervention approach. The wise clinician will use nonretarded development as a guide for creative programming.

The language intervention targets will differ with the language skills of the client. Initial training should focus on cognitive perceptual, social, and communicative skills and on the establishment of early communication. Early building blocks will be semantic and pragmatic. Once short multiword utterances are trained, the speech-language pathologist should target language rule systems. As the client becomes more capable in using language rules, language use becomes a tool for normalization training. Such training is particularly true of clients in vocational training programs.

We began this chapter with a quote from Nigel Hunt and will end with one as well:

Thank you ever so much for letting me write this book. I am most delightful. *(p. 124)*

Case Study

Catherine is a 33-year-old, severely retarded adult residing in a developmental center but attending a day training program in the community. She has been institutionalized since early childhood. The cause of retardation is unknown. Her mental age measured on the Wechsler Intelligence Scale for Children—Revised is slightly above age 6, although her language performance is lower. She experiences seizures, primarily of the petit mal type. During seizure activity, Catherine usually stares and her expression is blank. Such episodes are usually a few seconds in duration, although on a few occasions she has lost consciousness. Currently, her seizures are controlled through medication. At times, Catherine will become violent and strike other clients for no apparent reason. Her placement in a community residence is dependent upon control of this behavior. She has good self-help skills as evidenced on the AAMD Adaptive Behavior Scale.

Catherine's receptive vocabulary age is approximately 5 years, as measured on the Peabody Picture Vocabulary Test. Although she can point to pictures named, she has difficulty explaining word meanings. Her equivalent receptive language age as measured by the Test for Auditory Comprehension of Language—Revised (TACL—R) is 4 years 2 months. This score is corroborated by the Carrow Elicited Language Inventory. In this sentence imitation test, she received an age equivalent of 46 months. Her performance was characterized by sentence simplification, omission of articles, and difficulties with verb tensing and pronouns. On the TACL—R she also made several errors in verb tensing and pronouns. A free sample analyzed using Miller's Assigning Structural Stage indicated that her language skills are primarily those found in Brown's Stage IV Her MLU is approximately 3.67. Language is primarily responsive and characterized by short sentences, a scarcity of complex or compound sentences, little use of pronouns beyond *you, me, he, she,* and *him,* and absence of tensing markers. Some auxiliary verbs and modals are present, but there is some confusion with the verb *to be.* Most sentences are simple declaratives or negatives.

In the vocational training program, Catherine's communication behavior is mostly responsive, although staff report that she also exhibits perseverative verbal behavior. While in vocational training, she will continually repeat instructions she has been given or statements made to her. This behavior is whispered but still annoys others around her. Staff report that it is difficult to stop this behavior.

Catherine is seen by the speech-language pathologist twice weekly for individual programming and once a week for group training. Within the individual sessions, the speech-language pathologist works primarily on verb tensing, focusing on the regular and irregular past and the future tense. Once a correct response is given, the speech-language pathologist attempts to gain a longer verbalization. Group work attempts to encourage initiation of conversation and use of longer utterances. In her vocational training program, Catherine is expected by the staff to provide longer responses in conversation. A questioning technique is used to elicit expansions of previous utterances. In addition, she is reinforced for short periods without perseverative whispering.

Study Questions

1. What is the AAMD definition of mental retardation? Explain each portion of this definition.
2. How does cognitive functioning of the retarded population differ from that of the nonretarded population? How might these differences relate to overall intervention considerations?
3. Compare all aspects of the language abilities of the retarded and nonretarded populations.
4. Explain the developmental model of intervention and its relation to language training with persons who are mentally retarded.
5. What are some of the targets for language intervention with persons who are mentally retarded?

References

Abbeduto, L., Davies, B., & Furman, L. (1988). The development of speech act comprehension in mentally retarded individuals and nonretarded children. *Child Development, 59,* 1460–1472.

Abbeduto, L., Davies, B., Solesby, S., & Furman, L. (1991). Identifying the referents of spoken messages: Use of context and clarification requests by children with and without mental retardation.

American Journal on Mental Retardation, 95, 551–562.

Abbeduto, L., Furman, L., & Davies, B. (1989). Relation between the receptive language and mental age of persons with mental retardation. *American Journal on Mental Retardation,* 93, 535–543.

Abbeduto, L., & Rosenberg, S. (1980). The communicative competence of mildly retarded adults. *Applied Psycholinguistics,* 1, 405–426.

Abrahamsen, A., Romski, M., & Sevcik, R. (1989). Concomitants of success in acquiring an augmentative communication system: Changes in attention, communication, and sociability. *American Journal on Mental Retardation,* 93, 475–496.

Affleck, G. (1976). Role-taking ability and the interpersonal tactics of retarded children. *American Journal of Mental Deficiency,* 80, 667–670.

Affleck, G., Allen, D., McGrade, B., & McQueeney, M. (1982). Home environments of developmentally disabled infants as a function of parent and infant characteristics. *American Journal of Mental Deficiency,* 86, 445–452.

Ambron, S., & Irwin, D. (1975). Role-taking and moral judgment in 5- and 7-year olds. *Developmental Psychology,* 11, 102.

ASHA Ad Hoc Committee on Communication Processes and Nonspeaking Persons. (1980). Nonspeech communication: A position paper. *ASHA,* 22, 267–272.

Ashman, A. (1982). Coding, strategic behavior, and language performance of institutionalized mentally retarded young adults. *American Journal of Mental Deficiency,* 86, 627–636.

Baker, B. (1976). Parent involvement in programming for the developmentally disabled child. In L. Lloyd (Ed.), *Communication assessment and intervention.* Baltimore: University Park Press.

Balla, D., & Zigler, E. (1971). Luria's verbal deficiency theory of mental retardation and performance on sameness, symmetry and opposition tasks: A critique. *American Journal of Mental Deficiency,* 75, 400–413.

Balthazar, E., & Stevens, H. (1974). *The emotionally disturbed, mentally retarded: A historical and contemporary perspective.* Englewood Cliffs, NJ: Prentice Hall.

Bangs, T. (1961). Evaluating children with language delay. *Journal of Speech and Hearing Disorders,* 26, 6–18.

Bangs, T., & Dodson, S. (1979). *Birth to Three Developmental Scales.* Seattle: University of Washington Press.

Bates, E., Benigni, L., Bretherton, I., Camaioni, L., & Volterra, V. (1979). *The emergence of symbols: Cognition and communication in infancy.* New York: Academic Press.

Bedrosian, J., & Prutting, C. (1978). Communicative performance of mentally retarded adults in four conversational settings. *Journal of Speech and Hearing Research,* 21, 79–95.

Bee, H., Van Egeren, L., Streissguth, A., Nyman, B., & Leckie, M. (1969). Social class differences in maternal teaching strategies and speech patterns. *Developmental Psychology,* 1, 726–734.

Bellinger, D. (1980). Consistency in the pattern of change in mothers' speech: Some discriminant analysis. *Journal of Child Language,* 7, 469–487.

Belmont, J. (1967). Long-term memory in mental retardation. In N. Ellis (Ed.), *International review of research in mental retardation* (Vol. 1). New York: Academic Press.

Bender, N., & Carlson, J. (1982). Prosocial behavior and perspective-taking of mentally retarded and nonretarded children. *American Journal of Mental Deficiency,* 86, 361–366.

Berger, J., & Cunningham, C. (1983). The development of early vocal behaviors and interactions in Down syndrome and non-handicapped infant-mother pairs. *Developmental Psychology,* 19, 322–331.

Berko, J. (1958). The child's learning of English morphology. *Word,* 14, 150–177.

Berry, P., Groeneweg, G., Gibson, D., & Brown, R. (1984). Mental development of adults with Down's syndrome. *American Journal of Mental Deficiency,* 89, 252–256.

Bilsky, L., Walker, N., & Sakales, S. (1983). Comprehension and recall of sentences by mentally retarded and nonretarded individuals. *American Journal of Mental Deficiency,* 87, 558–565.

Birch, H., Richardson, S., Baird, D., Horobin, G., & Illsley, R. (1970). *Mental subnormality in the community: A clinical and epidemiological study.* Baltimore: Williams & Wilkins.

Blacher, J. (1982). Assessing social cognition of young mentally retarded and nonretarded children. *American Journal of Mental Deficiency,* 86, 473–484.

Bleile, K., & Schwartz, I. (1984). Three perspectives on the speech of children with Down's syndrome. *Journal of Communication Disorders,* 17, 87–94.

Blodgett, E., & Miller, V. (1981). *The facilitative language model.* Paper presented at the American Speech-Language-Hearing Association Annual Convention, Los Angeles.

Bloom, L. (1973). *One word at a time: The use of single-word utterances before syntax.* The Hague: Mouton.

Borkowski, J., & Cavanaugh, J. (1979). Maintenance and generalization of skills and strategies by the retarded. In N. Ellis (Ed.), *Handbook of mental deficiency: Psychological theory and research.* Hillsdale, NJ: Lawrence Erlbaum Associates.

Borkowski, J., & Wanschura, P. (1974). Mediational processes in the retarded. In N. R. Ellis (Ed.), *International review of research in mental retardation* (Vol. 7). New York: Academic Press.

Bottorf, L., & DePape, D. (1982). Initiating communication systems for severely speech-impaired persons. *Topics in Language Disorders,* 2, 55–72.

Bowler, D. (1991). Rehearsal training and short-term free-recall of sign and word labels by severely handicapped children. *Journal of Mental Deficiency Research,* 35, 113–124.

Bradbury, B., & Lunzer, E. (1972). The learning of grammatical inflections in normal and subnormal children. *Journal of Child Psychology and Psychiatry,* 13, 239–248.

Bray, N. (1979). Strategy production in the retarded. In N. Ellis (Ed.), *Handbook of mental deficiency: Psychological theory and research.* Hillsdale, NJ: Lawrence Erlbaum Associates.

Bricker, D. (1972). Imitative sign training as a facilitator of word-object association with low-functioning children. *American Journal of Mental Deficiency,* 76, 509–516.

Bricker, D. (1993). *Assessment, Evaluation, and Programming Systems: AEPS Measurement for Birth to Three Years* (Vol. 1). Baltimore, MD: Paul Brookes.

Bricker, D., Squires, J., & Mounts, L. (1995). *Ages and Stages Questionnaire (ASQ): A Parent-Completed Child-Monitoring System.*

Bricker, W., Heal, L., Bricker, D., Hayes, W., & Larsen, L. (1969). Discrimination learning and learning set with institutionalized retarded children. *American Journal of Mental Deficiency,* 74, 242–248.

Brightman, R., Ambrose, S., & Baker, B. (1980). Parent training: A school-based model for enhancing teaching performance. *Child Behavior Therapy,* 2, 35–47.

Brooks, P., & Baumeister, A. (1977). A plea for consideration of ecological validity in the experimental psychology of mental retardation: A guest editorial. *American Journal of Mental Deficiency,* 81, 407–416.

Brophy, J. (1970). Mothers as teachers of their own preschool children: The influence of socioeconomic status and task structure on teaching specificity. *Child Development,* 41, 79–94.

Brown, A. (1974). The role of strategic behavior in retardate memory. In N. Ellis (Ed.), *International review of research in mental retardation* (Vol. 7). New York: Academic Press.

Brown, A. (1978). Knowing when, where, and how to remember: A problem in meta cognition. In R. Glaser (Ed.), *Advances in instructional psychology.* Hillsdale, NJ: Lawrence Erlbaum Associates.

Brown, A., Campione, J., & Murphy, M. (1974). Keeping track of changing variables: Long-term retention of a trained rehearsal strategy by retarded adolescents. *American Journal of Mental Deficiency,* 78, 446–453.

Brown, R. (1973). *First language: The early stages.* Cambridge: Harvard University Press.

Brownell, M. D., & Whiteley, J. H. (1992). Development and training of referential communication in children with mental retardation. *American Journal on Mental Retardation,* 97, 161–172.

Bruner, J. (1974–1975). From communication to language—A psychological perspective. *Cognition,* 3, 255–287.

Bruner, J. (1977). Early social interaction and language acquisition. In R. Schaffer (Ed.), *Studies in mother-infant interaction.* New York: Academic Press.

Bryen, D., Goldman, A., & Quinlisk-Gill, S. (1988). Sign language with students with severe/profound mental retardation: How effective is it? *Education and Training in Mental Retardation,* 23, 129–137.

Bryen, D., & McGinley, V. (1991). Sign language input to community residents with mental retardation. *Education and Training in Mental Retardation,* 26, 207–214.

Buckhalt, J., Rutherford, R., & Goldberg, K. (1978). Verbal and nonverbal interaction of mothers with their Down's syndrome and nonretarded infants. *American Journal of Mental Deficiency,* 82, 337–343.

Buium, N., Rynders, J., & Turnure, J. (1974). Early maternal linguistic environment of normal and Down's syndrome language-learning children. *American Journal of Mental Deficiency,* 79, 52–58.

Bullowa, M. (Ed.). (1979). *Before speech: The beginning of interpersonal communication.* New York: Cambridge University Press.

Bunce, B., Ruder, K., & Ruder, C. (1985). Using the miniature linguistic system in teaching syntax: Two case studies. *Journal of Speech and Hearing Disorders,* 50, 247–253.

Burger, A., Blackman, L., & Clark, H. (1981). Generalization of verbal abstraction strategies by EMR children and adolescents. *American Journal of Mental Deficiency,* 85, 611–618.

Burger, A., Blackman, L., Clark, H., & Reis, E. (1982). Effects of hypothesis testing and variable format training on generalization of a verbal abstraction strategy by EMR learners. *American Journal of Mental Deficiency,* 86, 405–413.

Burger, A., Blackman, L., Holmes, M., & Zetlin, A. (1978). Use of active sorting and retrieval strategies as a facilitator of recall, clustering, and sorting by EMR and nonretarded children. *American Journal of Mental Deficiency,* 83, 253–261.

Burger, A., Blackman, L., & Tan, N. (1980). Maintenance and generalization of a sorting and retrieval strategy by EMR and nonretarded individuals. *American Journal of Mental Deficiency,* 84, 373–380.

Burggraf, A. (1972). *Sign language as a verbal-facilitator with mentally retarded children.* Master's thesis, Ohio State University, Columbus.

Burr, D., & Rohr, A. (1978). Patterns of psycholinguistic development in the severely mentally retarded: A hypothesis. *Social Biology,* 25, 15–22.

Butterfield, E., & Belmont, J. (1978). Assessing and improving the cognitive functions of mentally retarded people. In I. Bialer & M. Sternlicht (Eds.), *The psychology of mental retardation: Issues and approaches.* New York: Psychological Dimensions.

Butterfield, E., Wambold, C., & Belmont, J. (1973). On the theory and practice of improving short-term memory. *American Journal of Mental Deficiency,* 77, 654–669.

Bzock, K., & League, R. (1978). *Receptive Expressive Emergent Language Scale.* Austin, TX: Pro-Ed.

Calculator, S. N. (1988). Exploring the language of adults with mental retardation. In S. Calculator & J. Bedrosian (Eds.), *Communication assessment and intervention for adults with mental retardation* (pp. 95–106). San Diego: College-Hill.

Calculator, S., & Luchko, C. (1983). Evaluating the effectiveness of a communication board training program. *Journal of Speech and Hearing Disorders,* 48, 185–191.

Campione, J., & Brown, A. (1977). Memory and metamemory development in educable retarded children. In R. Kail & J. Hagen (Eds.), *Perspectives on the development of memory and cognition.* Hillsdale, NJ: Lawrence Erlbaum Associates.

Cardone, I., & Gilkerson, L. (1989). *Family Administered Neonatal Activities.* Washington, DC: Bulletin of the National Center for Clinical Infant Programs.

Cardosa-Martins, C., & Mervis, C. (1990). Mothers' use of substantive deixis and nouns with their children with Down syndrome: Some discrepant findings. *American Journal on Mental Retardation,* 94, 633–637.

Cardosa-Martins, C., Mervis, C., & Mervis, C. (1985). Early vocabulary acquisition by children with Down's syndrome. *American Journal of Mental Deficiency,* 90, 177–184.

Caro, P., & Snell, M. (1989). Characteristics of teaching communication to people with moderate and severe disabilities. *Education and Training in Mental Retardation,* 24, 63–77.

Caron, J. (1994). Male-female characteristics of Fragile X syndrome. Typescript.

Case, R. (1978). Intellectual development from birth to adulthood: A neo-Piagetian interpretation. In R. Siegler (Ed.), *Children's thinking: What develops?* Hillsdale, NJ: Lawrence Erlbaum Associates.

Cegelka, P., & Prehm, H. (1982). *Mental retardation: From categories to people.* Columbus, OH: Merrill/Macmillan.

Chandler, M., Greenspan, S., & Barenboim, C. (1974). Assessment and training of role-taking and referential communication skills in institutionalized emotionally disturbed children. *Developmental Psychology,* 10, 546–553.

Chaney, R., Eyman, R., & Miller, C. (1979). Comparison of respiratory mortality in the profoundly mentally retarded and the less retarded. *Journal of Mental Deficiency Research, 23,* 107.

Chapman, R. S., Kay-Raining Bird, E., & Schwartz, S. E. (1990). Fast mapping of words in event contexts by children with Down syndrome. *Journal of Speech and Hearing Disorders, 55,* 761–770.

Chapman, R. S., & Miller, J. (1980). Analyzing language and communication in the child. In R. Schiefelbusch (Ed.), *Nonspeech language and communication: Analysis and intervention.* Baltimore: University Park Press.

Cheseldine, S., & McConkey, R. (1979). Parental speech to young Down's syndrome children: An intervention study. *American Journal of Mental Deficiency, 83,* 612–620.

Clark, C. (1981). Learning words using traditional orthography and the symbols of Rebus, Bliss, and Carrier. *Journal of Speech and Hearing Disorders, 46,* 191–196.

Clark, D., Baker, B., & Heifetz, L. (1982). Behavioral training for parents of mentally retarded children: Prediction of outcome. *American Journal of Mental Deficiency, 87,* 14–19.

Cole, K. N., Dale, P. S., & Mills, P. E. (1992). Stability of intelligence quotient-language relation: Is discrepancy modeling based on a myth? *American Journal on Mental Retardation, 97,* 131–144.

Coleman, C., Cook, A., & Myers, L. (1980). Assessing non-oral clients for assistive communication devices. *Journal of Speech and Hearing Disorders, 45,* 515–526.

Connard, P. (1984). *Preverbal Assessment Intervention Profile,* Austin, TX: Pro-Ed.

Connor, F., Williamson, G., & Siepp, J. (1978). *Program guide for infants and toddlers with neuromotor and other developmental disabilities.* New York: Teachers College Press.

Conroy, J., Efthimiou, J., & Lemanowicz, J. (1982). A matched comparison of the developmental growth of institutionalized and deinstitutionalized mentally retarded clients. *American Journal of Mental Deficiency, 86,* 581–587.

Cook, D., & Seymour, H. (1980). *A comparison among three language elicitation procedures.* Paper presented at the American Speech-Language-Hearing Association Convention, Detroit.

Coplan, J. (1987). *Early Language Milestone Scale.* Tusla, OK: Modern Education Corporation.

Crais, E., & Roberts, J. (1991). Decision making in assessment and early intervention planning. *Language, Speech and Hearing Services in Schools, 22,* 19–30.

Cummins, J. (1979). Language functions and cognitive processing. In J. Das, J. Kirby, & R. Jarman (Eds.), *Simultaneous and successive cognitive processes.* New York: Academic Press.

Cummins, J., & Das, J. (1978). Simultaneous and successive synthesis and linguistic processes. *International Journal of Psychology, 13,* 129–138.

Dance, F. (1967). Toward a theory of human communication. In F. Dance (Ed.), *Human communication theory: Original essays.* New York: Holt, Rinehart & Winston.

Daniloff, J., Lloyd, L., & Fristoe, M. (1983). Amer-Ind transparency. *Journal of Speech and Hearing Disorders, 48,* 103–110.

Das, J. (1972). Patterns of cognitive ability in nonretarded and retarded children. *American Journal of Mental Deficiency, 77,* 6–12.

Das, J., Kirby, J., & Jarman, R. (1975). Simultaneous and successive synthesis: An alternative model for cognitive abilities. *Psychological Bulletin, 80,* 97–113.

Das, J., Kirby, J., & Jarman, R. (1979). *Simultaneous and successive cognitive processes.* New York: Academic Press.

Davis, H., Stroud, A., & Green, L. (1988). Maternal language environment of children with mental retardation. *American Journal on Mental Retardation, 93,* 144–153.

Day, J., & Hall, L. (1988). Intelligence-related differences in learning and transfer and enhancement of transfer among mentally retarded persons. *American Journal on Mental Retardation, 93,* 125–137.

Detterman, D. (1979). Memory in the mentally retarded. In N. Ellis (Ed.), *Handbook of mental deficiency: Psychological theory and research.* Hillsdale, NJ: Lawrence Erlbaum Associates.

Dever, R. (1978). *TALK—Teaching the American language to kids.* Columbus, OH: Merrill/Macmillan.

Dever, R., & Gardner, W. (1970). Performance of normal and retarded boys on Berko's test of morphology. *Language and Speech, 13,* 162–181.

Dore, J. (1974). A pragmatic description of early language development. *Journal of Psycholinguistic Research, 3,* 343–350.

Drash, P., Raver, S., Murrin, M., & Tudor, R. (1989). Three procedures for increasing vocal response to therapist prompt in infants and children with Down syndrome. *American Journal on Mental Retardation, 94,* 64–73.

Duhammel, T., Lin, S., Skelton, A., & Hantke, L. (1974). Early parental perceptions and the high risk neonate. *Clinical Pediatrics, 13,* 1052–1056.

Dunst, C. (1980). *A clinical and educational manual for use with the Uzgris and Hunt scales of infant psychological development.* Austin, TX: Pro-Ed.

Dwinell, M., & Connis, R. (1979). Reducing inappropriate verbalizations of a retarded adult. *American Journal of Mental Deficiency, 84,* 87–92.

Eheart, B. (1982). Mother-child interactions with nonretarded and mentally retarded preschoolers. *American Journal of Mental Deficiency, 87,* 20–25.

Ellis, N. (1963). Stimulus trace and behavioral inadequacy. In N. Ellis (Ed.), *Handbook of mental deficiency.* New York: McGraw-Hill.

Ellis, N. (1970). Memory processes in retardates and normals. In N. Ellis (Ed.), *International review of research in mental retardation* (Vol. 4). New York: Academic Press.

Ellis, N., Deacon, J., Harris, L., Poor, A., Angers, D., Diorio, M., Watkins, R., Boyd, B., & Cavalier, A. (1982). Learning, memory, and transfer in profoundly, severely, and moderately mentally retarded persons. *American Journal of Mental Deficiency, 87,* 186–196.

Ellis, N., Deacon, J., & Wooldridge, P. (1985). On the nature of short-term memory deficit in mentally retarded persons. *American Journal of Mental Deficiency, 89,* 393–402.

Ellis, N., Woodley-Zanthos, P., & Dulaney, C. (1989). Memory for spatial location in children, adults, and mentally retarded persons. *American Journal on Mental Retardation, 93,* 521–527.

Emery, G., & Ramey, C. (1976). *Maternal teaching styles as a function of mothers' level of education.* Paper presented at fourth biennial Southeastern Conference on Human Development.

Engle, R., & Nagle, R. (1979). Strategy training and semantic encoding in mildly retarded children. *Intelligence, 3,* 17–30.

Ervin-Tripp, S. (1973). Some strategies for the first two years. In T. Moore (Ed.), *Cognitive development and the acquisition of language.* New York: Academic Press.

Evans, D. (1977). The development of language abilities in Mongols: A correlational study. *Journal of Mental Deficiency Research, 21,* 103–117.

Evans, R., & Bilsky, L. (1979). Clustering and categorical list retention in the mentally retarded. In N. Ellis (Ed.), *Handbook of mental deficiency: Psychological theory and research.* Hillsdale, NJ: Lawrence Erlbaum Associates.

Ezell, H., & Goldstein, H. (1991). Comparison of idiom comprehension of normal children and children with mental retardation. *Journal of Speech and Hearing Research, 34,* 812–819.

Feldman, H. M., Evans, J. L., Brown, R. E., & Wareham, N. L. (1992). Early language and communicative abilities of children with periventricular leukomalacia. *American Journal on Mental Retardation, 97,* 222–234.

Fenson, L., Dale, P., Reznick, S., Thal, D., Bates, E., Hartung, J., Pethnick, S., & Reilly, J. (1993). *MacArthur Communicative Development Inventories.* San Diego: Singular Publishing.

Fewell, R., & Langley, M. (1984). *Developmental Activities Screening Inventory.* Austin, TX: Pro-Ed.

Forehand, R., & Atkeson, B. (1977). Generality of treatment effects with parents as therapists: A review of assessment and implementation procedures. *Behavior Therapy, 8,* 575–593.

Frailberg, S. (1979). Blind infants and their mothers: An examination of the sign system. In M. Bullowa (Ed.), *Before speech.* New York: Cambridge University Press.

Frank, H., & Rabinovitch, M. (1974). Auditory short-term memory: Developmental changes in rehearsal. *Child Development, 45,* 397–407.

Fristoe, M., & Lloyd, L. (1980). Planning an initial expressive sign lexicon for persons with severe communication impairment. *Journal of Speech and Hearing Disorders, 45,* 170–180.

Giattinno, J., Pollack, E., & Silliman, E. (1978). *Adult input in language impaired children.* Paper presented at the American Speech and Hearing Association Annual Convention, San Francisco.

Glidden, L. (1977). Stimulus relations, blocking, and sorting in the free recall and organization of EMR adolescents. *American Journal of Mental Deficiency, 82*, 250–258.

Glidden, L., & Warner, D. (1985). Semantic processing and serial learning by EMR adolescents. *American Journal of Mental Deficiency, 89*, 635–641.

Goetz, L., Gee, K., & Sailor, W. (1985). Using a behavior chain interruption strategy to teach communication skills to students with severe disabilities. *Journal of the Association for Persons with Severe Handicaps, 10*, 21–30.

Goldberg, S. (1977). Social competence in infancy: A model of parent-infant interaction. *Merrill-Palmer Quarterly, 23*, 163–177.

Goossens, C. (1984). *Assessment for nonspeech*. Paper presented at the annual conference of American Association on Mental Deficiency, Minneapolis, MN.

Graham, J., & Graham, L. (1971). Language behavior of the mentally retarded: Syntactic characteristics. *American Journal of Mental Deficiency, 73*, 623–629.

Greenfield, P., & Smith, J. (1976). *The structure of communication in early language development*. New York: Academic Press.

Greenspan, S. (1979). Social intelligence in the retarded. In N. Ellis (Ed.), *Handbook of mental deficiency: Psychological theory and research*. Hillsdale, NJ: Lawrence Erlbaum Associates.

Greenwald, C., & Leonard, L. (1979). Communicative and sensorimotor development of Down's syndrome children. *American Journal of Mental Deficiency, 84*, 296–303.

Grossman, H. (1983). *Classification in mental retardation*. Washington, DC: American Association on Mental Deficiency.

Guess, D., Koegh, W., & Sailor, W. (1978). Generalization of speech and language behavior: Measurement and training tactics. In R. Schiefelbusch (Ed.), *Bases of language intervention*. Baltimore: University Park Press.

Guess, D., Sailor, W., & Baer, D. (1976). *Functional speech and language training for the severely handicapped*. Lawrence, KS: H and H Enterprises.

Gullo, F., & Gullo, J. (1984). An ecological language intervention approach with mentally retarded adolescents. *Language, Speech and Hearing Services in Schools, 15*, 182–191.

Gutmann, A., & Rondal, J. (1979). Verbal operants in mothers' speech to nonretarded and Down's syndrome children matched for linguistic level. *American Journal of Mental Deficiency, 83*, 446–452.

Gutowski, W., & Chechile, R. (1987). Encoding, storage, and retrieval components of associative memory deficits of mildly mentally retarded adults. *American Journal of Mental Deficiency, 92*, 85–93.

Hagerman, R., Kemper, M., & Hudson, M. (1985). Learning disabilities and attentional problems in boys with the Fragile X syndrome. *American Journal of Diseases of Children, 139*, 674–678.

Halle, J., Alpert, C., & Anderson, S. (1984). Natural environment language assessment and intervention with severely impaired preschoolers. *Topics in Early Childhood Special Education, 4*, 36–56.

Hanley-Maxwell, C., Wilcox, B., & Heal, L. (1982). A comparison of vocabulary learning by moderately retarded students under direct instruction and incidental presentation. *Education and Training of Mentally Retarded, 3*, 214–221.

Hanna, R., & Lippert, E., & Harris, A. (1982). *Developmental Communication Curriculum Inventory*. San Antonio, TX: Psychological Corporation.

Hanzlik, J., & Stevenson, M. (1986). Interaction of mothers with their infants who are mentally retarded, with cerebral palsy, or nonretarded. *American Journal of Mental Deficiency, 90*, 513–520.

Harding, C. (1984). Acting with intention: A framework for examining the development of the intention to communicate. In L. Feagans, C. Garvey, & R. Golinkoff (Eds.), *The origins and growth of communication*. Norwood, NJ: Ablex.

Hargis, K., & Blechman, E. (1979). Social class and training of parents as behavior change agents. *Child Behavior Therapy, 1*, 69–74.

Haring, N., & Bricker, D. (1976). Overview of comprehensive services for the severely/profoundly handicapped. In N. Haring & L. Brown (Eds.), *Teaching the severely handicapped*. New York: Grune & Stratton.

Harris, D. (1982). Communicative interaction processes involving nonvocal physically handicapped children. *Topics in Language Disorders, 2*, 21–38.

Harris, D., Lippert, J., Yoder, D., & Vanderheiden, G. (1977). Blissymbolics: An augmentative symbol communication system for non-vocal severely handicapped children. In R. York & E. Edgat, (Eds.), *Teaching the severely handicapped* (Vol. 4). Seattle: Special Press.

Harris-Vanderheiden, D., Brown, W., MacKenzie, P., Reinen, S., & Schiebel, C. (1975). Symbol communication for the mentally handicapped. *Mental Retardation, 13*, 34–37.

Hayes, C., & Koch, R. (1977). Interpersonal distance behavior of mentally retarded and nonretarded children. *American Journal of Mental Deficiency, 82*, 207–209.

Heifetz, L. (1980). From consumer to middleman: Emerging roles for parents in the network of services for retarded children. In R. Abidin (Ed.), *Parent education and intervention handbook.* Springfield, IL: Charles Thomas.

Hess, R., & Shipman, V. (1965). Early experience and the socialization of cognitive modes in children. *Child Development, 36*, 886–896.

Hockey, R. (1973). Rate of presentation in running memory and direct manipulation of input processing strategies. *Quarterly Journal of Experimental Psychology, 25*, 104–111.

Hogg, J. (1975). Normative development and educational program planning for severely educationally subnormal children. In C. Kiennan & F. Woodford (Eds.), *Behavior modification with the severely retarded.* Amsterdam, The Netherlands: Associated Scientific Publishers.

Horstmeier, D., & MacDonald, J. (1978). *Environmental Prelanguage Battery.* San Antonio, TX: Psychological Corporation.

Houghton, J., Bronicki, G., & Guess, D. (1987). Opportunities to express preferences and make choices among students with sever disabilities in classroom settings. *Journal of the Association for Persons with Severe Handicaps, 12*, 18–27.

Hoy, E., & McKnight, J. (1977). Communication style and effectiveness in homogeneous and heterogeneous dyads of retarded children. *American Journal of Mental Deficiency, 81*, 587–598.

Humphreys, L., & Parsons, C. (1979). Piagetian tasks measure intelligence and intelligence tests assess cognitive development: A reanalysis. *Intelligence, 3*, 369–382.

Hunt, N. (1967). *The world of Nigel Hunt: The diary of a mongoloid youth.* New York: Garret.

Hunt, P., Goetz, L., Alwell, M., & Sailor, W. (1986). Using an interrupted behavior chain strategy to teach generalized communication responses. *Journal of the Association for Persons with Severe Handicaps, 11*, 196–204.

Ingalls, R. (1978). *Mental retardation: The changing outlook.* New York: Wiley.

Ingram, D. (1972). Transivity in child language. *Language, 47*, 888–910.

Jarman, R. (1978). Patterns of cognitive ability in retarded children: A reexamination. *American Journal of Mental Deficiency, 82*, 344–348.

Jarman, R., & Das, J. (1977). Simultaneous and successive synthesis and intelligence. *Intelligence, 1*, 151–169.

Johnson-Martin, N., Jens, K., Attermeier, S., & Hacker, B. (1991). *Carolina Curriculum for Infants and Toddlers with Special Needs.* Baltimore, MD: Paul Brookes.

Johnston, J., & Schery, T. (1976). The use of grammatical morphemes by children with communication disorders. In D. Morehead & A. Morehead (Eds.), *Normal and deficient child language.* Baltimore: University Park Press.

Jones, O. (1977). Mother-child communication with prelinguistic Down's syndrome and normal infants. In H. Schaffer (Eds.), *Studies in mother-infant interaction.* New York: Academic Press.

Jones, P. (1972). Home environment and the development of verbal ability. *Child Development, 43*, 1081–1086.

Kahn, J. (1975). Relationship of Piaget's sensorimotor period to language acquisition of profoundly retarded children. *American Journal of Mental Deficiency, 79*, 640–643.

Kahn, J. (1977). A comparison of manual and oral language training. *Mental Retardation, 15*, 21–23.

Kamhi, A. (1981). Developmental vs. different theories of mental retardation: A new look. *American Journal of Mental Deficiency, 86*, 1–7.

Kamhi, A., & Masterson, J. (1989). Language and cognition in mentally handicapped people: Last rites for the difference-delay controversy. In M. Beveridge, G. Conti-Ramsden, & I. Leudar (Eds.), *Language and communication in mentally handicapped people.* London: Chapman & Hall.

Kangas, K., & Lloyd, L. L. (1988). Early cognitive skills as prerequisites to augmentative and alternative communication use: What are we waiting for? *Augmentative and Alternative Communication, 4*, 211–221.

Karen, R., Astin-Smith, S., & Creasy, D. (1985). Teaching telephone-answering skills to mentally retarded adults. *American Journal of Mental Deficiency,* 89, 595–609.

Karrer, R., Nelson, M., & Galbraith, G. (1979). Psychophysiological research with the mentally retarded. In N. Ellis (Ed.), *International review of research in mental retardation* (Vol. 7). New York: Academic Press.

Kearsley, R. (1979). Latrogenic retardation: A syndrome of learned incompetence. In R. Kearsley & I. Sigel (Eds.), *Infants at risk: Assessment of cognitive functioning.* Hillsdale, NJ: Lawrence Erlbaum Associates.

Kellas, G., Ashcroft, M., & Johnson, N. (1973). Rehearsal processes in the short-term memory performance of mildly retarded adolescents. *American Journal of Mental Deficiency,* 77, 670–679.

Kendall, C., Borkowski, J., & Cavanaugh, J. (1980). Maintenance and generalization of an interrogative strategy by EMR children. *Intelligence, 4,* 255–270.

Kernan, K. (1990). Comprehension of syntactically indicated sequence by Down's syndrome and other mentally retarded adults. *Journal of Mental Deficiency Research, 34,* 169–178.

Kintsch, W., & van Dijk, T. (1978). Toward a model of text comprehension and productions. *Psychological Review, 85,* 363–394.

Klaus, M., & Kennell, J. (1976). *Maternal-infant bonding.* St. Louis: Mosby.

Klein, M., & Briggs, M. (1987). *Observation of Communicative Interactions.* Los Angeles: Mother-infant Communication Project, California State University.

Klink, M., Gerstman, L., Raphael, L., Schlanger, B., & Newsome, L. (1986). Phonological process usage by young EMR children and nonretarded preschool children. *American Journal of Mental Deficiency, 91,* 190–195.

Kogan, K., Wimberger, H., & Bobbitt, R. (1969). Analysis of mother-child interaction in young mental retardates. *Child Development, 40,* 799–812.

Kohl, F. (1981). Effects of motoric requirements on the acquisition of manual sign responses by severely handicapped students. *American Journal of Mental Deficiency, 85,* 396–403.

Kohl, F., Karlan, G., & Heal, L. (1979). Effects of pairing manual signs with verbal cues upon the acquisition of instruction-following behaviors and the generalization to expressive language with severely handicapped students. *AAESPH Review, 4,* 291–300.

Konstantases, M., Oxman, J., & Webster, C. (1917). Simultaneous communication with autistic and other severely dysfunctional nonverbal children. *Journal of Communication Disorders, 10,* 267–282.

Krupski, A. (1977). Role of attention in the reaction-time performance of mentally retarded adolescents. *American Journal of Mental Deficiency, 82,* 79–83.

Lackner, J. (1968) A developmental study of language behavior in retarded children. *Neuropsychologia, 6,* 301–320.

LaGreca, A., Stone, W., & Bell, C. (1983). Facilitating the vocational-interpersonal skills of mentally retarded individuals. *American Journal of Mental Deficiency, 88,* 270–278.

Lamberts, F. (1981). Sign and symbol in children's processing of familiar auditory stimuli. *American Journal of Mental Deficiency, 86,* 300–308.

Layton, T., & Sharifi, H. (1979). Meaning and structure of Down's syndrome and nonretarded children's spontaneous speech. *American Journal of Mental Deficiency, 83,* 439–445.

Leahy, R., Balla, D., & Zigler, E. (1982). Role-taking, self-image, and imitativeness of mentally retarded and nonretarded individuals. *American Journal of Mental Deficiency, 86,* 372–379.

Lee, L. (1974). *Developmental sentence analysis.* Evanston, IL: Northwestern University Press.

Leonard, L., Cole, B., & Steckol, K. (1979). Lexical usage of retarded children: An examination of informativeness. *American Journal of Mental Deficiency, 84,* 49–54.

Leonard, L., Steckol, K., & Panther, K. (1983). Returning meaning to semantic relations: Some clinical applications. *Journal of Speech and Hearing Disorders, 48,* 25–35.

Levine, H., & Langness, L. (1985). Everyday cognition among mildly mentally retarded adults: An ethno graphic approach. *American Journal of Mental Deficiency, 90,* 18–26.

Liebert, A., & Baumeister, A. (1973). Behavioral variability among retardates, children, and college students. *The Journal of Psychology, 83,* 57–65.

Lincoln, A., Courchesne, E., Kilman, B., & Galambos, R. (1985). Neuropsychological correlates of information-processing by children with Down syndrome. *American Journal of Mental Deficiency,* 89, 403–414.

Lobato, D., Barrera, R., & Feldman, R. (1981). Sensorimotor functioning and prelinguistic communication of severely and profoundly mentally retarded individuals. *American Journal of Mental Deficiency,* 85, 489–496.

Lobb, H. (1974). Effects of verbal rehearsal on discrimination learning in moderately retarded nursery-school children. *American Journal of Mental Deficiency,* 79, 449–454.

Longhurst, T., & Berry, G. (1975). Communication in retarded adolescents: Response to listener feedback. *American Journal of Mental Deficiency,* 80, 158–164.

Looney, P. (1980). Instructional intervention with language-disordered learners. *Directive Teacher,* 2, 30–31.

Luftig, R., & Johnson, R. (1982). Identification and recall of structurally important units in prose of mentally retarded learners. *American Journal of Mental Deficiency,* 86, 495–502.

Luria, A. (1975). Basic problems of language in the light of psychology and neurolinguistics. In E. Lenneberg & E. Lenneberg (Eds.), *Foundations of language development: A multidisciplinary approach.* New York: Academic Press.

MacDonald, J. (1978a). *Environmental Language Inventory.* San Antonio, TX: Psychological Corporation.

MacDonald, J. (1978b). *Environmental Language Intervention Program.* Columbus, OH: Merrill/Macmillan.

MacDonald, J. (1985). Language through conversation: A model for intervention with language-delayed persons. In S. Warren and A. Rogers-Warren (Eds.), *Teaching functional language* (pp. 89–122). Baltimore: University Park Press.

MacDonald, J., Blott, J., Gordon, K., Spiegal, B., & Hartmann, M. (1974). An experimental parent-assisted treatment program for preschool language-delayed children. *Journal of Speech and Hearing Disorders,* 39, 295–415.

MacDonald, J., & Gillette, Y. (1978). *Environmental Communication System (ECO).* San Antonio, TX: Psychological Corporation.

MacDonald, J., & Gillette, Y. (1982). *ECO, ecological communication system: A clinical handbook for parents and teachers.* Columbus, OH: Nisonger Center.

MacMillan, D. (1972). Paired-associate learning as a function of explicitness of mediational set by EMR and nonretarded children. *American Journal of Mental Deficiency,* 76, 686–691.

Macnamara, J. (1972). Cognitive basis of language learning in infants. *Psychological Review,* 79, 1–13.

Mahoney, G., Fors, S., & Wood, S. (1990). Maternal directive behavior revisited. *American Journal on Mental Retardation,* 94, 398–406.

Mahoney, G., Glover, A., & Finger, I. (1981). Relationship between language and sensorimotor development of Down syndrome and nonretarded children. *American Journal of Mental Deficiency,* 86, 21–27.

Mahoney, G., & Snow, K. (1983). The relationship of sensorimotor functioning to children's response to early language training. *Mental Retardation,* 21, 248–254.

Mahoney, G., & Weller, E. (1980). An ecological approach to language intervention. *New Directions for Exceptional Children,* 2, 17–33.

Malgady, R., Barcher, R., Towner, G., & Davis, J. (1979). Language factors in vocational evaluation of mentally retarded workers. *American Journal of Mental Deficiency,* 83, 432–438.

Manolson, A. (1983). *It takes two to talk.* Toronto: Hanen Early Language Resource Centre.

Marcell, M., & Armstrong, V. (1982). Auditory and visual sequential memory of Down syndrome and nonretarded children. *American Journal of Mental Deficiency,* 87, 86–95.

Marcell, M., & Jett, D. (1985). Identification of vocally expressed emotions by mentally retarded and nonretarded individuals. *American Journal of Mental Deficiency,* 89, 537–545.

Marcell, M., & Weeks, S. (1988). Short-term memory difficulties and Down's syndrome. *Journal of Mental Deficiency Research,* 32, 153–162.

Marshall, N., Hegrenes, J., & Goldstein, S. (1973). Verbal interactions: Mothers and their retarded children vs. mothers and their nonretarded children. *American Journal of Mental Deficiency,* 77, 415–419.

Maurer, H., & Sherrod, K. (1987). Context of directives given to young children with Down syndrome and nonretarded children: Development over two years. *American Journal of Mental Deficiency,* 91, 579–590.

McCarver, R., & Craig, E. (1974). Placement of the retarded in the community: Prognosis and outcome. In N. Ellis (Ed.), *International review of research in mental retardation* (Vol. 7). New York: Academic Press.

McCormick, L. (1986). Keeping up with language trends. *Teaching Exceptional Children,* 18, 123–129.

McLean, J., & Snyder-McLean, L. (1978). *A transactional approach to early language training.* Columbus, OH: Merrill/Macmillan.

McLeavey, B., Toomey, J., & Dempsey, P. (1982). Nonretarded and mentally retarded children's control over syntactic structures. *American Journal of Mental Deficiency,* 86, 485–494.

McNutt, J., & Leri, S. (1979). Language differences between institutionalized and noninstitutionalized retarded children. *American Journal of Mental Deficiency,* 83, 339–345.

Meador, D. (1984). Effects of color on visual discrimination of geometric symbols by severely and profoundly mentally retarded individuals. *American Journal of Mental Deficiency,* 89, 275–286.

Mehrabian, A., & Williams, M. (1971). Piagetian measures of cognitive development for children up to age two. *Journal of Psycholinguistic Research,* 1, 113–126.

Mental retardation: Definition, classification, and systems of support (ninth edition). (1992). Washington, DC: American Association on Mental Retardation.

Menyuk, P. (1974). Early development of receptive language: From babbling to words. In R. Schiefelbusch & L. Lloyd (Eds.), *Language perspectives—Acquisition, retardation and intervention.* Baltimore: University Park Press.

Mercer, C., & Snell, M. (1977). *Learning theory research in mental retardation.* Columbus, OH: Merrill/Macmillan.

Merrill, E. (1985). Differences in semantic processing speed of mentally retarded and nonretarded persons. *American Journal of Mental Deficiency,* 90, 71–80.

Merrill, E., & Bilsky, L. (1990). Individual differences in the representation of sentences in memory. *American Journal on Mental Retardation,* 95, 68–76.

Merrill, E. C., & Jackson, T. S. (1992). Degree of associative relatedness and sentence processing by adolescents with and without mental retardation. *American Journal on Mental Retardation,* 97, 173–185.

Merrill, E., & Mar, H. (1987). Differences between mentally retarded and nonretarded persons' efficiency of auditory sentence processing. *American Journal of Mental Deficiency,* 91, 406–414.

Miller, A., & Miller, F. (1973). Cognitive developmental training with elevated boards and sign language. *Journal of Autism and Childhood Schizophrenia,* 3, 65–68.

Miller, A., & Newhoff, M. (1978). *Language disordered children: Language disordered mothers?* Paper presented at the American Speech and Hearing Association Annual Conference, San Francisco.

Miller, J. (1980). *Assessing language production in children.* Baltimore: University Park Press.

Miller, J., Chapman, R., & MacKenzie, H. (1981). Individual differences in the language acquisition of mentally retarded children. *Proceedings from the second Wisconsin symposium on research in child language disorders.* Madison: University of Wisconsin.

Miller, J. F., Sedey, A. L., & Miolo, G. (1995). Validity of parent report measures of vocabulary development for children with Down syndrome. *Journal of Speech and Hearing Research,* 38, 1037–1044.

Miller, J., & Yoder, D. (1974). An ontogenetic language teaching strategy for retarded children. In R. Schiefelbusch & L. Lloyd (Eds.), *Language perspectives—Acquisition, retardation, and intervention.* Baltimore: University Park Press.

Miller, S., & Sloan, H. (1976). The generalization effects of parent training across stimulus settings. *Journal of Applied Behavior Analysis,* 9, 355–370.

Mindell, C., & Budd, K. (1977). *Issues in the generalization of parent training across settings.* Paper presented at the annual meeting of the American Psychological Association.

Mittler, P. (1974). Language and communication. In A. Clarke & A. Clarke (Eds.), *Mental deficiency: The changing outlook.* London: Methuen.

Mittler, P. (1976) Assessment for language learning. In P. Berry (Ed.), *Language and communication in the mentally handicapped.* Baltimore: University Park Press.

Montague, J., Hutchinson, E., & Matson, E. (1975). Comparative computer content analysis of the verbal behavior of institutionalized and noninstitutionalized retarded children. *Journal of Speech and Hearing Research,* 18, 43–57.

Moran, M., Money, S., & Leonard, D. (1984). Phonological process analysis of the speech of mentally retarded adults. *American Journal of Mental Deficiency,* 89, 304–306.

Muma, J. (1978). *Language handbook: Concepts, assessment, intervention.* Englewood Cliffs, NJ: Prentice Hall.

Musselwhite, C., & St. Louis, K. (1982). *Communication programming for the severely handicapped: Vocal and non-vocal strategies.* Houston: College-Hill Press.

Naremore, R., & Dever, R. (1975). Language performance of educable mentally retarded and normal children at five age levels. *Journal of Speech and Hearing Research,* 18, 82–95.

Newfield, M. (1966). *A study of the acquisition of English morphology by normal and EMR children.* Master's thesis, Ohio State University, Columbus.

Newfield, M., & Schlinger, B. (1968) The acquisition of English morphology in normal and educable mentally retarded children. *Journal of Speech and Hearing Research,* 11, 693–706.

Nigro, G., & Roak, R. (1987). Mentally retarded and nonretarded adults' memory for spatial location. *American Journal of Mental Deficiency,* 91, 392–397.

Nugent, P., & Mosley, J. (1987). Mentally retarded and nonretarded individuals' attention allocation and capacity. *American Journal of Mental Deficiency,* 91, 598–605.

Nussvaum, R., & Ledbetter, D. (1986). Fragile X syndrome: A unique mutation in man. *Annual Review of Genetics, 20,* 109–145.

O'Connor, N., & Hermelin, B. (1978). *Seeing and hearing and space and time.* New York: Academic Press.

Ogletree, B. T., Wetherby, A. M., & Westling, D. L. (1992). Profile of the prelinguistic intentional communicative behavior of children with profound mental retardation. *American Journal on Mental Retardation,* 97, 188–196.

Oller, D., & Seibert, J. (1988). Babbling of prelinguistic mentally retarded children. *American Journal on Mental Retardation,* 92, 369–375.

Olswang, L., Stoel-Gammon, C., Coggins, T., & Carpenter, R. (1987a). *Assessing Linguistic Behavior (ALB).* Seattle: University of Washington Press.

Olswang, L., Stoel-Gammon, C., Coggins, T., & Carpenter, R. (1987b). *Assessing Prelinguistic Behaviors in Developmentally Young Children.* Seattle: University of Washington Press.

O'Regan-Kleinert, J. (1980). *Pre-speech/language therapeutic techniques for the handicapped infant.* Paper presented at the American Speech-Language-Hearing Association Convention, Detroit.

O'Regan-Kleinert, J., Rosenwinkel, P., & Robbins, R. (1979). *Remediation of severe language disorders: A pre-speech sensorimotor developmental model.* Paper presented at the American Speech-Language-Hearing Association Convention, Atlanta.

Osofosky, J., & O'Connell, E. (1972). Daughter's effects upon mother's and father's behavior. *Developmental Psychology, 7,* 157–168.

Owens, R. E. (1978). *Speech acts in the early language of non-delayed and retarded children: A taxonomy and distributional study.* Unpublished doctoral dissertation, The Ohio State University.

Owens, R. (1982a). *Caregiver Interview and Environmental Observation.* San Antonio, TX: Psychological Corporation.

Owens, R. (1982b). *Developmental Assessment Tool.* San Antonio, TX: Psychological Corporation.

Owens, R. (1982c). *Diagnostic Interactional Survey.* San Antonio, TX: Psychological Corporation.

Owens, R. (1982d). *Program for the Acquisition of Language with the Severely Impaired* (PALS). San Antonio: Psychological Corp.

Owens, R. E. (1995). *Language disorders: A functional approach to assessment and intervention* (2nd ed.). Boston: Allyn & Bacon.

Owens, R. (1996). *Language development: An introduction* (4th ed.). Columbus, OH: Merrill/Macmillan.

Owens, R., & House, L. (1984). Decision-making processes in augmentative communication. *Journal of Speech and Hearing Disorders,* 49, 18–25.

Owens, R., & MacDonald, J. (1982). Communicative uses of the early speech of nondelayed and Down syndrome children. *American Journal of Mental Deficiency,* 86, 503–510.

Owens, R., McNerney, C., Bigler-Burke, L., & Lepre-Clark, C. (1987). The use of language facilitators with residential retarded populations. *Topics in Language Disorders,* 7(3), 47–63.

Owens, R. E., & Rogerson, B. S. (1988). Adults at the presymbolic level. In S. Calculator & J. Bedrosian (Eds.), *Communicative assessment and intervention for adults with mental retardation* (pp. 189–230). San Diego: College-Hill.

Owings, N., & Guvette, T. (1982). Communication behavior assessment and treatment with the adult retarded: An approach. In N. Lass (Ed.), *Speech and language: Advances in basic research and practice* (Vol. 7). New York: Academic Press.

Page, J., & Horn, D. (1987). Comprehension in developmentally delayed children. *Language, Speech and Hearing Services in Schools, 18*, 63–71.

Papania, N. (1954). A qualitative analysis of vocabulary responses of institutionalized mentally retarded children. *Journal of Clinical Psychology, 10*, 361–365.

Petersen, G., & Sherrod, K. (1982). Relationship of maternal language to language development and language delay of children. *American Journal of Mental Deficiency, 86*, 391–398.

Phillips, I., & Williams, N. (1975). Psychopathology and mental retardation: 1. Psychopathology. *American Journal of Psychiatry, 132*, 1265–1271.

Phillips, J., & Balthazar, E. (1979). Some correlates of language deterioration in severely and profoundly retarded long-term institutionalized residents. *American Journal of Mental Deficiency, 83*, 402–408.

Pickett, J., & Flynn, P. (1983). Language assessment tools for mentally retarded adults: Survey and recommendations. *American Journal of Mental Deficiency, 21*, 244–247.

Platt, J. & Coggins, T. (1990). Comprehension of social-action games in prelinguistic children. *Journal of Speech and Hearing Disorders, 55*, 315–326.

Polk, X., Schilmoeller, G., Embry, L., Holman, J., & Baer, D. (1976). *Prompted generalization through experimenters' instructions: A parent training study.* Paper presented at the annual meeting of the Midwestern Association of Behavior Analysis, Chicago.

Poulson, C. (1988). Operant conditioning of vocalization rate of infants with Down syndrome. *American Journal on Mental Retardation, 93*, 57–63.

Prater, R. (1982). Functions of consonant assimilation and reduplication in early word productions of mentally retarded children. *American Journal of Mental Deficiency, 86*, 399–404.

Prior, M., Minnes, P., Coyne, T., Golding, B., Hendy, J., & McGillivray, J. (1979). Verbal interactions between staff and residents in an institution for the young mentally retarded. *Mental Retardation, 17*, 65–70.

Pruess, J., Vadasy, P., & Fewell, R. (1987). Language development in children with Down syndrome: An overview of recent research. *Education and Training in Mental Retardation, 22*, 44–55.

Prutting, C. (1979). Process: The action of moving forward progressively from one point to another on the way to completion. *Journal of Speech and Hearing Disorders, 44*, 3–30.

Prutting, C., & Kirchner, D. (1983). Applied pragmatics. In T. Gallagher & C. Prutting (Eds.), *Pragmatic assessment and intervention issues in language.* San Diego: College-Hill Press.

Realon, R., Lewallen, J., & Wheeler, A. (1983). Verbal vs. verbal feedback plus praise: The effects on direct care staff's training behaviors. *Mental Retardation, 21*, 209–213.

Rees, N. (1978). Pragmatics of language: Applications to normal and disordered language development. In R. Schiefelbusch (Ed.), *Bases of language intervention.* Baltimore: University Park Press.

Rees, N., & Wollner, S. (1981). *Toward a taxonomy of pragmatic abilities in children.* Paper presented at the ASHA Northeast Regional Conference, Philadelphia.

Reese, R., & Serna, L. (1986). Planning for generalization and maintenance in parent training: Parents need IEPs too. *Mental Retardation, 24*, 87–92.

Reich, R. (1978). Gestural facilitation of expressive language in moderately/severely retarded preschoolers. *Mental Retardation, 16*, 113–117.

Reichle, J. (1990). *Intervention with presymbolic clients: Setting up an initial communication system.* Paper presented at the New York State Speech-Language-Hearing Association annual convention, Kiamesha Lake, NY.

Reichle, J., & Sigafoos, J. (1991). Establishing an initial repertoire of requesting. In J. Reichle, J. York, & J. Sigafoos (Eds.), *Implementing Augmentative and Alternative Communication.* Baltimore: Paul H. Brookes.

Reid, G. (1980). Overt and covert rehearsal in short-term motor memory of mentally retarded and non-retarded persons. *American Journal of Mental Deficiency, 85*, 69–77.

Rein, R., & Kernan, K. (1989). The functional use of verbal perseveratives by adults who are mentally retarded. *Education and Training in Mental Retardation,* 24, 381–389.

Reiss, S., Levitan, G., & Szyszko, J. (1982). Emotional disturbance and mental retardation: Diagnostic overshadowing. *American Journal of Mental Deficiency,* 86, 567–574.

Reiter, S., & Levi, A. (1980). Factors affecting social integration of noninstitutionalized mentally retarded adults. *American Journal of Mental Deficiency,* 85, 25–30.

Rescorla, L. (1989). The Language Development Survey: A screening tool for delayed toddlers. *Journal of Speech and Hearing Disorders,* 54, 587–599.

Rheingold, H., & Eckerman, C. (1975). Some properties for unifying the study of social development. In M. Lewis & M. Rosenblum (Eds.), *Friendship and peer relations.* New York: Wiley.

Richmond, G., & Lewallen, J. (1983). Facilitating transfer of stimulus control when teaching verbal labels. *Education and Training of Mentally Retarded,* 18, 111–115.

Riley, A. (1984). *Evaluating acquired skills in communication.* Tucson, AZ: Communication Skill Builders.

Robinson, L. A., & Owens, R. E. (1995). Functional augmentative communication and positive behavior change. *Augmentative and Alternative Communication,* 11, 207–211.

Robinson, N., & Robinson, H. (1976). *The mentally retarded child: A psychological approach* (2nd ed.). New York: McGraw-Hill.

Romer, L., & Schoenberg, B. (1991). Increasing requests made by people with developmental disabilities and deaf-blindness through the use of behavior chain interruption strategies. *Education and Training in Mental Retardation,* 26, 70–78.

Romski, M., Sevcik, R., Pate, J., & Rumbaugh, D. (1985). Discrimination of lexigrams and traditional orthography by nonspeaking severely mentally retarded persons. *American Journal of Mental Deficiency,* 90, 185–190.

Romski, M., Sevcik, R., & Rumbaugh, D. (1985). Retention of symbolic communication skills by severely mentally retarded persons. *American Journal of Mental Deficiency,* 89, 441–443.

Rondal, J. (1976). *Maternal speech to normal and Down's syndrome children matched for mean length of utterance* (Research Report No. 98). Washington, DC: BEH (Contract No. 300–76–0036).

Rondal, J. (1978). Maternal speech to normal and Down's syndrome children matched for mean length of utterances. In C. Meyers (Ed.), *Quality of life in severely and profoundly mentally retarded people.* Washington, DC: American Association on Mental Deficiency.

Rondal, J., Ghiotto, M., Bredart, S., & Bachelet, J. (1988). Mean length of utterance of children with Down syndrome. *American Journal on Mental Retardation,* 93, 64–66.

Ross, D., & Ross, S. (1979). Cognitive training for the EMR child: Language skills prerequisite to relevant-irrelevant discrimination tasks. *Mental Retardation,* 17, 3–7.

Rossetti, L. (1990). *Infant-Toddler Language Scale.* East Moline, IL: LinguiSystems.

Russell, A., & Tanquay, P. (1981). Mental illness and mental retardation: Cause or coincidence? *American Journal of Mental Deficiency,* 85, 570–574.

Ryan, J. (1975). Mental subnormality and language development. In R. Lenneberg & E. Lenneberg (Eds.), *Foundations of language development* (Vol. 2). New York: Academic Press.

Sacks, J., & Young, E. (1982). Infant Scale of Communication Intent. *Pediatrics Update,* 7, 1–5.

Salzberg, C., & Villani, T. (1983). Speech training by parents of Down syndrome toddlers: Generalization across settings and instructional contexts. *American Journal of Mental Deficiency,* 87, 403–413.

Schiefelbusch, R. (Ed.). (1963). Language studies in mentally retarded children. *Journal of Speech and Hearing Disorders, Monograph Supplement No. 10.*

Scruggs, T., Mastropieri, M., & Levin, J. (1985). Vocabulary acquisition of mentally retarded students under direct and mnemonic instruction. *American Journal of Mental Deficiency,* 89, 546–551.

Seitz, S., & Riedel, G. (1974). Parent-child interactions as the therapy target. *Journal of Communication Disorders,* 7, 295–304.

Semmel, M. (1967). Language behavior of mentally retarded and culturally disadvantaged children. In J. Magary & R. McIntyre (Eds.), *Distinguished lectures in special education.* Berkeley: University of California Press.

Semmel, M., Barritt, L., & Bennett, S. (1970). Performance of EMR and non-retarded children on a modified cloze task. *American Journal of Mental Deficiency,* 74, 681–688.

Semmel, M., & Herzog, B. (1966). The effects of grammatical form class on the recall of Negro and Caucasian educable retarded children. *Studies of Language and Language Behavior,* 3, 1–9.

Shane, H., & Bashir, A. (1980). Election criteria for the adoption of an augmentative communication system: Preliminary considerations. *Journal of Speech and Hearing Disorders,* 45, 408–414.

Shane, H., Lipshultz, R., & Shane, C. (1982). Facilitating the communicative interaction of nonspeaking persons in large residential settings. *Topics in Language Disorders,* 2, 73–84.

Shane, H., & Wilbur, R. (1980). Potential for expressive signing based on motor control. *Sign Language Studies,* 29, 331–347.

Sharav, T., & Shlomo, L. (1986). Stimulation of infants with Down syndrome: Long-term effects. *Mental Retardation,* 24, 81–86.

Share, J. (1975). Developmental progress in Down's syndrome. In R. Koch & F. de la Cruz (Eds.), *Down's syndrome.* New York: Bruner Mazel.

Shepard, G., & Marshall, J. (1976). Perceptions of interpersonal communication of EMR adolescents and their mothers. *Education and Training of Mentally Retarded,* 11, 106–111.

Shriberg, L., & Widder, C. (1990). Speech and prosody characteristics of adults with mental retardation. *Journal of Speech and Hearing Research,* 33, 627–653.

Siegel, G. (1975). The use of language tests. *Language, Speech and Hearing Services in Schools,* 6, 211–217.

Silverman, F. (1980). *Communication for the speechless.* Englewood Cliffs, NJ: Prentice Hall.

Simic, J., & Bucher, B. (1980). Development of spontaneous mending in language deficient children. *Journal of Applied Behavior Analysis,* 13, 523–528.

Skinner, B. F. (1957). *Verbal behavior.* New York: Appleton-Century-Crofts.

Smith, L., & Hagen, V. (1984). Relationship between the home environment and sensorimotor development of Down syndrome and nonretarded infants. *American Journal of Mental Deficiency,* 89, 124–132.

Snart, F., O'Grady, M., & Das, J. (1982). Cognitive processing of subgroups of moderately mentally retarded children. *American Journal of Mental Deficiency,* 86, 465–472.

Snell, M. (1979). Higher functioning residents as language trainers of the mentally retarded. *Education and Training of Mentally Retarded,* 14, 77–84.

Snow, C., & Ferguson, C. (1977). *Talking to children.* New York: Cambridge University Press.

Snyder, L. (1978). Communicative and cognitive abilities and disabilities in the sensorimotor period. *Merrill-Palmer Quarterly,* 24, 161–180.

Sokolov, J. L. (1992). Linguistic imitation in children with Down syndrome. *American Journal on Mental Retardation,* 97, 209–221.

Sommers, R., Patterson, J., & Wildgren, P. (1988). Phonology of Down syndrome speakers, ages 13–22. *Journal of Childhood Communication Disorders,* 12, 65–91.

Sommers, R., & Starkey, K. (1977). Dichotic verbal processing in Down's syndrome children having qualitatively different speech and language skills. *American Journal of Mental Deficiency,* 82, 44–53.

Spiegel, B. (1983). The effect of context on language learning by severely retarded young adults. *Language, Speech and Hearing Services in Schools,* 14, 252–259.

Spitz, H. (1966). The role of input organization in the learning and memory of mental retardates. In N. Ellis (Ed.), *International review of research in mental retardation* (Vol. 2). New York: Academic Press.

Spitz, H. (1979). Beyond field theory in the study of mental deficiency. In N. Ellis (Ed.), *Handbook of mental deficiency: Psychological theory and research.* Hillsdale, NJ: Lawrence Erlbaum Associates.

Spradlin, J. (1963). Language and communication of mental defectives. In N. Ellis (Ed.), *Handbook of mental deficiency.* New York: McGraw-Hill.

Spradlin, J., & Siegel, G. (1982). Language training in natural and clinical environments. *Journal of Speech and Hearing Disorders,* 47, 2–6.

Steffens, M. L., Kimbrough Oller, D., Lynch, M., & Urbano, R. C. (1992). Vocal development in infants with Down syndrome who are developing normally. *American Journal on Mental Retardation,* 97, 235–246.

Stephens, B., & McLaughlin, J. (1974). Two-year gains in reasoning by retarded and nonretarded persons. *American Journal of Mental Deficiency, 79,* 116–126.

Stephens, W. (1972). Equivalence formation by retarded and nonretarded children at different mental ages. *American Journal of Mental Deficiency, 77,* 311–313.

Sternberg, L., Pegnatore, L., & Hill, C. (1983). Establishing interactive communication behaviors with profoundly mentally handicapped students. *TASH Journal, 8,* 39–46.

Stevenson, M., & Lamb, M. (1979). Effects of infant sociability and the caretaking environment on infant cognitive performance. *Child Development, 50,* 340–349.

Stillman, R. (1978). *Callier-Azusa Scale.* Dallas: Callier Center, University of Texas.

Stoneman, Z., Brody, G., & Abbott, D. (1983). In-home observations of young Down syndrome children with their mothers and fathers. *American Journal of Mental Deficiency, 87,* 591–600.

Stowitschek, J., McConaughy, E., Peatross, D., Salzberg, C., & Lignngaris/Kraft, B. (1988). Effects of group incidental training on the use of social amenities by adults with mental retardation in work settings. *Education and Training in Mental Retardation, 23,* 202–212.

Sudhalter, V., Cohen, I., Silverman, W., & Wolf-Schein, E. (1990). Conversational analysis of males with Fragile X, Down syndrome, and autism: Comparison of the emergence of deviant language. *American Journal on Mental Retardation, 99,* 431–441.

Switsky, H., Rotatori, A., Miller, T., & Freagon, S. (1979). The developmental model and its implications for assessment and instruction for the severely/profoundly handicapped. *Mental Retardation, 17,* 167–170.

Szymanski, L., & Tanquay, P. (Eds.). (1980). *Emotional disorders of mentally retarded persons.* Baltimore: University Park Press.

Tannock, R. (1988). Mothers' directiveness in their interactions with their children with and without Down syndrome. *American Journal on Mental Retardation, 93,* 154–165.

Tannock, R., Girolametto, L., & Siegel, L. S. (1992). Language intervention with children who have developmental delays: Effects of an interactive approach. *American Journal on Mental Retardation, 97,* 145–160.

Taylor, A., & Turnure, J. (1979). Imagery and verbal elaboration with retarded children: Effects on learning and memory. In N. Ellis (Ed.), *Handbook of mental deficiency: Psychological theory and research.* Hillsdale, NJ: Lawrence Erlbaum Associates.

Tizard, B., Cooperman, O., Joseph, A., & Tizard, J. (1973). Environmental effects on language development: A study of young children in long stay residential nurseries. *Annual Progress in Child Psychiatry & Child Development, 13,* 705–728.

Trotter, R. (1983, August). Baby face. *Psychology Today,* pp. 14–20.

Turner, L., & Bray, N. (1985). Spontaneous rehearsal by mildly mentally retarded children and adolescents. *American Journal of Mental Deficiency, 90,* 57–63.

Ullman, D. (1974). Breadth of attention and retention in mentally retarded and intellectually average children. *American Journal of Mental Deficiency, 78,* 640–648.

Van Biervliet, A. (1977). Establishing words and objects as functionally equivalent through manual sign training. *American Journal of Mental Deficiency, 82,* 178–186.

Van Borsel, J. (1988). An analysis of the speech of five Down's syndrome adolescents. *Journal of Communication Disorders, 21,* 409–421.

Van Der Gagg, A. (1989). The view from Walter's window: Social environment and the communicative competence of adults with a mental handicap. *Journal of Mental Deficiency Research, 33,* 221–227.

Vanderheiden, G. (1982). *Computers can play a dual role for disabled individuals.* Madison: University of Wisconsin, Trace Center.

Variety Pre-Schooler's Workshop. (1987). *Parent/Professional Preschool Performance Profile (5Ps).* Syosset, NY: Variety Pre-Schooler's Workshop.

Varnhagen, C., Das, J., & Varnhagen, S. (1987). Auditory and visual memory span: Cognitive processing by TMR individuals with Down syndrome or other etiologies. *American Journal of Mental Deficiency, 91,* 398–405.

Vihman, M. (1978). Consonant harmony: Its scope and function in child language. In J. Greenberg (Ed.), *Universals of human language: Vol. 2. Phonology.* Stanford, CA: Stanford University Press.

Volpe, R. (1976). Orthopedic disability, restriction, and role-taking activity. *The Journal of Special Education, 10*, 371–381.

Watkins, O., & Watkins, M. (1980). The modality effect and echoic persistence. *Journal of Experimental Psychology: General, 109*, 251–278.

Weiss, B., Weisz, J., & Bromfield, R. (1986). Performance of retarded and non-retarded persons on information-processing tasks: Further tests of the similar structure hypothesis. *Psychological Bulletin, 100*, 157–175.

Welch, S., & Pear, J. (1979). Generalization by autistic-type children of verbal responses across settings. *Journal of Applied Behavior Analysis, 12*, 273–282.

Westby, C. (1980). Assessment of cognitive and language abilities through play *Language, Speech and Hearing Services in Schools, 11*, 154–168.

Wetherby, A., & Prizant, B. (1993). *Communication and Symbolic Behavior Scales.* Chicago: Riverside.

Whatmough, J. (1956). *Language: A modern synthesis.* New York: American Library.

White, B., Watts, J., Barnett, I., Kahan, B., Marmor, J., & Shapiro, B. (1973). *Experience and environment: Major influences on the development of the young child* (Vol. 1). Englewood Cliffs, NJ: Prentice Hall.

Wilcox, M., & Campbell, P. (1983). *Assessing communication in low-functioning multihandicapped children.* Paper presented at the American Speech-Language-Hearing Association Annual Convention, Cincinnati, OH.

Wilkinson, K. M., & Romski, M. A. (1995). Responsiveness of male adolescents with mental retardation to input from nondisabled peers: the summoning power of comments, questions, and direct prompts. *Journal of Speech and Hearing, 38*, 1045–1053.

Windle, C. (1962). Prognosis of mental subnormals. *American Journal of Mental Deficiency* (Monograph Supplement).

Winitz, H. (1983). Use and abuse of the developmental approach. In H. Winitz (Ed.), *Treating language disorders.* Baltimore: University Park Press.

Wolf-Schein, E., Sudhalter, V., Cohen, I., Fisch, G., Hansen, D., Pfadt, A., Hagerman, R., Jenkins, E., & Brown, W. (1987). Speech-language and Fragile X syndrome. *Asha, 29*, 35–38.

Wolfensberger, W. (1967). Counseling the parents of the retarded. In A. Baumeister (Ed.), *Mental retardation: Appraisal, education, and rehabilitation.* Chicago: Aldine.

Wolfensberger, W., Mein, R., & O'Connor, N. (1963). A study of the oral vocabularies of severely subnormal patients: III. Core vocabulary, verbosity and repetitiousness. *Journal of Mental Deficiency Research, 7*, 38–45.

Wolff, P., Gardner, J., Lappen, J., Paccia, J., & Meryash, D. (1988). Variable expression of the Fragile X syndrome in heterozygous females of normal intelligence. *American Journal of Medical Genetics, 30*, 213–225.

Woodward, M., & Stern, D. (1963). Developmental patterns of severely subnormal children. *British Journal of Educational Psychology, 33*, 10–21.

Wulbert, M., Inglis, S., Kreigsmann, E., & Mills, B. (1975). Language delay and associated mother-child interactions. *Developmental Psychology, 11*, 61–70.

Wulz, S., Hall, M., & Klein, M. (1983). A home-centered instructional communication strategy for severely handicapped children. *Journal of Speech and Hearing Disorders, 48*, 2–10.

Yoder, D., & Miller, J. (1972). What we may know and what we can do: Input toward a system. In J. McLean, D. Yoder, & R. Schiefelbusch (Eds.), *Language intervention with the retarded.* Baltimore: University Park Press.

Yoder, P. J., & Davies, B. (1992). Do children with developmental delays use more frequent and diverse language in verbal routines? *American Journal on Mental Retardation, 97*, 197–208.

Yoder, P. J. & Feagans, L. (1988). Mothers' attributions of communication to prelinguistic behavior of developmentally delayed and mentally retarded children. *American Journal on Mental Retardation, 93*, 36–43.

Zeaman, D., & House, B. (1963). The role of attention in retardate discrimination learning. In N. Ellis (Ed.), *Handbook of mental deficiency.* New York: McGraw-Hill.

Zeaman, D., & House, B. (1979). A review of attention theory. In N. Ellis (Ed.), *Handbook of mental deficiency: Psychological theory and research.* Hillsdale, NJ: Lawrence Erlbaum Associates.

Zetlin, A., & Gallimore, R. (1983). The development of comprehension strategies through the regulatory function of teacher questions. *Education and Training of Mentally Retarded,* 18, 176–183.

Zigler, E. (1967). Mental retardation technical comment. *Science,* 157, 578.

Zigler, E. (1971). The retarded person as a whole person. In H. Adams & W. Boardman (Eds.), *Advances in experimental clinical psychology.* New York: Pergamon Press.

Autism: Learning to Communicate

ELLENMORRIS TIEGERMAN-FARBER
School for Language and Communication Development
and
Adelphi University

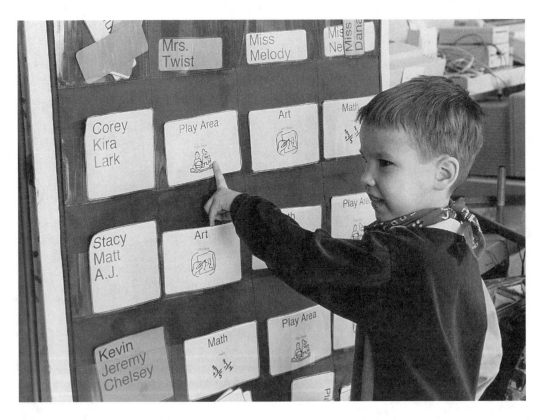

Each child who is autistic has unique learning needs. Just as there are differences in normal language learners, so there are individual differences in disordered language learners. It is unrealistic, therefore, to view a population of language-disordered children as a single entity. The autistic population includes such a broad range of children who evidence language, cognitive, communicative, behavioral, and social learning problems that many researchers have suggested that perhaps it is not a single group. Some researchers question whether there is a single cause or etiology for the disorder. The issue relates to how children are classified. Within the medical model, the underlying cause for a disorder is considered of primary importance. Historically, this point of view has carried over to the public school domain. As a result, children with disabilities are assigned to classes based upon etiological labels (mental retardation, autism, neurological impairment, and so on). Certainly there are advantages and disadvantages to both the etiological and the nonetiological models. One advantage to a nonetiological approach to disorders in the schools might be the classification of children by characteristics such as communication and language behaviors, the approach described in this chapter. These behaviors give insight into the unique educational needs of this population of individuals.

A discussion of autism research, more than research concerning any other population within the educational system, reveals the many theoretical and therapeutic changes that have occurred recently in the area of child language acquisition. In addition, it is my theoretical position that children with autism are severely language-disordered learners, rather than behaviorally impaired children. It should also be noted that the language learning characteristics of children with autism are also evident in the language patterns of other language-disordered children. To the extent that the language needs are the same, children with autism should be educated in the same manner as other language-disordered children. The discussion of autism research in this chapter highlights theoretical and therapeutic changes in the following areas:

1. The theoretical and etiological perceptions of the underlying cause(s) of autism
2. The therapeutic programming provided for children with autism
3. The setting(s) within which autistic children are trained—the possibility of inclusion
4. The role of the speech-language pathologist in serving children with autism
5. The role of the parent in serving the autistic child
6. Our expectations of how the autistic person can function within society
7. The relationship between autism and language acquisition theory

Theory and Terminological Issues

Psychiatrists who diagnose infantile autism are troubled by problems of agreement on terms and diagnostic reliability. The same difficulties confront neurologists and language pathologists who diagnose developmental aphasia or central language disorders. Diagnostic problems and terminological differences create formidable complications in placement and remediation. Specific theories relating to the cause of autism have been proposed but not proven. The range of etiological views of autism extends from a psychoanalytic perspective of the parent-child relationship to organic, genetic, and biochemical causes.

Coleman and Gillberg (1985) suggested that autism is a syndrome with a broad range of characteristics and a number of definable subgroups. Criteria for classifying children as autistic are not completely similar across authors and researchers. Rosenberger-Debiesse and Coleman (1986) provided evidence for multiple etiologies in autism. These researchers proposed that the subgroups must be more clearly defined by establishing the relationship between physiological characteristics and clinical symptomatology. The following descriptions of theories show how views of autism's underlying cause have changed in recent years. When reading about the theories, consider the therapeutic orientation that would result from each.

Etiology: A Psychological-Psychoanalytic Perspective

Kanner (1943) was the first to describe children with autism as being in a distinct category. Since that time, autism has been the subject of much clinical investigation and research; yet the nature of its causes, manifestations, and treatment remains in dispute. Kanner defined the cause as an innate inability to form biologically affective contact with people. He attributed this inability to an emotional deprivation resulting from rigidity of the parents. The parents of the children studied were characterized by obsessive meticulousness and intellectualization. This theory was supported by Eisenberg (1956), who categorized the mothers of autistic children as cold and distant.

Bettelheim, in *The Empty Fortress* (1967), proposed a similar perspective. He suggested that the mother does not produce autism, but, rather, that autism is the child's reaction to her attitudes. The child with autism fears maternal destruction and rejects the mother. When the child withdraws, the mother becomes indifferent or angry. The child retreats within himself even further, and reality becomes so fearful that inactivity is the only available response; autism develops. Thus, the symptoms of autistic children have been attributed to problems with early interpersonal relationships, motivation, and emotionality resulting in a diagnosis of emotional disturbance. Controlled studies have failed to demonstrate significant differences in parental psychopathology and early mother-child interaction between groups of psychotic and nonpsychotic brain-damaged children. For a long time, the psychoanalytic view that the mother-child relationship was the cause of autism was widely accepted; however, support for that view has gradually declined as newer research has uncovered evidence of an organic basis for the disorder.

Etiology: A Psychological-Cognitive Approach

This psychological-cognitive theoretical orientation suggests that the problems exhibited by autistic children extend beyond the linguistic area to more generalized cognitive difficulties. This perspective emphasizes the differences in the ways in which children with autism process and organize information. These generalized and more broad-based analytical differences can be used to explain the various types of deviant language behaviors in children with autism. The psychological-cognitive approach views the autistic child's language as a productive result of limited and less flexible processing abilities. Although different, the autistic child's idiosyncratic language behaviors should be addressed from the child's perspective of his or her environment. These language differences should provide a basis for developing therapeutic goals that generate from the child and his or her individual language needs. Perhaps a critical component to this theoretical approach is the utilization of the autistic child's language behavior in the therapy process rather than its elimination (Duchan & Palermo, 1982; Prizant, 1982).

Etiology: Central Language Disorder

Churchill (1978) presented a different theoretical model from which to analyze the child with autism. He hypothesized that psychotic children with a psychiatric diagnosis of autism have a central language deficit that is more severe than that found in children with central language disorders. In addition, the three most prominent and clinically significant features of childhood psychosis are impairment of communicative interaction, of social interaction, and of appropriate object manipulation. Churchill presented some general response similarities of the autistic children involved in his experimental language investigation. Some of the autistic children evidenced channel-specific deficits (i.e., they indicated a conditioning preference for one stimulus modality). Other children displayed a difficulty in responding to two familiar elements simultaneously. All the children displayed difficulties in generalizing, classifying, cross-referencing, and syntactic/linguistic manipulating. The most important information found was that each child was unique (i.e., children with autism are a heterogeneous group of disordered children). Churchill concluded that each child generated a different profile of linguistic abilities and disabilities. The population presents a level of heterogeneity that underscores scattered and idiosyncratic patterns of development.

Almost 60 percent of the children with autism have IQs in the severely retarded range; as a result mental retardation is often associated with this disorder. Wetherby and Gaines (1982) however, did not observe the similarity in level of cognitive and linguistic ability that is typical in mentally retarded children in the autistic children in their study; cognitive abilities exceeded linguistic abilities in several areas. The authors suggested that the relationship between cognition and language is dynamic rather than static; the interdependence varies over time with development. Whereas cognitive development may be necessary for intentional communication, "cognitive development may not be sufficient for more advanced language development" (p. 69).

Loveland, Landry, Hughes, Hall, and McEvoy (1988) described autism as a pervasive developmental disorder characterized by severe deficits in language, cognition, and social development. The language of children with autism is severely delayed and is often described as disordered. In many cases, functional language does not develop at all. Verbal language, when it does develop, is usually rigid, ritualistic, and stereotypical. Children with autism develop verbal routines that never change in form and are used over and over again in a variety of related and somewhat related contexts. Even though the language and gestures of autistic children are pragmatically deficient, they can be communicative despite the unconventional forms. Loveland and colleagues showed that, when compared to children of similar mental age and language level, children with autism present a different pattern of use of gesture and language. Autistic children produce fewer communicative acts than language-delayed children. In addition, the autistic group in the Loveland and colleagues research showed some performance heterogeneity in their ability to produce communicative acts. Some of the autistic children did not produce any communicative acts. The autistic children tended to produce acts that functioned only to continue interaction.

Loveland and colleagues (1988) suggested that although autistic children have difficulties initiating interaction, they seem to have less difficulty responding to the directions of another. Their data support the idea that children with autism are relatively poor at engaging another person's attention or introducing a topic or taking turns in an interaction. The authors hypothesized, "The ability to initiate communication is closely tied to underlying social-pragmatic skills that are impaired in autism. In the autistic child learning language, the degree of skill initiating may therefore reflect the degree of social-pragmatic impairment" (p. 600). Autistic children in the study had a lower level of pragmatic abilities than normally developing 2-year-olds. Language level, mental age, and IQ could not account for the autistic children's pragmatic interactional deficits. The authors suggested that there is an asynchrony in development between content areas (pragmatic and semantic) and structural areas (syntax and phonology). The language development of children with autism follows a sequence that is quite different from that of other children.

Related Factors

Four factors have contributed to the changing ways in which children with autism have been viewed in the past several years. First, the National Society for Autistic Children has heightened society's awareness of the needs of children with autism. This awareness has affected the direction of legislation in state and federal funding of educational programs. Second, Public Law 94-142 has had profound implications in the development of curricula due to its mandate that children with disabilities be educated in the least restrictive environment. As a result, there have been expanding funds available for the development of educational programs for autistic children, particularly in public school settings. Third, recent developments in research have suggested neurological differences in processing (visual, auditory, linguistic, and cognitive) between autistic children and other populations of children. Neurological differences suggest an etiological explanation other than emotional disturbance; specifically, that the underlying cause for the disorder relates to perceptual, cognitive, and information-processing differences. These characteristic differences result in language patterns that develop differently. The fourth and final factor involves the recent research in child language development. The changing perspectives in language theory and therapy have affected the view that the communication and language deficits in autistic children are of critical importance, suggesting that pragmatic deficits may serve to explain behavioral problems. The interplay among these factors has resulted in the progressive attempt to develop language and educational programs for the autistic within various learning contexts: home, school, and intermediate care facility (ICF).

Since the goal of this chapter is to describe children with autism in terms of characteristic behaviors, many aspects of developmental learning are presented: behavioral characteristics, language, cognition, play, social interaction, and so forth. These characteristics provide a comprehensive picture of the autistic child as one who has communication and language learning problems. The chapter compares the developmental differences between children with autism and children with normal language development. Adam, a 3-year-old autistic child, is described throughout the chapter in order to highlight the complex learning needs of the "whole child" in relation to his or her environment.

Behavioral Characteristics

The behavioral characteristics of children with autism were originally presented by Kanner (1943, 1944); many of these characteristics are still considered valid today. The classic autistic child, as described by Kanner (1943) and Bettelheim (1967), exhibits most or all of the characteristics. The population of individuals with autism, however, is very heterogeneous. Children vary in the number and severity of characteristics exhibited, and the "classic autistic child" is probably a rarity. For the sake of description, all of the characteristics presented in this chapter are discussed in terms of Adam, who has been diagnosed as a classic autistic child. As children exhibit fewer of the characteristics, they become more autisticlike than autistic. Some of these characteristics will be discussed more fully in later sections dealing with communication and language.

Gaze Aversion

Perhaps the most salient characteristic of autism is the lack of eye contact with other people during the communication exchange process. This characteristic more than any other has caused autistic children to be described as aloof, distant, withdrawn, and nonrelating. Children with autism do not look at or facially orient their gaze toward another person; they avert their eyes when someone talks to them. In fact, attempts by a communication partner to get the autistic child to look are met with physical resistance, particularly when that person is physically near the child. Hutt and Ounsted (1966) noted that as autistic children get farther away from another person, they exhibit a greater number of gazes oriented to that person. Another difference concerns the physical orientation of the child. Unless one is sneaking a look, the bodies of both speaker and listener are normally lined up shoulder to shoulder. Children with autism turn their entire body (and head) away from the speaker and emit infrequent, fleeting gazes from the corners of their eyes.

Consider Adam's gaze pattern during an interactional exchange. Even after having been trained to look at the speaker, Adam would change the orientation of his body. The more he focused on the speaker facially the more of his body was turned away when holding his head so that face-to-face interaction could take place, his eyes shifted from corner to corner (side to side).

Ritualistic Behavior

Rituals are a normal part of the daily routines and patterns of life. Most children and adults exhibit ritual patterns. There are, however, differences between the rituals exhibited by non-impaired children and those of autistic children. The autistic child's ritual is a sequence or pattern of behavior that must be exhibited in the same way and in the same order; there is little room for change. The chair must be placed just so in the living room. The child can only drink from the Snoopy cup. When there is a change in the environment, children with autism attempt to reorder and recreate the sameness they seek to maintain. Rituals also involve the ways in which children manipulate objects within the environment. Children with autism spin records, twirl wires, bang objects, and turn lights on and off incessantly. They do not manipulate objects appropriately in a functional way. Performances with an object are repeated for hours. There are also rituals in which the child rocks back and forth in a corner. These repetitive behaviors are frequently referred to as self-stimulatory behaviors. They are presumably the child's attempt to maintain sameness or to get attention. Let us consider several rituals:

- Jeremy's ritual: Take bottles and Binkys (pacifiers) upstairs. Put bottles and Binkys in bed. Put Superdog in bed. Cover Superdog. Give Superdog his bottle. Give Superdog his Binky. Jeremy drinks bottle. Jeremy takes Binky. (ritual pattern exhibited every night)
- Ellenmorris's ritual: "Hi, Adam. Come on, let's go play." Offers hand to Adam. Walk hand-in-hand to therapy room. (ritual pattern exhibited before every therapy session)

What are the differences between normal ritual patterns and those that characterize autism? First, with a child who is developing normally, the ritual pattern represents only a small part of the child's performance or interaction repertoire. Because children with autism have very restricted performance repertoires, their ritual pattern constitutes a much larger proportion. Much of what autistic children do involves performing or developing a ritualized pattern of some kind. "Everything becomes a ritual," noted Adam's mother.

The second difference is that it is very difficult to change the autistic child's ritualized patterns. Any minute change in a ritual can result in a catastrophic reaction from the child. Many parents note that the resulting violent temper tantrums are so aversive that they hesitate to, and often do not, change environmental sequences or events. Jeremy might balk a bit if something were performed differently or left out of their nightly sequence (e.g., not giving Superdog his Binky), but the result would not be a catastrophic reaction.

The third difference is that nonimpaired children's ritualized patterns, referred to as adultomorphisms by Piaget (1962), indicate the child's relational knowledge of experiences and events within the environment. The child's sequences show progressive and developmental changes. They incorporate the child's changing perceptions and conceptions of the world. Therefore, for the normally developing child, the ritual indicates an attempt to integrate and synthesize observed environmental sequences. For the child with autism, however, the ritualized pattern represents an attempt to maintain a systematic order within the environment.

Temper Tantrums

There are aspects of the natural environment that develop and maintain ritualized patterns. Let us reconsider Ellenmorris's ritual, described previously, with regard to temper tantrums.

Ellenmorris's ritual: One afternoon, therapy was running late. Because the clinician was getting ready to see Adam, a graduate student volunteered to meet Adam in the waiting room of the Speech and Hearing Center. A few minutes later, Adam was wildly screaming in the hall. The clinician walked into the hall to see Adam screaming and pounding the side of his head with his fists. The therapy session was, to say the least, difficult. Before Adam's mother left, she was asked if anything had happened on the way to the center, and if Adam were feeling all right. She said that he was perfectly all right until the graduate student had met him in the waiting room.

For the two years that Adam had been enrolled at the Speech and Hearing Center, the clinician herself had gone to the waiting room to bring him to the therapy room. In essence, a ritualized pattern had developed. As a result of this experience, the clinical staff attempted to identify the existence of other ritual patterns in their interactions with Adam. The purpose of the investigation was to identify and modify the clinician's and the child's patterns of ritualized interaction. Adam's response (a temper tantrum) was typical of how children with autism react to attempts to introduce change into their world. The temper tantrum is the autistic child's catastrophic reaction to change.

Temper tantrums can be either self-abusive or aggressive in form. Self-abusive and aggressive behaviors exhibited by autistic children can include any of the following: pulling hair, biting, scratching, head banging, pinching, head-butting, and so on. The difference between self-abusive and aggressive behaviors is the direction of the behavior—toward self or toward others. One of the difficulties related to temper tantrums is the intensity of the child's reaction to even a slight environmental change; a minute change in the environment or in a ritual can result in a violent outburst. Children with autism can become physically uncontrollable; obviously, the older and bigger they get, the harder it is for a parent or a teacher to manage them.

Self-Stimulatory Behavior

Self-stimulation includes high-frequency behaviors that have been traditionally described as noncommunicative and noninteractional. They are often emitted when the child seeks to withdraw from the environment. This withdrawal pattern occurs when an autistic child cannot cope with direct input from teaching or instruction. Self-stimulatory behaviors are nonprogressive. They interfere with the child's learning, especially in the classroom. What should the clinician or teacher do about these behaviors? Behavioral approaches to training children with autism have proposed eliminating or decreasing their frequency by means of aversive consequences. However, the autistic child's repertoire includes so many self-stimulatory behaviors that eliminating them would leave very little emitted behavior.

Hypo- versus Hypersensitivity to Stimuli

Children with autism do not indicate the same response threshold to environmental stimuli as do nonimpaired children. A reduced sensitivity to stimuli is called hyposensitivity. A parent might say, "I could clap a pair of cymbals next to my child's ear and he would not blink." Children with autism do not react to, or seem in any way to recognize, certain sounds consistently. It is not surprising that many autistic children at some point in their history have been identified as hearing impaired or deaf. Their general pattern of unawareness of environmental stimuli is inconsistent. Many parents describe the autistic child as being "here and there." Whenever Adam was responsive during a therapy session, his mother would say, "He's come in for a landing." The child's inconsistent responding is complicated by his inconsistent and often extreme reaction to even the slightest change in input. Heightened or excessive sensitivity to stimuli is called hypersensitivity. Adam would place his hands over his ears and eyes to block out input. The inconsistency in responding, with the ever present possibility of the catastrophic temper tantrum, reduces child assessment (i.e., determining how he is going to react) to a guessing game for parents, clinicians, and teachers.

Mutism

Mutism includes a range of behavior, from periods of total silence to the production of meaningless sounds (i.e., used for self-stimulatory rather than communicative purposes). Most, if not all, children with autism progress through a period of mutism. Some autistic children remain mute all their lives. Hurford (1991) posited that there is a critical period for language acquisition. The clinical and developmental concern is that if a functional system is not acquired by 5 years of age, there is little probability of it developing thereafter. Often when the autistic child becomes verbal, his initial words or phrases are quite intelligible. There seems to be a quantum leap or change in the child's performance that cannot as of yet be explained. The child with autism does not evidence the gradual developmental changes in pragmatics, phonology, semantics, and syntax during the first 36 months that are seen in the normally developing child. Fay and Schuler (1980) noted that most of the information accumulated about this period of time comes from parental reports, which are affected by "an emotional climate that can best be defined as a developmental hope countered by fear" (p. 22). We are not sure why some children progress to the next stage—echolalic behavior—and some do not; we are not sure what changes within the child result in transition to the next stage. For example, Adam's developmental history represents a dramatic and unexplainable change from one stage to another. Mute until the age of 4 years 3 months, Adam produced only meaningless grunts. When he started to speak, his productions were long, imitated utterances, such as "Open door please" and "Time go home now." His productions were, as his mother described, "as clear as a bell."

Some children with autism never develop speech or language. The incidence of muteness ranges from 28 percent (Lotter, 1967) to 61 percent (Fish, Shapiro, & Campbell, 1966); the variability being a function of the difficulties with terminology and the issues discussed at the beginning of this chapter. Bartak and Rutter (1976) found that approximately 80 percent of all autistic children were misdiagnosed as deaf at one time in their developmental history. DeMyer, Barton, DeMyer, Norton, Allen, and Steele (1973) noted that about 65 percent of the children who were mute at age 5 were still mute several years later. A large proportion of the autistic population never develops conventional communicative and/or linguistic interactions within the environment. Why do so many children with autism remain nonverbal?

Echolalia

Echolalia has been defined traditionally as the meaningless repetition of someone else's words. As a result, some researchers have advocated that the behavior should be eliminated or decreased through therapy. Echolalia also has been described traditionally as a transition period between muteness and the evidence of linguistic knowledge, but research on autistic children's progress through the various learning stages is limited. Is the autistic child's imitation meaningless? If not, what function does it serve? Prizant and Duchan (1981) noted that to determine what echolalic utterances mean, one must analyze them within a natural communicative environment. It is important to understand how the child functions within the communicative context; specifically, how children with autism use whatever behavior they have developed for the purpose of communication. In order to determine the communicative intent of the autistic child's message, the researcher and clinician must analyze the communicative context within which the utterance occurs. In such cases, eliminating echolalia would actually decrease the occurrence of communicative behavior. It thus becomes important to determine if the echolalic form represents the child's communicative intention. The following interactions illustrate that Adam's dramatic jump to an echolalic period revealed the need to assess the child's meaning within context. The examples indicate how this autistic child manipulated various linguistic and nonlinguistic behaviors to convey communicative intentions. Adam's mother was, to say the least, thrilled when her son started to "talk." However, her exuberance quickly wore away. She described Adam as her "talking shadow." A typical exchange between mother and child is presented to highlight the difficulty, confusion, and frustration in an exchange with a child who is echolalic.

Mother: Adam, are you ready?

Adam: Adam, are you ready?

Mother: Go open the door.

Adam: Go open the door.

Mother: Where is your coat?

Adam: Your coat.

To determine if Adam's imitations were meaningful, several aspects of his behavior could be analyzed within the context. For example, let us analyze the following exchange:

Mother: Go open the door.

Adam: Go open the door.

Nonverbal behavior: Adam looks at the door, then gets up and opens it.

Adam indicated by means of his behavior that, although he echoed his mother's production, he understood the meaning of her message and its related action. The nonverbal behavior (i.e., gaze behavior, gestures, and actions) of children with autism provides an indication of their understanding of the speech message and whether their echoic utterance was meaningful.

Mother: Where is your coat?

Adam: Your coat.

Nonverbal behavior: Adam looks at the coat, then goes to pull on the coat, which is lying across a chair.

In the second interchange, Adam's nonverbal behavior indicated his interpretation of the context. The interchange gives us additional information as well. First, the linguistic form of Adam's production was slightly different than that of his mother's utterance. Second, his intonation pattern, which was different from his mother's (upward inflection), indicated his ability to make changes in suprasegmental features. Third, he exhibited nonverbal behaviors that signaled he understood his mother's message. This interchange indicates several ways in which the child with autism can manipulate some of the components of the language process. These interchanges indicate how the form and function of the autistic child's communicative behavior can be analyzed within the ongoing natural context. But many questions about the echolalic period remain unanswered: Does the echolalic period incorporate several progressive stages? Does echolalic behavior change structurally and/or functionally over time? Does the echolalic period contribute to language and communication development in the child with autism?

Prizant and Wetherby (1987) proposed that ordinarily intentionality must combine with conventionality to develop communication. A close analysis of communicative intent might highlight the social and communicative dysfunctions in children with autism. Although they may not use conventional forms such as pointing or showing, children with autism may use idiosyncratic behaviors such as echolalia and self-stimulation to signal various communicative functions. One cannot assume that because the child with autism does not use conventional forms of communication, he or she cannot communicate. This position is as inappropriate as the one that assumes that the autistic child's use of conventional forms reflects an intention to communicate. The meaning of the child's interaction can be determined only by analyzing the child's behavior within the context. Such analyses of a child's unconventional communicative forms and functions require multiple observations across different contexts. The authors noted that the ultimate challenge in evaluating the autistic child is to determine if the unconventional forms actually express communicative intentions.

Prizant and Rydell (1984) investigated the functions of delayed echolalia in children with autism. In delayed echolalia, children repeat utterances long after they originally heard them. The authors noted that "echolalic behaviors, both immediate and delayed, are best described as a continuum of behaviors in regard to exactness of repetition, degree of comprehension, and underlying communicative intent" (p. 183). Delayed echolalia has also been referred to as old forms applied to new situations. The use of echolalia as a form of communication is an unusual strategy in the normally developing child, but it serves several important functions in a child with autism. The fact that the child with autism uses old forms in new contexts indicates that on some associative level he establishes a relationship between a linguistic form (as rigid as it is) and an event. That is, the production of a delayed echolalic response indicates that the child perceives a relationship between a verbal utterance and a context. As the child's linguistic abilities increase, he is able to substitute, delete, and/or conjoin elements in the echoed response (delayed mitigated echolalia).

The autistic child's unique ability to verbally imitate sophisticated linguistic sentences and paragraphs is often quite deceptive in terms of the child's actual spontaneous ability. In the Prizant and Rydell (1984) study, a production was considered a delayed echolalic utterance if it satisfied one or both of the following criteria: (a) the repetition was beyond the child's syntactic abilities and (b) the utterance consisted of a rigid and routinized string. The children in the Prizant and Rydell study showed a marked discrepancy between the mean length of utterance for echolalic and spontaneous productions. Whereas the children's spontaneous productions were primarily at a Phase 1 level of linguistic complexity, the echolalic utterances represented a much more sophisticated linguistic ability.

Whether the autistic child uses immediate or delayed echolalia, his or her productions are generated for interactive purposes. Echolalia is not a simplistic or unitary form; it represents a continuum of interaction and comprehension. The listener's interpretation of the echolalic utterance is going to be based on his or her knowledge of the child and characteristic of their shared context. One of the most interesting findings of the Prizant and Rydell (1984) study was that some of the noninteractive echolalic utterances—those produced without communicative intent by the child—did serve meaningful purposes. Although some of the utterances served no specific functions, others served cognitive and/or conversational or turn-taking functions. Echolalia has been described as a transitional phase of development that signals movement from (a) echolalia without communicative intent, to (b) echolalia with the intent but limited linguistic competence, to (c) echolalia with intent and linguistic ability. This developmental pattern of linguistic and comprehension changes is similar to the communicative sequence exhibited by the nonimpaired child as he or she learns language.

The perlocutionary, illocutionary, and locutionary stages of normal communication development (Bates, Camaioni, & Volterra, 1975; see Chapter 3) may also describe the use of echolalia by the autistic child. The child's early echolalia may be perlocutionary, that is, expressed without any awareness of the communicative impact of the behavior. When the child begins to realize that his or her utterances have an affect on the behavior of listeners, the nature of the act changes from perlocutionary to illocutionary. The final locutionary stage, however, is rarely achieved by autistic children; this stage represents the final stage of functional communication development. This is the stage in which conventional word forms are used. For the child with autism, the use of unconventional forms interferes with the development of language's conventional forms and higher-ordered metalinguistic abilities.

Socio-affective Deficits

In the chapter on social cognition (Chapter 2), it was emphasized that the child's experiences within the environment with agents, actions, and objects were important to the language learning process. Bryson, Landry, and Smith (1994) noted that children with autism exhibit deficits in social cognition, relationships with people and objects. These object deficits manifest themselves in a limited toy-play repertoire, self-stimulatory behavior, bizarre manipulation behaviors, and nonprogressive play skills. The interpersonal deficits manifest themselves as a lack of gaze interaction, decreased physical interaction, and severe limitations in cooperative play and social interaction. Children with autism have difficulty relating to and interacting with the environment. Many children with autism withdraw from the approach and touch of others and become rigid or stiff when held or cuddled. Considering that communication and social learning involve interactional exchanges with peers and adults in the environment, one can only wonder how the autistic child's behavior affects parents and peers. Interaction implies reciprocity; there must be some reaction or response from the child. When the autistic child does not respond to or withdraws from the adult's initiations, what is the adult's reaction? Is it a feeling of rejection? Is it a feeling of frustration? Consider how Adam's mother and Jeremy described their interaction with Adam.

Adam's mother: It is difficult to get close to a child who always pushes you away. Interaction is totally nonreinforcing.

Jeremy: Him no like me.

Notice that Adam's lack of responsiveness negatively affected the communicative initiations of these two individuals. Children with autism need to learn about the social context, yet their behavior leads to further isolation.

Shapiro, Sherman, Calamari, and Koch (1987) indicated that social and affective deficits were the most salient characteristics of the autistic population. Often a child with autism is described as aloof, withdrawn, and unresponsive to other people. Nevertheless, the findings demonstrate that children with autism are not uniformly aloof and isolated. For some children, the repertoire of behavior they use with their mothers is not the same as that used with strangers. The difference in behavioral responsiveness may be considered to be evidence of attachment. The authors suggested that most autism research focuses on developmental variables such as language and cognition; there should be greater attention paid to affective competence. Children with autism present discrete problems in comprehending affective responses in others; "it is not so much that autistic children do not make attachments but that they make attachments variably in accordance with their capacity for affective display and understanding" (p. 483).

Snow, Hertzig, and Shapiro (1987) reported that children with autism display specific deficits in the area of affective expression. Their results contradict the belief that autistic children have flat affective response patterns or that their affective responses are inappropriate and unrelated to the social context. The children in their study did occasionally display smiling and laughing behaviors that appeared to be appropriately related to the interpersonal situation. Although they did not occur often, these behaviors did occur. The children also showed through negative reactions their ability to differentially respond to various partners: "Young autistic children were able to distinguish among partners in a way that prompted differential negative reactions" (p. 838). Children with autism have difficulty analyzing the affective behaviors of social partners; they are severely impaired within the affective domain in the production and comprehension of emotional responses.

Onset before 30 Months

A child is usually identified as autistic before age 3. Some parents describe their early awareness of a problem during the infant's first months of life. They note that the infant "could not be comforted." The younger the infant, the more tenuous the determination of disorder, unless there are neurological signs of impairment. Generally, parents proceed through the frustrations of a diagnostic evaluation as their child approaches the second birthday. One of the most important diagnostic variables—language—is often difficult to evaluate by standardized means before 24 months. It has been only within the past few years that early identification, focusing on the child between 2 and 3 years of age, resulted in intervention. Educational options are still rather limited for the preschool child with autism (Wagner & Lockwood, 1994).

According to Short and Schopler (1988), the onset of autism before age 30 months has been a central criterion in the differential diagnosis of autism. Their study indicates that in 76 percent of autism cases, parents identified a problem before their child was 24 months of age. In 94 percent of cases, parents identified a problem before their child was 36 months old. Parents who recognized a problem earlier tended to seek help sooner. In addition, early onset also related to developmental severity, particularly in behavioral functioning. Children with later developmental onsets scored significantly higher on IQ tests than the early-onset children, suggesting that these "later" cases were less severe in terms of autistic symptomatology. The authors recommended the need for further research into the differential diagnosis of two distinct groups within the late-onset category: (a) autistic children who experience a developmental regression after 30 months of age and (b) autistic children who are identified at a much later developmental period because their symptomatology is relatively mild.

Short and Schopler (1988) also discussed the relationship between clinical diagnosis and parental perceptions of their child's development. The identified age of onset may only be the age of recognition: "The late onset cases with no evidence of regression may well have had an earlier onset, possibly from birth, but were not recognized as disordered until later" (p. 215). Early recognition of disorder requires further investigation because parents contribute significantly to this process. The language, communication, and behavioral symptoms identified by the parent before clinical diagnosis may be critical in clarifying the relation of autism to other developmental disorders such as schizophrenia and disintegrative psychoses.

Behavioral Characteristics: A Means of Discriminating between Children?

The nine characteristics of autism described previously can be used to differentiate between and among children. Table 13-1 highlights some of the performance differences between Adam's and Bryan's interactions within the environment.

There are some obvious developmental differences between the two children that might reflect language and processing differences. These differences are typical of children within the population and highlight the fact that autistic children have very individual interactional patterns and styles. Developmental differences in gaze interaction, joint attention, and orienting to speech suggest that children with autism can be identified as early as one year of age. In addition to behavioral characteristics, communication, play, and linguistic behaviors provide insight into the most critical variable in autism-language functioning. Children with autism indicate severe deficits in language development. This inability to interact and to communicate imposes a restriction on learning about language as a social process. Communication, play, and linguistic behaviors provide a more holistic picture of the autistic child's unique interactional style within a complex social environment as well as a means of identifying the disorder earlier (Osterling & Dawson, 1994).

Communication Behaviors

In the communication exchange between the adult and the child, the two are participants in an ongoing interactive event. A 30-month-old child with autism does not evidence many of the communication behaviors exhibited by a normally developing 6-month-old. The autis-

TABLE 13-1   A Comparison of Behavioral Performances

Behavior	Adam (40 mos.)	Bryan (40 mos.)
Gaze aversion	Gaze aversion	Gaze aversion, but does track a moving object
Imitation	Lack of motor and vocal imitation	Lack of vocal imitation, limited motor imitation
Ritualistic behavior	Feeding, dressing, and washing rituals	Constantly rearranging furniture in the room (and house)
Self-stimulatory behaviors	Walks on toes, flaps hands, rocks back and forth, makes grunting/guttural noises	Spins, opens and closes eyes rapidly, sticks finger down throat
Object performances	Nonfunctional and undifferentiated performances; spins, shakes, mouths, and bangs toys	Basically nonfunctional and undifferentiated; spins, shakes, mouths, and bangs toys. Some appropriate object-related performances: picks up telephone receiver and makes noises into receiver, puts baby in bed, stacks rings on stick, can replace pieces in Simplex puzzle
Temper tantrums	Self-abusive behavior: head-banging, handbiting. Aggressive behavior; pulls hair and scratches	No self-abusive behavior. Aggressive behavior; bites, scratches, pinches, kicks, bunts his head, pulls hair, punches
Speech	Mute	Echolalic
Relational behavior	Turns and moves away when approached, stiffens when touched	Approaches people (adults and children), requests hugs, kisses, and tickles
Onset	Mother noted that something was wrong at 3 months of age. Psychiatric evaluation and diagnosis at 24 months.	Mother states that child progressed "normally" until 12 months of age and then withdrew. Child's behavior deteriorated. Psychiatric evaluation and diagnosis at 30 months.

tic child does not exhibit the normal developmental progression in gaze, vocal, and gestural communication behaviors or the ability to coordinate these behaviors into complex patterns and sequences. Often we are not aware that the child is autistic until after infancy (between 18 and 36 months). By this time, it has become clear that the child has not developed early communication and linguistic behaviors. The information concerning behavioral and communication development before the time of diagnosis is subjective and a function of the parents' interpretation and memory of early experiences with the child.

The fact that communication behaviors are not present at 30 months of age does not mean that the behaviors were not present earlier. It is possible that early communication behaviors did develop during the first 9 to 12 months but due to neurological deficits deteriorated. Current diagnostic skills are not adequate to identify the deficits that occur during infancy and early childhood and result in the disorder of autism. Infancy can provide some important insights into the early appearance and progression of this disorder, however. Gaze, vocal, and gestural communication behaviors may be critical in the early identification of the autistic child. The expanding knowledge of developmental processes between birth and 12 months will ensure the identification and diagnosis of disorder in younger and younger children. The ability to understand disorder is inextricably tied to our understanding of normal development. For early identification to occur in infants between birth and 12 months of age, selected gaze, vocal, and gestural behaviors must be identified as prognostic indicators (Wagner & Lockwood, 1994).

Play

It is generally acknowledged that play is important to the development of adaptability, learning, cognition, and social behavior (Lifter, Sulzer-Azaroff, Anderson, & Cowdery, 1993). The function of play is to exercise and develop manipulative and interactional strategies that children will later integrate into more sophisticated task-oriented sequences. A more general theory suggests that in play, children learn to affect and control activities they are unable to execute or dominate in other contexts. In play, children develop control over animate and inanimate objects or contexts (Linder, 1990; Strain & Odom, 1986; Warren & Gazdag, 1990). Recent analyses of early social interactions suggest that play behavior influences the physical and interactional behaviors of all children involved in the experience (Fewell & Kaminski, 1988; Haring, 1985; Kennedy, Sheridan, Radlinski, & Beeghly, 1991). Thus, play has a cognitive, social, and integrative function in development.

The theory underlying play indicates that play begins with action manipulations directed by the child. As manipulative and physical abilities expand, children develop an increasing capacity to deal with objects more actively. Children with autism, however, are limited in their interaction with the environment. Because of their restricted experience, they share with other disordered children many behavioral and learning problems, whether the specific diagnosis is mental retardation, cerebral palsy, brain damage, or autism. Children with autism withdraw from interactional experiences and learn to manipulate by means of temper tantrums and disruptive behaviors. Withdrawal from the environment makes it difficult to determine if they do not know how to play, if they lack the opportunity to do so, or both. Many researchers have suggested that there is a cyclical relationship between autistic children's bizarre manipulative performance and their inability to integrate experiences within the environment, causing even further withdrawal. The child's creation of an inner world is an attempt to establish and maintain an internal order that he or she cannot establish in the outside world. Self-stimulatory and ritualistic behaviors might be a result of socio-affective deficits (Ozonoff, Pennington, & Rogers 1991).

Mundy, Sigman, Ungerer, and Sherman (1987) investigated the social and cognitive correlates of language acquisition in young children with autism. They found that functional and symbolic play skills were associated with language abilities. In addition, specific nonverbal communication skills such as gestures also correlated with language acquisition. The authors suggested that object manipulation skills may involve representational abilities—the child must be able to recognize that the toy object can represent the real object. The symbolic skills require that the child store and retrieve information on the relationships between agents and objects, actions and objects, and agents and actions. Object manipulation and symbolic play deficits represent a significant problem for children with autism (Jarrold, Boucher, & Smith, 1993).

Language Components

In describing autism as a communication and language-based disorder, several components of language will be discussed: pragmatics, semantics, syntax, phonology, and cognition. Cromer (1981) noted that it is important to understand these language components "as a means of focusing on the problems that may be faced by specific language-disordered groups" (p. 71). Studying the interrelationship among these components in children with autism can provide insight into the unique learning needs of these language-impaired children.

It has been suggested that semantic and syntactic development can progress independently from one another; a child may evidence more advanced or complex semantic skills while his or her syntactic abilities remain severely retarded, or more advanced syntactic skills with severe deficits in semantic development. This uneven developmental pattern across language components is linked to the structures and functions of the nervous system and their control of different language processes (Tager-Flusberg, Calkins, Nolin, Baumberger, Anderson, & Chadwick-Dias, 1990; Tager-Flusberg, 1989). Uneven development indicates that different areas within the central nervous system are more or less impaired, which determines the level of functioning and the language abilities developed within the child. Language represents an integrated system; every component contributes to the development of the whole. To understand the learning needs of children with language disorders, particularly autistic children, it is important to compare and contrast development within and across components. The language and communication deficits evidenced in autistic children might be caused by:

1. Uneven developments within and/or across the components of the learning system
2. An inability to interface and/or exchange developmental information across the components of the system

Social Cognition

The relationships among perception, language, and cognition remain rather controversial. Current trends have been influenced by cognitive theories that stress the importance of early social and interactional experiences within the environment. As discussed in earlier chapters, Piaget (1962) described language development as based within the sensorimotor period. Such cognitive theories have described the development of the child's conceptual knowledge and its changing effect on the development of language. In discussing cognitive development in children with autism, it is important to consider perceptual and cognitive processes as well as social interactional experiences.

Kanner (1952) indicated that children with autism evidence good motor dexterity, excellent rote memory, and an absence of physical stigmata and motor developmental delays.

These characteristics, in combination with nearly normal IQ scores, led Kanner to propose that intellectual deficits were a function of an affective disorder. Although Kanner's criteria are still used for diagnostic purposes, serious questions have been raised about the cognitive potential of these children. Most clinical research indicates that a majority of children with autism function within the mentally retarded range of intellectual skills (DeMyer, Barton, Alpern, Kimberlin, Allen, Yang, & Steele, 1974). However, unlike children who are mentally retarded, children with autism demonstrate a wide variability of skills. Autistic children display significantly higher abilities on tasks that require the discrimination of concrete visual spatial relations and significantly lower abilities on tasks that require abstraction or the ability to organize concrete information on the basis of subtle relationships between stimuli (Hermelin, 1978). Children with autism evidence integration deficits when stimuli increase in complexity and/or require cross-modal processing (Bryson, 1970). They have difficulties in identifying what is meaningful and relevant in a situation (Dalgleish, 1975). Children with autism use a rigid set of rules when interacting with the environment. In addition, they attend to, or fixate on, one aspect of a picture or story, often some irrelevant minutiae (Maltz, 1981). All of these examples serve to explain an idiosyncratic pattern of interaction within the environment.

Children with autism also have difficulty in generalizing learned behaviors from one context to another. Because these children cannot identify the relevant information within the complexities of a situation, they cannot identify what is important and what is not, creating a further problem in establishing conceptual or perceptual relationships. The ability to establish categories of any kind depends upon the ability to discriminate differences as well as to determine how stimuli are associated and related to one another. Children with autism tend to fixate on irrelevant aspects of a situation. As a result, their perceptions of the environment are rather distorted and limited. These deficits contribute to the failure to generalize learning and to develop strategies for adapting to continually changing social contingencies. Social rigidity limits their ability to adjust to changing social contingencies, and perseverative responses interfere with the development of problem-solving skills (Russell, Mauthner, Sharpe, & Tidswell, 1991; Prior & Hoffmann, 1990).

Fay and Schuler (1980) suggested that the deficits in generalization indicate a cognitive impairment in autistic children, a problem that seriously limits their ability to learn spontaneously and to benefit from more structured and formalized learning. The inability to identify the relationships among stimuli and to benefit from past learning experiences condemns autistic children to repeated learning experiences. These children are not able to extract and use the similarities across situations. Nonimpaired children search for rules. In order to establish rules, they identify relevant and related stimuli within conceptual categories. Generalization involves the ability to identify the relationship between situation A and situation B, and then to apply the rule to situations A' and B'. Without rule-governed behavior, children have difficulty processing, categorizing, and interpreting environmental stimuli.

The uneven developmental pattern in children with autism is difficult to explain. The autistic child's abilities (sometimes savant skills) are contrasted with extreme delays in other areas of skill acquisition. Adam, for example, had an excellent memory and rote recall. His ability, however, should be viewed in terms of his use of the skill within the social context. His remarkable recall was often used for noncommunicative and self-stimulatory purposes. Information was frequently extracted as a whole and not used for interactional purposes. Adam would sit in a corner of his room and recite verbatim the news report presented the previous night. Identifying strengths, skills, or abilities is only an initial step; it is important with autistic children, to determine how skills are used or applied within the learning context (see Hyperlexia).

Little is known about how children with autism perceive their environments. Assumptions are made on the basis of their patterns of interaction in the environment; that is, the way in which they relate to agents, actions, and objects. The behavioral characteristics described previously provide some indication of the child's internal operations and the resulting reactions to the impinging world. What is it that the autistic child sees and hears? One can only infer, on the basis of observed responses and reactions, the child's difficulties and confusions. The behavior of children with autism suggests that very little of what they see and hear makes sense to them. Words, voices, faces, and gestures are no more than rapidly changing stimuli, like changes in color that are transient and difficult to grasp. People handle the child and do things to him or her; what does it mean? All those faces and changing expressions; what do they mean? Little looks the same to the autistic child; everything is always changing. That the world appears confusing to the child with autism is not surprising. Nor is it surprising that the child maintains a ritualized, ordered environment and, indeed, struggles to continue that order and sameness. Finally, when the environment impinges beyond the management point, the child fights back and throws tantrums, which are the result of frustration and confusion. The child creates an inner world that is more understandable and consistent. Self-stimulation can be seen as an attempt to reestablish sameness. Many parents say that their autistic child exhibits self-stimulatory behavior when exposed to a new situation or experience. The perceptual deficits of the child with autism create further disturbance because they severely limit the child's interactional experiences within the environment. Children who see the world in a distorted manner interact with that world in a distorted manner. This cycle does not enable the child to experience the multiplicity of interactions that are the building blocks of conceptual development (Bee, 1992).

The roots of representational behavior are based on the child's interactional experiences within the environment, it is important therefore to examine the interrelationship between cognitive and communicative functioning. Research now supports the view that the unique acquisition and use of language by autistic children results from a cognitive processing style that differs from that of nonimpaired children. Children with autism have often been described as "language chunkers." Prizant (1982) suggested that the autistic characteristics of ritualistic behavior and echolalia indicate a gestalt processing style. As a result of this gestalt preference, children with autism produce whole phrases and sentences without understanding the individual linguistic elements. This means that autistic children cannot manipulate the building blocks of language to combine and recombine linguistic structures creatively. Although the gestalt processing mode occurs as a part of normal language development, it is integrated with an analytic processing strategy. The interface between these two processing approaches provides normal language learners with a creativity and flexibility that autistic learners do not indicate in their language productions.

Prizant (1983) suggested that echolalia and routinized rituals should be viewed as related to cognitive-linguistic processing styles in the autistic child rather than as deviant characteristics. Because they use a gestalt style of language processing, children with autism do not learn to break down long memorized strings into elemental units of language. Language development, production, and creativity depend on an analytic style of processing that offsets the gestalt processing style. To generate language, children must learn to use linguistic rules to combine and recombine the basic units. Without a working knowledge of the meaningful units of language, the child with autism can form only surface associations between long language chunks and contexts. Often the meaning relationship between the memorized chunk and the context is tangential. The discrepancy between form and function presents a serious strain on the communication process. The listener must attempt to derive the child's communicative intent based on what the listener thinks the child means.

In studying autistic, mentally retarded, and nonimpaired children, Sigman and Ungerer (1984) attempted to identify the early cognitive deficits specific to the syndrome of autism. As noted earlier, the majority of children with autism are also mentally retarded. With spontaneous play, autistic children demonstrated less diverse functional play performances than the mental-age-matched mentally retarded and nonimpaired children. The children with autism, however, were not deficient in sensorimotor skills. Functional and symbolic play were associated with more advanced receptive language, as was the ability to imitate gestures and vocalizations. Although sensorimotor skills and language were positively correlated in nonimpaired and mentally retarded children, they were unrelated in the children with autism. The authors suggested that sensorimotor knowledge may be necessary but not sufficient for language development. The marked discrepancy between the autistic children's sensorimotor abilities and language disabilities provides support for the argument that sensorimotor and symbolic knowledge may involve divergent development. The autistic children in the study presented with specific deficits in imitation, symbolic abilities, play, and language. Several hypotheses may explain the variation in deficits. The first theoretical possibility is that representational thought may require the interface of two subsystems. One such subsystem involves the development of sensorimotor skills with the ability to recall information for problem solving. The second subsystem involves the ability to translate experiences into symbols; it is with this area that the autistic children have difficulty. The second hypothesis is that cognitive deficits in children with autism are secondary to social deficits. The authors noted that "all the areas of specific cognitive deficit identified to date depend on social interaction for their development" (p. 301). This finding highlights the significance of the social learning context to other developmental areas. The social experience becomes the "field with developmental areas such as play, cognition, imitation, and language facilitated on this field."

Theory of Mind and Meta Abilities

Hughes and Russell (1993) indicate that the development of a "theory of mind" involves the ability to represent mental states. Research indicates that normal children realize that the actions of other people are related to what they think and believe and not necessarily to factual occurrences. A child's ability to take the perspective of another person to understand another's point of view, begins in early childhood (Flavell, Green, & Flavell, 1990). Theory of mind research in autistic children focuses on the ability to judge how false beliefs determine action and judgment; the understanding of false belief is crucial to the conceptualization underlying meta-representation. Holroyd and Baron-Cohen (1993), describe a shift in theoretical perspective concerning the underlying origin of autism as a deficit in metarepresentation. Given social and communicative deficits in autistic children, the concept of "theory of mind" may provide an explanation for social, behavioral, and pragmatic-communicative abnormalities. Their results indicated that the majority of autistic individuals (60–70 percent) presented limited development in the meta-representational area; a minority (20–30 percent) appear to develop to a level equivalent to 3- to 4-year-old normal children by the time they reach teenage years. Investigations related to research in the area of "theory of mind" propose that the communication, socialization, and mental imagery deficits characteristic of autistic individuals may be attributable to their inability to symbolize and conceptualize mental states (Perne, Frith, Leslie, & Leeham, 1989; Frith, 1989). Happe (1994) indicated that autistic individuals presented with conceptual difficulties in connected situations requiring judgments about joking, lying, persuasion, and pretense.

Autistic children may also have difficulty developing the behavioral strategies involving disengagement of attention from focal objects. The results of Hughes and Russell (1993) indicated that autistic subjects failed a test of strategic deception because they had difficulty mentally disengaging from a focal object and not because they were unable to perform a "theory of mind" task. The ability to disengage attention from a focal object is one of many mental operations referred to as executive functions. These functions "are separately necessary and jointly sufficient for volitional goal directed behavior; inhibition of perceptually triggered or inappropriate responses; planning and embedding of behavioral and cognitive sequences; maintaining an appropriate set; disengaging from an inappropriate one; and monitoring the success and failure of current strategies" (p. 507). The researchers further suggest that the results achieved from the tests traditionally used to assess "theory of mind" may have been confounded by the executive difficulties exhibited in autistic individuals.

Mundy and colleagues (1987) proposed that play may involve metacognitive abilities. The "meta" skills—metacognitive and metalinguistic skills—require intact production and comprehension abilities in the child. The metas involve the abilities to revise, reflect, and repair language rules. Metalinguistic skills represent a higher conceptual understanding of production and comprehension skills when the child can "talk about talking"; he or she is aware of language structures and can make judgments about their appropriateness. Metacognitive skills involve the ability to deal abstractly with one's thought processes in comprehension, memory, information processing, reasoning, and problem solving (Brown, 1978). For the child who is autistic, pervasive deficits in social interaction, language production, and comprehension limit the development of the more abstract meta skills.

Pragmatics

For children with autism, the use of language for communicative purposes remains severely impaired in spite of developments in other language areas. Part of the problem relates to the interrelationship between social interaction and communication. Most children with autism do not develop a range of communicative functions, and as a result their communicative and social interactions are limited. Whereas the social context facilitates learning in the normally developing child, this is the environment that presents the most difficulty for the child with autism, who removes himself or herself from the very context the child needs to learn about communication. Given the child's severe communication deficits, the social situation becomes of primary importance for further learning (Eales, 1993).

In addition, the few interactive behaviors exhibited by children with autism are often part of specific and unusual routines. As noted previously, the established routine allows children with autism to maintain some control within their rapidly changing environment. The routine establishes predictability by maintaining a contextual sameness. Although children with autism indicate a preference for building such routines, these ritualized patterns further restrict social interaction. This added social limitation maintains the communication deficit. By responding to a limited range of behaviors, children with autism selectively reinforce certain aspects of the adult's input. The adult's problem is the child's limited interactional responsiveness and tolerance for change. Frequently, for the sake of interaction, the adult continues to provide a highly restricted form of communication. As a result, social interaction tends to be inflexible, ritualistic, and rigidly routinized. In turn, these social and interactional patterns affect the communication behavior problems typically described in children with autism:

1. Initiating and terminating interaction
2. Maintaining conversational topics
3. Functioning within speaker and listener roles
4. Using behavior for the purpose of communication

In general, children with autism present the following pragmatic problems: (a) they do not develop a range of communicative functions, (b) they do not develop gaze interaction skills, (c) they do not develop prototypical behaviors such as protodeclaratives or protoimperatives, (d) they do not develop attention and joint action schemes, (e) they do not develop an awareness of agent, action, or object contingencies, (f) they do not develop turn-taking or reciprocal action skills, and (g) they do not develop gestures or imitation behaviors. Prelinguistic behaviors such as pointing, showing, or turn-taking typically are not present in children with autism. As a result, the development of communicative behavior in autistic children is different from the normal developmental sequence. The differential aspects of each child promotes different patterns of responding and contingencies for interaction in peers and adults within the child's environment.

Bernard-Opitz (1982) demonstrated that communicative performance is related to specific variables within the communicative context. The author analyzed how an autistic child used language with his mother, his clinician, and a stranger. The child's communicative style was different with each communication partner. With his mother, the child initiated communication by using requests as the primary speech act, whereas with the clinician the child used statements to interact. The communicative interaction with the stranger resulted in unintelligible and noncommunicative utterances. In addition, the adults had a tendency to use requests as the predominant speech act during interaction with the child. The author suggested that the differences in the child's communicative behavior might have been related to his familiarity with the listener. Also, the child did not typically respond to the requests of the adults but rather generated another request by imitating the adult's syntactic structure. Another interesting aspect was the difference between the mother's and the clinician's response to the child's echolalic behavior. The mother reinforced the echolalic pattern by answering or clarifying the child's behavior. The clinician's response to unrelated utterances was to introduce another topic, redirecting the discourse rather than responding directly to the child's utterance. The description of autistic children as noncommunicative and noninteractive is not borne out by the Bernard-Opitz investigation. The child in this study, even with a limited range of communicative behaviors within his repertoire, responded differently to different interactional partners. So it is not that a child with autism cannot interact but rather that his or her range of communicative options is limited.

Another factor that interferes with autistic children's communicative effectiveness involves idiosyncratic behaviors. The normal language learner develops conventional behaviors to communicate his or her needs; the child with autism uses behaviors that are not standard communication or linguistic forms. The result is that the social communicators in the child's environment may misinterpret and misunderstand the child's intentions and meaning. Beisler and Tsai (1983) studied the development of communicative functions in five children with autism. The authors noted that communication, rather than specific linguistic forms or structures, should be facilitated. One problem related to the learning style of children with autism is that forms are often acquired as routinized chunks. Historically, clinical and educational programs have focused on teaching specific linguistic structures or forms, the result being that children with autism learned to reproduce rigid or "frozen" strings without a semantic-syntactic understanding of these utterances. Programmatic and instructional goals should focus on teaching autistic children about the process of interactional communication rather than teaching them responses to specific questions or forms.

Wetherby (1986) also noted that children with autism have been stereotyped as noncommunicative and noninteractive. The reality, however, is that the autistic population is heterogeneous; it consists of individuals with a range of communication and language deficits. According to the author, children with autism should not be differentiated from other children with language disorders. As already noted, autistic children appear to use various strategies in an attempt to interact even with a limited repertoire of conventional forms. In addition, they develop a more limited range of communicative functions than nonimpaired children. Normal communicative development does not occur consecutively from one function to another; some functions emerge concurrently. Linguistic structures develop from the communicative functions; children talk about the interactional context and their manipulative experiences. It is the social context that provides the basis for the development of conventional forms. The synchronous development of communicative functions evident in nonimpaired children appears as a nonsequential pattern in children with autism. This suggests that the communicative pattern developed by autistic children is qualitatively, as well as quantitatively, different from the normal prelinguistic sequence. Children with autism acquire communicative functions in a different developmental sequence, and as a result their linguistic abilities will be different. The author described the following communicative characteristics:

1. Communicative intent in gestural and vocal areas develops asynchronously.
2. The communicative profile is different from profiles in other children with language disorders.
3. The sequence of communicative development is different from that nonimpaired children.

4. The profile of communicative functions is relatively homogeneous.
5. Communicative functions are limited.
6. Certain aberrant behaviors can be intentional, interactive, and communicative.
7. Autistic children develop many behaviors that result in an environmental consequence but few behaviors that result in a social consequence.

Finally, Wetherby suggested that educational techniques must take into consideration the communication learning style of the individual child. Children with autism do not readily develop the range of communicative intentions produced by nonimpaired children because of an inability to develop and coordinate the interactional behaviors described previously. If and when linguistic skills do develop, communicative deficits remain.

Communicative Acts

Do children with autism communicate? If yes, what is the nature of the interaction? The only way to determine intentional behaviors is to observe and analyze how children with autism behave within the social situation. What should the clinician look for in an autistic child's behavior? Even the most severely impaired child has behaviors that can be identified as communicative if they are analyzed within the context. Several incidents with Adam highlight this point.

Situation 1: Clinician places a tightly sealed container of vanilla ice cream on the table.
Adam: Adam walks over to the table, turns over the container, tries to pull open the top, bites on the container, and drops it on the table. He walks away for several moments. He walks back to the table and picks up the container. He brings the container to the clinician and puts it in her lap. He walks away from the clinician and looks at her from across the room. (The clinician, of course, does nothing.) Adam approaches the clinician from the side, takes her hand, and places it on the ice cream.
Interpretation: Adam is requesting that the clinician perform an action (open the ice cream) that he could not do himself.

Situation 2: Clinician approaches Adam and sits down next to him.
Adam: Adam gets up and moves away from the clinician.
Interpretation: Adam is rejecting interaction.

Situation 3: Clinician talks to Adam.
Adam: Adam puts his hands over his ears, turns away from the clinician, but does not move away. Periodically, he takes his hands off his ears. When the clinician stops talking, Adam turns back to the clinician.
Interpretation: Adam does not want to engage in verbal interaction. The clinician learned that during these periods, Adam would participate in activities that could be maintained without discourse (e.g., puzzles, blocks, coloring).

The preceding incidents can be identified in the repertoires of even the most impaired autistic children. Adam could communicate several different intentions and evidenced different combinations of behavior to indicate his response to input and stimuli from the environment. The clinician must learn to read the child's behaviors within the contextual framework before attempting to interpret the child's reactions to the environment. In fact, the maternal variable of rich interpretation—in which the mother assumes that her infant reacts to the environment and treats the infant as an active listener and communicator—facilitates the communication exchange process. The assumption that children with autism do not have the ability to communicate results in a self-fulfilling prophesy: Because it is believed they cannot communicate, they are not treated as communicators and their behaviors are not analyzed to identify communicative interactions.

Semantics

The linguistic term *semantics* refers to meaning as it is encoded in language. Semantic knowledge, therefore, refers to the meaning within a language that is linguistically coded. Conceptual knowledge affects the acquisition of the semantic component of language. Cromer (1981) suggested that conceptual knowledge in nonimpaired children is transformed into semantic knowledge. The difficult task for children is to determine which aspects of concepts are encoded within their particular linguistic system. The interactional experiences with agents, actions, and objects develop semantic relationships that code the content of language. Tager-Flusberg (1981) commented that there are "no systematic studies of semantic development in autistic children" (p. 49). This lack of research is rather unfortunate because an understanding of the semantic component in autistic children could describe how they develop and organize their conceptual experiences into progressively more sophisticated linguistic structures.

Baltaxe and Simmons (1975) collected speech samples and noted that the most frequent errors were violations of semantic constraints. The researchers hypothesized that autism involves a semantic deficit in language learning. Ricks and Wing (1975) suggested that autism involves a deficit in representational behavior and high-level abstractions. Children with autism have difficulty developing complex relationships and, as a consequence, establishing the underpinnings for symbolic forms of behavior, which provide the foundations for language. Menyuk (1978) suggested that the underlying deficit relates to an inability to establish meaningful and relevant perceptual-conceptual categories. These abilities and their interaction enable nonimpaired children to establish general categories; that is, to relate agents, actions, and objects to one another. The establishment of categories enables children to make some cohesive and consistent sense of an environment, stimuli in the environment, and experiences within the environment that would otherwise be continually novel and changing. The abilities identified by Menyuk provide nonimpaired children with the means of organizing what they see and experience into manageable and related categories. According to Schmidt (1976), autistic subjects could not understand how objects were functionally related or associated (e.g., needle–thread). Tager-Flusberg (1981) suggested that children with autism are not able to translate their real-world experiences into linguistic structures; they cannot make use of a semantically based processing strategy.

Table 13-2 describes Adam's development of lexical items to express his semantic knowledge and ideas about the world. Adam's semantic development at this time (4 years 9 months) indicates his limited or restricted developmental use of functions. Adam devel-

TABLE 13-2   Adam's Early Lexicon

Semantic Functions	Lexical Entries
Object	Car, cookie, pretzel, juice, ice cream, milk, chip, M&M, hot dog, lolly, soda, popcorn, puzzle, Slinky, block, shoe, raisin, grape
Action	Open, push, eat, drink, throw, give
Negation: rejection	No
cessation	No
Recurrence	(Repeat of item label)
Agent	—
Action + Object	—

oped lexical items within four semantic categories. Most of the lexical items were food related—specifically, desserts. There were fewer action performances than objects coded, and two of the action performances related to food (e.g., eat and drink). Analyzing the child's corpus in this way provides the clinician with insight into what is important to the child within the environment. The child's preferences can then be incorporated into therapeutic activities.

Old knowledge provides a framework for processing new information. With the analytic style, new information can be compared to old information to develop concepts, specifically semantic concepts. Prizant (1983) noted that semantic memory involves the ability to conceptualize beyond any single or specific context. Here the child abstracts relevant information across situations to organize concepts for long-term memory. This semantic ability would allow the child to symbolically represent and reconstruct an event. So, in order to learn language, a child must be able to reconstruct sentence elements, not merely imitate them. The analytic style allows for generation with an understanding of meaning and internal structure of utterances. Children with autism have a language pattern characterized by repetition of unanalyzed forms. This language pattern indicates an inability to use generative rules for production purposes and an inability to analyze the internal structure of another's production.

Prizant (1983) suggested that gestalt and analytic styles represent processing abilities on opposite ends of a continuum. Because autistic children have an extreme style of gestalt processing, generative language development becomes a very difficult process. In particular, "those who remain primarily echolalic demonstrate a failure to move along the continuum toward analytic processing due to cognitive imitations" (p. 303). The author proposed that as spontaneous utterances increase, echolalia decreases. Spontaneous productions appear to indicate more flexibility in the use of combinatorial rules. This movement toward the analytic end of the processing continuum is necessary for the development of semantic-syntactic relations. To understand further the impact of the autistic child's processing pattern on language learning, splinter abilities can be contrasted with idiosyncratic deficits. Children with autism have excellent memories, visual processing skills, visual-spatial abilities, numerical skills, and musical abilities. The gestalt learning style interferes with the analytic requirements for the development of semantic functions and semantic-syntactic relationships.

Hyperlexia

The term *hyperlexia* has been used to describe autistic children with highly developed word-recognition skills, with little or no comprehension of the words that they recognize. There appears to be a disparity between this site recognition ability and the underlying semantic comprehension that relates to the processing of meaning in language (O'Connor & Hermelin, 1994; Tirosh & Canby, 1993). Hyperlexia has been described as a savant skill in verbal autistic individuals. Why certain children acquire this splinter skill and its overall relationship to other developmental areas of learning continues to be perplexing and interesting from an educational perspective. Many of the characteristics of autism involve highly idiosyncratic and fragmented abilities including hyperlexia. These splinter skills present learning problems over time because they are not well integrated or cross referenced with other areas of the child's learning; these skills do not represent functional behaviors that serve a social or communicative process (Patti & Lupinetti, 1993; Treffert, 1988; Aram & Healy, 1988). Hyperlectic readers appear to be highly attuned to orthographic and phonological features; this visual–verbal decoding ability is not integrated with semantic and reading comprehension. As a result, the pervasive semantic deficits can be understood, given the hyperlectic process in autistic children. Savant abilities and splinter skills highlight uneven and nonintegrated aspects of developmental learning and appear to develop independently from areas of social communicative learning. Since the savant skill does not serve to facilitate communicative interaction, it poses an interesting problem for parents and teachers. In trying to understand an advanced reading ability or any savant skill in autistic children, the question becomes, how can this splinter skill be utilized educationally to facilitate the child's interactional abilities within the social context?

Phonology

Phonological development in children with autism or any savant skill seems to follow the same course as it takes in nonimpaired children (Paul, 1987). Few studies have been conducted investigating phonological abilities in autistic children possibly because speech-language production is so limited (Wolk & Edwards, 1993). The suprasegmental features of rate, prosody, rhythm, and quality, however, represent deviant aspects of autistic children's speech. Bartolucci, Pierce, Streiner, and Eppel (1976) suggested that the frequency of distribution of phonemes in autistic children was similar to that found in mentally retarded children. In both groups of children, the highest percentage of errors involved phonemes that were generally acquired later in nonimpaired children. The order of phonemic acquisition seems to follow the normal developmental pattern, in spite of the delay in the onset of speech. Fay and Schuler (1980) noted that the phonological ability of children with autism contrasted markedly with their developmental delays in the other linguistic and communicative areas.

Suprasegmental features such as stress and intonation are often described as deviant in autistic children. Many clinicians have noted that children with autism have peculiar voice quality and sometimes speak in a monotone. The stress and pitch patterns used by children with autism are often inappropriate to the meaning of the linguistic utterance and the context of the situation. In addition, autistic children's lack of affect may be explainable by the inability to process and use intonational features (environmental cues). This explanation of autistic children's speech behavior is more parsimonious than the suggestion of emotional impairment. The flat affect and monotonic pattern that is so typical of children with autism may be the result of an inability to process, register, and generate suprasegmental features within the linguistic message (Fay & Schuler, 1980).

Let's consider how these variables appeared in Adam's developmental pattern. Adam's progression from a period of muteness and virtual silence to a period of intelligible imitative productions was remarkable. There are many questions concerning this transition: Did the transition from muteness to echolalia result from the therapeutic and environmental experiences, neurological development, or both? As noted, Adam remained mute until the age of 4 years 3 months. The only sounds he produced were self-stimulatory sounds used to block out input from the environment. During these occurrences, Adam would raise the loudness of his own voice to block out various types of input: speakers' voices, music, and environmental noises such as those from a telephone, a fire engine, or an airplane. The only other sounds he uttered were whining and crying sounds of distress. When Adam started to speak, he evidenced echolalic behavior. Although the suprasegmental features were deviant, resulting in robotlike, wooden productions, his articulatory productions were extraordinarily intelligible. By 4 years 6 months, Adam's phonological development (a) had progressed further than any other language component and (b) followed the normal pattern or progression more closely than any other component.

Syntax

Curtiss (1981) proposed that language components emerge from developments in cognitive knowledge. The development of a normal linguistic system in which structure is related to meaning requires an interfacing of linguistic and nonlinguistic cognitive development. Curtiss suggested that lexical and relational semantic abilities are linked to broader conceptual development but that morphological and syntactic abilities are not. There are very few studies that provide detailed information about the syntactic developments in children with autism. Bartolucci and colleagues (1976) described the particular difficulty autistic children have with the developmental use of verb endings, such as past tense and present progressive. The researchers did not interpret these findings as a difficulty with grammatical structure, but rather as a difficulty with semantic development. The more basic problem for children with autism is that they do not understand underlying conceptual ideas such as past occurrence that contribute to the formulation of language. Children with autism have difficulties using or manipulating certain linguistic forms of language because they do not understand their semantic counterparts. Bartak, Rutter, and Cox (1975) compared autistic with dysphasic children. The researchers found both groups comparable in mean length of utterance (one of the major measures of productive language development) and grammatical complexity. On a test of comprehension, however, the children with autism performed more poorly than the children with dysphasia. It seems that the syntactic delays in children with autism are related to their general developmental delays. These children present syntactic processing skills similar to those evidenced by children with other types of disorders. Linguistic analyses indicate the use of rule-governed behavior in the autistic child's limited production and comprehension of language. Tager-Flusberg (1981) reported that "autistic subjects display mastery of a variety of grammatical rules, similar to matched groups of retarded, schizophrenic, or developmental aphasic subjects" (p. 49).

Adam's productions are analyzed within the framework of various contextual and interactional situations to highlight his limited linguistic processing abilities. Consider Adam's use of the following morphemes: present progressive, past tense, personal pronouns, relative pronouns, copula, articles, and plurals.

Clinician: What is Mommy doing?

Adam: Mommy is opening juice.

Within the framework of an interaction with the adult, Adam was able to use the copula and present progressive morphemes within his own speech. He also responded to the adult's question by altering the inflectional form of the adult's utterance (i.e., he did not imitate the question's inflectional pattern).

Clinician: What did you do?

Adam: Adam eat three cookie.

Within the framework of this interaction with the adult, Adam responded to the question by referring to himself as Adam; he did not use any of the personal pronouns. He was not able to code (or use) the past-tense form. When Adam was not able to code the morphemic structures presented within the adult's production, he reduced his own utterance or reverted to a string of content words. Plural forms were coded by the use of number without the plural -s. In the preceding examples, there was a structural relationship between the linguistic input provided by the adult and the child's linguistic response: Adam patterned his response on the structure of the adult's input. The following interaction shows what happened to Adam's linguistic structure when adult input was not provided:

Clinician: (has just poured Adam some juice)

Adam: Drink juice. (describing his own action)

Adam: More. (requesting more juice)

Adam: Pour juice. (directing clinician to perform an action)

Adam: Give. (requesting cup from clinician)

In this interaction, the clinician responded nonverbally to all of Adam's requests and directions. He did not, therefore, have the adult's linguistic input to rely on to structure his own utterances. The result was a reduction to the minimum use of forms that would "get the message across" effectively. This reduction process was quite typical of Adam's spontaneous, or self-initiated, speech. To understand the structural/syntactic abilities of children with autism, it is important to analyze if and how the language structure changes within various interactional situations. For Adam, the adult's input provided a syntactic framework for responses. Finally, Adam's productions required a close analysis of the context in order to disambiguate the meaning of his utterances. He rarely provided gestural support for his verbal productions.

During the third year of life, the normal language learner begins to encode meaning syntactically in the form of phrases, sentences, and finally, narratives. In the process of combining words, the child learns that words must be organized into sentences given specific linguistic rules. The normally developing child learns that ideas can be expressed by using sentence structures that express questions, negation, coordination, sequence, causality, and temporality. Conventional forms are important to the expression of ideas. By 3 years of age, the normal language learner has already integrated aspects of formal structure, semantic meaning, and communicative interaction. This can be contrasted with some striking statistics on autistic children. Newsom, Carr, and Lovaas (1979) estimated that 50 percent of all children with autism are mute and that 75 percent of those who become verbal are echolalic by 5 years of age.

Therapeutic Issues and Strategies

The clinical view of the child with autism has changed in the past several years. Theoretical changes in the area of child language development have dramatically affected the content and context of therapeutic programs. Children with autism now undergo communication training rather than speech training. With the focus on communication learning, several related issues have been investigated by speech-language pathologists: parent language training, home training, alternative language systems, and language socialization in inclusive classrooms. These components present a more holistic approach to the language learning experience for children with autism.

Therapeutic programming varies from child to child, family to family, and clinician to clinician. It is this variety in training approaches and styles that provides our profession with its clinical strength. Given their developmental differences and needs, children with autism present a number of challenges for educators, parents, and public officials. Autistic children require an integrated educational approach that facilitates the development of a life-cycle philosophical approach for home and school. Autism is, after all, a lifelong developmental disability. For a child with autism, each context represents an ecology with its place on life's learning continuum. Research in the area of therapeutic issues stresses the need for adaptive communication in multiple contexts, integration of services, and development of inclusive social learning models. This "systems" view establishes programming and decision making across a long term service continuum from birth through adulthood. In addition, the professional network must enhance the child's transition from one environmental context to another and from one developmental stage to another. Finally, programming itself should focus on the process of learning rather than specific content.

Social Problems and Behavioral Technology

Because of the extensive behavioral difficulties characteristic of children with autism, many clinicians use behavioral procedures to train targeted behaviors such as self-care and daily living skills, as well as speech behaviors. The behavioral approach is also used as part of an educational program to deal with inappropriate and injurious behaviors exhibited within the classroom (McEachlin, Smith, & Lovaas, 1993; Matson, Sevin, Box, Francis, & Sevin, 1993). The classroom teacher relies on the modification model because of the need to operationalize classroom procedures and training goals. Underlying the behavioral approach is the identification of an observable and measurable targeted performance (e.g., sitting, looking, or vocalizing). For example, rather than targeting attention as a training performance, the clinician or teacher would identify all of the descriptive behaviors of attention: sitting, physical orientation, eye contact, and so on. These identified behaviors are then trained by means of a successive approximation procedure.

The management difficulties presented by autistic children impact significantly upon the abilities of educators and parents to integrate these children within social contextual environments. The behavior problems often exhibited by autistic children: aggression, self-injurious behavior, unanticipated explosive behaviors, self-stimulation, and extraneous verbal-vocal behaviors often interfere with the child's acceptance by others within natural settings and complex community contexts. The management of severe behavior problems requires a combined treatment approach utilizing highly individualized training schedules by means of behavior analysis. Children's behavior must be assessed and functionally analyzed in order to determine the most appropriate management schedule within the educational setting at home and within the community (Carr & Carlson, 1993). The management of intrusive behaviors requires the identification of contingent stages that will be utilized by a multidisciplinary team of professionals across various learning settings. The combined behavioral approach emphasizes the identification of target behaviors and also emphasizes the need for developing appropriate social learning skills that will be maintained and reinforced by adults and peers. Gunter, Fox, McEvoy, Shores, and Denny (1993) describe the stigmatization that occurs when a child's behavior results in social rejection and ultimately interferes with the educational learning process that would naturally occur within the social environment. The identification of training procedures may vary from child to child, but the behavioral needs of autistic children suggest targeted programming and instruction within the special education classroom. This is necessary if this child is going to be ultimately mainstreamed to less restrictive educational and environmental placements. Research has documented that preschool special education programs are including many more children with autism, behavioral-emotional, and pervasive developmental disabilities.

Public Law 99-457 has created the legal and educational framework for early intervention services, and as a result, developmentally disabled children are being identified at a much earlier age. Inclusive programming during the preschool years in which handicapped and nonhandicapped children are integrated by means of socialization experiences may represent the best point in time to integrate and to manage behavioral-social problems in autistic children. The preschool special education curriculum focuses on daily living skills, language learning skills, play skills, peer interactions, self-awareness, and independence. The preschool process also provides an important link between educational programming between the classroom and the home environment. Preschool programs often coordinate their goals across educational and therapeutic services by collaborating with parents. Educational and instructional needs identified at home and at school provide the basis for parent-teacher coordination of social and behavioral planning (Ford, Riggs, Nissenbaum, & LaRaia, 1994).

Children with autism have great difficulty generalizing learned behaviors to new contexts and situations. Educational programming must begin early during the infant years. The focus of instructional goals on socialization, peer interactions, and communication behaviors will provide the autistic child with a repertoire of social skills. The child's ability to remain within the social context of the classroom, the restaurant, the playground, the mall, and other natural environments is based upon the generalized use of social-communicative behaviors. Early intervention programs emphasize the importance of social-communication behavior within the framework of a peer-mediated integrated classroom. The very nature of the early childhood curriculum reinforces these abilities (Wolfberg & Schuler, 1993).

Learning Contexts

Adam's training was changed to reflect the theoretical issues raised in the literature during the 1990s. In the following program, there was an attempt to incorporate each environment (school, after-school therapy, and home) within the educational process. A set of operating principles was developed to coordinate intervention goals and therapeutic programming with inclusive education in mind. The identified learning contexts represented a means of generalizing communication experiences for the child across the different educational environments. The communication behaviors learned in the classroom could be generalized across the curriculum to the home or the therapy room.

The following operating principles were used to develop Adam's learning contexts:

1. A learning context was defined as any activity that provided an interactional framework, that is, an opportunity for interchange between the adult and the child.
   The activity was then described in terms of the type of (a) interactions to be developed, (b) communicative behaviors to be learned, and (c) semantic functions to be coded (see Table 13-3).
2. Each learning context presented a format or routine.

TABLE 13-3   An Example of a Learning Context

Place	Activity/Context	Materials	Routine	Communicative Behavior
Therapy room	Making bubbles	Bubbles	Get Bubbles	Point to object
	Large bubble	Wand	Open bubbles	Gaze at object/adult
		Fan	Get wand	Sign for object
			Pour bubbles (or action)	
			Turn fan on	Consistent vocalization for object (or action)
			Make bubbles	Word
				Some combination of these behaviors

3. Each learning context established a task structure to develop an anticipation and sequence of events in the routine.
4. The learning context facilitated action and interaction; it allowed for the development of reversible role relationships between adult and child.
5. A core lexicon was developed within each learning context to consistently and systematically focus communication and language training across all the adults working with the child.
6. The core lexicon was based on the development of those communicative behaviors that appear earliest in child language. These communicative behaviors were used across a variety of learning contexts to generalize language and communication relations.
7. Communicative interaction was stressed above production of stereotypic/routinized utterances.
8. Learning contexts developed were relevant and functional to the child. To facilitate interaction and communication, the adult focused on activities that the child preferred.
9. Input to the child was limited in complexity and mean length of utterance. Adult input was functional and relevant to the immediate context and semantically related to the child's vocal, verbal, and nonlinguistic behavior.
10. The child was presented with a choice of learning contexts; at any time, the child could maintain or terminate an activity. Verbal, vocal, and nonverbal behaviors were analyzed within the learning contexts to determine communicative intentions.
11. The child was first trained to participate and interact within the context. Then the child was trained to produce behaviors that code the next occurrence in the routine.
12. Every adult working with the child was given a copy of the communication/language description of each learning context. Thus, each adult provided consistent input within and across activities (see Table 13-4).
13. Echolalic behavior was used to develop language behaviors. With the knowledge that the child would imitate, the adult would code, for instance, a nonlinguistic event:

Event: Adam opening the bubbles

Adult: Adam open bubbles.

Adam: Adam open bubbles.

The clinical goals identified for Adam's training included:

1. Development of imitative interaction skills
2. Expansion of object manipulation skills (semantic knowledge)
3. Development of sign/gesture forms
4. Use of interactional behaviors that signal communicative intentions
5. Generalization of communication behaviors

The goals and procedures described in this section should be considered, given the need to individualize language and communication programming. However, the following procedures and issues are related to interactional deficits that are characteristic of all autistic children.

Mirenda and Schuler (1988) noted that natural learning contexts and the underlying need to regulate the social environment should provide the scaffolding for therapeutic de-

TABLE 13-4　An Example of a Communication/Language Description of a Learning Context (Context: bubbles; Materials: bottle of bubbles, bubble maker, fan)

Semantic Functions	Forms Trained/Adult Input
1. Object	Bubbles, fan
2. Action	Open, blow, give, turn on
3. Agent	Ellen, Adam, Mommy, Daddy
4. Agent + Agent	Adam open, Ellen open Adam blow, Ellen blow
5. Action + Object	Make bubbles, pour bubbles, open bubbles
6. Recurrence	Bubbles . . . bubbles . . . bubbles, more, 　more bubbles
7. Negation 　Rejection 　Cessation (action)	No, no bubbles Stop, no more, no more bubbles No pour, no blow
8. Agent + Action + Object	Adam open bubbles Ellen open bubbles Mommy open bubbles Adam pour bubbles Ellen pour bubbles Adam blow bubbles Ellen blow bubbles Mommy blow bubbles

cision making. Communication interaction would be the result of "predictable interaction routines" between two or more people. Once the child learns to operate within these familiar contexts, event sequences can be altered and the child's expectations violated. The child's awareness of the environment can be determined by noting the child's awareness of the unanticipated change and his or her attempt to repair the situation. This provides prime opportunities to aid the development of communicative behaviors and interactions between adult and child or child and child interactants. The authors noted that it is important to provide autistic children with opportunities to initiate and to regulate actions, people, and events in their environment. Children with autism need to develop a contingency relationship between their behavior and that of other social interactants; reciprocal interaction is based on such a consequence-based conceptualization.

Echolalia and Communicative Intentions

Prizant (1983) suggested that echolalia should be viewed as a dynamic and integral part of autistic children's developmental pattern. Their echolalic behavior can provide a means for training communication interactions. Their imitative ability can be used to assimilate and coordinate a linguistic event with a related nonlinguistic event. By emphasizing the relationship between linguistic behavior and nonlinguistic environmental consequences, echolalic behavior can be embedded meaningfully within appropriate contexts. The development of communicative intentions should be actively stimulated by the adult initially using the child's echolalic tendencies to establish the relationship between language and environmental referents (objects, actions, and people). The adult language input model should be regulated in terms of linguistic complexity to the child's level of comprehension (Tiegerman-Farber & Cartusciello-King, 1995c). In addition, the adult's language model, which sets the occasion for the child's echolalic behavior, should always result in an immediate and observable environmental consequence. It is important to teach autistic children that language has an effect—it creates change. Whenever possible and relevant, the adult should manipulate the environment to produce the effect the child linguistically codes. The teacher's use of exaggerated gesture and intonation, linguistic simplification and repetition, and action repetition are helpful in focusing the child on language that is relevant to an activity.

In attempting to teach autistic children to express their needs, the clinician should manipulate contextual events to create the need and facilitate its expression.

Context: Ice cream container cannot be opened by the child.

Adult: Ellen open ice cream.

Adam: Ellen open ice cream.

Consequence: Ellen performs action.

It is important for the teacher to identify a number of situational contexts that create communicative need. These situations provide children who are autistic with the opportunity to intentionally direct the course of events within the environment. The ultimate goal is teaching autistic children that language is a tool, a vehicle, a means to affect the behavior of other interactants. To achieve this goal, autistic children must experience themselves as effective communicators within the social context.

In Adam's case, the transition from the use of sign language to oral language forms is difficult to explain. The end result of this period was echolalic behavior. Adam's "eureka" experience—as his mother called it—occurred one day when he came to language therapy producing (very clearly) a verbal label in place of a learned sign. In the next 4 weeks, he replaced his sign productions with verbal productions. In Adam's case, sign training seems to have facilitated his development of verbal production. Once a sign was replaced with a verbal production, the sign was never used again. His communication system, therefore, consisted of several forms: words, sign forms, and interchangeable sign/verbal forms. These interchangeable forms indicated a transition—a replacement of sign by word. Use of each new word form increased as use of the sign decreased. This replacement process emphasizes that even as an impaired learner, Adam indicated a systematic learning pattern. Perhaps the pattern represents a unique or idiosyncratic pattern of learning, but it was a pattern nonetheless, and when identified, provided some insight into how Adam learned.

The information-processing style of children with autism becomes an important issue when adaptive systems are being considered. Mirenda and Schuler (1988) noted that there are no clear-cut conclusions on the efficacy of any of the intervention systems: sign language, Blissymbols, pictorial and written words, communication boards, micro computers, and facilitated communication. The highly individualized learning styles of autistic children must be taken into consideration. The authors noted that the introduction of an adaptive learning system does not mean that the communication learning problems will be automatically resolved. The gestalt processing style in autistic children suggests that the way information is processed must be incorporated into therapeutic decision making. Mirenda and Schuler noted that "because of its dual spatial and temporal organization, sign language may have the potential to facilitate the transition from a simultaneous to a more sequential mode of processing" (p. 26). The communication difficulties of children with autism are often offset by extraordinary abilities in memory and visual processing. Some verbal autistic children present hyperlectic reading abilities; advanced word recognition without language comprehension. Given the marked discrepancy between "the form and the function:" the issue for educators becomes one of attempting to use and to integrate the autistic child's skills in teaching communication. The variability in the population is compounded by the highly individualized scatter of skills in each child. Intervention procedures must be matched to the child's learning style and needs.

Peer-Mediated Communicative Intervention

The integration of autistic children within less restrictive special education classrooms and general education classrooms requires a high degree of specialized programming and teacher training (Kames, Locke, Delguardri, & Hall, 1989; Odom, Chandler, Ostrosky, McConnell, & Reaney, 1992; Odom, McConnell, & McEvoy, 1992; Kohler & Greenwood, 1990). Researchers advocating for full inclusive programming propose peer-mediated social strategies as a mechanism for facilitating social skills and integration in autistic children. The process of teaching children to teach children provides the general education classroom with an opportunity to integrate autistic children. Cooperative learning and peer tutoring, in which handicapped and nonhandicapped learners are brought together to interact and socialize, provide an opportunity for students to develop a social awareness of peer roles, responsibilities, and skills as socialization becomes a primary focus for instruction (Tiegerman-Farber & Radziewicz, 1996).

The normal language learner can provide peer instruction and modeling for the autistic child. It becomes important, however, for teachers and adults to educate normal peers and ready them for this peer instructional opportunity (Tiegerman-Farber & Cartusciello-King, 1995c). The normal or regular environment plays an important role in the social learning process for all developmentally disabled students. The autistic child presents a rather unique set of learning needs in social and communicative areas. In the effort to improve peer acceptance, it becomes important for early intervention programs to develop a peer training program; normal learners must be instructed on how to teach and to facilitate their disabled peers. The integrated environment must be "readied" and modified to accept autistic learners. Activities, interactional experiences, learning contingencies and educational procedures must all be defined with peer partners in mind. The normal language peer and a more socially challenging environment provides an opportunity for language learning and natural environmental contingencies. The regular preschool classroom provides the opportunity for naturalistic learning. Warren and Gazdag (1990) suggested that milieu teaching approaches include naturalistic language intervention techniques: "Milieu teaching approaches are characterized by the use of dispersed training trials, attempts to baseline teaching of the child's attentional lead within the context of normal conversational interchanges, and an orientation toward teaching the form and content of language in the context of normal use" (p. 62). Clinical research has clearly evidenced a change in intervention technologies to focus on child specific, contextual, and interactional variables as underpinnings for teaching communication to the autistic child.

For the autistic child who presents with severe language and communication deficits, early peer experiences by means of dyadic and triadic interchanges provide an opportunity for social learning. Goldstein and Strain (1988) noted that peer-mediated communicative interventions provide a means of facilitating social interactions in disabled children who are withdrawn. Autistic children usually remain on the outside of the social play situations that would naturally provide them with the very learning stimulation they need. In addition, children with autism are provided with few opportunities to interact with nondisabled peers, given pervasive behavioral deficits. The authors suggested that normal peers can be trained to interact with autistic children. Normally developing children can be trained to use specific interactional strategies to engage disabled peers in various activities and thereby facilitate the social learning process.

Social scripts can provide the means for controlled interactions between disabled and nondisabled children. Each child learns about the script story and then his or her own role. The script provides the format and the structure for the social interactions among the "players" (Tiegerman-Farber & Cartusciello-King, 1995c). The rehearsal of the script is very similar to the early social games that mothers engage in with their infants. The game provides a limited semantic domain and clearly defined roles for the interactants. With the sociodramatic play scripts, nondisabled children can model for the autistic child and provide ongoing gestural and verbal cues.

The results of their investigation indicated:

1. Training peers to act as social agents resulted in higher rates of communicative interaction in preschoolers with disabilities.
2. Children with disabilities were equally responsive to teacher and peer input, suggesting that nondisabled children can take on more directive responsibility for facilitating intervention with autistic peers.

Early childhood programs and schools attempting to provide inclusive opportunities for handicapped children will require organizational efforts and funding support for the following (Tiegerman-Farber & Radziewicz, 1996):

- The collaborative development of an inclusion mission for parents and teachers
- Physical reconstruction of classrooms and buildings to remove structural barriers to inclusion
- Teacher training and staff development for regular education and special education teachers on instructional management of diverse learners
- Development of an inclusion curriculum that provides modified instruction for autistic learners in the general education classroom
- Parent education programs that incorporate families within the educational decision-making process

Facilitated Communication

A recent controversy within the clinical journals involves a therapeutic technique called facilitated communication. In facilitated communication, an adult facilitator provides physical support to help the child with autism overcome his or her neuromotor difficulties. This physical support may be provided by helping the child to isolate his or her index finger and/ or stabilizing his or her hand, wrist, or arm during a typing process. What is interesting about the technique is its underlying therapeutic premise. Basic to the use of facilitated communication is the supposition that the child with autism is not cognitively impaired but rather has a form of praxis. This motor processing disorder interferes with the expression of language and communication, and the underlying etiology is clearly different from anything discussed earlier within this chapter (Eberlin, McConnachie, Ibel, & Volpe, 1993; Cabey, 1994; Duchan, 1993).

Biklen (1992) described the use of facilitated communication with a number of autistic children. He detailed a series of steps, similar to a successive approximation procedure, that gradually allows the autistic child to become more independent in his or her use of this procedure. When facilitated communication was used with the subjects within his study, all demonstrated literacy skills. This suggests that children with autism have acquired a linguistic set of skills but cannot express the skills verbally. Facilitated communication provides a mechanism just as other alternative systems do to allow the developmentally disabled child to communicate by means of another system.

Facilitated communication represents a controversial form of therapeutic intervention for a number of reasons described by Calculator (1992). According to Calculator, "This communication technique remains one that is characterized by its ambiguity (e.g., lack of specific teaching process), mystique, recording anecdotes and spiritual underpinning" (p. 18). Calculator noted that facilitated communication exploded on the therapeutic scene before its efficacy had been experimentally investigated. Thus professionals and clinicians know little about how or why and/or with whom facilitated communication works or does not work. Calculator noted that experimental investigation is critical because this procedure suggests that we must reevaluate our perception of autism as a social, cognitive disability. This clearly has important implications for children with autism and other nonverbal developmentally disordered children. In the process of analyzing results, advocates for facilitated communication must be responsible for their claims of success. This cannot be another panacea that over time leads parents, teachers, and professionals "down a chaotic road." One important question involves how the autistic child has learned to be literate despite severe communicative, behavioral, and social difficulties. Researchers describe ongoing theoretical and clinical issues related to methodological problems in facilitated communication. There have been several attempts to replicate investigations reported in the literature to demonstrate the effectiveness of facilitated communication and the role of the facilitator in influencing the responses of the autistic individual. Duchan (1993) presents a comprehensive discussion of the collaborative view of communication; this view provides a general framework for understanding some of the problems related to facilitated communication. Analyzing the communication process in terms of interactional variables provides researchers and clinicians with possible explanations for some of the unusual phenomena associated with facilitated communication.

The Interdisciplinary and Transdisciplinary Educational Approaches

Due to Public Law 94-142 and the mandate of least restrictive environment, many public school districts have developed classes for the autistic within mainstreamed environments. New York State Education Department regulations require that children with autism be educated in classes with a 6:1:1 ratio (6 children for every one teacher and one aide) and be provided with 5 half hours of speech-language therapy per week. In addition, depending on the individual learning needs of the child, related services such as occupational therapy, physical therapy, and adaptive physical education can also appear on the individualized educational plan (IEP). Special education programming involves the assessment and intervention of many educational specialists. The primary classroom teacher has historically been the special education teacher. The speech-language pathologist only provides mandated related services by means of a pull-out process that removes the autistic child from the classroom. When an educational facility employs professionals to evaluate and remediate the child separately and independently, the educational model used is an interdisciplinary approach. Although it provides the child with many services, this model involves only limited interaction and interface among professionals. It is critical that educators network with each other on a regular and consistent basis. It has also been noted that this model does not adequately address the language learning needs of children with autism, a criticism relating specifically to the type of classroom teacher and the pull-out services.

Some educational facilities use a transdisciplinary educational model instead of an interdisciplinary approach. This involves the development of an educational or professional team that works together, as the same time, to evaluate a child with a disability. The evaluative reports and IEPs are then developed by the group of professionals as a whole. The transdisciplinary approach requires a collaborative educational effort. As a result, professionals work together more closely to generate a more holistic picture of the child. The transdisciplinary approach emphasizes professional collaboration in educational decision making as well, which presents an important alternative to the interdisciplinary model.

Given the fact that autism is now understood to be a severe language and communication disorder, the level of "speech therapy" services has been described as dramatically inadequate. Language learning must become the primary goal for classroom instruction and not just another related service. The educational curriculum and IEP should include language-communication goals and procedures. In addition, special education teachers have very limited academic training in language development and language disorders. Many educational programs are now placing speech-language pathologists in classrooms rather than only employing them as individual service providers. At the School for Language and Communication Development in New York, the speech-language pathologist is the primary classroom teacher. Clearly the language learning needs of children with autism require more than what the traditional education model has provided in the past.

Finally, the use of an etiological placement approach provides serious educational problems for children with autism. Adam's mother noted that a class of six autistic children is really six one-child classes. Six children who cannot interact and communicate also cannot serve as facilitators for one another. If the need is communication, children with autism must be provided with child models who can facilitate such interactional development. A nonetiological educational approach to placement would certainly address this issue. It would also provide autistic children with a less restrictive educational placement and the opportunity to interact with higher-functioning social peers. Peer facilitation would allow for language modelling in the special education classroom. The placement of autistic children should be based upon language level of functioning rather than etiological label. To make this a reality, however, state education departments across the United States would have to change their disability categories and their (etiologically based) educational placement processes. The enactment of PL 99-457 in 1986 mandated educational services for preschool children with disabilities. Preschoolers (ages 3 to 5 years) now can receive educational services. The need for early intervention has moved from a dream to a reality. Society will finally actualize the findings of research proving that children with disabilities have a better prognosis the earlier intervention occurs.

Generalization of Communication Behaviors through Home Training

A home training program can be used to help children generalize the language learning experience to various environments (Tiegerman-Farber, 1995a). In Adam's case, the home provided a training experience within a more natural learning environment. Part of the home training program developed for Adam included training parents and siblings as communication facilitators. In addition, a dedicated group of volunteers was trained to work within the framework of the program and to provide extensive training 7 days a week—after school and on weekends. The home training program can be contrasted to the more traditional therapy experience provided for Adam in school. Family members could not participate in sessions during the school day, whereas at home the parent training model incorporated everyone's participation. His mother was present and integrated into the framework of each session. She was carefully trained by the speech-language pathologist to work with Adam at home.

The home and school training experiences were different in terms of the amount of stimulation provided. The home-based program was developed to be a language training program for as long as Adam was awake. In school, the speech-language pathologist provided language training outside the classroom three times a week for 30 minutes. Coordinating training goals with the classroom teacher was possible but difficult. Another difference concerned the nature of the training experience itself. The home training program focused on the development of language and communication behaviors within all of the training contexts (see Table 13-3). Activities were identified to facilitate interaction and communication. The activity provided a means to an end: adult-child interaction. Nothing had to be simulated. Activities were meaningful and relevant to the child's daily living needs and the immediate context. The adult's input to the child and the child's language corpus were

1. Regulated to the child's level of communication functioning
2. Related semantically to the ongoing nonlinguistic experience
3. Sensitive to the child's interests and preferences

Traditional classroom activities with colors, shapes, numbers, beads, and pegs were never used because of their limited potential for facilitating communication and interaction.

As a language learning experience, the home training program presented certain advantages for Adam as a severely language-disordered child. First, family members were trained to function as communication facilitators. Second, various activities within the home provided the means to integrate language behavior with relevant nonlinguistic experiences. Third, the use of communicative behaviors was generalized across learning contexts. Fourth, the orientation of the program emphasized the child's language and communication needs. These components were not available to Adam within the traditional special education classroom. The home training program proved to be an important addition to traditional learning.

The educational setting has a responsibility to develop parent language training programs to formally provide parents with academic and procedural knowledge (Tiegerman-Farber, 1995b). Training parents to function as communication facilitators for their autistic children extends the educational process beyond 3 P.M. to the home context. Parents need to understand language development, language disorders, and language intervention issues if they are going to assist in the educational development of their children; teaching parents about language and the language needs of their children gives them the tools to do so. To teach parents to understand their children is the greatest responsibility and the greatest gift of education.

The Inclusion Mandate

There is a great deal of legal and social support for the inclusion of all students, including those with severe developmental disabilities, within regular classroom settings (Wisniewski & Alpert, 1994; Polansky, 1994; Rock, Rosenberg, & Carran, 1995). Several research studies support the notion that students with severe developmental disabilities can be provided with appropriate educational services in general education classrooms. These studies also document the fact that students with severe disabilities can benefit from an inclusive setting, given the expanded opportunities for communication and social interactions between handicapped and nonhandicapped learners. Children with severe developmental disabilities can be provided with appropriate social and language models from age appropriate peers. Students without disabilities have the humanistic opportunity to acquire an understanding of social values that relate to learning differences between people. Nonhandicapped children need to be provided with a curriculum that addresses positive attitudes about a variety of multicultural learners—disabled and nondisabled.

The failure to include students with severe disabilities underscores the complications within the public school system to implement and to achieve full inclusion. What is the least restrictive environment for an autistic child (Tiegerman-Farber & Radziewicz, 1996)? Autistic children present with severe language and communication deficits, social relational problems, and behavioral management needs. The principle of normalization that is often raised about inclusive education suggests that the autistic child would benefit from the regular education experience provided by nondisabled peers. Although there may be an attempt to maintain the autistic child within ongoing regular academic activities such as reading, math, social studies, and science, the differences in learning require major modifications in teacher instruction, classroom procedures, and peer sensitivity-awareness. Part of the decision making concerning the appropriateness of a regular classroom for an autistic child involves, therefore, the issue of resources in personnel and in instructional time.

If the autistic child is nonverbal, several alternative systems of communication may be necessary within the classroom. Each of these alternative systems requires techniques, time, and professional expertise if the autistic child is going to be appropriately maintained within the dynamics of the regular classroom. One criticism of the regular classroom may involve the fact that the autistic child's education may not be individualized to the same degree as it would be in a special education classroom. Can the regular classroom be redesigned and restructured as a learning environment that can handle the diverse needs of severely behaviorally impaired children? Gerrard (1994) suggests that education must focus on identifying what is in the best interest of the child. The integration and inclusion of an autistic child within a regular classroom requires a great deal of reorganization and commitment from parents, teachers, and administrators. As professionals, the more we understand about the autistic child's language development and learning, the greater the opportunities for designing an appropriate inclusive setting for this population.

Summary

This chapter has emphasized the unique language learning problems presented by children with autism. Autistic children have traditionally been described as a single population, but the research cited in this chapter has stressed the heterogeneity exhibited within this group, suggesting that the etiological label is misleading. In addition, the use of this label detracts from the central problem related to the disorder: the inability to integrate communicative function with other aspects of language. The research describes a schism between "form and function" in autistic children with basic language disturbances in pragmatic and semantic skills; phonological and syntactic skills develop relatively intact. In fact, literature describing the language of higher-functioning autistic individuals indicates severe communicative deficits in contrast to the almost normal acquisition of structural linguistic skills. Such communicative incompetence includes ongoing problems with initiating and terminating interaction deficits in topic maintenance, and speaker/listener roles.

Autism (as a disorder) requires language-based educational programming during the infant and preschool years; the earlier, the better! The changes in child language theory have contributed greatly to the new therapeutic approaches used with autistic children such as Adam. In a way, Adam is a product of the pragmatic era and the communication revolution. At this point, the impact of these theoretical and therapeutic changes on children with autism can only be imagined. Finally, the speech-language pathologist has a central role to play in the educational programming developed for autistic children. There is no other professional who can better understand the language and communication deficits underlying this disorder.

Case Study

Adam was evaluated at the School for Language and Communication Development. Following is a condensed summary of his language and communication report, which was sent to his school district. At the time of this evaluation, Adam was 5.4 years of age. Adam was eventually placed by his school district in a class for children with autism.

Summary of Abilities

Adam displays a severe and pervasive language disorder involving the pragmatic, semantic, and syntactic components of language. He also presents with severe deficits in social interactional skills. Adam is highly routinized and perseverative in his behavioral and play patterns. He uses developed language scripts to respond to social contexts. He does not have the conceptual and/or linguistic ability to modify these scripts. As a result, there are times when the content of Adam's production is tangential or unrelated to the environmental context. It is difficult for Adam to incorporate new information into his knowledge base. Adam does not use a range of communicative, linguistic, or social responses. He is confined to learning and relearning because he cannot generalize his knowledge from one situation to another.

Pragmatic Abilities

Adam does not maintain appropriate gaze interaction behaviors with peers and adults. He will often verbalize without looking directly at a listener. He will often stand sideways when he is communicating with someone. He does not comprehend or produce a range of pragmatic functions. He requires verbal prompts and models from the adult to appropriately code the functions of requesting, regulating, rejecting, and calling attention. He does not comment or request information. Adam inconsistently responds to requests, comments and *wh-* questions presented to him. Even now he inconsistently responds to his name. He has difficulty attending to tasks and engaging in social interactional exchanges. Discourse skills are severely limited to two exchanges on any given topic; the result is a conversation with many topics and very few turns on any one topic. The quality of his verbal productions during conversations is limited to a statement of the object label, function, and color. Adam requires highly structured activities with simple response requirements. In unstructured situations such as free play, Adam remains on the perimeter of the social group. He does not initiate interaction with any of his peers and begins to self-stimulate by flapping his hands when a peer approaches him. He exhibits a monotonic intonational pattern during verbal production. Adam does not use any formal gestures to initiate interaction or communication. He signals requests by moving the adult's hand to a specific object. When encouraged to interact with peers, his body becomes rigid, he self-stimulates, and/or he verbally perseverates.

Semantic Abilities

Adam codes through Phase III of Bloom and Lahey's developmental paradigm with scattered abilities in Phases IV and V. He is a gestalt language user, or "chunker." He can recite entire commercials and news reports without an analytic understanding of the linguistic elements. His seemingly spontaneous utterances are routinized and perseverative in nature. Spontaneously, he is at a single-word level with some inconsistent productions of agent + object, action + object, and agent + action. Adam's narratives are chunked, unanalyzed scripts often tangential to the ongoing context. When confronted with a new learning situation, he will produce fragmented sentences with jargon and/or perseverative phrases. He is able to follow one-step directions if the adult regulates down to a two- or three-word phrase.

Syntactic Abilities

Adams echolalic MLU is greater than 10.0. This contrasts with his spontaneous MLU, which is 1.0. Adam is inconsistently beginning to alter his echolalic responses by changing his inflectional intonation.

Phonological Abilities

Adam does not demonstrate any deficits in phonological processing; however, stimulability and intelligibility are judged to be poor in general.

Integration of Language Components

Adam displays significant difficulty integrating the linguistic components of form, content, and use. He also has difficulties integrating linguistic structures with nonlinguistic experiences. He exhibits difficulty linking ideas to their appropriate linguistic form and channeling those forms into cohesive sequential structures. Adam does not use language creatively. As the linguistic complexity increases during communication and response demands increase, organizational problems increase and Adam begins to self-stimulate.

Learning Style

Adam inconsistently responds to auditory input; he responds more consistently to information presented visually. He is highly echolalic and therefore relies on routinized structures to communicate. Adam has excellent memory skills and as a result he can recall chunks of information. He attempts to relate these learned chunks to various contexts. His relatedness, however, varies from tangential to completely unrelated, depending on his ability more or less to associate the chunk to the situation.

Metalinguistic Ability

Adam has not acquired the more sophisticated meta skills. Since he has not acquired the foundation production and comprehension abilities, he does not have the conceptual ability to talk about language rules. He is not aware of himself as a speaker-initiator or speaker-responder. He is not aware of the communication process and he does not acknowledge the need to repair communicative breakdowns.

Academic Learning

Adam is able to identify, match, and sort colors, shapes, letters, and numbers. He inconsistently demonstrates the ability to categorize objects by class and/or function. His visual discrimination skills involve inconsistent figure-ground abilities. He exhibits poor sound-symbol relationships. He can print his name. He has excellent sensorimotor skills. Adam can manipulate objects but he cannot describe those manipulations. He has not developed the symbolic representational skills necessary for language and communication development. Adam also appears to have hyperlectic reading skills that are not comprehension based and are more advanced than his linguistic abilities. Any academic skills that require language abilities are likely to be delayed, if ever acquired. Subjects such as science, social studies, and reading will be based on Adam's ability to process information and extract meaning.

Play Skills
Adam's object manipulations are isolated. Often his object manipulations are not functionally related to the object. He does not show objects to acquire attention or initiate interaction. He does not exhibit what is described as integrative, facilitative, or progressive play. Nor does he exhibit parallel, representational, symbolic, or functional play. He does not learn by observing the actions of others and he cannot imitate the behaviors of others.

Management Needs
Adam requires a highly structured learning environment. When placed in an unstructured situation, he begins to self-stimulate. Adam is adult dependent on support, direction, regulation, and input. He demonstrates deficits in establishing and maintaining interaction with people, events, and objects. His inability to maintain interaction results in highly fragmented information being processed. He requires a high degree of individualized attention and instruction. The teacher must regulate the level of linguistic and semantic input to his level of comprehension within a social context. Adam requires a small self-contained special education classroom with peers who can provide appropriate social models.

Study Questions

1. How has the definition of autism changed since Kanner in 1944 described the population and its characteristics?
2. Describe the language learning characteristics of the autistic child.
3. How do severe pragmatic deficits interfere with the autistic child's social interactions with peers?
4. Discuss the advantages and disadvantages of educating the autistic child in an inclusive preschool setting.
5. Discuss the advantages and disadvantages of educating an autistic child within a general education classroom. What kinds of instructional and social modifications would have to be made to maintain the autistic child within a regular classroom setting?
6. Describe various kinds of therapeutic and educational techniques that are presently being utilized with autistic children.
7. The autistic child presents with a pervasive language disorder; (a) discuss the characteristics that the child shares with other language-disordered children, and (b) discuss the characteristics that set the child apart as a highly individualized learner.
8. Early intervention provides an extraordinary opportunity for the autistic child. Discuss the role of early intervention services for autistic children.
9. What purpose does the ritual serve? How do ritualized patterns affect the language of children with autism?
10. How could the speech-language pathologist analyze the interactional behaviors of autistic children to determine their communicative intentions?

11. Why should the speech-language pathologist play a central role in the educational programming of autistic children in inclusive classrooms?
12. Discuss the changing role of parents in collaborative decision making.

References

Aram, D. M., & Healy, J. M. (1988). Hyperlexia: A review of extraordinary word recognition. In L. K. Obler & D. Fein (Eds.), *The exceptional brain: Neuropsychology of talent and special abilities* (pp. 70–102). New York: Guilford.

Baltaxe, C., & Simmons, J. (1975). Language in childhood psychosis: A review. *Journal of Speech and Hearing Disorders, 40,* 439–458.

Bartak, L., & Rutter, M. (1976). Differences between mentally retarded and normally intelligent autistic children. *Journal of Autism and Childhood Schizophrenia, 6,* 109–120.

Bartak, L., Rutter, M., & Cox, A. (1975). A comparative study of infantile autism and specific developmental receptive language disorder. 1. The children. *British Journal of Psychiatry, 126,* 127–145.

Bartolucci, G., Pierce, S., Streiner, D., & Eppel, P. T. (1976). Phonological investigation of verbal autistic and mentally retarded subjects. *Journal of Autism and Childhood Schizophrenia, 6,* 303–316.

Bates, E., Camaioni, L., & Volterra, V. (1975). The acquisition of performatives prior to speech. *Merrill-Palmer Quarterly, 21,* 205–226.

Bee, H. (1992). *The developing child* (6th ed.). New York: HarperCollins College Publishers.

Beisler, J., & Tsai, L. (1983). A pragmatic approach to increase expressive language skills in young autistic children. *Journal of Autism and Developmental Disorders, 13,* 287–303.

Bernard-Opitz, V. (1982). Pragmatic analysis of the communicative behavior of an autistic child. *Journal of Speech and Hearing Disorders, 47,* 99–109.

Bettelheim, B. (1967). *The empty fortress: Infantile autism and the birth of the self.* New York: Free Press.

Biklen, D. (1992). Typing to talk: Facilitated communication. *American Journal of Speech Language Pathology,* January, 15–18.

Brown, A. L. (1978). Knowing when, where, and how to remember: A problem of metacognition. In R.

Glaser (Ed.), *Advances in instructional psychology* (vol. 1). Hillsdale, NJ: Lawrence Erlbaum.

Bryson, C. (1970). Systematic identification of perceptual disabilities in autistic children. *Perceptual and Motor Skills, 31,* 239–246.

Bryson, S. E., Landry, R., & Smith, I. M. (1994). Brief report: A case study of literacy and socioemotional development in a mute autistic female. *Journal of Autism and Developmental Disorders, 24* (2), 225–230.

Cabey, M. (1994). Brief report: A controlled evaluation of facilitated communication using open-ended and fill-in questions. *Journal of Autism and Developmental Disorders, 24* (4), 517–526.

Calculator, S. (1992). Perhaps the emperor has clothes after all: A response to Biklen (1992). *American Journal of Speech Language Pathology,* January, 18–20.

Carr, E. G., & Carlson, J. I. (1993). Reduction of severe behavior problems in the community using a multicomponent treatment approach. *Journal of Applied Behavior Analysis, 26* (2), 157–172.

Churchill, D. (1978). *Language of autistic children.* New York: Wiley.

Coleman, M., & Gillberg, G. (1985). *The biology of the autistic syndromes.* New York: Praeger Scientific.

Cromer, R. (1981). Developmental language disorders: Cognitive processes, semantics, pragmatics, phonology and syntax. *Journal of Autism and Developmental Disorders, 11,* 57–74.

Curtiss, S. (1981). Dissociations between language and cognition: Cases and implications. *Journal of Autism and Developmental Disorders, 11,* 15–30.

Dalgleish, B. (1975). Cognitive processing and linguistic reference in autistic children. *Journal of Autism and Childhood Schizophrenia, 5,* 353–361.

DeMyer, M., Barton, S., Alpern, G., Kimberlin, C., Allen, J., Yang, E., & Steele, R. (1974). The measured intelligence of autistic children. *Journal of Autism and Childhood Schizophrenia, 4,* 42–60.

DeMyer, M., Barton, S., DeMyer, E., Norton, J., Allen, J., & Steele, R. (1973). Prognosis in autism: A follow-up study. *Journal of Autism and Childhood Schizophrenia, 3*, 199–216.

Duchan, J. F. (1993). Issues raised by facilitated communication for theorizing and research on autism. *Journal of Speech and Hearing Research, 36*, 1108-1119.

Duchan, J., & Palermo, J. (1982). How autistic children view the world. *Topics in Language Disorders, 3*, 10–16.

Eales, M. J. (1993). Pragmatic impairments in adults with childhood diagnoses of autism or developmental receptive language disorder. *Journal of Autism and Developmental Disorders, 23* (4), 593–616.

Eberlin, M., McConnachie, G., Ibel, S., & Volpe, L. (1993). Facilitated communication: A failure to replicate the phenomenon. *Journal of Autism and Developmental Disorders, 23* (3), 507–530,

Eisenberg, L. (1956). The autistic child in adolescence. *American Journal of Psychiatry, 112*, 607–612.

Fay, W., & Schuler, A. (1980). Emerging language in autistic children: Language intervention series. Baltimore: University Park Press.

Fewell, R. R., & Kaminski, R. (1988). Play skills development and instruction for young children with handicaps. In S. L. Odom & M. B. Karnes (Eds.), *Early intervention for infants and children with handicaps: An empirical base* (pp. 145–158). Baltimore: Paul H. Brookes.

Fish, B., Shapiro, T., & Campbell, M. (1966). Long-term prognosis and the response of schizophrenic children to drug therapy: A controlled study of trifluoperazine. *American Journal of Psychiatry, 123*, 32–39.

Flavell, J. H., Green, F. L., & Flavell, E. R. (1990). Developmental changes in young children's knowledge about the mind. *Cognitive Development, 5*, 1–27.

Ford, L., Riggs, K. S., Nissenbaum, M., & LaRaia, J. (1994). Facilitating desired behavior in the preschool child with autism: A case study. *Contemporary Education, 65* (3), 148–151.

Frith, U. (1989). A new look at language and communication in autism. *British Journal of Disorders of Communication, 24*, 123–150.

Gerrard, L. (1994). Inclusive education: An issue of social justice. *Equity and Excellence in Education, 27*, 1, 58–67.

Goldstein, H., & Strain, P. (1988). Peers as communication intervention agents: Some new strategies and research findings. *Topics on Language Disorders, 9*, 44–57.

Gunter, P. L., Fox, J. J., McEvoy, M. A., Shores, R. E., & Denny, R. K. (1993). A case study of the reduction of aberrant, repetitive responses of an adolescent with autism. *Education and Treatment of Children, 16* (2), 187–197.

Happe, F. (1994). An advanced test of theory of mind: Understanding of story characters' thoughts and feelings by able autistic, mentally handicapped, and normal children and adults. *Journal of Autism and Developmental Disorders, 24* (2), 129–154.

Haring, T. G. (1985). Teaching between-class generalization of toy play behavior to handicapped children. *Journal of Applied Behavior Analysis, 18*, 127–139.

Hermelin, B. (1978). Images and language. In M. Rotter & E. Schopler (Eds.), *Autism: A reappraisal of concepts and treatment*. New York: Plenum Press.

Holroyd, S., & Baron-Cohen, S. (1993). Brief report: How far can people with autism go in developing a theory of mind? *Journal of Autism and Developmental Disorders, 23* (2), 379–384.

Hughes, C., & Russell, J. (1993). Autistic children's difficulty with mental disengagement from an object: Its implications for theories of autism. *Developmental Psychology, 29* (3), 498–510.

Hurford, J. (1991). The evolution of the critical period for language acquisition. *Cognition, 40*, 159–201.

Hutt, C., & Ounsted, C. (1966). The biological significance of gaze aversion with particular reference to the syndrome of infantile autism. *Behavioral Science, 11*, 346–356.

Jarrold, C., Boucher, J., & Smith, P. (1993). Symbolic play in autism: A review. *Journal of Autism and Developmental Disorders, 23* (2), 281–306.

Kames, D., Locke, P., Delguardri, J., & Hall, R. V. (1989). Increasing academic skills of students with autism using fifth grade peers as tutors. *Education and Treatment of Children, 12*, 38–51.

Kanner, L. (1943). Autistic disturbances in affective contact. *Nervous Child, 2*, 217–250.

Kanner, L. (1944). Early infantile autism. *Journal of Pediatrics, 25*, 211–217.

Kanner, L. (1952). Emotional interference with intellectual functioning. *American Journal of Mental Deficiency, 56*, 701–707.

Kennedy, M. D., Sheridan, M. K., Radlinski, S. H., & Beeghly, M. (1991). Play-language relationships in young children with developmental delays: Implications for assessment. *Journal of Speech and Hearing Research, 34,* 112–122.

Kohler, F. W., & Greenwood, C. R. (1990). Effects of collateral peer supportive behaviors with the classwide peer tutoring program. *Journal of Applied Behavior Analysis, 23,* 307–322.

Lifter, K., Sulzer-Azaroff, B., Anderson, S. R., Cowdery, G. E., (1993). Teaching play activities to preschool children with disabilities: The importance of developmental considerations. *Journal of Early Intervention,* 17 (2), 139–159.

Linder, T. W. (1990). *Transdisciplinary play-based assessment: A functional approach to working with young children.* Baltimore: Paul H. Brookes.

Lotter, V. (1967). Epidemiology of autistic conditions in young children: Some characteristics of parents and children. *Social Psychiatry,* 1, 163–181.

Loveland, K., Landry, S., Hughes, S., Hall, S., & McEvoy, R. (1988). Speech acts and the pragmatic deficits of autism. *Journal of Speech and Hearing Research,* 31, 593–604.

Maltz, A. (1981). Comparison of cognitive deficits among autistic and retarded children on the Arthur Adaption of the Leiter International Performance Scales. *Journal of Autism and Developmental Disorders,* 11, 413–426.

Matson, J. L., Sevin, J. A., Box, M. L., Francis, K. L., & Sevin, B. M. (1993). An evaluation of two methods for increasing self-initiated verbalizations in autistic children. *Journal of Applied Behavior Analysis,* 26 (3), 389–398.

McEachin, J. J., Smith, T., & Lovaas, O. I. (1993). Long-Term outcome for children with autism who received early intensive behavioral treatment. *American Journal on Mental Retardation,* 97 (4), 359–372.

Menyuk, P. (1978). Language: What's wrong and why. In M. Rutter & E. Schopler (Eds.), *Autism: A reappraisal of concepts and treatment.* New York: Plenum Press.

Mirenda, P., & Schuler, A. (1988). Augmenting commenting for persons with autism: Issues and strategies. *Topics in Language Disorders,* 9, 24–43.

Mundy, P., Sigman, M., Ungerer, J., & Sherman T. (1987). Nonverbal communication and play correlates of language development in autistic children. *Journal of Autism and Developmental Disorders,* 17, 349–364.

Newsom, C. D., Carr, E. G., & Lovaas, O. I. (1979). The experimental analysis and modification autistic behavior. In R. S. Davidson (ed.), *Modification of Pathological Behavior.* New York: Gardener Press.

O'Connor, N., & Hermelin, B. (1994). Two Autistic Savant Readers. *Journal of Autism and Developmental Disorders,* 24 (4), 501–514.

Odom, S. L., Chandler, L. K., Ostrosky, M., McConnell, S. R., & Reaney, S. (1992). Fading teacher prompts from peer-initiation interventions for young children with disabilities. *Journal of Applied Behavior Analysis,* 25, 307–317.

Odom, S. L., McConnell, S., & McEvoy, M. (1992). *Social competence of young children with disabilities: Issues and strategies for intervention.* Baltimore: Brookes.

Osterling, J., & Dawson, G. (1994). Early recognition of children with autism: A study of first birthday home videotapes. *Journal of Autism and Developmental Disorders,* 24 (3), 247–256.

Ozonoff, S., Pennington, B. F., & Rogers, S. J. (1991). Executive function deficits in high-functioning autistic individuals: Relationship to theory of mind. *Journal of Child Psychology and Psychiatry,* 32, 1081–1105.

Patti, P. J., & Lupinetti, L. (1993) Brief report: Implications of hyperlexia in an autistic savant. *Journal of Autism and Developmental Disorders,* 23 (2), 397–404.

Paul, (1987). Communication. In D. J. Cohen, A. M. Donnellan, & R. Paul (Eds.), *Handbook of autism and pervasive developmental disorders* (Ch. 4). New York: John Wiley and Sons.

Perne, J., Frith, U., Leslie, A., & Leekam, S. (1989). Exploration of the autistic child's theory of mind: Knowledge, belief and communication. *Child Development,* 60, 689–700.

Piaget, J. (1962). *Play, dreams, and imitation in childhood.* New York: Norton.

Polansky, H. B. (1994). The meaning of inclusion. Is it an option or a mandate? *School Business Affairs,* 27–29.

Prior, M., & Hofmann, W. (1990). Brief report: Neuropsychological testing of autistic children through an exploration with frontal lobe tests. *Journal of Autism and Developmental Disorders,* 20, 581–590.

Prizant, B. (1982). Gestalt language and gestalt processing in autism. *Topics in Language Disorders, 3,* 16–24.

Prizant, B. (1983). Language acquisition and communicative behavior in autism: Toward an understanding of the "whole" of it. *Journal of Speech and Hearing Disorders, 46,* 241–249.

Prizant, B., & Duchan, J. (1981). The functions of immediate echolalia in autistic children. *Journal of Speech and Hearing Disorders, 46,* 241–249.

Prizant, B. M., & Rydell, P. (1984). Analysis of functions of delayed echolalia in autistic children. *Journal of Speech and Hearing Research, 27,* 183–192.

Prizant, B. M., & Wetherby, A. M. (1987). Communicative intent: A framework for understanding social-communicative behavior in autism. *Journal of the American Academy of Child and Adolescent Psychiatry, 26,* 472–479.

Prizant, B. M., & Wetherby, A. M. (1988). Providing services to children with autism (ages 0 to 2 years) and their families. *Topics in Language Disorders, 9,* 1–23.

Ricks, D., & Wing, L. (1975). Language, communication and the use of symbols in normal and autistic children. *Journal of Autism and Childhood Schizophrenia, 5,* 191–220.

Rock, E. E., Rosenberg, M. S., & Carran, D. T. (1995). Variables affecting the reintegration rate of students with serious emotional disturbance. *Exceptional Children, 61* (3), 254–268.

Rosenberger-Debiesse, J., & Coleman, M. (1986). Brief report: preliminary evidence for multiple etiologies in autism. *Journal of Autism and Developmental Disorders, 16*(3), 385–391.

Russell, J., Mauthner, N., Sharpe, S., & Tidswell, T. (1991). The "window task" as a measure of strategic deception in preschoolers and autistic subjects. *British Journal of Developmental Psychology, 9,* 331–349.

Schmidt, J. (1976). Relations between paired-associate learning and utterance patterns in children with echolalia. Doctoral dissertation, Boston University School of Education.

Shapiro, T., Sherman, M., Calamari, G., & Koch, D. (1987). Attachment in autism and other developmental disorders. *Journal of the American Academy of Child and Adolescent Psychiatry, 26,* 480–484.

Short, A., & Schopler, E. (1988). Factors relating to age of onset in autism. *Journal of Autism and Developmental Disorders, 18,* 207–216.

Sigman, M., & Ungerer, J. A. (1984). Cognitive and language skills in autistic, mentally retarded, and normal children. *Developmental Psychology, 20,* 293–302.

Snow, M. E., Hertzig, M. E., & Shapiro, T. (1987). Expression of emotion in young autistic children. *Journal of the American Academy of Child and Adolescent Psychiatry, 26,* 836–838.

Strain, P. S., & Odom, S. L. (1986). Peer social initiations: Effective intervention for social skills development of exceptional children. *Exceptional Children, 52,* 543-552.

Tager-Flusberg, H. (1981). On the nature of linguistic functioning in early infantile autism. *Journal of Autism and Developmental Disorders, 11,* 45–56.

Tager-Flusberg, H. (1989). A psycholinguistic perspective on language development in the autistic child. In G. Dawson (Ed.), *Autism: Nature, diagnosis and treatment.* New York: Guilford.

Tager-Flusberg, H., Calkins, S., Nolin, T., Baumberger, T., Anderson, M., & Chadwick-Dias, A. (1990). A longitudinal study of language acquisition in autistic and Down syndrome children. *Journal of Autism and Developmental Disorders, 20,* 1–22.

Tiegerman-Farber, E. (1995a). Training the parent as facilitator. In *Language and Communication Intervention in Preschool Children.* Needham Heights, MA: Allyn & Bacon.

Tiegerman-Farber, E. (1995b). The changing role of the family. In *Language and Communication Intervention in Preschool Children.* Needham Heights, MA: Allyn & Bacon.

Tiegerman-Farber, E., & Cartusciello-King, R. (1995c). The classroom as language laboratory. In E. Tiegerman-Farber (Ed.), *Language and Communication Intervention in Preschool Children.* Needham Heights, MA: Allyn & Bacon.

Tiegerman-Farber, E., & Radziewicz, C. (1996). *Collaborative mainstreaming: The Pathway to Inclusion.* Englewood Cliffs, NJ: Prentice Hall.

Tirosh, E., & Canby, J. (1993). Autism with hyperlexia: A distinct syndrome? *American Journal on Mental Retardation, 98* (1), 84–92.

Treffert, D. A. (1988). The idiot savant: A review of the syndrome. *American Journal of Psychiatry, 145,* 563–572.

Wagner, A. E., & Lockwood, S. L. (1994). Pervasive developmental disorders: Dilemmas in diagnosing very young children. *Infants and Young Children,* 6 (4), 21–32.

Warren, S., & Gazdag, G. (1990). Facilitating early language development with milieu intervention procedures. *Journal of Early Intervention,* 14, 62–86.

Wetherby, A. M. (1986). Ontogeny of communicative functions in autism. *Journal of Autism and Developmental Disorders,* 16, 295–316.

Wetherby, A. M., & Gaines, B. H. (1982). Cognition and language development in autism. *Journal of Speech and Hearing Research,* 47, 63–71.

Wisniewski, L., & Alpert, S. (1994). Including students with severe disabilities in general education settings. *Remedial and Special Education,* 15 (1), 4–13.

Wolfberg, P. J., & Schuler, A. L. (1993). Integrated play groups: A model for promoting the social and cognitive dimensions of play in children with autism. *Journal of Autism and Developmental Disorders,* 23 (3), 467–488.

Wolk, L., & Edwards, M. L. (1993). The emerging phonological system of an autistic child. *Journal of Communication Disorders,* 26, 161–177.

Considerations and Implications for Habilitation of Hearing-Impaired Children

CHRISTINE RADZIEWICZ
School for Language and Communication Development

SUSAN ANTONELLIS
St. John's University

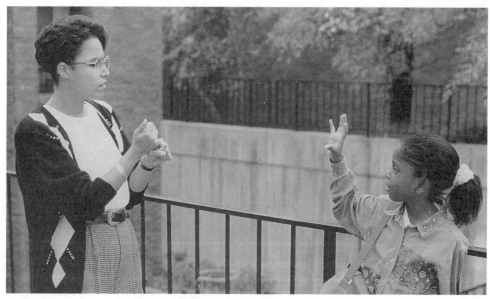

The identification and rehabilitation of a child with a hearing impairment is an enormous and important task. Research has certainly confirmed the importance of early identification along with the profound effects of chronic otitis media on speech and language.

Rehabilitating children with hearing impairments encompasses the instrumentation, the methods, and the follow-up. Technology has miniaturized the amplification systems available. We have gone from the bulky body aid to the tiny canal aid, from the hardwire induction loop to the personal FM unit, and from the preschool screening to the pediatric evaluation with aural acoustic immittance testing. More sophisticated objective testing has arisen, such as auditory brainstem response and the most current otoacoustic emissions.

The educational setting has also changed for hearing-impaired children. In the past, education routinely took place in residential schools for the deaf. Today, children with hearing impairments are more often educated in regular classrooms, exercising the mainstreaming option.

Educating children with hearing impairments has been accomplished through either an aural/oral approach or an approach incorporating manually coded English. Over the last thirty years a tremendous body of research has been accumulated highlighting the advantages of each. An aural/oral approach incorporates speech and speechreading as the primary communication channels. The total communication approach incorporates manual communication or sign language with speech and speechreading. It appears that for those children with severe to profound hearing losses the total communication approach is preferred—Jordan, Gustason, and Rosen (1979) reported that approximately 65 percent of deaf children in the United States are taught using some combination of manual and oral communication.

Objectives

The objectives of this chapter are as follows:

1. To define and explore the type, classification and degree of hearing loss
2. To discuss the efforts of the government and professionals toward early identification of hearing loss and the parent's role in this cause
3. To explore the intricate details of an audiological evaluation and discuss each parameter that encompasses it, including aural acoustic immittance testing
4. To consider the adjustments and special tests needed in preparing for the pediatric evaluation
5. To be able to identify the proper management needed after diagnosis of hearing loss, whether it be a permanent sensorineural hearing loss or a temporary conductive hearing loss
6. To understand the educational needs of the hearing impaired, including reading, written language, whole language, sign language, and bilingualism
7. To discuss the mainstreaming option and its impact on the hearing-impaired child
8. To identify several techniques that facilitate successful inclusion of preschool hearing-impaired children with normal hearing peers
9. To identify challenges to family—professional collaboration related to cultural diversity and socioeconomic status

10. To identify those factors that facilitate successful inclusion of school-aged hearing-impaired children in regular educational settings
11. To identify those factors that put hearing-impaired children at educational risk
12. To identify the differences between mainstreaming and inclusion

Type, Classification, and Degree of Hearing Loss

Hearing loss should be considered in terms of type, classification, and degree. Hearing loss falls into three types: the conductive hearing loss, the sensorineural hearing loss, and the mixed hearing loss. This section describes each of these types, then presents a classification system used to define degree of loss.

Conductive Hearing Loss

The conductive hearing loss results from interference of any sort in the transmission of sound from the external auditory canal to the inner ear (Northern & Downs, 1984); the inner ear functions normally. Conductive hearing loss never exceeds a hearing threshold of 60 dB (hearing thresholds are discussed shortly) and is generally medically treatable. A common disorder found in children associated with conductive impairment is otitis media. Otitis media is defined as the presence of inflammation in the middle ear cavity (Scheidt & Kavanagh, 1986). Medically, otitis media needs to be looked at more specifically. **Acute otitis media** is an active inflammation and/or infection of the middle ear space. The presence of a bulging tympanic membrane and/or pus behind the tympanic membrane are evidence of acute otitis media. **Serous otitis media** is the presence of a thin, watery clear fluid in the middle ear space and is usually an early sign of eustachian tube dysfunction. **Chronic otitis media** is an infection of the middle ear space with purulent fluid (pus) persisting beyond the time limit of acute otitis media. Also, whereas acute otitis media can be quite painful and develops over a short period of time, chronic otitis media is not generally accompanied by pain and therefore can go untreated. **Secretory otitis media** refers to a condition associated with a thick, glue-like fluid found in the middle ear space.

Pashley (1984) classified these changes in otitis media according to stages: acute, which lasts up to 5 weeks; subacute, which begins at 6 weeks and lasts up to 11 weeks; and chronic, which occurs from 12 weeks onward.

Chronic otitis media has its effects in the early childhood years, most often during the critical years of speech and language development. Chronic otitis media is linked with fluctuating hearing loss ranging anywhere from 10 to 40 dB. Presumably, hearing will return to normal after the episode is over. Because otitis media occurs most frequently during the first 3 years of life, it can have a dramatic effect on speech and language during these years. It is during these years that "the infant moves from being a communicator to being a competent (although not fully competent) user of the speech and language categories of the language" (Menyuk, 1986). Kaplan, Fleishman, Bender, and Clark (1973) studied the incidence of otitis media in Eskimo children and its effect on their speech and language development. This longitudinal study of approximately 500 children traced their development from birth to 7 through 10 years of age. All the children were assessed using the Wechsler

Intelligence Scale for Children (WISC), the Bender-Gestalt Test for Perceptual Problems, the Metropolitan Achievement Test, and the Draw-A-Person Test. Results of this study demonstrated that those children who had a history of otitis media before age 2 had suffered 5 to 7 attacks, had hearing thresholds of 26 dB or greater, evidenced a significant loss of verbal ability, and had deficits in reading, math, and language. From this study, it can be concluded that children who have recurrent episodes of otitis media beginning before the age of 2 are likely to be delayed in speech and language development. This delay can result later in poor academic performance and/or behavioral/attention deficits.

Conductive hearing loss can also occur as a result of a totally blocked air conductive pathway as in atresia, stenosis, complete stapes fixation, or ossicular discontinuity.

Sensorineural Hearing Loss

The sensorineural hearing loss results from damage to the sensory end organ, the cochlear hair cells, or the auditory nerve (damage may have occurred during development of the ear, from injury or infection, from individual environment, or from the degenerative effects of aging). Sensorineural hearing losses may easily be overlooked upon physical examination, because the external auditory canal and tympanic membrane will appear normal. This type of hearing loss is not medically treatable and almost always irreversible.

Mixed Hearing Loss

The mixed hearing loss can occur in children as well as adults. It is a problem that occurs simultaneously in both the conductive and sensorineural mechanisms. This results in a loss via bone conduction due to the sensorineural component and an even greater loss of sensitivity by air conduction.

Classification System

The following is an audiometric classification system, suggested by Bess and McConnell (1981), for defining hearing loss. The classifications also can be used to describe the degree of hearing loss.

Hearing Threshold Level	Classification
26–40 dB	Mild
41–55 dB	Moderate
56–70 dB	Moderately severe
71–95 dB	Severe
96 dB +	Profound

Intensity of sound is measured in decibels (dB). Hearing is also affected by the frequency of the sound wave; higher pitched sounds have higher frequencies (measured in hertz, Hz). This classification system is based on a pure tone average; that is, the average of the thresholds of 500 Hz, 1,000 Hz, and 2,000 Hz, respectively. These frequencies, commonly known as the speech frequencies, are known to be important for hearing speech. Pure tone thresholds are discussed more fully later in this chapter.

Hearing Loss and Language Development

Describing the speech and language behaviors of children with hearing impairments is a difficult task. Various factors influence the development of language in the presence of hearing loss (Quigley & Kretschmer, 1982). These variables include

- Degree of hearing loss
- Age of onset of loss
- Slope of hearing loss
- Age of identification of hearing loss
- Age of habilitation
- Amount of habilitation
- Type of habilitation

As noted, degree of hearing loss refers to the severity of the hearing loss and is easily measured. According to Knauf (1972), the hearing threshold is frequently the first measurement available for estimating the impact of the child's hearing impairment. In the past, it had generally been assumed that the greater the hearing loss, the greater the impact on speech and language development. Although a severe hearing loss of 71 dB to 90 or 95 dB does have a devastating effect on speech and language development, we cannot assume that a mild hearing loss of 26 to 40 dB will always have a minimal effect or that a profound loss of 96 dB or above will have the most detrimental effect on speech and language development.

To emphasize this point, Northern (1984) referred to the case report of a 13-year-old patient who had suffered from frequent bouts of otitis media. Over a period of 7 years, from age 6 to age 13, the air conduction thresholds fluctuated from normal to mild to moderate levels. Over the 7 years, five myringotomies were performed. However, the child's repeated attacks of serous otitis media resulted in a progressive sensorineural hearing loss. The condition was identified as an underlying mild to moderate sloping sensorineural hearing loss with bone conduction thresholds of 25 dB at 4,000 Hz in one ear and of 30 and 45 dB at 2,000 Hz and 4,000 Hz in the other ear. In this case, not only the degree of hearing loss but also the age of onset, the age of identification, and the type of habilitation were critical factors affecting the severity of the language deficit. Although this child's loss was not discovered until the age of 6, he probably had suffered from chronic otitis media earlier in his life. Age of onset could have occurred more than 5 years before age of identification and therefore could have included the critical language learning years. Furthermore, habilitation involved surgical myringotomies without habilitative speech and language therapy. Northern concluded his description of this case by stating that when the 13-year-old patient was given a hearing aid for habilitation, it was already 13 years too late. This child was evidencing a delay in speech and language that was irreversible.

The degree of hearing loss, although the most salient variable, is not necessarily the most critical. The combination and interplay of all the aforementioned variables determine the effect of hearing loss on speech and language development. Because of the interdependency of variables, one can never predict with certainty the detrimental effects of hearing loss on speech and language from degree of impairment alone. The only certainty is that hearing loss in any form (conductive, sensorineural, or mixed) and of any degree (mild to profound) can have a devastating effect on speech and language development.

Identification and Habilitation

Early identification of hearing loss and the delivery of appropriate services are critical factors in the habilitation of children with hearing impairments. Because language development begins at the time a child is born, there is an urgent need for an organized infant screening procedure to identify those infants who may have hearing losses. Identification of hearing impaired infants can be facilitated through neonatal screenings of infants with a high risk of hearing loss. The National Joint Committee of Newborn Screening in 1973 (Bess & McConnell, 1981) compiled these high-risk criteria:

1. History of hereditary childhood hearing impairment
2. Rubella or other nonbacterial intrauterine fetal infection (e.g., herpes virus infection)
3. Defects of ear, nose, or throat
4. Birth weight less than 1,500 grams
5. Bilirubin level greater than 20 mg/100 ml serum

An infant demonstrating any of these criteria should be referred for a complete audiological evaluation within the first 2 months of life.

In 1977, to further delineate the follow-up procedures for a high-risk register, the National Maternal Child Health Conference generated the following guidelines for early screening (Northern & Downs, 1978, p. 207):

1. Audiological follow-up of high-risk infants should be made as soon as possible, certainly by 7 months.
2. The mother-child relationship in the first 4 months should be safeguarded by education and careful information.
3. Informed consent should be obtained.
4. Information on what to look for in later infancy should be given to the parents.
5. Development and implementation of adequate identification and diagnostic procedures related to hearing impairments should be undertaken by public health agencies.

Early Parent-Infant Interaction

Early language development of the infant with normal hearing has been of great interest to researchers. These investigations have shown that normal hearing children have a basic capacity for perceiving speech behaviors in the environment and also are sensitive to the social and affective aspects of the context of language (Eimas, 1974; Miller & Morse, 1976; Miller, Morse, & Dorman, 1977; Morse, 1972). Bloom and Lahey (1978) have stated that one of the precursors of language use occurs when infants begin to exchange gaze and vocalizations with their mothers. Bateson (1975) also described this mutual gaze or eye contact between mother and infant and called it protoconversation. Jaffe, Stern, and Peery (1973) studied the infant-mother dyad and found mother-infant gazing to be analogous to the rhythms of adult dialogue. Behaviors such as these are all continuous with the eventual development of speech and language that begins in the second year of life. Although infants with hearing impairments do not have the perceptual capabilities to receive and discriminate speech sounds as well as children with normal hearing, they do have a residual amount of hearing that allows for some discrimination when amplification is used. In addition, they are able to extract the social and affective aspects of the context of language (Bloom & Lahey, 1978).

Brown (1975) stated that the most important form of concept learning for the infant is probably socially mediated. The first social contact of the infant is the parents. They are the most responsible for the development of the behaviors that lead to language growth in the normally developing child, and they are the major forces in the habilitation of the hearing impaired child. Because studies have demonstrated that mothers of normal hearing children play a vital role in the development in speech and language, it becomes obvious that mothers of hearing impaired infants play an even more crucial role.

Greenstein, Bush, McConville, and Stellini (1977) examined the mother-infant communication dyad and its effect on language acquisition in infants with hearing impairments. They found that affective aspects of mother-infant interaction were central to the language acquisition of the hearing impaired child. All other aspects of the mother's language input to the child were far less significant than the existence of a good mother-infant bond. This bond frequently was broken by the mother's discovery of the child's hearing impairment. Vorce (1974) believed that the social relationships that exist between the mother and child stimulate the infant's early vocalizations, and therefore this relationship should be emphasized.

Snow (1972) proposed two models of early parent-child communication. The feedback model states that mothers' speech input to their infants provides the ideal context for facilitating the development of speech and language through the use of consistency, redundancy, and simplicity of utterances. In addition, the speech and language capabilities of the infant influence the stylistic features of the mother's speech. Based on feedback from the child, mothers alter their speech forms to accommodate to the linguistic needs of the child.

The conversational model (Snow, 1977) explains the distinctive features of mothers' speech to infants in relation to the development of discourse strategies. Mothers use certain stylistic features (e.g., repetition, use of interrogative, etc.) to initiate, repair, and maintain conversations. Other research suggests that the same strategies are used by normal hearing mothers in interactions with their hearing-impaired infants (Cross, Johnson-Moores, & Nienhuys, 1980). It should be noted, however, that these mothers tended to be more physically manipulative, more conversationally dominant, and more verbally controlling.

In addition, their speech input was characterized by a reduced MLU, less complex syntactic structures, less referencing to absent objects, and more repetitions (Goss, 1970; Wedell-Monnig, & Westerman, 1977). These findings suggest that it is the nature of the disability that results in these parental interactive behaviors.

Because speech and language development begins with the earliest social exchanges between mother and infant, and because the affective aspects of mother-infant interaction are crucial to future language acquisition, programs that enhance mother-infant communication are invaluable in effective intervention for children with hearing impairments. Parent-infant programs, first developed during the 1970s, educate parents about their critical role in the development of their hearing impaired child. Parents are taught to make everyday experiences language-enhancing experiences. They learn to understand the implications of hearing impairment on speech and language development and how to deal with their feelings about the hearing loss in their child. Furthermore, they are taught how to incorporate auditory training into the child's daily life and how to employ language learning strategies when they are interacting with their child. Parent and infant come to the parent-infant center at least once a week for training, and the teacher/speech-language pathologist makes weekly visits to the home. Parents frequently meet with other professionals such as psychologists and audiologists for additional training and support.

The teacher/speech-language pathologist employs a variety of training techniques. For example, videotapes have been used in many ways to enhance communication between parents and hearing-impaired infants. Cole and St. Clair-Stokes (1984) analyzed videotaped caregiver-child interactions to identify interactive behaviors promoting development of early language. Radziewicz (1985) used videotapes as a technique to train parents to incorporate more effective communicative behaviors in their interactions with their infants. The use of videotapes has resulted in clearer understanding of hearing loss and more appropriate communicative interactions.

When hearing impaired children and their parents are enrolled in a parent-infant program, that child's education begins during the critical speech and language learning years. Intervention before the age of 3 increases the child's chances of developing more normal speech and language. Parents can gain insights into management and effective communication behaviors that will facilitate language development in their child. They can be trained to model and develop interactive language learning opportunities during all their parent-child interactions. The parent-infant program also bridges the gap between early identification of hearing impairment and enrollment of the child into a preschool educational program (Elwood, Johnson, & Mandell, 1977).

In today's multicultural society, the children from diverse cultural communities are frequently identified as having language disorders. It is important that bilingual evaluators and interpreters be used when evaluating these children. However, once these children are identified, it is imperative that the parents and professionals participate when developing the IEP and IFSP. When large differences—such as socioeconomic status and differences in values and beliefs—exist between families and professionals, this collaborative partnership becomes more fragile and poses challenges to all team members. For early intervention to be successful, the early interventionist must work on everyday activities that are part of the family's cultural customs and must be viewed by the family as appropriate. The extent to which the family has been exposed to the customs of the dominant society will determine the level of conflicts that may occur between the family and the professionals working with them (Hanson, Lynch, & Wayman, 1990). A recent study by DeGangi, Wietlisbach, Poisson, Stein, and Royeen (1994) identified the challenges to family-professional collaboration related to cultural diversity and socioeconomic status (SES). It was found that families from lower SES and educational backgrounds often were concerned with basic survival needs and deferred to professional judgments when setting goals; had difficulty identifying their child's needs; and showed reluctance in sharing information. With all this in mind it is imperative that professionals working collaboratively with families recognize the impact of culture and socioeconomic status on the collaborative process.

Audiological Assessment

The routine audiological evaluation consists of pure tone findings, speech audiometry yielding speech reception thresholds and speech discrimination scores, and aural acoustic immittance testing. Because not all testing procedures can be used with very young children, pediatric evaluation is considered separately.

Pure Tone Findings

The search for accurate pure tone thresholds is no small feat, particularly with small children. Before the options and procedures for finding threshold are discussed, it is necessary to define threshold. A **pure tone threshold** is the faintest tone a person can hear 50 percent of the time. We find threshold in order to (a) diagnose hearing loss and/or ear pathology and (b) acquire information that may be used in obtaining appropriate remediation for the hearing impaired individual (Green, 1978).

Two techniques are used to measure threshold. In the ascending method, the person being tested is exposed to stimuli that range from inaudible to audible. In the descending method, the stimuli go from audible to inaudible. In determining pure tone threshold by air conduction, proper earphone placement is essential. The diaphragm of the earphone must be placed directly over the opening of the external canal. If placement is not secure, test results could be invalid.

Having discussed threshold and the method for obtaining the result, consider the step-by-step procedure in obtaining the pure tone findings:

1. Instruct patient to respond when a tone is heard, even if the tone is very soft.
2. Place the earphones on the head of the patient with proper positioning as previously discussed. A specific earphone is used for the right and left ear.
3. Test the better ear first, in case masking is needed.
4. Start with a 1,000 Hz tone and allow the patient to hear what it sounds like; that is, present the tone at an audible level for the patient.
5. Find threshold at 1,000 Hz by presenting the signal in an "up 5 down 10" method.
6. Use the same procedure for the other audiometric frequencies, following this order: 2,000, 4,000, 8,000, 500, and 250 Hz.
7. Follow the same procedure for the second ear, but do not start at 1,000 Hz.
8. Plot each threshold obtained on the audiogram (see Figure 14-1).
9. Find the pure tone average of each ear (average 500, 1,000, and 2,000 Hz).
10. Conduct bone conduction testing in the same manner, using the bone oscillator. Proper placement of the oscillator on the mastoid process is important for accuracy.

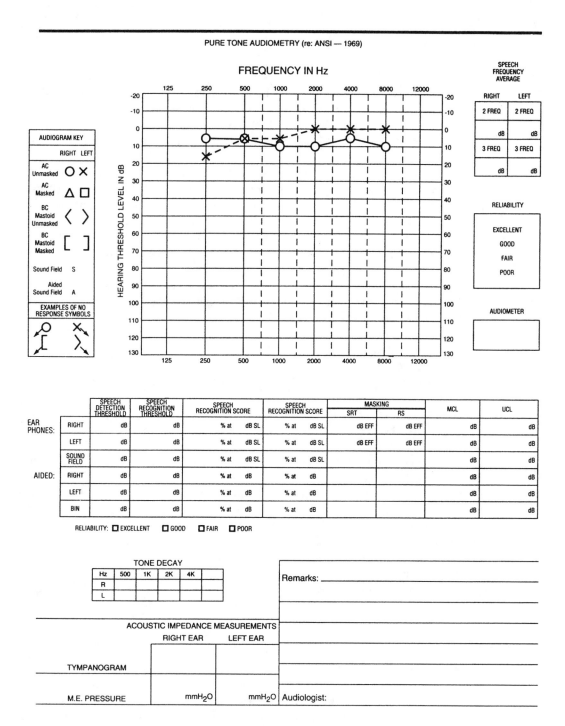

FIGURE 14-1   Pure tone thresholds plotted on audiogram.

Speech Audiometry

The speech audiometry portion of the audiological evaluation consists primarily of determining the speech recognition threshold and the speech recognition score.

The **speech recognition threshold** (SRT) typically refers to the threshold of intelligibility, which is the lowest level (in dB) at which the listener is able to identify approximately 50 percent of spondaic bisyllabic words (Hopkinson, 1978).

The SRT is administered by having the patient hear examples of test words through the earphones. This test can be performed with live voice or a recorded speech signal. The pure tone thresholds of each ear allow the technician to choose an audible level to begin the test procedure. Chaiklin and Ventry (1964) recommended the following method:

1. Set the hearing level dial 25 dB above the average of the best two thresholds already obtained at 500, 1,000, and 2,000 Hz.
2. Present one spondee (bisyllabic) word at that level, and then decrease the level by 5 dB and present another spondee. Attenuate the signal level in 5-dB steps, presenting a single word at each level.
3. Continue this procedure until
   A. The patient fails to respond
   B. The patient responds incorrectly
   C. The minimum level of the audiometer is reached (in this event, the value is recorded as the SRT for that ear)

If the patient fails to respond or responds incorrectly before the lower limit of the testing range is reached, raise the single level 5 dB until a correct response is obtained.

The second portion of speech testing is the evaluation of the speech recognition score. This test is a significant one, because a common complaint is "I hear, but I don't understand." **Speech recognition** is a measure of the ability to differentiate between various speech sounds, such as nonsense syllables, monosyllabic words, and multisyllabic words (Nicolosi, Harryman, & Krescheck, 1978). Use the following procedure to obtain a speech recognition score via earphones:

1. Conduct the test at 35–40 dB above the speech reception threshold.
2. Present phonetically balanced word lists (monosyllabic words, equal in stress) via earphones. Calculate the percent of correct answers in the test for each ear.

Aural Acoustic Immittance Testing

In view of the major role the middle ear plays in audiological diagnosis, the importance of aural acoustic immittance testing must be considered.

Aural acoustic immittance testing is an essential piece of the audiological assessment. It consists of tympanometry, acoustic reflexes, and eustachian tube evaluation. For our purposes, we will not discuss eustachian tube evaluation at this time.

Tympanometry is the measurement of the resistance to the flow of acoustical energy at the tympanic membrane during various pressure changes (Nicolosi et al., 1978). Tympanometry testing produces a chart of results called a tympanogram. Figure 14-2 illustrates several possible tympanogram results:

1. Type A tympanogram—normal tympanic membrane.
2. Type B tympanogram—middle ear effusion, patent ventilating tubes, or perforation.
3. Type C tympanogram—eustachian tube dysfunction, retracted tympanic membrane; effusion may be present.
4. Type A_s tympanogram—stiff tympanic membrane.
5. Type A_d tympanogram—flaccid tympanic membrane or ossicular discontinuity.

It is important in looking at a tympanogram that we observe three parameters: pressure (x-axis), amplitude (y-axis), and shape. Pressure is measured in milliliters of H_2O, which creates either positive or negative pressure within the canal (see Figure 14-2).

The **acoustic reflex** is the bilateral contraction of the intra-aural muscles (tensor tympani and stapedius) in response to sound (Nicolosi et al., 1978). In this test, the reflex stimulus (tone or noise) is introduced at varied levels and the response is monitored on the meter of the tympanometer or through some form of a written display (Woodford, Feldman, & Wright, 1975). The diagnostic significance of the acoustic reflex lies in helping detect the presence or absence of pathology. One pathology to consider is middle ear pathology, which is the most common. Others are central pathology and nonorganic hearing loss,

It is apparent in this discussion of pure tone findings, speech audiometry, and aural acoustic immittance testing that the audiological evaluation consists of a network of intricate pieces that produce a holistic picture of the auditory system of an individual.

Pediatric Evaluation

Early detection of hearing loss in an infant is imperative, yet this is not an easy task. Although the audiological evaluation can yield a wealth of information about an individual's auditory system, many of the tests described cannot be successfully administered to the infant or preschooler. In view of this, it is necessary to discuss options in the evaluation process for the young pediatric population.

First and foremost, a discussion with the parents before actual testing plays an important role in the audiological assessment. Secondly, the clinician needs to establish a pleasant relationship with the child.

Because testing procedures change with the age of the child, it is best to discuss audiological procedures in terms of age. In the pediatric evaluation procedures described, accuracy, consistency, and reliability are of utmost importance.

Infant (Birth to Age 2).   Obviously an infant cannot raise her finger to indicate when she hears a tone; therefore, a keen observer/clinician is needed to watch an infant's responses. Visual reinforcement audiometry (VRA) should be used routinely. VRA is a procedure using lighted toys that are activated simultaneously with the introduction of the auditory signal during a conditioning period. As the evaluation continues, the light is flashed following an appropriate response.

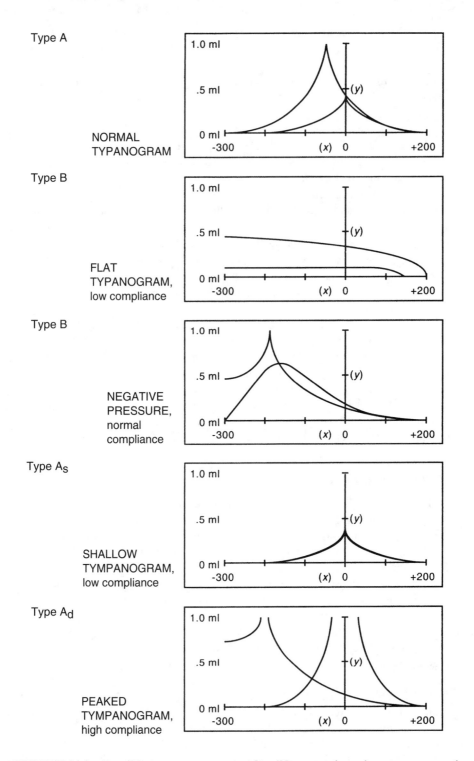

FIGURE 14-2   **Possible tympanogram results.** (*Note:* x-axis = air pressure; y-axis = compliance)

Testing of infants requires an adequate sound room, a quiet state, and measured noises (Northern & Downs, 1984). It is visually appropriate to seat the mother with the baby in her lap in the middle of the sound room. The audiologist should get the baby's attention straight ahead by moving a toy back and forth. Next, a noisemaker is introduced without the baby seeing it. Responses to watch for are eye widening, eyes turning, a rapid eye blink, and, if the child is at least 4 months old, a rudimentary head turn. At about 5 to 7 months, the infant will turn her head toward the side of a signal. The audiologist continues this procedure using speech stimuli and warble tones. As the child reaches 9 months, the audiologist can obtain a speech awareness threshold by repeating a phrase such as "Bye-bye Amy," slowly reducing the level of presentation until the child ceases to respond. As the child's age increases, additions are made to the evaluation process. For example, the child may be asked to recognize or point to familiar pictures.

Child (Ages 2 to 5).   The procedure known as play conditioning can be used for children 2 to 5 years old. The 2-year-old will probably need to sit in mother's lap for the procedure, but the 4- or 5-year-old most likely can sit alone. The audiologist introduces the procedure as a game, using motivational toys such as pegs or building blocks. The peg or block is placed in the child's hand, and the child is instructed to listen for a little sound (presented in the sound field). When a sound is heard, the child is guided in putting the peg into a bucket or box. Once the child can do the task alone, the sounds can be presented to the child through earphones. This procedure is followed for pure tones, as discussed in the "Audiological Assessment" portion of this chapter. It is necessary to move rapidly with small children because their attention span is generally short.

Speech audiometry can be accomplished through various picture pointing tasks. Objective testing, such as evoked response audiometry (ERA), is most assistive in diagnosing the difficult-to-test child. This testing includes responses observed by way of electrical impulses of the cerebral cortex. Responses are recorded on a graph.

Otoacoustic Emissions.   The twentieth century has brought with it the birth of otoacoustic emissions. In 1978, Kemp made an extraordinary discovery, using the simple technique of coupling a small microphone to the external ear canal and recording the sound present in the canal during and after the presentation of click stimuli. Kemp's microphone system was similar to that used in clinical immittance instruments. Kemp's observations revealed that low-intensity sounds could be detected in the ear canal for several milliseconds after the presentation of each click. The procedure is similar to the way auditory brainstem responses are obtained. These sounds provided a quick view of the cochlea's active response to sound, a response that involves the addition of energy to that provided by the stimulus arriving at the ear. Outer hair cells are thought to play a major role. Kemp's recordings represent one form of *emission* of acoustic energy from the cochlea. Collectively, these sounds are known as *otoacoustic emissions* (OAE) (Glattke and Kujawa, 1991).

One of the most significant and promising clinical applications of evoked otoacoustic emissions (EOAE) is in the pediatric population and its contribution in pediatric audiology. Among the applications are: (1) screening for hearing impairment in neonates and infants, (2) separating peripheral hearing loss and central auditory dysfunction in infants and young children, particularly those with multiple disabilities, and (3) monitoring cochlear status in infants and young children receiving ototoxic drugs (Norton, 1993).

It is not known at this time how successful OAEs are at detecting permanent hearing impairment, but it is encouraging that the OAE screen (transient) is able to detect most of the infants who failed the ABR test at 3 months of age. Because transient-evoked OAE testing takes a shorter amount of time to complete (9 minutes less than ABR), it has the potential to become a primary screening tool (Prieve, 1992).

Audiological Management

Diagnosis of a child with a hearing loss is only the beginning. A child with a hearing impairment must have adequate audiological management to be successful educationally, psychologically, and socially.

Amplification Devices

When a family first learns that their child is hearing impaired, the primary concern is: "What can be done? What physician do we see?" The child first must be seen by an otolaryngologist to provide medical clearance for amplification. The audiologist then conducts an ongoing evaluation to find the appropriate type of amplification for the individual child. In the young child, it can take anywhere from 6 months to 1 year before a final fitting is decided. In the interim, the child may be fitted with a loaner hearing aid.

Hearing aids are devices in which a microphone picks up auditory signals that are then routed to an amplifier (Berger & Millin, 1989). The amplifier boosts the energy of the signal and sends it to the receiver, which acts as a miniature speaker to transform the signal from electrical to acoustical energy (Berger & Millin, 1989). All hearing aids are activated by a battery.

There are various types of amplification, ranging from the body aid to the canal aid.

Body Aid.   About the size of a pocket radio, the body aid is connected to an earmold in the ear by a receiver wire. In the past, only a body aid could provide adequate power to benefit those with more than a moderate hearing loss. Today, amplifiers with high power can be fit into a small space and the body aid is used rarely; however, due to its large size, it still provides more power than other hearing aid types and more flexibility as far as circuitry and controls. Most people who use a body aid are fitted monaurally (one ear).

Behind-the-Ear-Aid.   The behind-the-ear (BTE) hearing aid is also known as the postauricular hearing aid. This type of aid rests over and behind the pinna and has a plastic earhook at one end near the receiver. A small piece of plastic tubing connects the hook to the earmold. The BTE hearing aid also provides flexibility as far as circuitry and control options.

Eyeglass Aid.   The eyeglass aid is not as popular as it was years back. In fact, it accounts for few hearing aid sales today. The components of the hearing aid are built in the temples of the eyeglasses, and a small metal pin holds the plastic tubing connected to the earmold.

CROS Aid (Contralateral Routing of Signal). These hearing aids perform with sounds originating on the side of the impaired ear, picked up by a microphone mounted near that ear, amplified slightly, and routed across the head to a receiver mounted near the good ear (Nicolosi et al., 1978). The CROS aid can be obtained as an in-the-ear aid, a behind-the-ear aid, or an eyeglass aid. These instruments are recommended for people who have an ear that is unaidable. A variation of this aid is the BiCROS (Bilateral Contralateral Routing of Signal).

In-the-Ear/Canal Aid. The in-the-ear aid is the most popular in the 1990s. Modem technology and miniaturization have allowed for more power in a small space. This type of hearing aid holds all components in one shell. Many people choose this type of hearing aid for cosmetic reasons. Mahon (1987) reported that in-the-ear devices account for about 80 percent of total U.S. hearing aid sales. In-the-ear instruments are not always the best choice for small children, however, because the ear grows rapidly and modifications are needed more often.

Completely-in-the-Canal Aid. As the in-the-ear hearing aid and the canal hearing aid have been the most popular amplification used, we now have the emergence of the CIC hearing aid. This type of hearing aid requires a deep ear impression and produces a hearing aid that is completely in the canal and virtually invisible.

Hearing aids open a new world to the hearing-impaired child, but some problems can occur with the use of a hearing aid. Common problems are acoustic feedback, distorted signal, intermittent signal, noisy sound, or hearing aid dysfunction. Because these problems do exist, audiological follow-up is important.

Cochlear Implants. In considering amplification devices, it is important to include a brief discussion of cochlear implants. It has been nearly thirty years since the publication of the first reports on patients fitted with cochlear implants (Doyle, Doyle, & Turnbull, 1964; Simmons, 1966). The first reports were not promising; the most encouraging results were that speech signals were perceived as speech, but were not intelligible. As research progressed, however, and as the sophistication of signal processing increased, reports of patients with good—sometimes markedly improved—speech recognition abilities surfaced.

Cochlear implants provided auditory sensations by electrically stimulating residual nerve fibers in the ears of the profoundly deaf, and the most important function is to provide some level of speech recognition for the user. There are various available designs that perform the task of representing speech signals as electrical stimuli (Tartter, Hellman, & Chute, 1992).

In addition to the hearing aid and cochlear implants, there are various other assistive devices that can give extra help to a child with a hearing loss, particularly in the educational setting. The auditory trainer operates like a hearing aid and is used in the classroom or at a particular site as a training device. Because they are used collectively on site, size and appearance are not important considerations. Their large size enables them to be equipped with larger components and special circuitry that produce better fidelity.

There are four basic auditory trainer systems: desk trainers, hardwire units, induction loop units, and FM units.

Desk Trainers.   The desk trainer is built in a case and is usually found on the student's desk. The components are distributed in the case. The child can carry the desk trainer from one location to another. A disadvantage of the device is that its signal-to-noise ratio (the ratio between the intensity of the signal and the intensity of the noise present) is poor if there is a distance between teacher and student. These trainers are beneficial in training sessions with one child but are not particularly recommended in a classroom of hearing impaired children.

Hardwire Unit.   Hardwire units are also placed on children's desks, and each child has an individual volume control. The signal-to-noise ratio is good because the teacher speaks directly into a microphone. A disadvantage of hardwire units is that they are not portable.

Induction Loop Unit.   The loop system involves a wire loop around the room, installed under carpeting or under the floor. A current of electromagnetic force runs through the loop. Audio input from the teacher's microphone alters the force and creates a magnetic field around the loop (Berger & Millin, 1989). Each child in the room wears a hearing aid in the telephone position. The telephone coil in the hearing aid will pick up the signal and present it to the ear. The signal-to-noise ratio is excellent, but children can hear only the teacher and not the other children or themselves. Today, there are hearing aids available with a switch in which the microphone and telephone setting can be used simultaneously The loop system is flexible within the room itself.

FM Unit.   A wireless unit, the FM auditory trainer is the most widely used trainer. The teacher wears a microphone-transmitter, and the child wears an FM receiver with the hearing aid. The teacher transmits directly to the child's unit on a frequency-modulated radio carrier wave. The signal-to-noise ratio is generally good. Ross (1987) stated: "In my judgement, the advent of the FM Auditory Training System has been the most significant educational tool for the average hearing-impaired child since the initial appearance of modern hearing aids. Indeed, historically, they may be the most powerful such tool we've ever had."

Other Considerations in Audiological Management

Audiological management does not end with the fitting of a hearing aid or the use of an auditory trainer. The child who is hearing impaired needs to be monitored and followed throughout the educational years.

The child suffering from conductive hearing loss due to acute otitis media needs to be monitored as well as the child exhibiting a sensorineural hearing loss. Because of the high incidence of otitis media in young children, Feagans (1986) recommended that day care centers be places for early intervention and follow-up. The model she recommended contains four components:

1. Workshops for staff to educate them on the high incidence and long-term effects of otitis media
2. Routine hearing screenings to determine thresholds, in addition to ear checks by professionals

3. Routine developmental assessments, including a battery of cognitive, attention, and language measures, for children who have persistent recurrences of otitis media
4. Intervention, including training in sustained attention to language, and reorganization of day care setting and structure, including modification of classrooms to permit smaller groups and thus reduce noise characteristics

The child with sensorineural hearing loss who is fitted with amplification needs to be followed routinely. Once the child has been fitted with hearing aids, monitoring techniques must be implemented. First, the parents of the young child should be trained in use, care, and maintenance of the instruments. Secondly, the child needs to be seen by the audiologist at least every 6 months to be sure the earmolds are still secure and do not need to be remade. The tubing in the earmolds may need to be replaced or cleaned. Moisture, dirt, and wax buildup can cause the hearing aid to be dysfunctional. Thirdly, the child should receive an audiological assessment at least once a year. Lastly, the teachers of the hearing impaired child must be made aware of the child's needs and issues involving the hearing aid.

Education of the Hearing Impaired

The educational performance of hearing impaired children in the United States has been a cause of concern to educators for some time. In 1921, Reamer reported on the educational achievement of 2,500 deaf students. He found that they were academically delayed on an average of four to five years when compared with hearing peers. A 1968–1970 annual survey (Gentile & DiFrancesca) gathered statistical information on the educational performance of hearing impaired persons in preschool through college. This survey revealed that on the whole, children and youth with hearing impairments demonstrated an average educational lag of four years. Their highest levels of performance were in the areas of spelling and arithmetic computation (Bess & McConnell, 1981). However, it must be noted that arithmetic concepts and performance on word problems still presented much difficulty, as they inherently included the ability to decode written language. The area of greatest lag in achievement was reading, with the average reading comprehension for 15- to 16-year-olds at the 3.5 grade level. Later studies by the Office of Demographic Studies at Gallaudet confirmed this delay in reading achievement (King & Quigley, 1985). Specifically, Trybus and Karchmer (1977) reported that the median reading level for deaf students at age 20 was grade 4.5.

Poor performance in most academic subjects is not surprising, considering that reading comprehension plays a major role in academic learning and that the understanding of written language relates directly to the understanding of spoken language. From about the third or fourth grade, students are expected to read to learn; this task becomes extremely difficult for the hearing impaired child who does not have an adequate language base. In fact, the majority of children with severe hearing impairments do not develop the adequate language skills that would make them efficient decoders of written language. Because of this, their comprehension of written language is significantly delayed when compared with that of normal hearing children (Robbins, 1986). This is probably related to the fact that hearing impaired children take longer to reach the final stage of comprehension development of spoken language, in which they attend to syntactic and morphological aspects of sentences rather than to paralinguistic cues (Robbins, 1986). Furthermore, it has been suggested that children with hearing impairments use different strategies for comprehension of verbal language (Davis & Blasdell, 1975).

Reading

Learning to read is a complex task that requires the integration of syntactic, semantic, and pragmatic skills, as well as the ability to decode words. Once words are decoded, the reader must translate them into a more usable form. For the person with normal hearing, this form consists of phonetic elements. For the person who is hearing impaired, this form depends on the language input model and may be either phonetic forms, signs, fingerspelling, or visual orthography. In addition, the reader must have the ability to abstract both explicit and implicit meaning from the text through inferencing and hypothesizing (Kretschmer, 1989). This is further complicated by text variables such as vocabulary, syntax, figurative language, and discourse.

There are four basic approaches to teaching reading in programs for children with hearing impairments: the basal reader approach, the language experience approach (LEA), the programmed instruction approach, and an individualized approach. In the LEA, the most frequently used approach in primary grades, children use their own language to write stories; that is, a child dictates a story and the teacher writes it. The story is then used in reading instruction. The LEA has been expanded to include modifying the child's dictated story in order to model and incorporate English syntactical forms. Once the child has achieved some writing skills, these written samples are incorporated into the reading program. The stories that children either dictate or write are based on personal interaction and represent the children's experiences with their social environment. This approach is most interesting in that it bridges the processes of reading and writing (King & Quigley, 1985).

Computer-based instruction has also been used to facilitate development of reading skills. Unfortunately there have been relatively few studies that clearly support the use of computers with hearing-impaired children. However, a study by Prinz, Nelson, and Stedt (1982) highlighted improvement in word recognition and identification for 3- to 6-year-old deaf children who were trained to use the ALPHA Program, a sight word computer program. This program utilized words, pictures, and manual sign representations and therefore could be used by children whose primary form of communication was sign language. Further studies (Nelson, Prinz, & Dalke, 1989; Prinz & Nelson, 1985) on deaf children 3 and 11 years old supported the use of computer-based instruction for reading and writing. More recently Prinz, Nelson, Loncke, Geysels, and Willems, 1993 have continued to support computer-based instruction with elementary-age hearing-impaired children. Basically all of these above-mentioned studies espoused the use of multimodality and multimedia reading programs for young deaf children.

Before formal training in reading begins, hearing-impaired children must have developed language skills. An excellent way to develop language is through storytelling, which exposes children to story structure, print, and common cultural themes (Snow, 1983: Wells, 1985). A recent study by Schick and Gale (1995) examined storytelling with preschool deaf and hard-of-hearing children who used some form of manually coded English during three different language conditions: using pure ASL, using pure SEE2, and using SEE2 with ASL features and ASL structures. SEE2 is a form of manually coded English, while ASL is a sign language that is typically used by deaf adults. Interestingly, it was found that children participated more and initiated more interactions when stories contained ASL signing. This study is important when considering educational approaches for children using manually coded English. It suggests that including ASL in the deaf child's programming may promote more interest in communication and increase incidents of child-initiated interactions.

Written Language

Written language demands that the writer not only have intact language abilities but also be able to retrieve conceptual schemata and translate it into meaningful propositions that are coherent. Research studies examining the written language of children with hearing impairments highlight their lack of syntactic and semantic knowledge. The written compositions of severely to profoundly hearing impaired children lacked complexity; were marked by frequent grammatical errors, such as additions, substitutions, and deviant word order; had shorter sentence and clause length; contained pronouns, prepositions, adjectives, and adverbs; and demonstrated a lesser degree of abstraction than that of normal hearing children (Yoshinaga-Itano, 1986).

Academic knowledge is gained through the comprehension of written narrative discourse. Deficits in the production and understanding of discourse undoubtedly have a detrimental effect on academic learning. Yoshinaga (1983) hypothesized that examination of the written language of severely hearing impaired children might provide insights into the comprehension strategies of hearing impaired readers. In turn, knowledge of these strategies has important implications for remediation. Based on research of the semantic and syntactic characteristics of the written language of the deaf, she speculated that hearing impaired children's deficient narrative skills might be due to an undeveloped concept of story (Yoshinaga-Itano & Snyder, 1985). Remediation techniques for such children would include frequent opportunities to hear stories read and to observe them in plays or films.

Over the last decade there has been a "pragmatic explosion." What we have learned during this period is that language development cannot be compartmentalized, with each component taught in isolation with no relationship to other components. Language and communication must occur in context. With this in mind, one can understand why the acquisition of reading and writing skills is so difficult for children with hearing impairments. They must integrate a variety of linguistic and communicative skills in order to master the ancillary skills of reading and writing.

Whole Language

Most recently, a whole-language methodology has gained acceptance among teachers of the nondisabled population. Whole language is an educational philosophy that incorporates all areas of language in the acquisition process. It is based on a developmental view of language acquisition (Schory, 1990). Advocates of whole language propose that children fail to become facile readers and writers because reading and writing have traditionally been taught as discrete skills separate from language. They espouse the integration of speaking, reading, and writing in the learning process and consider learning to be an active, constructive process during which new information is continuously incorporated into existing knowledge (Norris & Damico, 1990).

This philosophy can be incorporated into habilitative strategies when working with children who are hearing impaired. Intervention should incorporate the following whole-language assumptions (Norris & Damico, 1990):

1. Language exists in order to comprehend our environmental interactions and to convey meaning about ourselves and our world.
2. All components of language simultaneously interact (phonology, syntax, morphology, pragmatics, semantics) and cannot be parceled out and taught as separate units.
3. Language occurs in context—without context there is no meaning.
4. Language learning is an active process that incorporates new knowledge with existing knowledge in order to develop complex schemata of knowing.

With these premises in mind, the speech-language pathologist/teacher must carefully organize and plan language learning activities that promote the discovery of various communication functions. Activities must be interesting and meaningful to the child as she relates to her environment, and they must encourage and optimize opportunities for social interaction (for specific teaching strategies, see Krashen, 1982; Norris & Damico, 1990; Sulzby, 1985).

Sign Language and Bilingualism

As already noted, children with hearing impairments have generally been educated via either an aural/oral program, emphasizing speechreading and speech and using no sign systems, or a total communication program, using signs, speechreading, and speech. A variety of sign systems have been used to educate children who are deaf. For example, Signing Essential English (Anthony, 1971) and Signing Exact English (Gustason, Pfetzing, & Zawolkow, 1972) consist of manual productions of spoken English and adhere to the syntactical and grammatical forms of spoken English. Educators who use this type of sign system are actually attempting to teach English as a first language through the use of a visual system.

During the 1970s a body of research evolved around American Sign Language (ASL), the sign language used by deaf adults (Bellugi & Fischer, 1972; Bellugi & Klima, 1975; Bellugi, Klima, & Siple, 1974; Wilbur, 1979). ASL is a language in its own right with its own syntax and idioms. ASL is just as different from English as is Spanish or Russian or any other language. Thus, researchers have suggested that hearing-impaired/deaf children born to hearing-impaired/deaf parents who use ASL at home should be taught spoken and written English in a different manner than hearing-impaired/deaf children born to parents with normal hearing. The premise is that the children exposed to ASL have already achieved a primary language base—ASL. When they are exposed to English in the educational setting, English is their second language, and therefore the educational approach must be a bilingual one. In addition, these hearing-impaired/deaf children have also been exposed to a deaf culture with its traditions and customs. This makes them bicultural and strengthens the position for teaching them with an ASL/ESL (English as a Second Language) approach.

Today, a bilingual approach to educating children who are deaf or hearing impaired has not been implemented to any great extent. Reasons for this include the following:

1. ASL is not the native language of the majority of deaf children.
2. ASL has no written form.
3. There are few trained teachers who know ASL.
4. Bilingual education in general is controversial.
5. Few ASL curricula have been published.
6. Some educators question the true language status of ASL (Strong, 1988).

In spite of these obstacles, there have been attempts to document and justify the use of a bilingual approach in education. An experimental curriculum described by Michael Strong (1988) uses a storytelling format to introduce ASL into the classroom setting. English is then taught via ASL. This program is particularly interesting because it emphasizes metalinguistic awareness.

Hanson and Padden (1989) designed an instructional approach that uses computers to present video instructional materials for teaching written English to deaf children fluent in ASL. In experimental trials, the approach was well received by teachers and students alike. Consequently, the authors are developing more software for this approach (Hanson & Padden, in press).

Considering the difficulty with which hearing impaired/deaf children acquire language and the poor academic performance common among many of these children, it seems possible and practical to adopt a second language acquisition approach in the educational setting. However, much more careful and systematic research is needed before extensive use of such an approach can be recommended.

Inclusionary Education

Today, many educational options are available for the young child who is hearing impaired. Whereas the choice was once limited to segregated settings such as residential schools for the deaf and day schools for the hearing impaired, changes in federal legislation have brought forth new options, including day classes, resource rooms, itinerant programs, and team teaching.

As discussed in other chapters, the Education of All Handicapped Children Act (PL 94-142) ensures that all children with disabilities, ages 3–21, receive appropriate special education services. PL 99-457, passed in 1986, mandates these services to children from birth through 2 years of age. Much discussion has centered around the least restrictive environment (LRE) concept, which includes educating children with disabilities together with nondisabled children to the greatest extent possible (Moores & Moores, 1989), and ultimately ties in with the concept of inclusion for deaf children.

Early inclusion of deaf and hard-of-hearing children with normal hearing peers provides considerable educational benefits for the hearing-impaired child. There are three types of preschool integration placement options available today (Luetke-Stahlman, 1994):

1. Enrolling normal-hearing preschoolers in early childhood programs specifically set up for children who are deaf or hard of hearing (reverse mainstreaming)

2. Placing children who are deaf or hard of hearing in self-contained early intervention programs for part of the day and then in child care centers for additional socialization experiences
3. Placing children who are deaf or hard of hearing in preschool classes comprised of normal-hearing peers, with sufficient support services that will enable the hearing-impaired child to participate fully in all activities with the other preschoolers throughout the day

Clearly, integrating hearing-impaired preschoolers into mainstreamed environments poses considerable challenges. Peer interactions between hearing-impaired and normal-hearing children is generally limited because the communication attempts of the hearing-impaired child are often inadequate and ineffective (Vendell & George, 1981). Children who are hearing impaired learn language by participating in conversational exchanges (Kretschmer & Kretschmer, 1989). If their conversational attempts are unreinforced due to unresponsive peers, placement in integrated settings will have little benefit unless specific facilitative strategies are employed to ensure rich reciprocal conversation. Such conversations will result not only in language learning, but also in socially interactive complex play as well. In order to facilitate good interaction between hearing-impaired children and their normal-hearing peers, several strategies can be employed, such as encouraging hearing-impaired children to articulate more clearly, encouraging hearing peers to increase their communicative interactions with the hearing-impaired children, and, if the hearing-impaired children sign, to insist that they utilize simultaneous speech and sign (Luetke-Stahlman, 1991).

In the 1980s the main thrust of special education was to facilitate mainstreaming, which is an educational attempt to serve children with disabilities in a regular school environment with the aid of supportive personnel (Nicolosi et al., 1978). Supportive personnel can include the speech-language pathologist, the audiologist, the teacher of the hearing impaired, and others. Birch (1976) recommended that children who are deaf should be mainstreamed only after thorough preparation, with sensitivity to the needs of all parties, and with careful monitoring and support. Inherent in the concept of mainstreaming is the expectation that the student can perform at the regular classroom educational level.

For mainstreaming to be successful, the child placed in a regular classroom must also receive personalized instruction and supportive services necessary to benefit from an individualized educational plan, known as the IEP. The IEP is confirmation for children with hearing impairments that a more objective and scientific educational decision-making process will be followed (Northern & Downs, 1984).

Bricker (1978) suggested that "integration is a means of eliminating the deleterious effects of segregation and the stigma often attached to the handicapped student." Flexer, Wray, and Ireland (1989) reported that for a hearing-impaired child to be able to survive in a regular classroom, three issues must be addressed: understanding the nature of hearing and consequences of hearing loss, the essential use of technology to enhance the signal-to-noise ratio, and educational management strategies.

Mainstreaming of a child who is hearing impaired can take several forms. Complete mainstreaming occurs when the child remains in the regular classroom for all academic instruction, which is given by the regular classroom teacher. In this instance, the child relies on speechreading and amplification for instructional input. A modification of this complete mainstreaming option includes the use of a sign language interpreter in the classroom. In 1982, this type of educational support option was challenged by the Hendrick Hudson Board of Education. The case was heard by the Supreme Court in Rowley v. Hendrick Hudson Board of Education. The court ruled that Amy did not need an interpreter; however, it upheld the argument that PL 94-142 entitled students with disabilities to personalized instruction such as interpreter services.

Other mainstreaming options include part-time placement in regular classes with some special classes, and part-time placement in a resource room with some regular classes (McCortney, 1984).

Once a mainstreaming option is selected for a child, it is necessary to consider what factors will lead to success. Reynolds and Birch (1977) highlight the following as necessary components for mainstreaming success:

1. The regular classroom teacher is given a choice as to whether he or she wants to have the hearing impaired child in the class.
2. Mainstreaming begins early, at the preschool level.
3. The educational setting has a teacher of the hearing impaired on staff.
4. In-service training is provided for all the staff who work with the hearing impaired child.
5. The classroom environment is well equipped with necessary amplification units.
6. Separation of the hearing impaired child from the regular educational setting is minimal.
7. All the professionals who work with the mainstreamed child meet regularly to review the child's progress and make modifications as needed.

More recently educators have been considering the concept of inclusion. In its purest form inclusion is the meaningful involvement of all students in their neighborhood, school, and community (Progorzelski & Kelly, 1995). For the most severely handicapped student the emphasis of inclusion is socialization, not academics, and academics are modified for the special needs student. For hearing-impaired children who are capable of acquiring age-appropriate academics, the concept of inclusion must not erode the integrity of academic programming and expectations. If hearing-impaired students require presentation of academic material via sign language such as ASL, then full inclusion would mean that both a regular education teacher and an ASL-proficient teacher of the deaf collaborative within the regular education classroom.

Summary

The acquisition of literacy skills, reading and writing, involves the complex integration of many areas of learning, including speaking, listening, and critical thinking. An oral or manual language system must be intact if a hearing impaired child is to learn to read and write. Learning to read and write involves the ability to store up word meanings, remember vocabulary, and make abstract judgments about causal relationships (Streng, 1964). A solid language foundation is a prerequisite for literacy skills.

Individuals with hearing impairments have the same innate abilities to develop speech and language as persons in the normal-hearing population. However, often times, because of the severity of their hearing loss they cannot acquire language through audition alone. Consequently, overall delays in language development can result, and hearing impaired children are at a great educational disadvantage. Only through application of normal language development theory can educators devise more effective methodology for educating students with hearing impairments. Their challenge is to be creative as well as effective. In addition, passage of PL 94-142 and the mandate for the least restrictive environment further challenge the professional working with hearing-impaired children in the mainstreamed setting. Children who are hearing impaired should not necessarily be segregated. Instead, they should be educated in the LRE with normal hearing peers. It is up to the educator to ensure that children who are hearing impaired benefit from instruction in the mainstreamed setting. Only through careful planning, monitoring, and a team approach can that occur.

In diagnosing hearing impairments in the pediatric population, the clinician needs to remember the importance of early detection and intervention. The complete audiological assessment needs to include pure tone findings, speech findings, and aural acoustic immittance testing. Appropriate test parameters must be based on the age of the child. Accuracy and reliability are significant variables. The objective tests available and their use as a screening tool is inevitable in assisting to ensure early detection.

Each child with a hearing impairment has unique management needs. In general, children suffering from chronic otitis media need routine medical and audiological follow-up. Children exhibiting sensorineural hearing loss have different management needs. These children must be fitted properly with amplification, appropriate assistive devices must be selected for the school setting, and an appropriate educational setting must be considered.

Major changes have taken place in the education of children who are hearing impaired. Continual research and application of effective rehabilitive and educational theory will ensure that professionals can continue to meet the challenges of educating the children with hearing impairments.

Study Questions

1. What are the three types of hearing loss?
2. What are the effects of chronic otitis media on speech and language?
3. What is the speech recognition threshold?
4. What is tympanometry?
5. What are the benefits of the FM auditory trainer unit?
6. What are three types of preschool integration placement options available today?
7. What activity is most beneficial in developing language skills in young hearing impaired children? Why?
8. How does a hearing loss affect educational achievement?
9. What are the reasons that a bilingual educational approach is not routinely used when educating children with severe hearing impairments?

10. What impact has the cochlear implant had on children in the educational setting?
11. How have otoacoustic emissions affected the early detection of hearing loss in neonates?

Glossary

Acoustic reflex   The bilateral contraction of the intra-aural muscles (tensor tympani and stapedius) in response to sound.

Acute otitis media   An active inflammation and/or infection of the middle ear space.

ASL (American Sign Language)   Typically used by deaf adults, ASL has its own syntax and grammar and is recognized as a language separate from English.

Chronic otitis media   An infection of the middle ear space with purulent fluid (pus) persisting beyond the time limit of acute otitis media.

Conductive hearing loss   Interference of any sort in the transmission of sound from the external auditory canal to the inner ear.

IEP (Individual Education Plan)   A plan generated by a Committee for Special Education for eligible children ages 3 years through age 21.

IFSP (Individualized Family Service Plan)   A plan for providing services to an eligible child, birth up to age 3, and the child's family.

Inclusion   The legal right of handicapped children to be accommodated in the natural school environment regardless of their physical or educational limitations.

Mainstreaming   An educational attempt to serve children with disabilities in a regular school environment; students who are mainstreamed should be able to handle academics in a manner comparable to their regular education classmates.

Mixed hearing loss   A problem that occurs simultaneously in both the conductive and sensorineural mechanisms.

Otoacoustic emissions   The low-intensity sounds detected in the ear canal, which represent the cochlea's active response to sound, a response involving the addition of energy to that provided by the stimulus arriving at the ear.

Pure tone average   The average of the thresholds of 500 Hz, 1,000 Hz, and 2,000 Hz.

Pure tone threshold   The faintest tone a person can hear 50 percent of the time.

Secretory otitis media   A condition associated with a thick, gluelike fluid found in the middle ear space.

SEE2 (Signing Exact English 2)   A manually coded English sign system.

Sensorineural hearing loss   Damage to the sensory end organ, the cochlear hair cells, or the auditory nerve.

Serous otitis media   The presence of a thin, watery clear fluid in the middle ear space, usually an early sign of eustachian tube dysfunction.

Speech recognition   A measure of the ability to differentiate between various speech sounds, such as nonsense syllables, monosyllabic words, and multisyllabic words.

Speech recognition threshold   The threshold of intelligibility, which is the lowest level (in Db) at which the listener is able to identify approximately 50 percent of spondiac bisyllabic words.

Tympanometry   The measurement of the resistance to the flow of acoustical energy at the tympanic membrane during various pressure changes.

Suggested Reading

Glattke, T. J., & Kujawa, S. (1991, November). Otoacoustic emissions. *American Journal of Audiology.* 2, 29–37.

Greenberg, J. (1985). *What is the sign for friend?* New York: F. Watts.

Kavanagh, J. F. (Ed.) (1986). *Otitis media and child development.* Parkton, MD: York Press.

Kretschmer, R. (1989). Pragmatics, reading, and writing: Implications for hearing impaired individuals. *Topics in Language Disorders,* 9(4) 17–32.

Northern, J. (Ed.). (1984). *Hearing disorders* (2nd ed.). Boston: Little, Brown.

Prieve, B. A. (1992) Otoacoustic emission in infants and children: Basic characteristics and clinical application. *Seminars in Hearing,* 13(1), 37–52.

Schow, R., & Nerbonne, M. (Eds.) (1989). *Introduction to aural rehabilitation* (2nd ed.). Baltimore: University Park Press.

References

Anthony, D. (1971). *Signing Essential English* (vols. 1 and 2). Anaheim, CA: Educational Division, Anaheim Union School District.

Bateson, M. C. (1975). Mother-infant exchanges: The epigenesis of conversational interaction. In M. Aaronson & R. Reiber (Eds.), *Annals of the New York Academy of Sciences:* Developmental psycholinguistics and communication disorders.

Bellugi, U., & Fischer, S. (1972). A comparison of sign language and spoken language. *Cognition,* 1, 173–200.

Bellugi, U., & Klima, E. (1975). Aspects of sign language and its structure. In J. Kavanagh and J. Cutting (Eds.), *The role of speech in language* (pp. 171-203). Cambridge: MIT Press.

Bellugi, U., Klima, E., & Siple, P. (1974). Remembering in signs. *Cognition,* 3, 93–125.

Berger, K., & Millin, J. (1989). Amplification/assistive devices for the hearing impaired. In R. Schow & M. Nerbonne (Eds.), *Introduction to aural rehabilitation* (2nd ed.) (pp. 31–80). Austin, TX: Pro-Ed.

Bess, F. H., & McConnell, F. E. (1981). *Audiology, education and the hearing impaired child.* St. Louis, MO: Mosby.

Birch, J. W. (1976). Mainstream education for hearing impaired pupils: Issues and interviews. *American Annals of the Deaf,* 121, 69–71.

Blennerhasset, L. (1984). Communicative styles of a 13-month-old hearing impaired child and her parents. *Volta Review,* 86, 217–228.

Bloom, L., & Lahey, M. (1978). *Language development and language disorders.* New York: Wiley.

Bricker, D. D. (1978). A rationale for the integration of handicapped and non-handicapped preschool children. In N. J. Guralnich (Ed.), *Early intervention and the integration of handicapped and non-handicapped children.* Baltimore: University Park Press.

Brown, R. (1975). *Social psychology.* New York: Free Press.

Bruner, J. (1975). The ontogenesis of speech acts. *Journal of Child Language,* 2, 1–19.

Chaiklin, J. B., & Ventry, I. M., (1964). Spondee threshold measurement: Comparison of 2 and 5 dB methods. *Journal of Speech and Hearing Disorders,* 2, 47–59.

Cole, E. B., & St. Clair-Stokes, J. (1984). Caregiver-child interactive behaviors: A videotape analysis procedure. *Volta Review,* 86, 200–216.

Cross, T. G., Johnson-Moores, J. E., & Nienhuys, T. G. (1980). Linguistic feedback and maternal speech: Comparisons of mothers addressing hearing and hearing-impaired children. *First Language,* 1, 163–189.

Davis, J. M., & Blasdell, R. (1975). Perceptual strategies by normal hearing and hearing-impaired children in the comprehension of sentences containing relative clauses. *Journal of Speech and Hearing Research,* 18, 281–295.

DeGangi, G., Wietlisbach, S., Poisson, S., Stein, E., & Royeen, C. (1994). The impact of culture and socioeconomic status on family–professional collaboration: Challenges and solutions. *Topics in Early Childhood Special Education,* 14(4), 503–520.

Doyle, J., Doyle, J., & Turnbull, F. (1964). Electrical stimulations of the eight cranial nerve. *Archives of Otolaryngology,* 80, 388–391.

Eimas, P. (1974). Auditory and linguistic processing cues for place of articulation by infants. *Perceptual Psychology,* 16, 513–521.

Elwood, P. C., Johnson, W. L., & Mandell, J. (Eds.). (1977). *Parent-infant program for the hearing impaired: A research guide.* Washington, DC: Bureau of Education of the Handicapped, Department of Health, Education, and Welfare/Office of Education.

Feagans, L. (1986). Otitis media: A model for long-term effects with implications for intervention. In J. F. Kavanagh (Ed.), *Otitis media and child development* (pp. 192–210). Parkton, MD: York Press.

Flexer, C., Wray, D., & Ireland, J. (1989). Preferential seating is not enough: Issues in classroom management of hearing impaired students. *Language, Speech and Hearing Services in Schools,* 20(1), 11–21.

Geers, A., Moog, J., & Schick, B. (1984). Acquisition of spoken and signed English by profoundly deaf children. *Journal of Speech and Hearing Disorders,* 49, 378–388.

Gentile, A., & DiFrancesca, S. (1969, Spring). *Academic achievement test performance of hearing impaired students: United States* (Series D, No. 1). Washington, DC: Gallaudet College, Office of Demographic Studies.

Glattke, T. J., & Kujawa, S. (1991, November). Otoacoustic emissions. *American Journal of Audiology.* 2, 29–37.

Goss, R. N. (1970). Language used by mothers of deaf children and mothers of hearing children. *American Annals of the Deaf,* 115, 93–96.

Green, D. (1978). Pure tone air conduction testing. In J. Katz (Ed.), *Handbook of clinical audiology* (2nd ed.) (pp. 98–109). Baltimore: Williams & Wilkins.

Greenstein, J. M., Bush, B., McConville, K., & Stellini, L. (1977). *Mother-infant communication and language acquisition in deaf infants.* New York: Lexington School for the Deaf.

Gustason, G., Pfetzing, D., & Zawolkow, E. (1972). *Signing Exact English.* Rossmoor, CA: Modern Sign Press.

Hanson, M., Lynch, E. W., & Wayman, K. I. (1990). Honoring the culture diversity of families when gathering data. *Topics in Early Childhood Education,* 10(1), 112–131.

Hanson, V. L., & Padden, C. A. (1989). Interactive video for bilingual ASL/English instruction of deaf children. *American Annals of the Deaf,* 134, 209–213.

Hanson, V. L., & Padden, C. A. (in press). Computers and videodisc technology for bilingual ASL/English instruction of deaf children. In D. Nix & R. Spiro (Eds.), *Cognition, education, and multimedia: Exploring ideas in high technology.* Hillsdale, NJ: Lawrence Erlbaum Associates.

Hopkinson, N. (1978). Speech reception threshold. In J. Katz (Ed.), *Handbook of clinical audiology* (2nd ed.) (pp. 141–148). Baltimore: Williams & Wilkins.

Jaffe, J., Stern, D., & Peery, J. (1973). "Conversational" coupling of gaze behaviors in prelinguistic human development. *Journal of Psycholinguistic Research,* 2, 321–328.

Jordan, I., Gustason, G., & Rosen, R. (1979). Current communication trends at programs for the deaf. *American Annals of the Deaf,* 124, 350–357.

Kaplan, G. K., Fleishman, J. K., Bender, T. R., & Clark, P. (1973). Long term effects of otitis media: A 10 year cohort study of Alaskan Eskimo children. *Pediatrics,* 52, 577–585.

Kemp, D. T. (1978). Stimulated acoustic emissions from within the human auditory system. *Journal of the Acoustic Society of America,* 64, 1386–1391.

King, C. M., & Quigley, S. P. (1985). *Reading and deafness.* San Diego: College-Hill Press.

Knauf, V. H. (1972). Meeting speech and language needs for the hearing impaired. In J. Katz (Ed.), *Handbook of clinical audiology* (2nd ed.) (pp. 733–777). Baltimore: Williams & Wilkins.

Krashen, S. (1982). *Principles and practices in second language acquisition.* New York: Pergamon.

Kretschmer, R. (1989). Pragmatics, reading, and writing. *Topics in Language Disorders,* 9(4) 17–32.

Kretschmer, R., & Kretschmer, L. (1989). Communication Competence: Impact of the pragmatics revolution on education of hearing impaired individuals. *Topics in Language Disorders,* 9(4), 1–16.

Luetke-Stahlman, B. (1991). Hearing impaired students in integrated child care. *Perspectives,* 9(1), 8–11.

Luetke-Stahlman, B. (1994). Procedures for socially integrating preschoolers who are hearing, deaf, and hard of hearing. *Topics in Early Childhood Special Education,* 14(4), 472–487.

Mahon, W. (1987). U.S. hearing aid sales summary. *The Hearing Journal,* 40, 9–14.

Mavilya, M. (1969). *Spontaneous vocalization and babbling in hearing-impaired infants.* Doctoral dissertation, Teacher's College, Columbia University, New York.

McCortney, B. (1984). Education in the mainstream. In R. Stoker & J. Spear (Eds.), *Hearing-impaired perspectives on living in the mainstream* (pp. 41–52). Washington, DC: Alexander Graham Bell Association for the Deaf.

Menyuk, P. (1986). Predicting speech and language problems with persistent otitis media. In James F. Kavanagh (Ed.), *Otitis media and child development* (pp. 83–98). Parkton, MD: York Press.

Miller, C., & Morse, P. (1976). The "heart" of categorical speech discrimination in young infants. *Journal of Speech and Hearing Research, 19,* 578–589.

Miller, C., Morse, P., & Dorman, N. (1977). Cardiac indices of infants' speech perception: Orienting and burst discrimination. *Quarterly Journal of Experimental Psychology, 29,* 533–545.

Moores, J. M., & Moores, D. (1989). Educational alternatives for the hearing impaired. In R. Show & M. Nerbonne (Eds.), *Introduction to aural rehabilitation* (2nd. ed.) (pp. 271–294). Austin, TX: Pro-Ed.

Morse, P. (1972). The discrimination of speech and speech stimuli in early infancy. *Journal of Experimental Psychology, 14,* 477–492.

Myklebust, H. R. (1960). *The psychology of deafness.* New York: Grune & Stratton.

Nelson, K., Prinz, P., & Dalke, D. (1989). Transitions from sign language to text via an interactive microcomputer system. In B. Woll (Ed.), *Papers from the Seminar on Language Development and Sign Language,* (Monograph 1, International Sign Linguistics Association). Bristol, UK: Centre for Deaf Studies, University of Bristol.

Nicolosi, L., Harryman, E., & Kresheck, J. (1978). *Terminology of communication disorders— speech—language—hearing.* Baltimore: Williams & Wilkins.

Norris, J., & Damico, J. (1990). Whole language in theory and practice: Implications for language intervention. *Language, Speech and Hearing Services in Schools, 21,* 212–220.

Northern, J. (Ed.). (1984). *Hearing disorders* (2nd ed.). Boston: Little, Brown.

Northern, J., & Downs, M. (1978). *Hearing in children.* Baltimore: Williams & Wilkins.

Northern, J., & Downs, M. (1984) *Hearing in children.* Baltimore: Williams & Wilkins.

Padden, C. (1980). The deaf community and the culture of deaf people. In C. Baker & R. Battison (Eds.), *Sign language and the deaf community.* Washington, DC: National Association for the Deaf.

Pashley, N. R. T. (1984). Otitis media. In J. Northern (Ed.), *Hearing disorders* (pp. 103–110). Boston: Little, Brown.

Prieve, B. A., (1992) Otoacoustic emission in infants and children: basic characteristics and clinical application. *Seminars in Hearing, 13*(1), 37–52.

Prinz, P. & Nelson, K. (1985). Alligator eats cookie: Acquisition of writing and reading skills by deaf children using the microcomputer. *Applied Psycholinguistics, 6,* 283–306.

Prinz, P., & Nelson, K., Loncke, F., Geysels, G., & Willems, C. (1993). A multimodality and multimedia approach to language, discourse and literacy development. In F. Coninx & B. Elsendoorn (Eds.), *Interactive learning technology for the deaf.* New York: Springer-Verlag.

Prinz, P., & Nelson, K. A. & Stedt, J. (1982). Early reading in young deaf children using microcomputer technology. *American Annals of the Deaf, 127,* 529–535.

Progorzelski, G., & Kelly, B. (1995). *Inclusion: The Collaborative Process.* Buffalo, NY: United Educational Services, Inc.

Quigley, S. P., & Kretschmer, R. E. (1982). *The education of deaf children.* Baltimore: University Park Press.

Radziewicz, C. (1985). *The use of videotapes as a means of parent training for parents of hearing-impaired infants.* Unpublished doctoral dissertation, Adelphi University, Garden City, New York.

Reamer, J. C. (1921). Mental and educational measurement of the deaf. *Psychological Monographs* (No. 132).

Reynolds, M. C., & Birch, J. W. (1977). *Teaching exceptional children in all America's schools.* Reston, VA: Council for Exceptional Children.

Robbins, A. M. (1986). Language comprehension in young children. *Topics in Language Disorders, 6,* 12–23.

Ross, M. (1987). FM auditory training systems as an educational tool. *Hearing Rehabilitation Quarterly, 12*(4), 4–6.

Scheidt, P., & Kavanagh, J. (1986). Common terminology for conditions of the middle ear. In J. J. Kavanagh (Ed.), *Otitis media and child development* (pp. XV–XVII). Parkton, MD: York Press.

Schick, B., & Gale, E. (1995). Preschool deaf and hard of hearing students' interactions during ASL and English storytelling. *American Annals of the Deaf,* 140, 363–370.

Schory, M. E. (1990). Whole language and the speech-language pathologist. *Language, Speech and Hearing Services in Schools,* 21, 206–211.

Simmons, B. (1966). Electrical stimulation of the auditory nerve in man. *Archives of Otolaryngology,* 84, 2–54.

Snow, C. (1972). Mothers' speech to children learning language. *Child Development,* 43, 549–565.

Snow, C. E. (1977). The development of conversation between mothers and babies. *Journal of Child Language,* 4, 1–22.

Snow, C. (1983). Literacy and language relationships during the preschool years. *Harvard Educational Review,* 53, 165–189.

Streng, A. (1964). *Reading for deaf children.* Washington, DC: Alexander Graham Bell Association for the Deaf.

Strong, M. (Ed.). (1988). *Language learning and deafness.* New York: Cambridge University Press.

Sulzby, E. (1985). Children's emergent reading of favorite storybooks: A developmental study. *Reading Research Quarterly,* 20, 45–81.

Tartter, V. C., Hellman, S. A., & Chute, P. M. (1992). Vowel perception strategies of normal-hearing subjects and patients using Nucleus Multichannel and 3M/house cochlear implants. *Journal of Acoustical Society of America,* 92, 1269–1283.

Trybus, R., & Karchmer, M. (1977). School achievement scores of hearing impaired children: National data on achievement status and growth patterns. *American Annals of the Deaf Directory of Programs and Services,* 122, 62–69.

Vendell, D. L., & George, L. B. (1981) Social interaction in hearing and deaf students: Successes and failures in initiations. *Child Development,* 52, 627–635.

Vorce, E. (1974). *Teaching speech to deaf children.* Washington, DC: Alexander Graham Bell Association for the Deaf.

Wedell-Monnig, J., & Westerman, T. B. (1977, September). *Mothers' language to deaf and hearing infants: Examination of the feedback model.* Paper presented at the Second Annual Boston University Conference on Language Development, Boston.

Wells, G. (1985). Preschool literacy related activities and success in school. In Dr. Olson, N. Torrance, & A. Hildyard (Eds.). *Literacy, language and learning: The nature and consequences of reading and writing* (pp. 229–255) New York: Cambridge University Press.

Wilbur, R. B. (1979), *American Sign Language and sign systems.* Baltimore: University Park Press.

Woodford, C. M., Feldman, A. S., & Wright, H. N. (1975) Stimulus parameters, the acoustic reflex and clinical implications. *NYS Speech and Hearing Review,* 7, 29–37.

Yoshinaga, C. (1983). *Syntactic and semantic characteristics in the written language of hearing impaired and normally hearing school-aged children.* Unpublished doctoral dissertation, Northwestern University, Evanston, IL.

Yoshinaga-Itano, C. (1986). Beyond the sentence level: What's in a hearing impaired child's story? *Topics in Language Disorders,* 6(3), 71–83.

Yoshinaga-Itano, C., & Snyder, L. (1985). Form and meaning in the written language of hearing impaired children. In R. R. Kretschmer (Ed.), *Learning to write and writing to learn* [Monograph]. *Volta Review,* 87(5), 75–90.

Index